a LANGE medical book

AF521760

CURRENT CONSULT
SURGERY

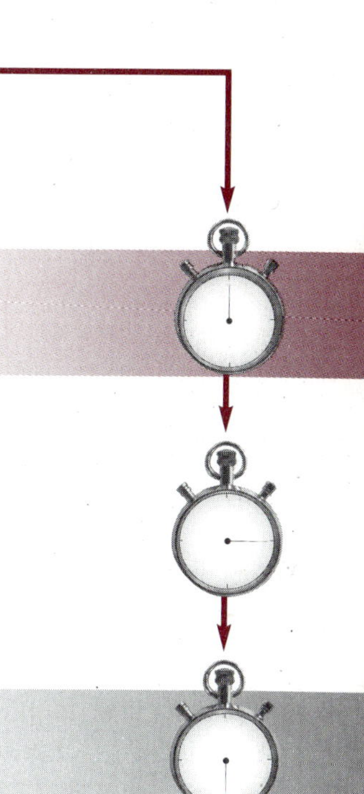

Diagnostic Index

A—Z Dx and Tx

Cancer Staging Tables

a LANGE medical book

CURRENT CONSULT
SURGERY

Edited by

Gerard M. Doherty, MD
N.W. Thompson Professor of Surgery
Section Head, General Surgery
University of Michigan Medical School
Ann Arbor

Gorav Ailawadi, MD
Department of Surgery
University of Michigan
Ann Arbor

Charles E. Binkley, MD
Department of Surgery
University of Michigan
Ann Arbor

Derek A. DuBay, MD
Department of Surgery
University of Michigan
Ann Arbor

Theodore R. Lin, MD
Department of Surgery
University of Michigan
Ann Arbor

John W. McGillicuddy, MD
Department of Surgery
University of Michigan
Ann Arbor

Brian D. Saunders, MD
Department of Surgery
University of Michigan
Ann Arbor

Theodore H. Welling III, MD
Department of Surgery
University of Michigan
Ann Arbor

Lange Medical Books/McGraw-Hill
Medical Publishing Division

New York Chicago San Francisco Lisbon London
Madrid Mexico City Milan New Delhi San Juan
Seoul Singapore Sydney Toronto

The McGraw-Hill Companies

Current Consult: Surgery

Copyright © 2005 by The McGraw-Hill Companies, Inc. All rights reserved. Printed in the United States of America. Except as permitted under the United States Copyright Act of 1976, no part of this publication may be reproduced or distributed in any form or by any means, or stored in a data base or retrieval system, without the prior written permission of the publisher.

1 2 3 4 5 6 7 8 9 0 QPDQPD 0 9 8 7 6 5 4 3 4

ISBN: 0-07-142313-3

ISSN: 1551-191X

Notice

Medicine is an ever-changing science. As new research and clinical experience broaden our knowledge, changes in treatment and drug therapy are required. The authors and the publisher of this work have checked with sources believed to be reliable in their efforts to provide information that is complete and generally in accord with the standards accepted at the time of publication. However, in view of the possibility of human error or changes in medical sciences, neither the authors nor the publisher nor any other party who has been involved in the preparation or publication of this work warrants that the information contained herein is in every respect accurate or complete, and they disclaim all responsibility for any errors or omissions or for the results obtained from use of the information contained in this work. Readers are encouraged to confirm the information contained herein with other sources. For example and in particular, readers are advised to check the product information sheet included in the package of each drug they plan to administer to be certain that the information contained in this work is accurate and that changes have not been made in the recommended dose or in the contraindications for administration. This recommendation is of particular importance in connection with new or infrequently used drugs.

This book was set in Adobe Garamond by Pine Tree Composition, Inc.
The editors were Shelley Reinhardt, Marc Strauss, Harriet Lebowitz, and Peter J. Boyle.
The production supervisor was Philip Galea.
The art manager was Charissa Baker.
The text was designed by Eve Siegel.
The index was prepared by Kathrin Unger.

Quebecor Dubuque was printer and binder.

This book is printed on acid-free paper.

INTERNATIONAL EDITION ISBN: 0-07-111470-X
Copyright © 2005. Exclusive rights by The McGraw-Hill Companies, Inc. for manufacture and export. This book cannot be re-exported from the country to which it is consigned by McGraw-Hill. The International Edition is not available in North America.

Current Consult Surgery: 3 Parts

CONTENTS: Alphabetical

CONTENTS: Topical

Adult Cardiac Surgery

Congenital Cardiac Surgery

Arteries

Veins & Lymphatics

Upper Gastrointestinal Surgery

Esophagus & Diaphragm

CONTENTS: Cancer Staging Tables

Preface

Current Consult: Surgery is designed to provide rapid, efficient access to the exact information you need when you only have a few minutes to review. Compiled by a select group of residents from the General Surgery Program at the University of Michigan, it covers the salient points relevant to surgical care. The 3 parts of *Current Consult: Surgery,* which are color coded, are

Diagnostic Index: THE RED PAGES
A–Z Diagnosis and Treatment: THE WHITE PAGES
Cancer Staging Tables: THE GRAY PAGES

The **DIAGNOSTIC INDEX** is a unique and valuable feature that groups disease topics according to related signs, symptoms, and patient presentations. It thereby offers differential diagnoses for patient evaluation, along with an immediate connection to the appropriate disorders included in the book.

A–Z DIAGNOSIS AND TREATMENT presents carefully selected information on essential surgical topics in a convenient two-page format for each disorder. Perfect as a reference when a rapid review of practical points is needed, the WHITE PAGES are not only organized alphabetically, but also are accompanied by an additional Contents list that categorizes the topics by subject area (for example, trauma, hepatobiliary, and pediatric groupings). Each disease entry in the A–Z section highlights

- Essential Features, including epidemiology
- Clinical Findings, such as symptoms and signs, laboratory findings, and imaging findings
- Diagnostic Considerations, including differential diagnosis and diseases to rule out
- Work-Up, including when to admit and when to refer
- Treatment and Management, such as surgery, medications, treatment monitoring, complications, prognosis, and prevention
- Resources, such as references, practice guidelines, and cancer staging.

The GRAY PAGES of *Current Consult: Surgery* allow easy access to **CANCER STAGING TABLES** by providing selected American Joint Committee on Cancer staging information relevant to the disease entries in the book. These tables are excerpted in the associated topics, and the full tables are available in this final section.

We hope that *Current Consult: Surgery* will be a useful and handy resource, providing the guidance that you need—when you need it—to enhance the care of your patients.

Gerard M. Doherty, MD
Ann Arbor, Michigan

Diagnostic Index

Abdominal Pain

Adult, Diffuse

More Common

- Acidosis, metabolic
- Appendicitis, acute
- Colitis, ischemic
- Ectopic pregnancy, ruptured
- Intra-abdominal abscess
- Mesenteric vascular occlusion, acute
- Pain, abdominal, nonspecific
- Pancreatitis, acute
- Pelvic inflammatory disease
- Peptic ulcer perforation
- Pyelonephritis, acute
- Small intestine, obstruction
- Ureteral or renal calculi

Less Common

- Abdominal aortic aneurysm
- Colitis, ulcerative
- Mesenteric ischemia
- Pancreatitis, chronic
- Peritonitis, bacterial
- Porphyria, acute
- Retroperitoneal abscess
- Small intestine, infectious diseases
- Volvulus

Abdominal Pain: Adult, Right Lower Quadrant

More Common

- Appendicitis, acute
- Cholecystitis (acute and chronic)
- Diverticulitis
- Ectopic pregnancy, ruptured
- Endometriosis
- Pelvic inflammatory disease
- Peptic ulcer perforation
- Pyelonephritis, acute
- Small intestine, obstruction
- Ureteral or renal calculi

Less Common

- Abdominal aortic aneurysm
- Crohn disease
- Retroperitoneal abscess
- Small intestine diverticula
- Small intestine, infectious diseases

Abdominal Pain: Adult, Right Upper Quadrant

More Common

- Appendicitis, acute
- Cholecystitis (acute & chronic)
- Cholelithiasis
- Cholelithiasis, rare complications
- Duodenal ulcer
- Gastric ulcer
- Hepatitis (acute & chronic)
- Pancreatitis, acute
- Peptic ulcer perforation
- Pneumonia
- Pyelonephritis, acute

Less Common

- Empyema
- Hepatic abscess
- Herpes zoster
- Pancreatic neoplasms, cystic
- Retroperitoneal abscess
- Small intestine, infectious diseases

Abdominal Pain: Adult, Left Lower Quadrant

More Common

- Appendicitis, acute
- Diverticulitis
- Ectopic pregnancy, ruptured
- Endometriosis
- Pelvic inflammatory disease
- Small intestine, obstruction
- Ureteral or renal calculi

Less Common

- Abdominal aortic aneurysm
- Retroperitoneal abscess
- Small intestine diverticula
- Small intestine, infectious diseases

Abdominal Pain: Adult, Left Upper Quadrant

More Common

- Empyema
- Gastric ulcer
- Gastroesophageal reflux disease & hiatal hernia
- Pancreatic abscess
- Pancreatic adenocarcinoma
- Pancreatitis, acute
- Peptic ulcer perforation
- Pneumonia
- Small intestine, obstruction

Less Common

- Gastric volvulus
- Herpes zoster
- Islet cell tumors, nonfunctioning
- Retroperitoneal abscess
- Small intestine, infectious diseases
- Splenic abscess
- Splenic cysts and tumors
- Splenic neoplasms
- Visceral aneurysms

Abdominal Pain: Adult, Flank

More Common

- Duodenal ulcer
- Empyema
- Hepatitis (acute & chronic)
- Pancreatitis, acute
- Peptic ulcer perforation
- Pneumonia
- Pyelonephritis, acute
- Ureteral or renal calculi

Less Common

- Adrenocortical carcinoma
- Hepatic abscess
- Retroperitoneal abscess
- Retroperitoneal hemorrhage
- Splenic abscess
- Splenic cysts & tumors
- Visceral aneurysms

Abdominal Pain: Adult, Periumbilical

- Appendicitis, acute
- Duodenal ulcer
- Ectopic pregnancy, ruptured
- Small intestine, infectious diseases
- Small intestine, obstruction
- Umbilical hernia

Abdominal Pain: Child, Diffuse

More Common

- Appendicitis, acute
- Crohn disease
- Inguinal hernia
- Intussusception, pediatric
- Pediatric intestinal obstruction, miscellaneous
- Small intestine, obstruction

Less Common

- Colitis, ulcerative
- Cystic fibrosis

Abdominal Pain: Post-traumatic

More Common

- Acidosis, metabolic
- Diaphragmatic hernia, traumatic
- Inguinal hernia
- Intra-abdominal abscess: hepatic abscess
- Pancreatitis, acute
- Pneumonia
- Small intestine, obstruction

Less Common
- Mesenteric vascular occlusion, acute
- Small intestine, infectious diseases
- Splenic vein thrombosis

Abdominal Pain: Postoperative

More Common
- Acidosis, metabolic
- Inguinal hernia
- Intra-abdominal abscess: hepatic abscess
- Pancreatitis, acute
- Pneumonia
- Small intestine, obstruction
- Surgical site infections

Less Common
- Mesenteric vascular occlusion, acute
- Small intestine, infectious diseases
- Splenic vein thrombosis

Abdominal Pain: Jaundice

More Common
- Ampulla of vater tumors
- Biliary atresia
- Biliary neoplasms, benign
- Biliary obstructions, benign
- Cholangiocarcinoma
- Cholecystitis (acute & chronic)
- Choledocholithiasis & gallstone pancreatitis
- Cholelithiasis
- Cholelithiasis, rare complications
- Cirrhosis
- Cirrhosis, primary biliary
- Gallbladder adenocarcinoma
- Hepatic failure, acute
- Hepatitis (acute & chronic)
- Jaundice
- Pancreatic adenocarcinoma
- Pancreatitis, chronic

Less Common
- Cholangitis, primary sclerosing
- Choledochal cyst
- Duodenal tumors, malignant
- Pancreatic neoplasms, cystic

Abdominal Pain: Vomiting

More Common
- Abdominal wall hernias, noninguinal
- Appendicitis, acute
- Cholecystitis (acute & chronic)
- Hypercalcemia
- Ileus
- Incisional (ventral) hernia
- Inguinal hernia
- Intussusception, adult
- Pancreatitis, acute
- Small intestine, infectious diseases
- Small intestine, obstruction
- Umbilical hernia

Less Common
- Achalasia
- Duodenal tumors, benign
- Duodenal tumors, malignant
- Pyloric obstruction
- Superior mesenteric artery obstruction of the duodenum

Abdominal Pain: Sudden Onset

More Common
- Appendicitis, acute
- Ectopic pregnancy, ruptured
- Mesenteric vascular occlusion, acute
- Peptic ulcer perforation
- Thoracic aortic dissection

Less Common
- Cholecystitis (acute & chronic)
- Diverticulitis
- Small intestine, infectious diseases
- Small intestine, obstruction

Abdominal Pain: Postprandial

More Common
- Abdominal wall hernias, noninguinal
- Cholelithiasis
- Incisional (ventral) hernia
- Inguinal hernia
- Mesenteric ischemia
- Pancreatitis, chronic
- Small intestine, obstruction

Less Common
- Intussusception, adult
- Pyloric obstruction
- Superior mesenteric artery obstruction of the duodenum

Abdominal Pain: Free Intraperitoneal Air

- Diverticulitis
- Peptic ulcer perforation
- Pneumatosis Intestinalis

Abdominal Pain: Constipation

More Common
- Anal fissure & ulcer
- Anorectal abscess & fistula
- Colorectal adenocarcinoma
- Colorectal tumors, uncommon
- Hemorrhoids
- Rectal fixation, abnormal
- Rectal ulcer, solitary

Less Common
- Anal canal cancer
- Anal margin cancer
- Hirschsprung disease
- Pediatric intestinal obstruction, miscellaneous

Abdominal Pain: Obstipation

More Common
- Anal canal cancer
- Anal margin cancer
- Colorectal adenocarcinoma
- Colorectal tumors, uncommon
- Intussusception, pediatric
- Rectal ulcer, solitary
- Volvulus

Less Common
- Hirschsprung disease
- Imperforate anus
- Intussusception, adult
- Pediatric intestinal obstruction, miscellaneous
- Small intestine, obstruction

Abdominal Pain: Fever

More Common
- Appendicitis, acute
- Cholecystitis (acute & chronic)
- Diverticulitis
- Empyema
- Pancreatitis, acute
- Pelvic inflammatory disease
- Peritonitis, bacterial
- Pneumonia
- Pyelonephritis, acute
- Small intestine, infectious diseases
- Small intestine, obstruction

Less Common
- Acidosis, metabolic
- Colitis, ischemic
- Hepatic abscess
- Hepatitis (acute & chronic)
- Peptic ulcer perforation
- Volvulus

Abdominal Pain: Blood in Stool

More Common
- Anal canal cancer
- Anal margin cancer
- Anorectal abscess & fistula
- Colitis, antibiotic-associated

- Colorectal adenocarcinoma
- Colorectal tumors, uncommon
- Diverticulitis
- Duodenal ulcer
- Gastric adenocarcinoma
- Hemorrhoids
- Peptic ulcer hemorrhage

Less Common

- Colitis, ischemic
- Colitis, ulcerative
- Small intestine diverticula

Abdominal Pain: Pneumaturia

- Colovesical fistula
- Diverticulitis
- Appendicitis, acute
- Pyelonephritis, acute

Abdominal Pulsation

More Common

- Abdominal aortic aneurysm
- Hepatic tumor, metastatic
- Iliac aneurysms
- Pancreatic adenocarcinoma
- Renal artery aneurysm
- Thoracic aortic aneurysms
- Visceral aneurysms

Less Common

- Adrenocortical carcinoma
- Gastrointestinal stromal tumor, leiomyomas, & leiomyosarcoma
- Hepatic neoplasms, benign
- Islet cell tumors, nonfunctioning
- Retroperitoneal hemorrhage
- Retroperitoneal sarcoma

Axillary Swelling

More Common

- Breast cancer, female
- Breast lesions, benign
- Carcinoma, inflammatory
- Deep venous thrombosis, upper extremity
- Furuncle, carbuncle & hidradenitis suppurativa

Less Common

- Breast cancer, male
- Chest wall tumors, benign soft tissue
- Chest wall tumors, malignant skeletal
- Chest wall tumors, malignant soft tissue
- Chest wall tumors, benign skeletal
- Desmoid tumor

Back Pain

More Common

- Abdominal aortic aneurysm
- Empyema
- Endometriosis
- Intra-abdominal abscess
- Lung abscess
- Lung cancer, primary
- Pancreatic abscess
- Pancreatic adenocarcinoma
- Pancreatitis, acute
- Pancreatitis, chronic
- Pleural tumors
- Pneumonia
- Pneumothorax
- Pulmonary thromboembolism
- Pyelonephritis, acute
- Retroperitoneal abscess
- Thoracic aortic aneurysms
- Thoracic aortic dissection
- Ureteral or renal calculi

Less Common

- Chest wall osteomyelitis
- Chest wall tumors, benign soft tissue
- Chest wall tumors, malignant skeletal
- Chest wall tumors, malignant soft tissue
- Chest wall tumors: benign skeletal
- Esophageal carcinoma
- Esophageal perforation
- Esophageal spasm, diffuse
- Esophagitis, corrosive
- Islet cell tumors, nonfunctioning
- Mediastinal masses
- Mediastinitis
- Osteitis fibrosa cystica
- Paget disease
- Pancreatic neoplasms, cystic
- Pancreatic pseudocyst
- Paraesophageal hiatal hernia
- Pleural effusion
- Renal artery aneurysm
- Retroperitoneal fibrosis
- Retroperitoneal hemorrhage
- Splenic abscess
- Visceral aneurysms

Bone/Extremity Mass

- Aneurysms, peripheral
- Desmoid tumor
- Lipoma
- Melanoma
- Soft tissue sarcoma
- Thrombophlebitis, superficial
- Varicose veins

Breast Lump

Male

More Common

- Gynecomastia
- Lipoma

Less Common

- Breast cancer, male
- Chest wall tumors, benign skeletal
- Chest wall tumors, benign soft tissue
- Chest wall tumors, malignant skeletal
- Chest wall tumors, malignant soft tissue

Breast Lump: Female

More Common

- Breast cancer, female
- Breast lesions, benign
- Carcinoma, inflammatory

Less Common

- Chest wall tumors, benign skeletal
- Chest wall tumors, benign soft tissue
- Chest wall tumors, malignant skeletal
- Chest wall tumors, malignant soft tissue
- Gynecomastia
- Lipoma
- Paget disease of breast

Breast Lump: Pain

- Breast cancer, female
- Breast lesions, benign
- Carcinoma, inflammatory
- Mondor disease (thrombophlebitis of the thoracoepigastric vein)
- Paget disease of breast

Breast Lump: Nipple Bleeding

- Breast cancer, female
- Breast lesions, benign
- Carcinoma, inflammatory
- Paget disease of breast

Breast Lump: Cyclical

- Breast cancer, female
- Breast lesions, benign
- Carcinoma, inflammatory
- Paget disease of breast

Breast Pain

Fever

More Common

- Breast lesions, benign
- Cellulitis

- Mondor disease (thrombophlebitis of the thoracoepigastric vein)

Less Common
- Breast cancer, female
- Carcinoma, inflammatory
- Necrotizing fasciitis

Breast Pain: Postpartum

More Common
- Breast cancer, female
- Breast lesions, benign
- Cellulitis
- Mondor disease (thrombophlebitis of the thoracoepigastric vein)

Less Common
- Carcinoma, inflammatory
- Necrotizing fasciitis

Breast Pain: Chronic

- Breast cancer, female
- Breast lesions, benign
- Mondor disease (thrombophlebitis of the thoracoepigastric vein)

Burns

- Burns
- Burns, respiratory injury
- Electrical injury

Chest Pain

Cough

More Common
- Aspiration
- Barrett esophagus
- Empyema
- Esophageal carcinoma
- Gastroesophageal reflux disease & hiatal hernia
- Head & neck squamous cell cancer
- Lung cancer, primary
- Lung lesions, metastatic
- Lung neoplasms, benign
- Mediastinal masses
- Pneumonia
- Pneumothorax
- Pulmonary edema, cardiogenic
- Pulmonary embolism
- Thoracic aortic aneurysms

Less Common
- Achalasia
- Bronchial adenomas & carcinoid tumors of lung
- Bronchiectasis
- Broncholithiasis
- Cystic diseases of lungs, congenital
- Cystic fibrosis
- Lung abscess
- Lung infection, aspergillosis
- Lung infection, blastomycosis
- Lung infection, coccidioidomycosis
- Lung infection, cryptococcosis
- Lung infection, histoplasmosis
- Lung infection, mucormycosis
- Pharyngoesophageal (Zenker) diverticulum
- Pleural tumors
- Sarcoidosis
- Thymic carcinoma
- Tuberculosis: pulmonary

Chest Pain: Fever

More Common
- Acute respiratory distress syndrome (ARDS)
- Aspiration
- Atelectasis
- Bronchiectasis
- Cellulitis
- Cholecystitis (acute & chronic)
- Empyema
- Esophageal perforation
- Hodgkin lymphoma
- Lung abscess
- Lung infections, fungal
- Pneumonia
- Pulmonary embolism
- Tuberculosis: pulmonary

Less Common
- Carcinoma, inflammatory
- Chest wall osteomyelitis
- Cystic diseases of lungs, congenital
- Cystic fibrosis
- Hepatic abscess
- Hodgkin lymphoma
- Lung infection, aspergillosis
- Lung infection, blastomycosis
- Lung infection, coccidioidomycosis
- Lung infection, cryptococcosis
- Lung infection, histoplasmosis
- Lung infection, mucormycosis
- Mediastinal masses
- Mediastinitis
- Pancreatic ascites & pancreatic pleural effusion

Chest Pain: Blood in Sputum

More Common
- Aspiration
- Bronchial adenomas & carcinoid tumors of lung
- Bronchiectasis
- Broncholithiasis
- Head & neck squamous cell cancer
- Lung abscess
- Lung cancer, primary
- Lung lesions, metastatic
- Lung neoplasms, benign
- Pneumonia
- Pneumothorax
- Pulmonary embolism
- Tuberculosis: pulmonary

Less Common
- Anaplastic (undifferentiated) thyroid cancer
- Cystic diseases of lungs, congenital
- Cystic fibrosis
- Empyema
- Lung infection, aspergillosis
- Lung infection, blastomycosis
- Lung infection, coccidioidomycosis
- Lung infection, cryptococcosis
- Lung infection, histoplasmosis
- Lung infection, mucormycosis
- Pulmonary edema, cardiogenic

Chest Pain: Post-traumatic

More Common
- Acute respiratory distress syndrome (ARDS)
- Aspiration
- Atelectasis
- Cardiac compressive shock
- Cardiogenic shock
- Empyema
- Lung abscess
- Pneumonia
- Pneumothorax
- Pulmonary contusion
- Pulmonary edema, cardiogenic
- Pulmonary embolism
- Thoracic injuries
- Volume overload

Less Common
- Lung infection, aspergillosis
- Lung infection, blastomycosis
- Lung infection, coccidioidomycosis
- Lung infection, cryptococcosis
- Lung infection, histoplasmosis

- Lung infection, mucormycosis
- Chest wall osteomyelitis
- Hepatic abscess
- Mediastinitis
- Pancreatic ascites & pancreatic pleural effusion
- Thoracic aortic dissection

Chest Pain: Dyspnea

More Common

- Aspiration
- Barrett esophagus
- Bronchial adenomas & carcinoid tumors of lung
- Bronchiectasis
- Esophageal carcinoma
- Gastroesophageal reflux disease & hiatal hernia
- Lung cancer, primary
- Lung lesions, metastatic
- Lung neoplasms, benign
- Pneumonia
- Pneumothorax
- Pulmonary contusion
- Pulmonary edema, cardiogenic
- Pulmonary embolism
- Tuberculosis: pulmonary

Less Common

- Achalasia
- Alkalosis, respiratory
- Cardiogenic shock
- Cystic diseases of lungs, congenital
- Cystic fibrosis
- Empyema
- Head & neck squamous cell cancer
- Lung abscess
- Lung infection, aspergillosis
- Lung infection, blastomycosis
- Lung infection, coccidioidomycosis
- Lung infection, cryptococcosis
- Lung infection, histoplasmosis
- Lung infection, mucormycosis
- Mediastinal masses
- Pleural tumors
- Pulmonary edema, neurogenic
- Sarcoidosis
- Thoracic aortic aneurysms
- Thymic carcinoma

Chest Pain: Palpable Mass

More Common

- Breast cancer, female
- Breast cancer, male
- Breast lesions, benign
- Chest wall tumors, benign skeletal
- Chest wall tumors, benign soft tissue
- Lipoma
- Lung cancer, primary
- Mondor disease (thrombophlebitis of the thoracoepigastric vein)

Less Common

- Chest wall osteomyelitis
- Chest wall tumors, malignant skeletal
- Chest wall tumors, malignant soft tissue

Chest Pain: Acute

More Common

- Aspiration
- Pneumonia
- Pneumothorax
- Pulmonary contusion
- Pulmonary edema, cardiogenic
- Pulmonary embolism
- Thoracic aortic aneurysms

Less Common

- Cardiogenic shock
- Empyema
- Esophageal carcinoma
- Lung abscess
- Lung cancer, primary
- Lung infection, aspergillosis
- Lung infection, blastomycosis
- Lung infection, coccidioidomycosis
- Lung infection, cryptococcosis
- Lung infection, histoplasmosis
- Lung infection, mucormycosis
- Lung lesions, metastatic
- Lung neoplasms, benign
- Pulmonary edema, neurogenic
- Tuberculosis: pulmonary

Chest Pain: Chronic

More Common

- Esophageal carcinoma
- Gastroesophageal reflux disease & hiatal hernia
- Lung cancer, primary
- Lung lesions, metastatic
- Pneumonia
- Sarcoidosis
- Tuberculosis: pulmonary

Less Common

- Achalasia
- Barrett esophagus
- Bronchial adenomas & carcinoid Tumors of lung
- Bronchiectasis
- Broncholithiasis
- Chest wall osteomyelitis
- Chest wall tumors, benign skeletal
- Chest wall tumors, benign soft tissue
- Chest wall tumors, malignant skeletal
- Chest wall tumors, malignant soft tissue
- Cystic diseases of lungs, congenital
- Cystic fibrosis
- Empyema
- Lung abscess
- Lung infection, aspergillosis
- Lung infection, blastomycosis
- Lung infection, coccidioidomycosis
- Lung infection, cryptococcosis
- Lung infection, histoplasmosis
- Lung infection, mucormycosis
- Lung neoplasms, benign
- Mediastinal masses
- Pleural tumors
- Thoracic aortic aneurysms
- Thymic carcinoma

Chest pain: Vomiting/Regurgitation

More Common

- Achalasia
- Cholecystitis (acute & chronic)
- Epiphrenic diverticulum
- Esophageal carcinoma
- Esophageal obstruction
- Esophageal sphincter dysfunction, upper
- Gastric adenocarcinoma
- Gastroesophageal reflux disease & hiatal hernia
- Goiter, simple or nontoxic (diffuse & multinodular)
- Mediastinal masses
- Pancreatitis, acute
- Paraesophageal hiatal hernia
- Pharyngoesophageal (Zenker) diverticulum

Less Common

- Abdominal wall hernias, noninguinal
- Barrett esophagus
- Duodenal tumors, benign
- Duodenal tumors, malignant
- Esophageal perforation
- Esophageal spasm, diffuse
- Esophageal tumors, benign
- Gastric bezoar
- Gastric lymphoma
- Gastric volvulus
- GIST, leiomyomas & lieomyosarcoma
- Hypercalcemia
- Parathyroid carcinoma

- Pediatric thoracic masses
- Pyloric obstruction
- Superior mesenteric artery obstruction of the duodenum

Constipation

Child

More Common

- Inguinal hernia
- Intussusception, pediatric
- Pediatric intestinal obstruction, miscellaneous
- Proctitis & anusitis, infectious
- Proctitis, inflammatory and radiation
- Pruritus ani
- Small intestine, obstruction
- Umbilical hernia

Less Common

- Cystic fibrosis
- Hirschsprung disease
- Imperforate anus
- Malrotation
- Mesenteric & omental cyst
- Rectal fixation, abnormal

Constipation: Adult, Pain

More Common

- Anal fissure & ulcer
- Anorectal abscess & fistula
- Colorectal adenocarcinoma
- Colorectal tumors, uncommon
- Hemorrhoids
- Proctitis & anusitis, infectious
- Proctitis, inflammatory & radiation
- Pruritis ani
- Rectal fixation, abnormal
- Rectal ulcer, solitary

Less Common

- Anal canal cancer
- Anal margin cancer
- Hirschsprung disease

Constipation: Adult, Chronic

More Common

- Anal canal cancer
- Anal fissure & ulcer
- Anal margin cancer
- Colorectal adenocarcinoma
- Colorectal tumors, uncommon
- Hemorrhoids
- Proctitis & anusitis, infectious
- Proctitis, inflammatory and radiation
- Pruritus ani
- Rectal fixation, abnormal
- Rectal ulcer, solitary

Less Common

- Anorectal abscess & fistula
- Hirschsprung disease

Constipation: Adult, Acute

More Common

- Colorectal adenocarcinoma
- Intussusception, pediatric
- Small intestine, obstruction
- Volvulus

Less Common

- Anal canal cancer
- Anal margin cancer
- Colorectal tumors, uncommon
- Hirschsprung disease
- Imperforate anus
- Pediatric intestinal obstruction, miscellaneous

Cough

Child

More Common

- Aspiration
- Cystic diseases of lungs, congenital
- Cystic fibrosis
- Empyema
- Gastroesophageal reflux disease & hiatal hernia
- Lung lesions, metastatic
- Lung neoplasms, benign
- Pneumonia
- Pneumothorax
- Pulmonary edema, cardiogenic
- Pulmonary embolism
- Tuberculosis: pulmonary

Less Common

- Bronchial adenomas & carcinoid tumors of lung
- Bronchiectasis
- Broncholithiasis
- Lung abscess
- Lung infection, aspergillosis
- Lung infection, blastomycosis
- Lung infection, coccidioidomycosis
- Lung infection, cryptococcosis
- Lung infection, histoplasmosis
- Lung infection, mucormycosis
- Mediastinal masses
- Pleural tumors
- Sarcoidosis

Cough: Adult, Chest Pain

More Common

- Aspiration
- Bronchiectasis
- Empyema
- Esophageal carcinoma
- Gastroesophageal reflux disease & hiatal hernia
- Lung abscess
- Lung cancer, primary
- Lung lesions, metastatic
- Mediastinal masses
- Pneumonia
- Pneumothorax
- Pulmonary embolism

Less Common

- Achalasia
- Barrett esophagus
- Bronchial adenomas & carcinoid tumors of lung
- Broncholithiasis
- Cystic diseases of lungs, congenital
- Cystic fibrosis
- Head & neck squamous cell cancer
- Lung infection, aspergillosis
- Lung infection, blastomycosis
- Lung infection, coccidioidomycosis
- Lung infection, cryptococcosis
- Lung infection, histoplasmosis
- Lung infection, mucormycosis
- Lung neoplasms, benign
- Pharyngoesophageal (Zenker) diverticulum
- Pleural tumors
- Pulmonary edema, cardiogenic
- Sarcoidosis
- Thoracic aortic aneurysms
- Thymic carcinoma
- Tuberculosis: pulmonary

Cough: Adult, Fever

More Common

- Acute respiratory distress syndrome (ARDS)
- Aspiration
- Atelectasis
- Bronchiectasis
- Empyema
- Lung abscess
- Mediastinitis
- Pneumonia
- Pulmonary embolism
- Tuberculosis: pulmonary

Less Common

- Cholecystitis (acute & chronic)
- Cystic diseases of lungs, congenital
- Cystic fibrosis
- Esophageal perforation
- Hodgkin lymphoma
- Lung infection, aspergillosis
- Lung infection, blastomycosis
- Lung infection, coccidioidomycosis
- Lung infection, cryptococcosis
- Lung infection, histoplasmosis
- Lung infection, mucormycosis
- Mediastinal masses
- Pancreatic ascites & pancreatic pleural effusion

Cough: Adult, Bloody Sputum

More Common

- Aspiration
- Bronchial adenomas & carcinoid tumors of lung
- Bronchiectasis
- Broncholithiasis
- Lung cancer, primary
- Lung neoplasms, benign
- Pneumonia
- Pulmonary edema, cardiogenic
- Pulmonary embolism
- Tuberculosis: pulmonary

Less Common

- Anaplastic (undifferentiated) thyroid cancer
- Cystic diseases of lungs, congenital
- Cystic fibrosis
- Empyema
- Head & neck squamous cell cancer
- Lung abscess
- Lung infection, aspergillosis
- Lung infection, blastomycosis
- Lung infection, coccidioidomycosis
- Lung infection, cryptococcosis
- Lung infection, histoplasmosis
- Lung infection, mucormycosis
- Lung lesions, metastatic
- Pneumothorax

Cough: Adult, Post-traumatic

More Common

- Aspiration
- Atelectasis
- Empyema
- Lung abscess
- Pneumonia
- Pneumothorax
- Pulmonary contusion
- Pulmonary edema, cardiogenic
- Pulmonary embolism
- Thoracic injuries
- Volume overload

Less Common

- Acute respiratory distress syndrome (ARDS)
- Cardiac compressive shock
- Cardiogenic shock
- Lung infection, aspergillosis
- Lung infection, blastomycosis
- Lung infection, coccidioidomycosis
- Lung infection, cryptococcosis
- Lung infection, histoplasmosis
- Lung infection, mucormycosis
- Mediastinitis
- Pancreatic ascites & pancreatic pleural effusion

Cough: Adult, Chronic

More Common

- Bronchiectasis
- Gastroesophageal reflux disease & hiatal hernia
- Lung cancer, primary
- Lung lesions, metastatic
- Lung neoplasms, benign
- Mediastinal masses
- Pulmonary edema, cardiogenic
- Pulmonary embolism
- Sarcoidosis
- Tuberculosis: pulmonary

Less Common

- Achalasia
- Aspiration
- Barrett esophagus
- Bronchial adenomas & carcinoid tumors of lung
- Broncholithiasis
- Cystic diseases of lungs, congenital
- Cystic fibrosis
- Empyema
- Esophageal carcinoma
- Head & neck squamous cell cancer
- Lung abscess
- Lung infection, aspergillosis
- Lung infection, blastomycosis
- Lung infection, coccidioidomycosis
- Lung infection, cryptococcosis
- Lung infection, histoplasmosis
- Lung infection, mucormycosis
- Pharyngoesophageal (Zenker) diverticulum
- Pleural tumors
- Pneumonia
- Pneumothorax
- Thoracic aortic aneurysms
- Thymic carcinoma

Cough: Adult, Nocturnal

More Common

- Achalasia
- Aspiration
- Esophageal carcinoma
- Gastroesophageal reflux disease & hiatal hernia
- Mediastinal masses
- Pharyngoesophageal (Zenker) diverticulum
- Pulmonary edema, cardiogenic
- Thymic carcinoma

Less Common

- Bronchial adenomas & carcinoid tumors of lung
- Bronchiectasis
- Broncholithiasis
- Cystic diseases of lungs, congenital
- Cystic fibrosis
- Empyema
- Head and neck squamous cell cancer
- Lung cancer, primary
- Lung infection, aspergillosis
- Lung infection, blastomycosis
- Lung infection, coccidioidomycosis
- Lung infection, cryptococcosis
- Lung infection, histoplasmosis
- Lung infection, mucormycosis
- Lung lesions, metastatic
- Lung neoplasms, benign
- Pleural tumors
- Pneumonia
- Pneumothorax
- Pulmonary embolism
- Thoracic aortic aneurysms

Cough: Adult, Postprandial

More Common

- Achalasia
- Aspiration
- Barrett esophagus
- Esophageal carcinoma
- Gastroesophageal reflux disease & hiatal hernia
- Pharyngoesophageal (Zenker) diverticulum

Less Common
- Head & neck squamous cell cancer
- Pulmonary edema, cardiogenic

Diarrhea

Child

More Common
- Appendicitis, acute
- Colitis, antibiotic-associated
- Crohn disease
- Intussusception, pediatric
- Pediatric intestinal obstruction, miscellaneous
- Short bowel syndrome
- Small intestine enteropathies, , noninfectious
- Small intestine, infectious diseases
- Small intestine, obstruction

Less Common
- Colitis, ischemic
- Colitis, ulcerative
- Proctitis & anusitis, infectious
- Proctitis, inflammatory & radiation
- Pyelonephritis, acute

Diarrhea: Adult

More Common
- Appendicitis, acute
- Colitis, antibiotic-associated
- Colitis, ischemic
- Colitis, ulcerative
- Crohn disease
- Small intestine enteropathies, , noninfectious
- Small intestine, infectious diseases
- Small intestine, obstruction

Less Common
- Endometriosis
- Intra-abdominal abscess
- Intussusception, adult
- Proctitis & anusitis, infectious
- Proctitis, inflammatory & radiation
- Pyelonephritis, acute
- Retroperitoneal abscess
- Short bowel syndrome

Diarrhea: Adult, Bloody
- Colitis, antibiotic-associated
- Colitis, ischemic
- Colitis, ulcerative
- Crohn disease
- Intussusception, adult
- Proctitis & anusitis, infectious
- Proctitis, inflammatory & radiation
- Small intestine, infectious diseases

Diarrhea: Adult, Abdominal pain

More Common
- Appendicitis, acute
- Colitis, antibiotic-associated
- Colitis, ischemic
- Colitis, ulcerative
- Crohn disease
- Intussusception, adult
- Small intestine, infectious diseases
- Small intestine, obstruction

Less Common
- Endometriosis
- Intra-abdominal abscess
- Proctitis & anusitis, infectious
- Proctitis, inflammatory & radiation
- Pyelonephritis, acute
- Retroperitoneal abscess

Diarrhea: Adult, Chronic
- Colitis, antibiotic-associated
- Colitis, ischemic
- Colitis, ulcerative
- Crohn disease
- Endometriosis
- Proctitis & anusitis, infectious
- Proctitis, inflammatory & radiation
- Short bowel syndrome
- Small intestine enteropathies, noninfectious
- Small intestine, infectious diseases
- Small intestine, obstruction

Diarrhea: Adult, Fever

More Common
- Appendicitis, acute
- Colitis, antibiotic-associated
- Colitis, ischemic
- Colitis, ulcerative
- Crohn disease
- Intussusception, adult
- Small intestine, infectious diseases
- Small intestine, obstruction

Less Common
- Intra-abdominal abscess
- Proctitis & anusitis, infectious
- Proctitis, inflammatory & radiation
- Pyelonephritis, acute
- Retroperitoneal abscess

Diarrhea: Adult, Postoperative
- Colitis, antibiotic-associated
- Colitis, ischemic
- Intra-abdominal abscess
- Intussusception, adult
- Proctitis & anusitis, infectious
- Proctitis, inflammatory & radiation
- Pyelonephritis, acute
- Retroperitoneal abscess
- Small intestine, infectious diseases
- Small intestine, obstruction

Dysphagia

More Common
- Achalasia
- Esophageal carcinoma
- Esophageal obstruction
- Esophageal sphincter dysfunction, upper
- Gastroesophageal reflux disease & hiatal hernia
- Goiter, simple or nontoxic (diffuse and multinodular)
- Hashimoto thyroiditis
- Head & neck squamous cell cancer
- Hürthle cell neoplasms
- Paraesophageal hiatal hernia
- Pharyngoesophageal (Zenker) diverticulum
- Thyroid cancer, papillary
- Thyroid nodule

Less Common
- Carotid aneurysm, extracranial
- Carotid body tumor
- Esophageal perforation
- Esophageal spasm, diffuse
- Esophageal tumors, benign
- Esophagitis, corrosive
- Graves disease
- Hypercalcemia
- Hypocalcemia
- Mediastinal masses
- Mediastinitis
- Parathyroid carcinoma
- Salivary gland infections
- Salivary gland tumors
- Sialolithiasis
- Superior vena cava syndrome
- Thymic carcinoma
- Thymoma and myasthenia gravis
- Thyroid cancer, anaplastic
- Thyroid cancer, follicular
- Thyroid cancer, medullary

- Thyroid lymphoma
- Thyroid metastasis
- Thyroiditis, acute suppurative
- Thyroiditis, de Quervain subacute
- Thyroiditis, Riedel

Fatigue

Acute

More Common

- Cardiac compressive shock
- Cardiogenic shock
- Cellulitis
- Hemolytic anemia, acquired
- Hepatic failure, acute
- Hypercalcemia
- Hypercalcemia of malignancy, humoral
- Hyperparathyroidism, primary
- Hypokalemia
- Hyponatremia
- Hypophosphatemia
- Intra-abdominal abscess
- Pelvic inflammatory disease
- Pulmonary edema, cardiogenic
- Pulmonary thromboembolism
- Pyelonephritis, acute
- Retroperitoneal abscess
- Septic shock
- Surgical site infections
- Volume overload

Less Common

- Empyema
- Endocarditis
- Heat stroke
- Hepatic abscess
- Hypovolemic shock
- Lung abscess
- Mechanical pulmonary failure
- Pleural effusion
- Pulmonary edema, neurogenic
- Superior vena cava syndrome

Fatigue, Chronic

More Common

- Adrenocortical carcinoma
- Breast cancer, female
- Carcinoma, inflammatory
- Cardiomyopathy, idiopathic
- Cardiomyopathy, ischemic
- Cholangiocarcinoma
- Colorectal adenocarcinoma
- Colorectal cancer, hereditary nonpolyposis
- Esophageal carcinoma
- Gastric adenocarcinoma
- Gastric lymphoma
- Hashimoto thyroiditis
- Head and neck squamous cell cancer
- Hemolytic anemia, acquired
- Hodgkin lymphoma
- Hyperadrenocorticism (Cushing disease/syndrome)
- Lung cancer, primary
- Lung lesions, metastatic
- Pancreatic adenocarcinoma
- Renal failure
- Superior vena cava syndrome
- Tuberculosis, pulmonary

Less Common

- Actinomycosis & nocardiosis
- Anal canal cancer
- Anal margin cancer
- Ascites
- Breast cancer, male
- Bronchial adenomas & carcinoid tumors of lung
- Bronchiectasis
- Chest wall osteomyelitis
- Colorectal tumors, uncommon
- Duodenal tumors, malignant
- Endocarditis
- Gastrointestinal stromal tumor, leiomyomas, & leiomyosarcoma
- Herpes zoster
- Islet cell tumors, nonfunctioning
- Lung infection, aspergillosis
- Lung infection, blastomycosis
- Lung infection, coccidioidomycosis
- Lung infection, cryptococcosis
- Lung infection, histoplasmosis
- Lung infection, mucormycosis
- Melanoma
- Retroperitoneal sarcoma
- Small intestine tumors, malignant
- Soft tissue sarcoma
- Thyroid cancer, anaplastic
- Thyroid cancer, follicular
- Thyroid cancer, medullary
- Thyroid cancer, papillary
- Thyroid lymphoma
- Thyroid metastasis

Fever

Postoperative

More Common

- Aspiration
- Atelectasis
- Cellulitis
- Colitis, antibiotic-associated
- Deep venous thrombosis
- Intra-abdominal abscess
- Pneumonia
- Pulmonary thromboembolism
- Pyelonephritis, acute
- Retroperitoneal abscess
- Septic shock
- Surgical site infections
- Thrombophlebitis, superficial

Less Common

- Anorectal abscess & fistula
- Deep venous thrombosis, upper extremity
- Empyema
- Lung abscess
- Necrotizing fasciitis

Fever: Post-traumatic

More Common

- Aspiration
- Atelectasis
- Cellulitis
- Colitis, antibiotic-associated
- Deep venous thrombosis
- Intra-abdominal abscess
- Pneumonia
- Pulmonary thromboembolism
- Pyelonephritis, acute
- Retroperitoneal abscess
- Septic shock
- Surgical site infections
- Thrombophlebitis, superficial

Less Common

- Anorectal abscess & fistula
- Deep venous thrombosis, upper extremity
- Empyema
- Lung abscess

Fever: Abdominal Pain

More Common

- Appendicitis, acute
- Cholecystitis (acute & chronic)
- Colitis, ischemic
- Diverticulitis
- Hepatic abscess
- Hepatitis (acute & chronic)
- Pancreatitis, acute
- Pelvic inflammatory disease
- Peritonitis, bacterial
- Pneumonia
- Pyelonephritis, acute
- Small intestine, infectious diseases

Less Common

- Acidosis, metabolic
- Empyema
- Peptic ulcer perforation
- Small intestine, obstruction
- Volvulus

Fever: Cough

More Common

- Acute respiratory distress syndrome (ARDS)
- Aspiration
- Atelectasis
- Bronchiectasis
- Cellulitis
- Empyema
- Lung abscess
- Lung infections, fungal
- Mediastinal masses
- Pneumonia
- Pulmonary embolism
- Tuberculosis: pulmonary

Less Common

- Chest wall osteomyelitis
- Cystic diseases of lungs, congenital
- Cystic fibrosis
- Esophageal perforation
- Lung infection, aspergillosis
- Lung infection, blastomycosis
- Lung infection, coccidioidomycosis
- Lung infection, cryptococcosis
- Lung infection, histoplasmosis
- Lung infection, mucormycosis
- Mediastinitis
- Pancreatic ascites & pancreatic pleural effusion

Groin Pain/Swelling

More Common

- Abdominal wall mass
- Aneurysms, peripheral
- Femoral hernia
- Furuncle, carbuncle & hidradenitis suppurativa
- Iliac aneurysms
- Inguinal hernia
- Lipoma
- Varicose veins

Less Common

- Anal canal cancer
- Anal margin cancer
- Hodgkin lymphoma
- Non-Hodgkin lymphoma
- Peritoneal neoplasms
- Retroperitoneal abscess
- Retroperitoneal sarcoma
- Thrombophlebitis, superficial

Heartburn/Indigestion

Chronic

More Common

- Achalasia
- Barrett esophagus
- Duodenal tumors, benign
- Duodenal tumors, malignant
- Epiphrenic diverticulum
- Esophageal carcinoma
- Esophageal obstruction
- Esophageal perforation
- Esophageal tumors, benign
- Gastric adenocarcinoma
- Gastric lymphoma
- Gastroesophageal reflux disease & hiatal hernia
- GIST, leiomyomas & leiomyosarcoma
- Hypercalcemia
- Mediastinal masses
- Paraesophageal hiatal hernia
- Pyloric obstruction

Less Common

- Esophageal spasm, diffuse
- Esophageal sphincter dysfunction, upper
- Gastric bezoar
- Gastric volvulus
- Goiter, simple or nontoxic (diffuse & multinodular)
- Pancreatitis, acute
- Parathyroid carcinoma
- Pediatric thoracic masses
- Pharyngoesophageal (Zenker) diverticulum
- Superior mesenteric artery obstruction of the duodenum

Heartburn/Indigestion: Acute

More Common

- Esophageal carcinoma
- Esophageal obstruction
- Esophageal perforation
- Gastroesophageal reflux disease & hiatal hernia
- Paraesophageal hiatal hernia

Less Common

- Hypercalcemia
- Pharyngoesophageal (Zenker) diverticulum
- Pyloric obstruction
- Superior mesenteric artery obstruction of the duodenum

Heartburn/Indigestion: Weight Loss

More Common

- Esophageal carcinoma
- Esophageal obstruction
- Gastric adenocarcinoma
- Gastric lymphoma
- GIST, leiomyomas & leiomyosarcoma
- Pyloric obstruction

Less Common

- Duodenal tumors, malignant
- Esophageal spasm, diffuse
- Esophageal tumors, benign
- Mediastinal masses
- Parathyroid carcinoma
- Superior mesenteric artery obstruction of the duodenum

Hematemesis

More Common

- Duodenal ulcer
- Gastric ulcer
- Peptic ulcer hemorrhage
- Portal hypertension
- Stress ulcer

Less Common

- Ascites
- Duodenal tumors, benign
- Duodenal tumors, malignant
- Gastric adenocarcinoma
- Gastric lymphoma
- Gastric volvulus
- Gastrinoma (Zollinger-Ellison syndrome)
- Small intestine tumors, benign
- Small intestine tumors, malignant
- Splenic vein thrombosis

Hypercalcemia

More Common

- Hypercalcemia
- Hypercalcemia of malignancy, humoral
- Hyperparathyroidism, primary
- Hyperparathyroidism, secondary
- Tertiary hyperparathyroidism

Less Common

- Hypercalcemia, familial hypocalciuric
- Multiple endocrine neoplasia I (MEN I)
- Multiple endocrine neoplasia II (MEN II)
- Osteitis fibrosa cystica

- Paget disease
- Parathyroid carcinoma

Hyperthyroidism

More Common
- Graves disease
- Hyperthyroidism, non-Graves

Less Common
- Hashimoto thyroiditis
- Thyroiditis, acute suppurative
- Thyroiditis, de Quervain subacute
- Thyroiditis, Riedel

Jaundice

More Common
- Ampulla of vater tumors
- Biliary neoplasms, benign
- Biliary obstructions, benign
- Cholangiocarcinoma
- Cholangitis, primary sclerosing
- Cholecystitis (acute & chronic)
- Choledocholithiasis & gallstone pancreatitis
- Cholelithiasis
- Cholelithiasis, rare complications
- Cirrhosis
- Hepatic failure, acute
- Hepatitis (acute & chronic)
- Jaundice
- Pancreatic adenocarcinoma
- Pancreatitis, chronic

Less Common
- Biliary atresia
- Choledochal cyst
- Cirrhosis, primary biliary
- Duodenal tumors, malignant
- Gallbladder adenocarcinoma
- Pancreatic neoplasms, cystic

Leg Pain

Chronic

More Common
- Deep venous thrombosis
- Lymphedema & lymphangitis
- Popliteal artery diseases
- Varicose veins
- Vascular occlusive disease, peripheral
- Venous insufficiency, chronic

Less Common
- Aneurysms, Peripheral
- Buerger disease
- Iliac aneurysms

Leg Pain: Acute

More Common
- Arterial occlusion, acute
- Arterial trauma, iatrogenic
- Cellulitis
- Deep venous thrombosis
- Lymphedema & lymphangitis
- Popliteal artery diseases
- Thrombophlebitis, superficial
- Varicose veins
- Vascular occlusive disease, peripheral

Less Common
- Aneurysms, peripheral
- Buerger disease
- Iliac aneurysms

Leg Ulcer

More Common
- Bites, arthropod
- Cellulitis
- Deep venous thrombosis
- Furuncle, carbuncle & hidradenitis suppurativa
- Lymphedema & lymphangitis
- Vascular occlusive disease, peripheral
- Venous insufficiency, chronic

Less Common
- Aneurysms, peripheral
- Melanoma
- Necrotizing fasciitis
- Popliteal artery diseases
- Snakebite
- Soft tissue sarcoma
- Vasoconstrictive disorders

Liver Enlargement

- Gallbladder adenocarcinoma
- Hepatic abscess
- Hepatic failure, acute
- Hepatic neoplasms, benign
- Hepatic tumor, metastatic
- Hepatic tumor, uncommon primary
- Hepatitis (acute & chronic)
- Hepatocellular carcinoma

Lung Cancer

More Common
- Lung cancer, primary
- Lung lesions, metastatic

Less Common
- Bronchial adenomas & carcinoid tumors of lung

Neck Mass

Central

More Common
- Esophageal carcinoma
- Goiter, simple or nontoxic (diffuse & multinodular)
- Graves disease
- Hashimoto thyroiditis
- Head & neck squamous cell cancer
- Hürthle cell neoplasms
- Pediatric neck masses
- Thyroglossal cyst
- Thyroid cancer, follicular
- Thyroid cancer, papillary
- Thyroid nodule

Less Common
- Parathyroid carcinoma
- Thyroid cancer, anaplastic
- Thyroid cancer, medullary
- Thyroid lymphoma
- Thyroid metastasis
- Thyroiditis, acute suppurative
- Thyroiditis, de Quervain, subacute
- Thyroiditis, Riedel

Neck Mass: Lateral

More Common
- Esophageal carcinoma
- Head & neck squamous cell cancer
- Hodgkin lymphoma
- Hürthle cell neoplasms
- Non-Hodgkin lymphoma
- Pediatric neck masses
- Salivary gland tumors
- Thyroid cancer, follicular
- Thyroid cancer, papillary

Less Common
- Carotid aneurysm, extracranial
- Carotid body tumor
- Thyroid cancer, anaplastic
- Thyroid cancer, medullary

Neck Mass: Child

- Pediatric neck masses

Oliguria

More Common
- Cardiac compressive shock
- Cardiogenic shock

- Dehydration (volume & electrolyte depletion)
- Hypovolemic shock
- Renal failure
- Septic shock

Less Common

- Arterial occlusion, acute
- Arterial trauma, iatrogenic
- Renal artery aneurysm
- Retroperitoneal abscess
- Retroperitoneal fibrosis
- Retroperitoneal hemorrhage
- Retroperitoneal sarcoma
- Thoracic aortic dissection
- Ureteral or renal calculi

Pancreas Cancer

More Common

- Pancreatic adenocarcinoma
- Pancreatic neoplasms, cystic

Less Common

- Gastrinoma (Zollinger-Ellison syndrome)
- Glucagonoma
- Insulinoma
- Islet cell tumors, nonfunctioning
- Somatostatinoma
- VIPoma

Pancreatitis

- Choledocholithiasis & gallstone pancreatitis
- Pancreatic abscess
- Pancreatic ascites & pancreatic pleural effusion
- Pancreatic insufficiency
- Pancreatitis, acute
- Pancreatitis, chronic

Pelvic Pain

Fever

More Common

- Appendicitis, acute
- Colitis, ischemic
- Diverticulitis
- Pelvic inflammatory disease
- Peptic ulcer perforation
- Peritonitis, bacterial
- Pyelonephritis, acute
- Small intestine, infectious diseases

Less Common

- Cholecystitis (acute & chronic)
- Colitis, antibiotic-associated
- Proctitis & anusitis, infectious
- Proctitis, inflammatory & radiation

Pelvic Pain: Postoperative

More Common

- Appendicitis, acute
- Colitis, antibiotic-associated
- Colitis, ischemic
- Diverticulitis
- Intra-abdominal abscess
- Mesenteric vascular occlusion, acute
- Pancreatitis, acute
- Pelvic inflammatory disease
- Peritonitis, bacterial
- Pyelonephritis, acute
- Small intestine, infectious diseases
- Small intestine, obstruction
- Surgical site infections

Less Common

- Cholecystitis (acute & chronic)
- Hepatic abscess
- Inguinal hernia
- Peptic ulcer perforation
- Proctitis & anusitis, infectious
- Proctitis, inflammatory and radiation

Pelvic Pain: Post-traumatic

More Common

- Appendicitis, acute
- Colitis, antibiotic-associated
- Colitis, ischemic
- Diverticulitis
- Intra-abdominal abscess
- Mesenteric vascular occlusion, acute
- Pancreatitis, acute
- Pelvic inflammatory disease
- Peritonitis, bacterial
- Pyelonephritis, acute
- Small intestine, infectious diseases
- Small intestine, obstruction
- Surgical site infections

Less Common

- Cholecystitis (acute & chronic)
- Hepatic abscess
- Inguinal hernia
- Peptic ulcer perforation
- Proctitis & anusitis, infectious
- Proctitis, inflammatory and radiation

Pulmonary Nodule

More Common

- Empyema
- Lung abscess
- Lung cancer, primary
- Lung lesions, metastatic
- Lung neoplasms, benign
- Pleural tumors
- Pneumonia
- Tuberculosis, pulmonary

Less Common

- Bronchial adenomas & carcinoid tumors of lung
- Bronchiectasis
- Broncholithiasis
- Chest wall osteomyelitis
- Chest wall tumors, benign skeletal
- Chest wall tumors, benign soft tissue
- Chest wall tumors, malignant skeletal
- Chest wall tumors, malignant soft tissue
- Lung infection, aspergillosis
- Lung infection, blastomycosis
- Lung infection, coccidioidomycosis
- Lung infection, cryptococcosis
- Lung infection, histoplasmosis
- Lung infection, mucormycosis

Rectal/Perianal Pain

More Common

- Anal fissure & ulcer
- Anorectal abscess & fistula
- Condylomata acuminata
- Hemorrhoids
- Proctitis & anusitis, infectious
- Pruritus ani
- Rectal ulcer, solitary

Less Common

- Anal canal cancer
- Anal margin cancer
- Colorectal adenocarcinoma
- Colorectal tumors, uncommon
- Proctitis, inflammatory & radiation

Rectal Tenesmus

- Anal canal cancer
- Anal fissure & ulcer
- Anal margin cancer
- Anorectal abscess & fistula
- Condylomata acuminata
- Hemorrhoids
- Proctitis & anusitis, infectious
- Proctitis, inflammatory & radiation
- Pruritus ani
- Rectal ulcer, solitary

Splenomegaly

- Hemolytic anemia, acquired
- Hemolytic anemias, miscellaneous hereditary (elliptocytosis, nonspherocytic, thalassemia)
- Hodgkin lymphoma
- Immune thrombocytopenic purpura (ITP)
- Non-Hodgkin lymphoma
- Spherocytosis
- Splenic abscess
- Splenic cysts & tumors
- Splenic neoplasms
- Thrombotic thrombocytopenic purpura

Swollen Legs

Acute

- Arterial occlusion, acute
- Cellulitis
- Deep venous thrombosis
- Lymphedema & lymphangitis
- Popliteal artery diseases
- Thrombophlebitis, superficial
- Varicose veins

Swollen Legs: Chronic

More Common

- Deep venous thrombosis
- Lymphedema & lymphangitis
- Popliteal artery diseases
- Thrombophlebitis, superficial
- Varicose veins
- Vascular occlusive disease, peripheral
- Venous insufficiency, chronic

Less Common

- Aneurysms, peripheral
- Buerger disease
- Iliac aneurysms

Swollen Legs: Postoperative

- Arterial occlusion, acute
- Cellulitis
- Deep venous thrombosis
- Lymphedema & lymphangitis
- Popliteal artery diseases
- Thrombophlebitis, superficial
- Varicose veins

Swollen Legs: Post-traumatic

- Arterial injuries
- Arterial occlusion, acute
- Blast injury
- Cellulitis
- Deep venous thrombosis
- Lymphedema & lymphangitis
- Popliteal artery diseases
- Thrombophlebitis, superficial
- Varicose veins

Testicular Pain

- Appendicitis, acute
- Femoral hernia
- Inguinal hernia
- Intra-abdominal abscess
- Pyelonephritis, acute
- Retroperitoneal abscess
- Retroperitoneal fibrosis
- Retroperitoneal hemorrhage
- Ureteral or renal calculi

Thyroid Cancer

More Common

- Hürthle cell neoplasms
- Thyroid cancer, follicular
- Thyroid cancer, papillary

Less Common

- Multiple endocrine neoplasia II (MEN II)
- Thyroid cancer, anaplastic
- Thyroid cancer, medullary
- Thyroid lymphoma
- Thyroid metastasis

Thyroid Enlargement

More Common

- Goiter, simple or nontoxic (diffuse & multinodular)
- Graves disease
- Hashimoto thyroiditis
- Hürthle cell neoplasms
- Thyroid cancer, follicular
- Thyroid cancer, papillary
- Thyroid nodule

Less Common

- Multiple endocrine neoplasia II (MEN II)
- Thyroid cancer, anaplastic
- Thyroid cancer, medullary
- Thyroid lymphoma
- Thyroid metastasis
- Thyroiditis, acute suppurative
- Thyroiditis, de Quervain subacute
- Thyroiditis, Riedel

Thyroid Pain

- Hashimoto thyroiditis
- Thyroglossal cyst
- Thyroiditis, acute suppurative
- Thyroiditis, de Quervain subacute
- Thyroiditis, Riedel

Trauma

- Abdominal injuries
- Arterial injuries
- Blast injury
- Diaphragmatic hernia, traumatic
- Drowning
- Hepatic trauma
- Neck injuries
- Pleural space trauma
- Pulmonary contusion
- Thoracic injuries
- Tracheobronchial injuries
- Trauma evaluation

Weight Gain

More Common

- Hashimoto thyroiditis
- Pulmonary edema, cardiogenic
- Volume overload

Less Common

- Adrenal tumors, sex hormone-producing
- Adrenocortical carcinoma
- Hyperadrenocorticism (Cushing disease/syndrome)
- Insulinoma

Weight Loss

More Common

- Blind loop syndrome
- Breast cancer, female
- Colorectal adenocarcinoma
- Colorectal cancer, hereditary nonpolyposis
- Dehydration (volume & electrolyte depletion)
- Duodenal tumors, malignant
- Esophageal carcinoma
- Esophageal obstruction
- Gastric adenocarcinoma
- Gastric lymphoma
- Graves disease
- Hepatic tumor, metastatic
- Hepatocellular carcinoma
- Hodgkin lymphoma

- Hyperthyroidism, non-Graves
- Melanoma
- Mesenteric ischemia
- Pain, abdominal, nonspecific
- Pancreatic adenocarcinoma
- Pancreatitis, chronic
- Pneumonia
- Retroperitoneal abscess
- Small intestine enteropathies, noninfectious
- Small intestine, infectious diseases
- Tuberculosis, pulmonary

Less Common

- Adrenocortical carcinoma
- Ampulla of vater tumors
- Anal canal cancer
- Anal margin cancer
- Annular pancreas
- Appendiceal neoplasms
- Bronchiectasis
- Cholangiocarcinoma
- Colitis, ulcerative
- Crohn disease
- Endometriosis
- Esophageal spasm, diffuse
- Esophageal tumors, benign
- Gallbladder adenocarcinoma
- Gastric bezoar
- Glucagonoma
- Hepatic tumor, uncommon primary
- Islet cell tumors, nonfunctioning
- Lung infection, aspergillosis
- Lung infection, blastomycosis
- Lung infection, coccidioidomycosis
- Lung infection, cryptococcosis
- Lung infection, histoplasmosis
- Lung infection, mucormycosis
- Mediastinal masses
- Non-Hodgkin lymphoma
- Pancreatic ascites and pancreatic pleural effusion
- Pancreatic insufficiency
- Pancreatic neoplasms, cystic
- Pancreatic pseudocyst
- Peritoneal neoplasms
- Pleural tumors
- Pyloric obstruction
- Retroperitoneal fibrosis
- Retroperitoneal sarcoma
- Small intestine carcinoid
- Small intestine tumors, malignant
- Soft tissue sarcoma
- Superior mesenteric artery obstruction of the duodenum
- Thymic carcinoma
- Thymoma and myasthenia gravis
- Thyroid cancer, anaplastic
- Thyroid lymphoma
- Vipoma
- Visceral aneurysms

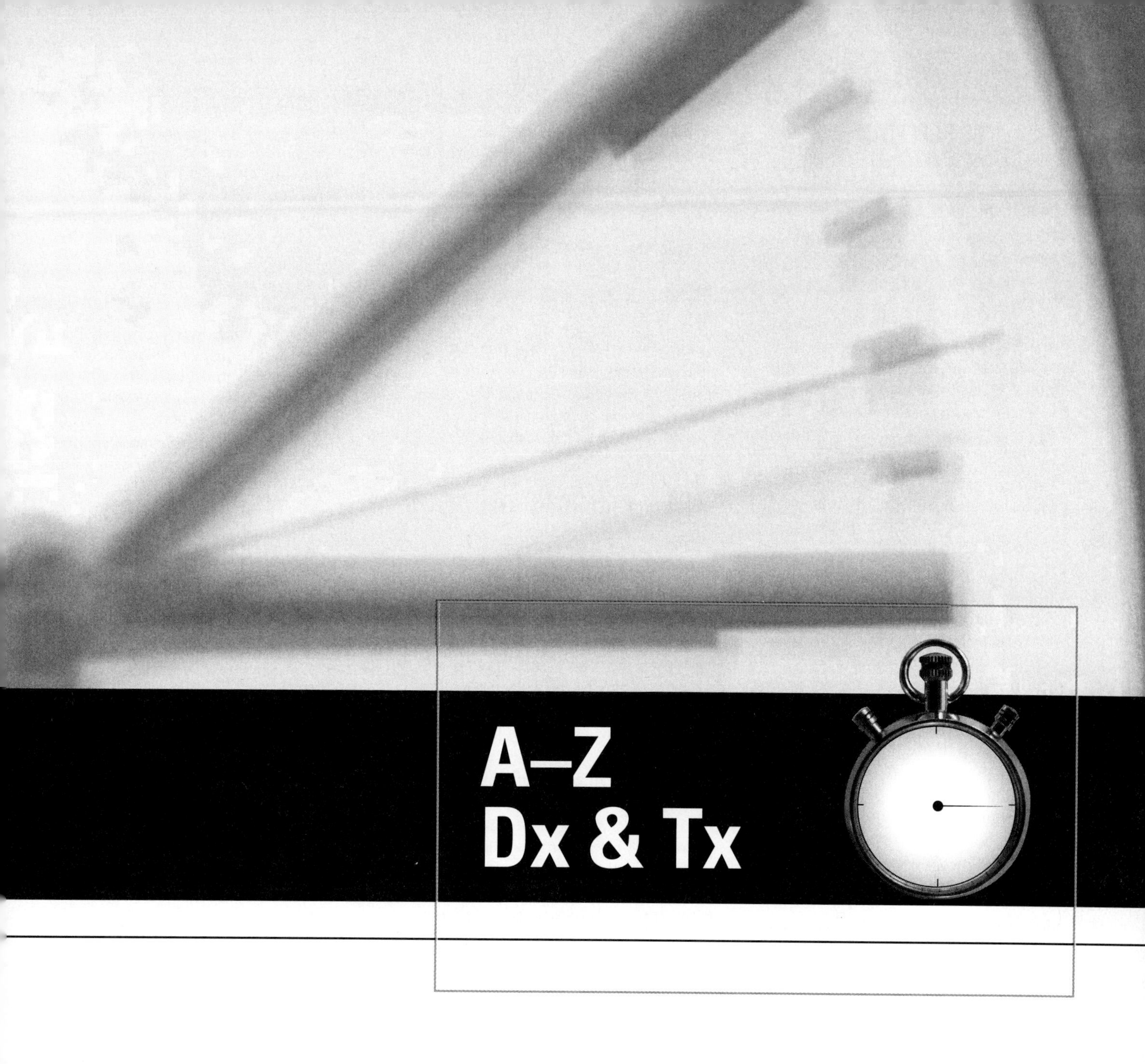

A–Z Dx & Tx

Abdominal Aortic Aneurysm (AAA)

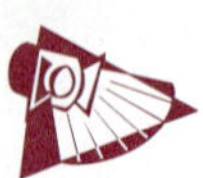

ESSENTIAL FEATURES

- Permanent aortic dilation (at least 50%)
- Classified by etiology (degenerative, inflammatory, mechanical, congenital, dissecting) and by shape (saccular, fusiform)
- Up to 25% of patients have symptoms of aortoiliac occlusive disease as well
- Most are infrarenal; decreased vasa vasorum and elastic lamellae may predispose to aneurysm formation
- Rupture risk correlates with size, following law of Laplace
- Average expansion rate of 0.4 cm/y depends on aneurysm size, diastolic blood pressure, and chronic obstructive pulmonary disease (COPD)
- For AAA measuring 5.0–5.5 cm, rupture risk is 40% at 5 years
- **Suprarenal:** Uncommon; extends proximal to renal arteries; low risk for rupture until exceeds 6–7 cm
- **Ruptured:** Most often ruptures posterolaterally to left; if short window present, likely contained rupture that eventually becomes free rupture
- **Inflammatory:** Characterized by inflammatory response external to aneurysmal wall, with inflammation usually confined to anterior aorta; 25% have ureteral obstruction, which results in dense, shiny fibrotic reaction enveloping adjacent viscera
- **Infected (mycotic):** Bacterial contamination of preexisting aneurysm (different from *Salmonella* causing false aneurysm); gram-negative infections result in higher rupture rates

EPIDEMIOLOGY

- Ruptured AAA is the 13th leading cause of death in the United States (15,000 deaths yearly)
- Present in 2% of population and incidence is increasing
- More men affected than women (4:1)
- 5% of patients with coronary artery disease have AAA
- 50% of patients with femoral or popliteal aneurysms have AAA
- 19% incidence among first-degree relatives
- **Rare causes:**
  - Marfan syndrome
  - Ehlers-Danlos syndrome
  - Behçet disease
  - Syphilis
  - Long-term sequelae of aortic dissection
- **Risks:**
  - Smoking
  - Hypertension (HTN)
  - COPD
- Diabetes appears to exert protective effect
- Increased incidence of rupture during fall and winter months
- *Strep, Haemophilus, Staph, E coli,* other gram-negative pathogens, and fungi identified in infected AAA

CLINICAL FINDINGS

SYMPTOMS AND SIGNS

- Rarely produces symptoms if intact
- Painless, pulsatile abdominal mass above umbilicus; may be uncomfortable on palpation
- Palpation may be difficult in obese patients
- Rarely produces back pain from pressure on nerves
- Severe pain caused by inflammatory or ruptured AAA or acute expansion
- Congestive heart failure from aortocaval fistula, GI bleed from duodenal erosion, and pyelonephritis from ureteral obstruction are rare
- Rupture causes sudden, severe abdominal/back pain radiating to back or inguinal area, faintness or syncope, shock; often tender pulsatile mass present
- **Triad for rupture:** Pain, pulsatile abdominal mass, hypotension found in < 67% of patients
- **Inflammatory:** Abdominal pain, tender AAA
- **Infected:** Rapidly enlarging tender pulsatile mass, fever

LABORATORY FINDINGS

- Infected AAA graft

IMAGING FINDINGS

- **Abdominal x-ray:** 20% calcifications in outer aortic wall on lateral view
- **US**
  - Inexpensive screening test, measures size and position
  - Used in cases of groin pseudoaneurysm to evaluate proximal anastomosis in abdomen
- **CT scan**
  - Diagnostic, accurate sizing, and provides information about anatomy: renal anomalies, retroaortic renal veins, circumaortic renal veins, duplicated vena cava, left-sided vena cava, other masses
  - Diagnoses inflammatory AAA
- **Aortogram**
  - Done only when mesenteric ischemia, renal vascular disease, horseshoe or pelvis kidney, unexplained impairment of renal function, coexistent occlusive disease is suspected
  - Infected AAA may have saccular component where infection is causing wall necrosis

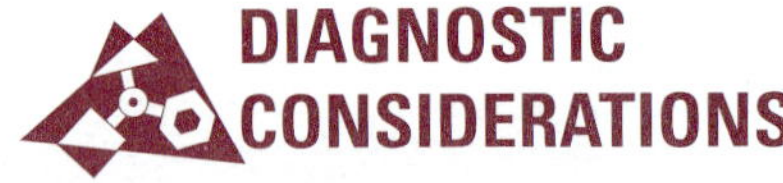

DIAGNOSTIC CONSIDERATIONS

- Consider inflammatory AAA when patient has severe pain without rupture

RULE OUT

- Ruptured AAA

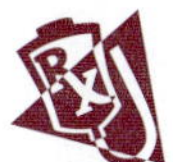

WORK-UP

- Maintain high suspicion for diagnosis of rupture
- If stable, can perform US to confirm diagnosis of AAA
- CT scan can diagnose rupture, but may be costly in terms of time

WHEN TO ADMIT

- Infected AAA: 50% of patients have positive blood cultures

WHEN TO REFER

- Consider referral if:
  - Suprarenal AAA
  - Concomitant renovascular or mesenteric disease

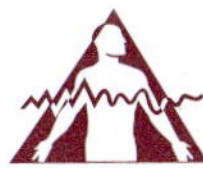

TREATMENT AND MANAGEMENT

- **Open repair options:** Tube graft, bifurcated graft (aortobiiliac, aortobifemoral)
- **Endovascular repair:** Evolving anatomic criteria; performed via open cutdown of femoral arteries
- **Suprarenal AAA:** Via thoracoabdominal approach with reimplantation of celiac, superior mesenteric artery (SMA), and renal arteries
- **Ruptured AAA:** To surgery immediately, prep patient before induction, immediate control of proximal aorta needed
- **Inflammatory AAA:** Clamp aorta at diaphragm, do not dissect duodenum from AAA, consider retroperitoneal approach
- **Infected AAA:** Excision of AAA and extra-anatomic bypass with prolonged antibiotics

SURGERY

Indications

- AAA size > 5–5.5 cm, depending on individual patient risk
- AAA expansion > 0.5–1 cm/y regardless of size

MEDICATIONS

- Prolonged antibiotics for infected AAA

TREATMENT MONITORING

- **Endovascular repair:** Serial CT scans necessary to rule out endoleak
- Monitor patients who have small AAA not large enough to warrant repair with serial US every 6–12 months

COMPLICATIONS

- 5–10% of open repair cases associated with complications, including bleeding, renal failure, myocardial infarction, limb loss, erectile dysfunction, paraplegia, and 2–4% operative mortality
- Risk is higher for suprarenal repair
- Malignant tumor found during surgery in 4% of cases
- Operative mortality from ruptured AAA > 60%; overall mortality, 90%

PROGNOSIS

- Graft failure rate low
- Long-term is excellent
- Determined by other cardiovascular disease
- Gram-positive infected AAA: 70% survival
- Gram-negative infected AAA: 25% survival

RESOURCES

REFERENCES

- Becquemin J et al. Mid-term results of endovascular versus open repair for abdominal aortic aneurysm in patients anatomically suitable for endovascular repair. *Eur J Vasc Endovasc Surg.* 2000;19:656.
- Beebe HG et al. Results of an aortic endograft trial: impact of device failure beyond 12 months. *J Vasc Surg.* 2001;33(2 Suppl):S55.
- Dardik A et al. Results of elective abdominal aortic aneurysm repair in the 1990s: a population-based analysis of 2335 cases. *J Vasc Surg.* 1999;30:985.
- Moore WS et al. Abdominal aortic aneurysm: a 6-year comparison of endovascular versus transabdominal repair. *Ann Surg.* 1999;230:298.

Abdominal Injuries

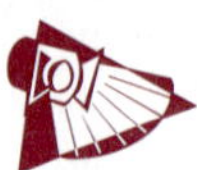

ESSENTIAL FEATURES

- Mechanism of injury in blunt trauma is rapid deceleration with noncompliant organs most at risk (kidney, liver, spleen, pancreas)

Penetrating Injuries

- May cause sepsis if a hollow viscus is penetrated
- Severe and early shock if major vessel or liver is involved
- Injuries of the kidney, spleen, or pancreas do not usually bleed massively unless a major vessel is involved

Blunt Injuries

- Focused Assessment with Sonography for Trauma (FAST) exam is important management tool
- Nonsurgical therapy used in more than 80% of blunt liver and spleen injuries

EPIDEMIOLOGY

- 30% of patients with "seatbelt signs" have internal injury
- 85% of patients with blunt liver injury stabilize with resuscitation alone

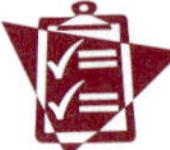

CLINICAL FINDINGS

SYMPTOMS AND SIGNS

- 35% of patients with hemoperitoneum may not manifest clinical signs of peritoneal irritation
- Elevated WBC count and fever appearing several hours later

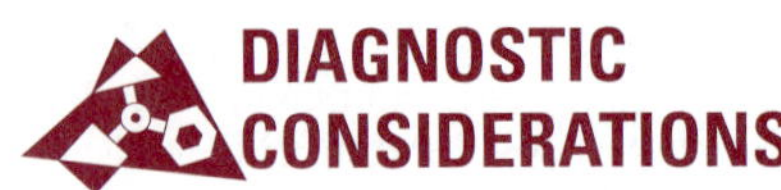

DIAGNOSTIC CONSIDERATIONS

- Do not obtain CT scan in an unstable patient
- CT has primary role in defining the location and magnitude of intra-abdominal injuries related to blunt trauma
- Diagnostic laparoscopy has an important role in cases of penetrating abdominal trauma
- Exploratory laparotomy has 3 main indications following blunt injury: peritonitis, unexplained hypovolemia, and the presence of other injuries know to be associated with intra-abdominal injuries

WORK-UP

- Local wound exploration may rule out peritoneal penetration
- FAST exam used to identify abnormal collections of blood or fluid and obviates need for diagnostic peritoneal lavage (DPL)
- CT is noninvasive, qualitative, sensitive, and accurate for the diagnosis of intra-abdominal injury

TREATMENT AND MANAGEMENT

Abdominal Wall Injuries

- Caused by blunt trauma are most often due to shear forces that devitalize the subcutaneous tissue and skin; debridement is necessary to avoid serious infection
- Caused by penetrating trauma, debridement and irrigation may be necessary

Liver Injuries

- Control hemorrhage at laparotomy
- Initial techniques to control hemorrhage include manual compression, perihepatic packing, and Pringle maneuver
- Do not use Pringle maneuver for more than 1 hour
- Hepatic bleeding can be controlled by suture ligation or clip application
- Electrocautery or the argon beam coagulator can be used to control bleeding from the raw surface of the liver
- Microfibrillar collagen or hemostatic thrombin soaked gel foam can be applied to bleeding areas with pressure
- Fibrin glue can be used to treat superficial and deep liver lacerations
- If massive blood loss has already occurred at time of surgery, consider packing the liver and reexploring in 24–48 hrs
- Rarely, selective hepatic artery ligation, resectional debridement, or hepatic lobectomy may be required to control hemorrhage
- Drains should always be used
- Decompression of the biliary system is contraindicated
- Suspect hepatic vein injuries when the Pringle maneuver fails to stop hemorrhage; mortality is very high
- Nonoperative management is superior in the hemodynamically stable patient and is successful in more than 90% of cases

Biliary Tract Injuries

- Treat gallbladder injuries with cholecystectomy, except when minor lacerations can be primary closed
- Most injuries to the common bile duct (CBD) can be treated by suture closure and insertion of a T tube
- Avulsion of the CBD due to duodenal or ampullary trauma may require choledochojejeunosotomy with total or partial pancreatectomy, duodenectomy, or other diversion procedures

Splenic Injuries

- Most common in blunt abdominal trauma
- 50–80% can be managed nonoperatively
- Severity of splenic injury evident on CT staging is used to guide nonoperative management
- High-grade injuries are better managed with surgery

Pancreatic Injuries

- May present with few clinical manifestations

- Suspect injury when upper abdomen has been traumatized, especially when serum amylase remains persistently elevated
- CT is best diagnostic method
- Minor injuries not involving the duct can be managed nonoperatively
- Moderate injuries usually require operative exploration, debridement, and the placement of external drains
- Severe injuries may require distal resection or external drainage
- Traumatic injuries to the pancreatic head often associated with vascular injury and carry high mortality; in most cases pancreaticoduodenectomy should not be attempted

GI Tract Injuries

- Most injuries of the **stomach** can be repaired; some large injuries may require subtotal or total resection
- **Duodenal injury** may not be evident on initial exam or x-ray studies
- Abdominal films will show retroperitoneal air within 6 hrs in most cases
- CT with oral contrast will often identify site of perforation
- Most injuries can be treated with lateral repair but some require resection with end-to-end anastamosis
- Pancreaticoduodenectomy may rarely be required to manage a severe injury
- Duodenal hematomas usually resolve with nonoperative management
- Large hematomas causing obstruction for more than 10–14 days may require operative evacuation
- Most **small bowel** injures can be treated with a 2-layer sutured closure
- The standard approach for **colon** injuries has been to divert the fecal stream or exteriorize the injury
- Consider primary closure for wounds that involve less than 50% of colon circumference
- Primary repair should not be done in hypotensive patients, those requiring multiple transfusions, or if there has been a delay of more than 6 hrs after injury or in the face of gross contamination
- Wounds extensive enough to require resection should not be closed primarily
- Small, clean **rectal** injuries may be closed primarily if conditions are favorable
- Treat large rectal wounds with diversion and insertion of presacral drains
- Irrigation of the distal stump should be done unless it would further contaminate the pelvic space

Genitourinary Injuries

- Most commonly injured organs are male genitalia, uterus, urethra, bladder, ureters, and kidneys
- **Male genitalia** injuries usually limited to skin loss only and should be treated with primary skin graft
- Treat scrotal skin loss with delayed reconstruction; testis can be temporarily protected by placing it subcutaneously in the thigh
- **Uterine** injuries are infrequent and can usually be repaired with absorbable suture; drainage is not necessary
- Hysterectomy may be necessary in more extensive injuries
- **Urethral** injuries associated with pelvic fractures or deceleration injuries
- Blood at the meatus is classic sign of injury
- Prostate may be elevated superiorly by hematoma and will be free-riding and high on rectal examination; urethrography should be performed before Foley placement
- Penetrating injuries are best treated with primary repair
- Suprapubic bladder drainage and delayed reconstruction of blunt urethral disruption injuries are safe and effective in most cases
- Major injuries to the bulbous or penile urethra should be managed by suprapubic urinary diversion
- **Bladder** rupture is frequently associated with pelvic fractures
- 75% of ruptures are extraperitoneal, and 25% are intraperitoneal
- Repair should be done through a midline abdominal incision
- Divert urine postoperatively for at least 7 days via a suprapubic cystostomy
- More than 50% of **kidney** injuries can be treated nonoperatively
- Nonoperatiave treatment of penetrating renal lacerations is appropriate in stable patients without other injuries
- Severe injuries carry high risk of delayed bleeding and should be treated operatively
- Consider renal exploration if laparotomy is indicated for associated injuries
- Renal vascular injuries require immediate operation to save the kidney
- Perirenal hematomas found incidentally at laparotomy should be explored if they are expanding, pulsatile, or not contained by retroperitoneal tissues or if preexploration urogram shows extensive urinary extravasation
- **Ureteral** injuries are easily missed; most can be reconstructed by primary repair, ureteroureterostomy, or ureteral reimplantations

SURGERY

Indications

- If the abdomen is likely source of exsanguinating hemorrhage, immediate laparotomy is indicated
- Most stab wounds of the lower chest or abdomen should be explored
- All gunshot wounds of lower chest and abdomen should be explored as incidence of injury to major structures exceeds 90%
- Patients in shock after 4 L crystalloid resuscitation with penetrating abdominal injury requires emergent laparotomy
- Unstable patients with positive FAST

PROGNOSIS

- Deaths principally from hemorrhage or sepsis

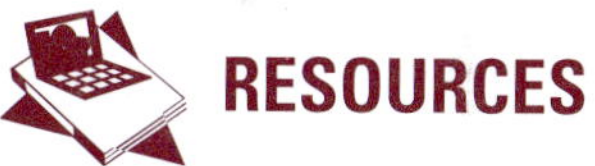

RESOURCES

REFERENCES

- Sartorelli KH et al. Nonoperative management of hepatic, splenic, and renal injuries in adults with multiple injuries. *J Trauma.* 2000;49:56.
- Shapiro MB et al. Damage control: collective review. *J Trauma.* 2000;49:969.
- Jacobs IA et al. Nonoperative management of blunt splenic and hepatic trauma in the pediatric population: significant differences between adult and pediatric surgeons? *Am Surg.* 2001;67:149.

Abdominal Wall Hernias, Noninguinal

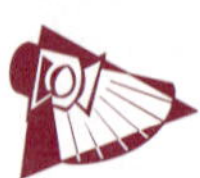

ESSENTIAL FEATURES

- Typically manifests clinically with an asymptomatic bulge or small bowel obstruction
- The abdominal wall defects are sometimes discovered during radiographic evaluation for vague abdominal discomfort or an unrelated condition
- Incarceration and strangulation are frequently presenting symptoms due to the elusive nature of these fascial defects

EPIDEMIOLOGY

- Noninguinal abdominal wall hernias are much less common than inguinal or incisional hernias
- Littre and Richter hernias occur in the setting of other hernia and are not an anatomically distinct hernia type (ie, a hernia subtype)
- Lumbar hernias occur most frequently in young athletic women

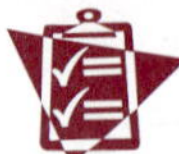

CLINICAL FINDINGS

SYMPTOMS AND SIGNS

- **Spigelian hernia:** Pain and abdominal wall bulge at the lateral edge of the rectus muscle at the level of the umbilicus
- **Lumbodorsal hernia:** Persistent flank bulge (hernia sac usually filled with retroperitoneal fat)
  - Grynfeltt: Superior lumbar triangle
  - Petit: Inferior lumbar triangle
- **Obturator hernia:** Pelvic sidewall mass appreciated on rectal or pelvic exam; pain extending down medial aspect of the thigh on abduction, extension, or internal rotation of the knee indicates a positive **Howship-Romberg sign**
- **Perineal hernia:** Typically manifests as easily reducible perineal bulges but may also include pain, dysuria, bowel obstruction, or perineal skin breakdown
- **Interparietal hernia:** Abdominal wall mass that occurs primarily or in the setting of a muscle-splitting appendectomy incision; this hernia defect is often confused with an abdominal wall tumor
- **Sciatic hernia:** Rarely appreciated externally; bowel obstruction is usually presenting symptom, and the hernia defect is discovered during abdominal exploration
- **Traumatic hernia:** Ecchymosis and abdominal wall bulge detected in the setting of significant blunt abdominal trauma
- **Supravesicular hernia:** Laterally displaced suprapubic mass associated with urinary or bowel obstruction symptoms

IMAGING FINDINGS

- Imaging findings specific to type of hernia
- US can detect an abdominal wall mass and differentiate between tumor, abscess, and hernia
- CT scan most useful method for identifying noninguinal abdominal wall hernias and differentiating between tumor, abscess, hematoma, and hernia

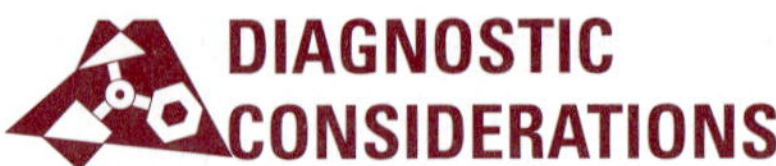

DIAGNOSTIC CONSIDERATIONS

- **Richter hernia:** Any strangulated hernia in which only part of the bowel wall becomes ischemic and gangrenous, thus complete bowel obstruction does not occur; typically occurs in the setting of a ventral hernia
- **Littre hernia:** A hernia that contains Meckel diverticulum in the hernia sac
- **Spigelian hernia:** Acquired ventral hernia through the linea semilunaris, located at the junction between the rectus abdominals muscle and the abdominal oblique musculature
- **Lumbodorsal hernia:** Hernia defects through the posterior abdominal wall at different levels in the lumbar region
  - Grynfeltt: Superior lumbar triangle
  - Petit: Inferior lumbar triangle
- **Obturator hernia:** Herniation through the obturator canal
- **Perineal hernia:** Myofascial defects of the perineum, usually following perineal surgery
- **Interparietal hernia:** Hernia between the layers of the abdominal wall
- **Sciatic hernia:** Outpouching of the intra-abdominal contents through the greater sciatic foramen
- **Traumatic hernia:** Direct blunt traumatic abdominal injury with resulting myofascial defect
- **Supravesicular hernia:** Myofascial defect adjacent to Cooper's ligament with visceral herniation anterior to the urinary bladder

RULE OUT

- Incarcerated or strangulated hernia
- Abdominal wall metastasis
- Primary abdominal wall tumor
- Abdominal wall abscess

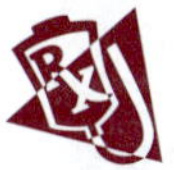

WORK-UP

- Thorough history and physical exam
- US or CT scan if clinical diagnosis is in question

WHEN TO ADMIT

- Presence of acute complications from the noninguinal abdominal wall hernia (namely bowel obstruction)

WHEN TO REFER

- Large, complex perineal or traumatic hernia defects best managed with native tissue reconstruction in conjunction with reconstructive plastic surgery

TREATMENT AND MANAGEMENT

- Uncomplicated abdominal wall defects can be approached electively, typically as an outpatient
- Patients with bowel obstruction require resuscitation and urgent operative reduction and repair

SURGERY

Indications

- All hernia defects should be repaired in the medically fit patients due to the high incidence of incarceration and bowel obstruction

TREATMENT MONITORING

- Recurrence of hernia bulge

COMPLICATIONS

- Hernia incarceration and strangulation
- Small bowel obstruction
- Progressive increase in size
- Recurrence

PROGNOSIS

- Mortality rate 13–40% with obturator hernias, making them the most lethal
- Patients frequently have complicated hernia defects, making postoperative complications more common

RESOURCES

REFERENCES

- Trupo FJ et al. Meckel's diverticulum in femoral hernia: a Littre's hernia. *South Med J.* 1987;80:655.
- Thor K. Lumbar hernia. *Acta Chir Scand.* 1985;151:389.
- Naude G et al. Obturator hernia is an unsuspected diagnosis. *Am J Surg.* 1997;174:72.

Abdominal Wall Mass

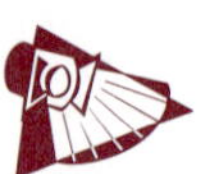

ESSENTIAL FEATURES

- Myriad of conditions manifest clinically with a palpable abdominal wall mass
- Key to diagnosis is careful history and physical exam
- Asymptomatic deep abdominal wall mass may be incidentally discovered on imaging studies

EPIDEMIOLOGY

- Rectus hematomas may arise following abdominal wall trauma or occur spontaneously in patients receiving anticoagulant therapy
- Spontaneous abdominal wall metastases are most commonly associated with lung and pancreatic adenocarcinoma
- Any intra-abdominal malignancy can extend into the abdominal wall or secondarily seed laparotomy incisions

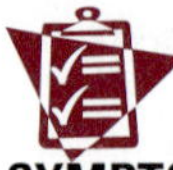

CLINICAL FINDINGS

SYMPTOMS AND SIGNS

- **Rectus hematoma:** An exquisitely tender mass that becomes more painful with flexion of the abdominal wall with surrounding ecchymosis is the classic finding
- **Deep wound infection or abdominal wall abscess:** Signs of infection or inflammation (erythema, induration, tenderness, exudate)
- **Abdominal wall hernia:** A reducible bulge that develops with the Valsalva maneuver
- **Soft-tissue neoplasms:** Most are asymptomatic with a slow growth pattern

LABORATORY FINDINGS

- Coagulopathy may be present in patients with rectus sheath hematoma
- Leukocytosis with deep wound infection or abdominal wall abscess

IMAGING FINDINGS

- Plain abdominal films are usually normal
- US can differentiate between a solid and a fluid-filled mass and reliably demonstrate the presence of abdominal viscera in the case of an incarcerated abdominal wall hernia
- CT will characterize the mass and differentiate between hematoma, fat, soft-tissue, and fluid-density lesions
- MRI is best method to evaluate soft-tissue masses suspicious for sarcoma

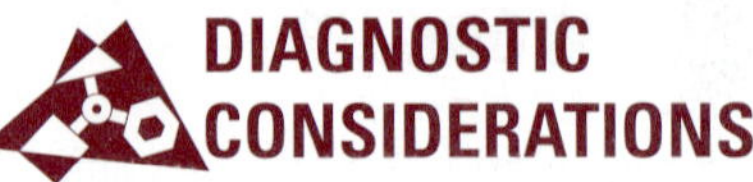

DIAGNOSTIC CONSIDERATIONS

- Rectus hematoma
- Tumor metastasis
- Desmoid tumor
- Deep wound infection
- Abdominal wall abscess
- Soft-tissue sarcoma
- Incisional hernia
- Interparietal hernia
- Spigelian hernia
- Lipoma
- Hemangioma
- Fibroma
- Endometrioma
- Stitch abscess
- Stitch granuloma

RULE OUT

- Tumor metastasis
- Hernia
- Soft-tissue sarcoma

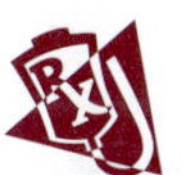

WORK-UP

- Careful history
  - Malignancy (metastasis)
  - Constitutional symptoms (metastasis)
  - Trauma (hematoma)
  - Cesarean section (desmoid tumor, endometrioma)
  - Familial adenomatous polyposis (desmoid tumor)
  - Prior laparotomy (incisional hernia)
  - Fever and chills (deep wound infection or abdominal wall abscess)
- Careful physical exam
  - Mass reducible (hernia)
  - Mass expanding (hematoma)
  - Pain, erythema, and induration (deep wound infection or abdominal wall abscess)
- Obtain CT or MRI when solid mass is suspicious for abdominal wall metastasis, soft-tissue sarcoma, or desmoid tumor
- Perform percutaneous biopsy for solid mass

WHEN TO ADMIT

- Uncomplicated abdominal wall mass work-up may be performed as an outpatient
- Patients with deep wound infection or abdominal wall abscess need to be admitted for drainage and antibiotic therapy
- Patients with complicated hernia (incarcerated, strangulated, small bowel obstruction) require admission for urgent surgical treatment

TREATMENT AND MANAGEMENT

- **Rectus sheath hematoma:** Correct coagulopathy, avoid antiplatelet medications, control pain, and provide expectant management
- **Soft-tissue mass:** Radiographic characterization with percutaneous or incisional biopsy to establish the diagnosis followed by definitive surgical excision
- **Deep wound infection or abdominal wall abscess:** Surgical debridement with serial dressing changes
- **Abdominal wall hernias:** Surgical repair
  - Uncomplicated hernia: Elective repair
  - Incarcerated or strangulated hernia: Emergent repair

SURGERY

Indications

- Diagnosis of soft-tissue mass
- Excision of a soft-tissue mass
- Repair of abdominal wall hernia
- Debridement of deep wound infection
- Removal of stitch abscess or granuloma

Contraindications

- Widespread metastatic disease in the case of abdominal wall metastases

TREATMENT MONITORING

- Depends on etiology of abdominal wall mass

COMPLICATIONS

- Depends on etiology of abdominal wall mass and treatment given

RESOURCES

REFERENCES

- Doherty GM, Boey JH. The acute abdomen. In: Way LW, Doherty GM (editors). *Current Surgical Diagnosis & Treatment,* 11e. New York: McGraw-Hill; 2003:503–516.

Achalasia

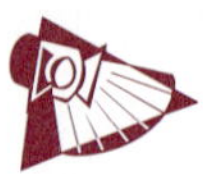

ESSENTIAL FEATURES

- Dysphagia
- Retention of ingested food in the esophagus
- Radiologic evidence of absent primary peristalsis, dilated body of the esophagus, and a conically narrowed cardioesophageal junction
- Absent primary peristalsis by manometry and cineradiography

EPIDEMIOLOGY

- Achalasia is a neuromuscular disorder; esophageal dilation and hypertrophy occur without organic stenosis
- Primary peristalsis is absent and the cardioesophageal sphincter fails to relax in response to swallowing; the circular muscle layer hypertrophies
- There is absence, atrophy, or disintegration of the ganglion cells of Auerbach myenteric plexuses and a reduction in nerve fibers within the wall of the esophagus
- The cause is unknown, but 2 theories exist:
  1. A degenerative disease of the neurons
  2. Infection of neurons by a virus (eg, herpes zoster) or other infectious pathogen
- Achalasia affects males more often than females and may develop at any age; peak incidence ranges from 30 to 60 years

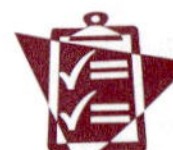

CLINICAL FINDINGS

SYMPTOMS AND SIGNS

- Dysphagia is dominant symptom
- Weight loss is not usually marked despite the functional obstruction
- Pain is infrequent
- Regurgitation of retained esophageal contents is common, especially during the night while the patient sleeps in a recumbent position
- A variant called **vigorous achalasia** is characterized by chest pain and esophageal spasms that generate nonpropulsive high-pressure waves in the body of the esophagus

IMAGING FINDINGS

- **Contrast radiography and endoscopy**
  - Narrowing at the cardia
  - The dilated body of the esophagus blends into a smooth cone-shaped area of narrowing 3–6 cm long
  - As the disease progresses, the esophagus dilates further and becomes tortuous
- **Manometry**
  - The body of the esophagus is devoid of primary peristaltic waves, but simultaneous disorganized muscular activity may be present
  - Pressure in the gastroesophageal sphincter is increased; relaxation after swallowing is incomplete or absent

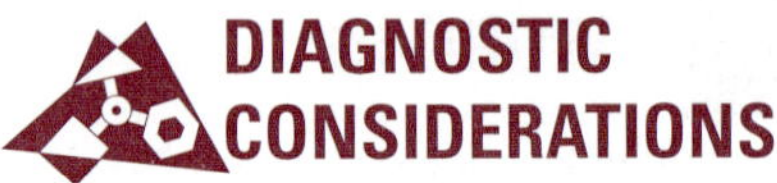

DIAGNOSTIC CONSIDERATIONS

- Symptoms should prompt contrast radiographic or endoscopic studies
- Endoscopy is essential for establishing the diagnosis and excluding other causes of symptoms
- Manometry is useful for confirming diagnosis

RULE OUT

- Benign strictures of the lower esophagus
- Carcinoma at or near the cardioesophageal junction
- Diffuse esophageal spasm

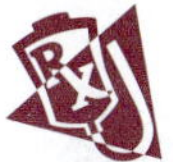

WORK-UP

- Gastroesophageal contrast radiography
- Upper GI endoscopy
- Esophageal manometry
- pH study, particularly if symptoms of reflux are present or fundoplication is planned

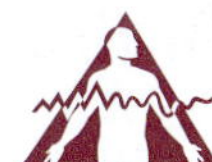

TREATMENT AND MANAGEMENT

- Goal is to relieve the functional obstruction either by pneumatic dilation or longitudinal division of all the esophageal muscular layers (Heller myotomy).

SURGERY

Indications

- Advanced disease
- Failed dilation
- If no reflux symptoms exist, the need to add an antireflux procedure has not been established

TREATMENT MONITORING

- Measure rate of esophageal passage of a technetium Tc 99m-labeled solid meal
- Periodic esophagoscopy; treatment of achalasia does not lessen the increased risk of squamous cell carcinoma

COMPLICATIONS

- Aspiration leading to pneumonitis
- Small mucosal ulcerations
- Squamous cell carcinoma of the esophagus in 3–5% of patients

PROGNOSIS

- **Dilation:** Long-term results are good in only 50%
- **Surgery:** Results are good to excellent in 90% of patients

RESOURCES

REFERENCES

- Finley RJ et al. Laparoscopic Heller myotomy improves esophageal emptying and the symptoms of achalasia. *Arch Surg.* 2001;136:892.
- Ben-Meir A et al: Quality of life before and after laparoscopic Heller myotomy for achalasia. *Am J Surg.* 2001;181:471.

Acidosis, Metabolic

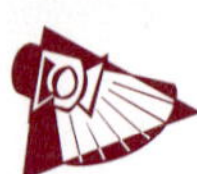

ESSENTIAL FEATURES

- Decreased serum pH (< 7.35)
- Decreased serum HCO_3

EPIDEMIOLOGY

- Etiologies include:
  - Diarrhea
  - Diuretics
  - Renal tubular disease
  - Ureterosigmoidostomy
  - Lactic acidosis
  - Diabetic ketoacidosis
  - Uremia

CLINICAL FINDINGS

LABORATORY FINDINGS

- Decreased serum pH (< 7.35)
- Decreased serum HCO_3

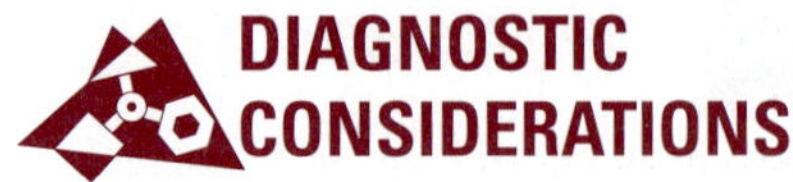

DIAGNOSTIC CONSIDERATIONS

- Differentiate between anion gap or hyperchloremic causes

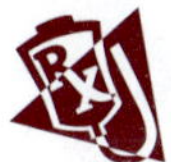

WORK-UP

- Serum electrolytes
- ABG measurements
- Calculate anion gap: Na – (Cl + HCO_3)
- Anion gap > 15: H^+ excess, lactic acidosis, diabetic ketoacidosis, uremia, methanol ingestion, salicylate intoxication, ethylene glycol ingestion
- Anion gap < 15: HCO_3 loss, diarrhea, renal tubular disease, ureterosigmoidostomy, acetazolamide, NH_4 Cl administration

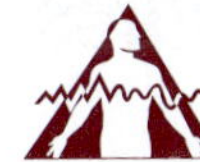

TREATMENT AND MANAGEMENT

- Treat underlying condition
- **Conservative HCO_3 administration:** Estimate need by multiplying base deficit by one half total body water

MEDICATIONS

- Sodium bicarbonate as needed

TREATMENT MONITORING

- Serial ABG measurements

COMPLICATIONS

- Hypotension
- Death

PROGNOSIS

- Varies with etiology

RESOURCES

REFERENCES

- Adrogue HJ et al. Management of life-threatening acid-base disorders. (Two parts.) *N Engl J Med.* 1998;338:26, 107.
- Ishihara K et al. Anion gap acidosis. *Semin Nephrol.* 1998;18:83.

Acidosis, Respiratory

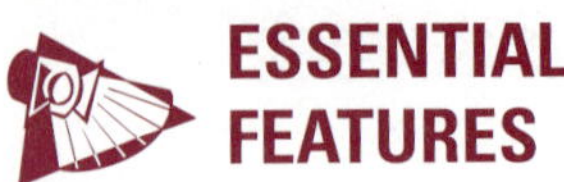

ESSENTIAL FEATURES

- Inadequate respiration
- Carbon dioxide accumulation

EPIDEMIOLOGY

- Etiologies include:
  - Acute airway obstruction
  - Aspiration
  - Respiratory arrest
  - Pulmonary infections
  - Pulmonary edema
  - Over sedation
  - Chronic respiratory failure

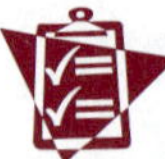

CLINICAL FINDINGS

SYMPTOMS AND SIGNS

- Somnolence
- None if chronic and well compensated

LABORATORY FINDINGS

- Decreased serum pH (< 7.35)
- Increased P_{CO_2}

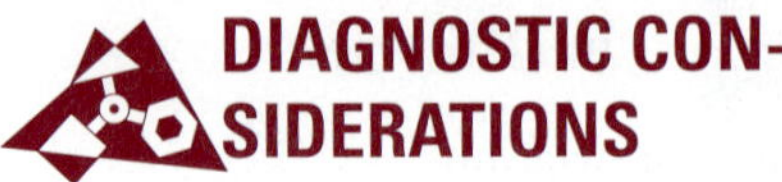

DIAGNOSTIC CONSIDERATIONS

- Causes may be neurologic, mechanical, or rarely from diffusion abnormality
- May be acute or chronic

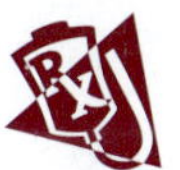

WORK-UP

- ABG measurements
- Plain chest film if pneumothorax is suspected or if endotracheal tube malposition or other anatomic consideration is of concern

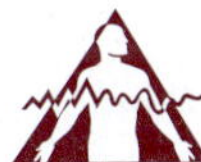

TREATMENT AND MANAGEMENT

- Restoration of adequate ventilation
- Intubation, if necessary
- Chronic-rapid correction may lead to severe metabolic alkalosis (post-hypercapneic metabolic alkalosis)

SURGERY

Indications

- If unable to intubate, cricothyroidotomy may be necessary

MEDICATIONS

- Sodium bicarbonate (rarely)
- Narcotic antagonists
- Benzodiazepine antagonists

TREATMENT MONITORING

- Serial ABG measurements

COMPLICATIONS

- Coma
- Death

PROGNOSIS

- Excellent if reversed quickly
- Varies with etiology

PREVENTION

- Avoid over sedation

RESOURCES

REFERENCES

- Adrogue HJ et al. Management of life-threatening acid-base disorders. (Two parts.) *N Engl J Med.* 1998;338:26, 107.

Actinomycosis & Nocardiosis

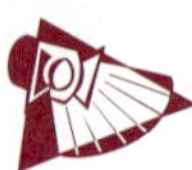

ESSENTIAL FEATURES

- Actinomycosis and nocardiosis are not communicable

Actinomycosis

- *Actinomyces israelii*
  - Gram-positive, non–acid-fast, filamentous organism that usually shows branching and may break up into short bacterial forms
  - Anaerobe, part of the normal flora of the human oropharynx and upper intestinal tract
- Chronic, slowly progressive infection that may involve many tissues, resulting in the formation of granulomas and abscesses that drain through sinuses and fistulas
- Lesions resemble those produced by mycobacteria, fungi, and cancer, although the causative organisms are bacteria
- Sinus tracts or fistulas usually become secondarily infected with other bacteria
- Abdominal infection may produce an abdominal mass mimicking a malignant process or may give rise to appendicitis

Nocardiosis

- *Nocardiae* are gram-positive, aerobic, branching, filamentous organisms that may be acid-fast
- *Nocardia asteroides* is the most common isolate
- May present in 2 forms:
  1. Localized, chronic granuloma with suppuration, abscess, and sinus tract formation resembling actinomycosis
  2. Systemic infection, usually beginning as pneumonitis with suppuration and progressing via the bloodstream to involvement of other organs

EPIDEMIOLOGY

Actinomycosis

- Inflammatory nodular masses, abscesses, and draining sinuses occur most commonly in the head and neck (50%)
- 20% of patients have primary lesions in the chest and an equal proportion in the abdomen, most commonly involving the appendix and cecum
- Pelvic actinomycosis can occur in women with prolonged use of an intrauterine device

Nocardiosis

- More apt to occur as a complication of immunodeficiency in patients with chronic obstructive pulmonary disease, cancer, HIV-associated disease, or corticosteroid-induced immunosuppression

CLINICAL FINDINGS

SYMPTOMS AND SIGNS

Actinomycosis

- Multiple draining sinuses with pus containing "sulfur granules"
- Lesions are often hard and relatively painless and nontender
- Systemic symptoms, including fever, are variably present
- Abdominal actinomycosis may mimic appendicitis
- Thoracic actinomycosis may give rise to cough, pleural pain, fever, and weight loss

Nocardiosis

- Systemic nocardiosis produces fever, cough, and weight loss and resembles mycobacterial or mycotic infections

LABORATORY FINDINGS

Actinomycosis

- Culture reveals gram-positive branching rods, with sulfur granules
- Organisms may be identified by immunofluoresence

Nocardiosis

- Culture reveals branching rods or filaments that are gram-positive or acid-fast

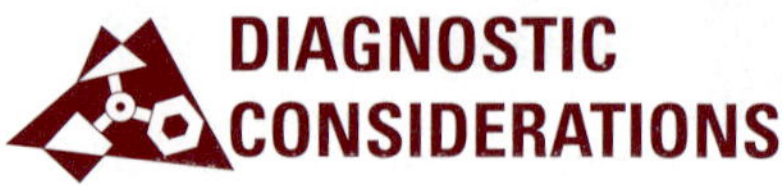

DIAGNOSTIC CONSIDERATIONS

Actinomycosis

- Abdominal neoplasm
- Appendicitis
- Mycobacterial or mycotic infection

Nocardiosis

- Systemic infection resembles mycobacterial or mycotic infections

RULE OUT

- Mycobacterial and mycotic infection
- Appendicitis
- Neoplasms

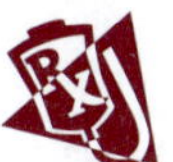

WORK-UP

- Complete history and physical exam
- Culture draining sinus tracts
- CT scanning and needle aspiration may be helpful diagnostically

WHEN TO ADMIT

- Since both nocardiosis and actinomycosis mimic symptoms of other potentially severe diseases, patients should be admitted to rule out other causes such as appendicitis or mycobacterial infection

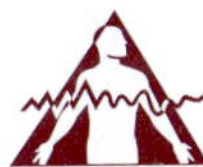

TREATMENT AND MANAGEMENT

- Actinomycosis is treated with penicillin G for many weeks
- Nocardiosis is best treated with sulfonamides or, when severe, with imipenem plus amikacin for many weeks

SURGERY

Indications

- Preoperative exclusion of other diagnoses may be difficult, leading to operation
- Surgery may be indicated to:
  - Drain abscesses
  - Excise fistulas
  - Repair defects or involved organs

MEDICATIONS

Actinomycosis

- Penicillin G

Nocardiosis

- Sulfonamides or imipenem plus amikacin

COMPLICATIONS

Actinomycosis

- Abdominal infection: Mimics appendicitis; if allowed to perforate, produces multiple lesions and forms sinuses of the abdominal wall
- Thoracic infection: Later in the course of the disease, the sinuses perforate the pleural cavity and the chest wall, often involving ribs or vertebrae

Nocardiosis

- Systemic infection with progression via the bloodstream to involve other organs (meningitis, encephalitis)

PROGNOSIS

- Mortality rate of nocardial bacteremia is as high as 50%

PREVENTION

- No vaccine or prophylactic drugs available

RESOURCES

REFERENCES

- Lerner PI. Nocardiosis. *Clin Infect Dis.* 1996;22:891.
- Smego R Jr et al. Actinomycosis. *Clin Infect Dis.* 1998;26:1255.

Acute Respiratory Distress Syndrome (ARDS)

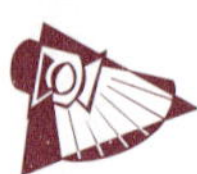

ESSENTIAL FEATURES

- Hypoxemia
- Hypercarbia
- Pulmonary edema (pulmonary capillary wedge pressure < 18 mm Hg)
- Absence of other causes

EPIDEMIOLOGY

- Often follows shock/trauma/sepsis

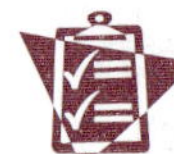

CLINICAL FINDINGS

SYMPTOMS AND SIGNS

- Hypoxemia
- Hypercarbia

IMAGING FINDINGS

- Diffuse bilateral pulmonary infiltrates

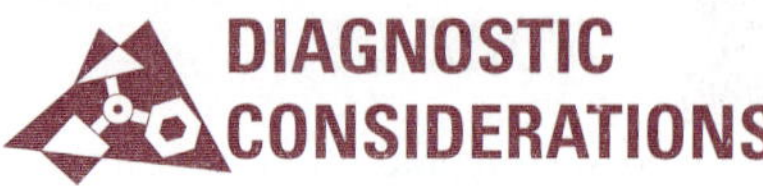

DIAGNOSTIC CONSIDERATIONS

- Typically follows shock and either trauma or sepsis
- ARDS typically develops 24 h after the resuscitation from the initial insult
- Diagnosis may be complicated by the presence of other potential causes of hypoxemia

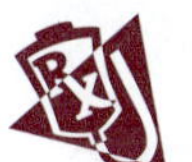

WORK-UP

- ABG measurements
- Chest films

TREATMENT AND MANAGEMENT

- Ventilator management (positive end-expiratory pressure, inspiratory reserve volume)
- Diuresis
- Treatment of inciting cause
- Transfusion
- Proning

TREATMENT MONITORING

- Invasive monitoring (pulmonary artery catheter)
- Serial arterial blood gas measurements

PROGNOSIS

- Determined by etiology

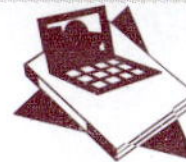

RESOURCES

REFERENCES

- Bulger EM et al. Current clinical options for the treatment and management of acute respiratory distress syndrome. *J Trauma.* 2000;48:562.

Adrenal Incidentaloma

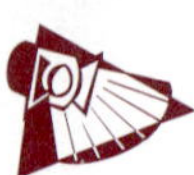

ESSENTIAL FEATURES

- Incidence of diagnosis has increased with use of ultrasonography, CT, and MRI for various, nonrelated diseases of the abdomen
- Diagnosis includes such conditions as nonfunctioning adrenocortical adenoma, functioning adenoma, pheochromocytomas with subclinical secretion of hormones, and adrenocortical carcinomas
- Major issue to determine is whether the tumor is hormonally active or whether it is a carcinoma

EPIDEMIOLOGY

- Found in 1–4% of CT scans
- Found in 6% of random autopsies
- Incidence increases with age
- Over 80% are nonfunctioning cortical adenomas
- 5% each are preclinical Cushing syndrome, pheochromocytoma, and adrenocortical carcinoma
- 2% are metastatic carcinoma
- 1% are aldosteronoma
- 25% of pheochromocytomas are found incidentally

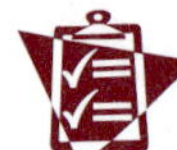

CLINICAL FINDINGS

SYMPTOMS AND SIGNS

- Asymptomatic; discovered on imaging study done for nonrelated disease process

LABORATORY FINDINGS

- Depends on type of tumor; nonfunctional adenoma will have no laboratory abnormalities

IMAGING FINDINGS

- Most pheochromocytomas are over 2 cm in diameter and characteristically bright on T2-weighted MRI
- CT scan findings of heterogeneity or irregular borders are suspicious for malignancy
- Adrenal scintigraphy with iodocholesterol derivatives (NP-59 scans) suggest a benign lesion with demonstration of normal uptake
- PET scans may be useful in detecting malignant lesions

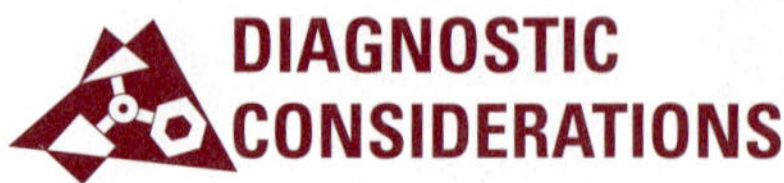

DIAGNOSTIC CONSIDERATIONS

- Simple adrenal cysts, myelolipomas, and adrenal hemorrhages can be identified by the CT characteristics alone
- Adrenal cysts can be very large but are very rarely malignant
- Since most tumors are nonfunctioning adenomas, the work-up should avoid unnecessary procedures and expense
- Nonfunctioning adrenal tumors that are greater than 5 cm have a high risk of cancer (up to 33%)
- An adrenal mass > 3 cm in a patient with a previously treated malignancy is very likely a metastasis
- Tumors that metastasize to the adrenal gland include: lung, breast, colon, hypernephroma, malignant melanoma, uterine, and prostate

WORK-UP

- Complete history and physical exam, with specific reference to previous malignancies, symptoms of Cushing syndrome, hypertension, virilization, or feminization
- All patients, even those without hypertension, should have plasma metanephrines and 24-hour urinary fractionated catecholamines determined to evaluate for pheochromocytoma
- All patients should have a serum cortisol, 24-hour urine collection for cortisol, and an overnight dexamethasone suppression test
- Patients who are hypertensive should have serum potassium and plasma aldosterone and renin activity measured
- Consider obtaining a dehydroepiandrosterone (DHEA) level (potential marker for adrenocortical carcinoma)
- If above studies show the tumor to be nonfunctional, the size of the tumor and the patient's overall medical condition determine management
- If metastasis is suspected and pheochromocytoma is ruled out, then CT-guided fine-needle aspiration can be useful

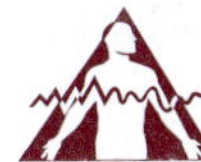

TREATMENT AND MANAGEMENT

- Management depends on functional status and size of the tumor
- Metastatic adrenal lesions should be treated appropriately in concert with the underlying primary cancer

SURGERY

Indications

- Hormonally active tumor
- Adrenocortical carcinoma
- Nonfunctional tumors > 4 cm
- Solitary adrenal metastasis

TREATMENT MONITORING

- Small, nonfunctioning tumors are almost always benign adenomas and can be followed with serial CT scans checking for changes in size

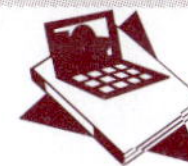

RESOURCES

REFERENCES

- Herrera MF et al. Incidentally discovered adrenal tumors: an institutional perspective. *Surgery.* 1991;110:1014.
- Gajraj H, Young AE. Adrenal incidentaloma. *Br J Surg.* 1993;80:422.
- Ross NS et al. Hormonal evaluation of the patient with an incidentally discovered adrenal mass. *N Engl J Med.* 1990;323:1401.
- Young WF et al. Management approaches to adrenal incidentalomas: a review from Rochester, Minnesota. *Endocrinol Metab Clin North Am.* 2000;29:159.

Adrenal Tumors, Sex Hormone-Producing

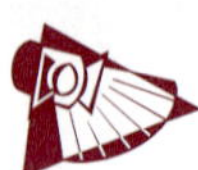

ESSENTIAL FEATURES

- 2 types: virilizing and feminizing
- Virilization is due to hypersecretion of adrenal androgens, mainly dehydroepiandrosterone (DHEA), its sulfate derivative (DHEAS), and androstenedione. All of these are converted peripherally to testosterone and 5α-dihydrotestosterone
- Very rarely do virilizing adrenal tumors secrete only testosterone
- Estrogens are not normally synthesized by the adrenal cortex

EPIDEMIOLOGY

- These tumors are rare
- 70% of virilizing adrenal tumors exhibit malignant behavior
- Virilizing adrenal tumors in children are less likely to be malignant

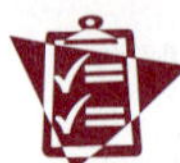

CLINICAL FINDINGS

SYMPTOMS AND SIGNS

- Virilization includes hirsutism, male pattern baldness, acne, deep voice, male musculature, irregular menses or amenorrhea, clitoromegaly, and increased libido
- Rapid linear growth with advanced bone age is common in children with virilizing tumors
- Feminization in men (bilateral gynecomastia, accelerated growth rate, female hair distribution, advanced bone age), or precocious puberty in women
- Feminizing adrenal tumors may present with vaginal bleeding in adult women

LABORATORY FINDINGS

- **Virilizing adrenal tumors:** Elevated DHEA, DHEAS, androstenedione, and testosterone
- **Feminizing adrenal tumors:** Elevated plasma or urine estrogens

IMAGING FINDINGS

- Adrenal cortical mass on CT or MRI

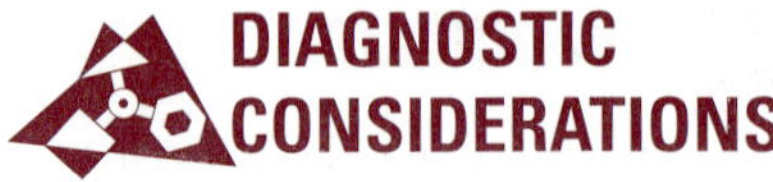

DIAGNOSTIC CONSIDERATIONS

- Differentiating between benign and malignant virilizing adrenal tumors, even with histopathology, is very difficult
- Feminizing adrenal tumors are almost always carcinomas

RULE OUT

- Congenital adrenal hyperplasia
- Ovarian tumors
- Testicular feminization
- Exogenous estrogen administration

Adrenal Tumors, Sex Hormone-Producing

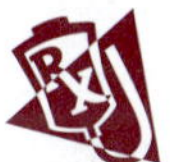

WORK-UP

- Complete history and physical exam
- Plasma androgen levels; urine and plasma estrogen levels
- Localization with CT or MRI

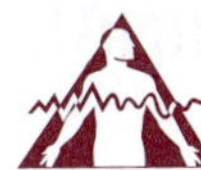

TREATMENT AND MANAGEMENT

- Resection is the only successful treatment

SURGERY

Indications

- All virilizing adrenal tumors should be resected
- All feminizing adrenal tumors should be excised

PROGNOSIS

- Worse for large virilizing tumors (> 100 g)
- Guarded for feminizing adrenal tumors

RESOURCES

REFERENCES

- Del Gaudio AD et al. Virilizing adrenocortical tumors in adult women. *Cancer.* 1993;72:1997.
- Goto T et al. Oestrogen producing adrenocortical adenoma: clinical, biochemical, and immunohistochemical studies. *Clin Endocrinol.* 1996;45:643.

Adrenocortical Carcinoma

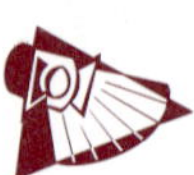

ESSENTIAL FEATURES

- Variety of clinical symptoms through excess production of adrenal hormones
- Complete surgical removal of the primary lesion and any resectable metastatic sites has been the mainstay of treatment

EPIDEMIOLOGY

- These tumors are rare; 1–2 cases per million persons in the United States
- Less than 0.05% of newly diagnosed cancers per year
- Bimodal occurrence, with tumors developing in children < 5 years of age and in adults in their fifth through seventh decade of life
- Male:female ratio is 2:1, with functional tumors being more common in women
- Left adrenal involved slightly more often than the right (53% vs 47%); bilateral tumors are rare (2%)
- 50–60% of patients have symptoms related to hypersecretion of hormones (most commonly Cushing syndrome and virilization)
- Feminizing and purely aldosterone-secreting carcinomas are rare
- 50% of patients have metastases at the time of diagnosis

CLINICAL FINDINGS

SYMPTOMS AND SIGNS

- Symptoms of specific hormone excess (cortisol excess, virilization, feminization)
- Palpable abdominal mass
- Abdominal pain
- Fatigue, weight loss, fever, hematuria

LABORATORY FINDINGS

- All laboratory abnormalities depend on hormonal status of tumor
- Elevated urinary free cortisol or steroid precursors
- Loss of normal circadian rhythm for serum cortisol
- Low serum adrenocorticotropic hormone (ACTH)
- Abnormal dexamethasone suppression test
- Elevated serum testosterone, estradiol, or aldosterone levels

IMAGING FINDINGS

- Evaluation of adrenal glands with CT or MRI (adrenocortical carcinomas are typically isodense to liver on T1-weighted MRI, and hyperdense relative to liver on T2-weighted MRI images)
- MRI more accurately gauges the extent of any intracaval tumor thrombus

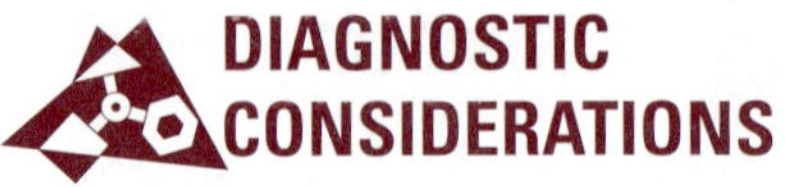

DIAGNOSTIC CONSIDERATIONS

- Mean diameter of adrenal carcinoma at diagnosis is 12 cm
- Radiographic evaluation of suspected metastatic sites for purposes of staging should be undertaken prior to thought of any surgery

RULE OUT

- Pheochromocytoma

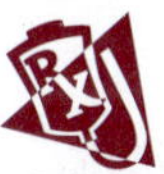

WORK-UP

- History and physical exam may reveal evidence of hormonal function, particularly the development of cushingoid, masculinizing, or feminizing features
- Imaging should include detailed anatomic imaging of both adrenal glands (CT or MRI) and potential sites of intra-abdominal metastasis (especially liver)
- Plasma metanephrines to rule out medullary tumor (pheochromocytoma)
- ACTH, serum cortisol urine free cortisol, aldosterone, and sulfate derivative of dehydroepiandrosterone (DHEAS) in all patients
- Testosterone or estrogen in patients with suggestive symptoms or signs

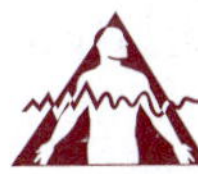

TREATMENT AND MANAGEMENT

- Surgery is the only treatment that can cure or prolong survival
- Laparoscopic surgery not recommended because of spread of tumor, fragility of tumor, and the possible need to resect adjacent involved organs
- For local recurrent disease, reoperation is the only effective therapy and may prolong life

SURGERY

Indications

- Disease localized to the adrenal, or local spread

Contraindications

- Widely metastatic disease

MEDICATIONS

- Mitotane (an adrenolytic agent) can be used as adjuvant therapy; controls endocrine symptoms in 50% of patients but does not generally affect survival

TREATMENT MONITORING

- Physical exam
- Chest radiograph
- Abdominal CT scan
- Biochemical testing when clinically indicated

COMPLICATIONS

- Recurrence is common despite an apparently complete resection

PROGNOSIS

- Tumor stage at the initial operation predicts survival
- Median survival is 25 months
- 5-year actuarial survival is 25%
- 5-year survival with grossly complete surgical resection is 50%

RESOURCES

REFERENCES

- Icard P et al. Adrenocortical carcinoma in surgically treated patients. *Surgery.* 1992;112:972.
- Icard P et al. Survival rates and prognostic factors in adrenocortical carcinoma. *World J Surg.* 1992;16:753.
- Luton JP et al. Clinical features of adrenocortical carcinoma, prognostic factors, and the effect of mitotane therapy. *N Engl J Med.* 1990;322:1195.
- Stratakis CA et al. Adrenal cancer. *Endocrinol Metab Clin North Am.* 2000;29:15.
- Wajchenberg BL et al. Adrenocortical carcinoma-clinical and laboratory observations. *Cancer.* 2000;88:711.

CANCER STAGING

MacFarlane System

Stage 1: T < 5 cm without local invasion

Stage 2: T > 5 cm without local invasion

Stage 3: Local invasion or + nodes

Stage 4: Distant metastases

PRACTICE GUIDELINES

- The National Comprehensive Cancer Network http://www.nccn.org/

Aldosteronoma (Primary Hyperaldosteronism)

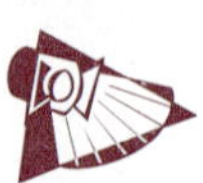

ESSENTIAL FEATURES

- Hypertension with or without hypokalemia
- Elevated aldosterone secretion and suppressed plasma renin activity
- Metabolic alkalosis, relative hypernatremia
- Weakness, polyuria, paresthesias, tetany, cramps due to hypokalemia
- **Common subtypes of primary hyperaldosteronism:** aldosteronoma (75%) and bilateral adrenal hyperplasia (25%)
- **Rare subtypes of primary hyperaldosteronism:** unilateral primary adrenal hyperplasia, aldosterone producing adrenocortical carcinoma, glucocorticoid-remediable hyperaldosteronism (familial hyperaldosteronism type 1)

EPIDEMIOLOGY

- 1% of patients with hypertension
- 8% of normokalemic hypertensive patients

CLINICAL FINDINGS

SYMPTOMS AND SIGNS

- Hypertension
- Headaches
- Malaise
- Muscle weakness
- Polyuria
- Polydipsia
- Cramps
- Paresthesias
- Hypokalemic paralysis (rare)

LABORATORY FINDINGS

- Hypokalemia
- Hypernatremia
- Metabolic alkalosis
- Elevated plasma aldosterone to renin ratio (> 20)
- Elevated plasma aldosterone concentration (> 15 ng/dL)
- Elevated urine/serum aldosterone level with PO or IV sodium challenge

IMAGING FINDINGS

- CT scan with thin sections through adrenals can identify most adenomas
- Adrenal vein sampling if CT is equivocal
- MRI can be used as well to identify an adrenal tumor

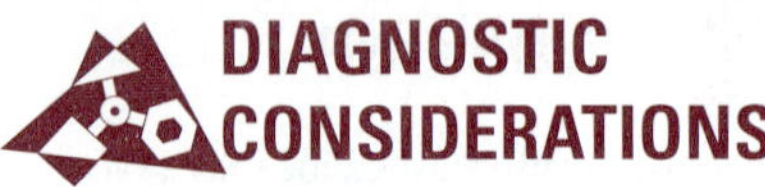

DIAGNOSTIC CONSIDERATIONS

- Aldosteronoma and rare unilateral primary adrenal hyperplasia are the most amenable types of primary hyperaldosteronism to surgical correction

RULE OUT

- Pheochromocytoma

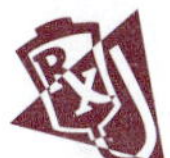

WORK-UP

- Thorough history and physical exam
- Confirmed hypertension (multiple measurements)
- Laboratory evaluation (electrolytes, serum aldosterone, and renin levels)
- Cross sectional imaging (CT, MRI)
- Possible bilateral adrenal vein sampling

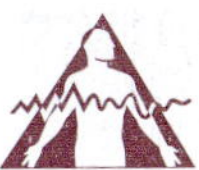

TREATMENT AND MANAGEMENT

- Goal is to prevent illness associated with hypertension and hypokalemia
- Surgical therapy for patients with aldosteronoma and unilateral primary adrenal hyperplasia
- Medical therapy for bilateral adrenal hyperplasia, or poor surgical candidates
- Preoperative preparation is key, with control of blood pressure and serum potassium

SURGERY

- Nearly always laparoscopic approach

Indications

- Unilateral aldosteronoma
- Unilateral primary adrenal hyperplasia

Contraindications

- Bilateral adrenal hyperplasia

MEDICATIONS

- **Spironolactone:** Competitive aldosterone antagonist
- **Amiloride:** Potassium-sparing diuretic
- Other antihypertensive agents such as ACE inhibitors and calcium channel blockers

TREATMENT MONITORING

- Monitor blood pressure

COMPLICATIONS

- Uncontrolled hypertension can lead to renal failure, stroke, or myocardial infarction
- Severe hypokalemia can lead to paralysis; risk of cardiac dysrhythmia increases in combination with digitalis

PROGNOSIS

- Removal of aldosteronoma normalizes potassium, but hypertension is not always cured
- 33% of patients have persistent, mild hypertension (easier to control than before operation)

RESOURCES

REFERENCES

- Bravo EL. Primary aldosteronism. Issues in diagnosis and management. *Endocrinol Metab Clin North Am.* 1994;23:271.
- Ghose RP et al. Medical management of aldosterone-producing adenomas. *Ann Intern Med.* 1999;131:105.
- Weinberger MH, Fineberg NS. The diagnosis of primary aldosteronism and separation of two major subtypes. *Arch Intern Med.* 1993;153:2125.

Alkalosis, Metabolic

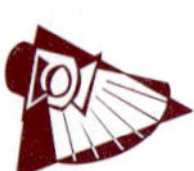

ESSENTIAL FEATURES

- Elevated serum pH (> 7.45)
- Increased serum HCO_3

EPIDEMIOLOGY

- Most common acid-base disturbance in surgical patients
- Pathogenesis involves loss of H^+ via NG suction, volume depletion, and hypokalemia

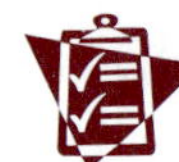

CLINICAL FINDINGS

LABORATORY FINDINGS

- Elevated serum pH
- Increased serum HCO_3
- Paradoxical aciduria
- Hypokalemia

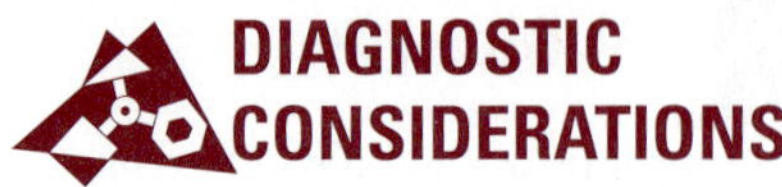

DIAGNOSTIC CONSIDERATIONS

- May be mixed, most commonly with respiratory acidosis, but ventilatory compensation is limited
- Usually marked volume depletion

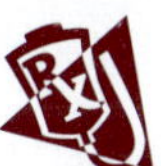

WORK-UP

- Serum electrolytes
- ABG measurement
- Urine electrolytes
- Urine pH

TREATMENT AND MANAGEMENT

- Fluid resuscitation (usually with normal saline)
- Potassium repletion as KCl

TREATMENT MONITORING

- Serial ABG measurement

PROGNOSIS

- Excellent

PREVENTION

- Maintain euvolemia
- Potassium supplementation

RESOURCES

REFERENCES

- Adrogue HJ et al. Management of life-threatening acid-base disorders. (Two parts.) *N Engl J Med.* 1998;338:26, 107.

Alkalosis, Respiratory

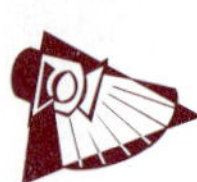

ESSENTIAL FEATURES

- Acute hyperventilation lowers $PaCO_2$ without concomitant changes in plasma bicarbonate concentration
- Chronic respiratory alkalosis occurs in pulmonary and liver disease

EPIDEMIOLOGY

- May be early sign of sepsis

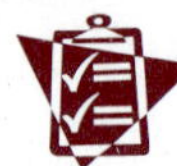

CLINICAL FINDINGS

SYMPTOMS AND SIGNS

- Paresthesias
- Carpopedal spasm
- Positive Chvostek sign

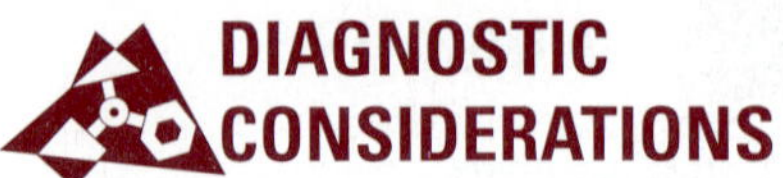

DIAGNOSTIC CONSIDERATIONS

- Electrolyte pattern of chronic respiratory alkalosis is the same as hyperchloremic acidosis; they can only be distinguished by ABG pH measurement

WORK-UP

- ABG measurement
- Serum electrolytes

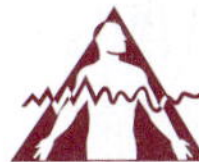

TREATMENT AND MANAGEMENT

- Chronic respiratory alkalosis does not generally require treatment

COMPLICATIONS

- Treatment of chronic respiratory alkalosis may lead to metabolic acidosis and hyperchloremia

RESOURCES

REFERENCES

- Adrogue HJ et al. Management of life-threatening acid-base disorders. (Two parts.) *N Engl J Med.* 1998;338:26, 107.

Ampulla of Vater Tumors

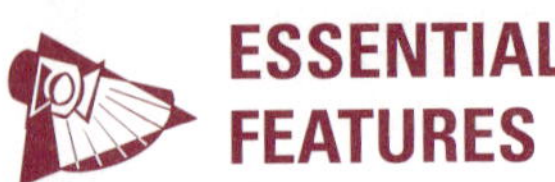

ESSENTIAL FEATURES

- Partial or complete obstruction of the common bile duct and pancreatic duct at the ampulla of Vater
- Exophytic mass at the ampulla visible on endoscopy
- Jaundice, abdominal pain, and weight loss may be presenting symptoms

EPIDEMIOLOGY

- Adenoma and adenocarcinoma of the ampulla of Vater account for about 10% of neoplasms that obstruct the distal bile duct
- Of primary tumors of the ampulla of Vater, 33% are adenomas and 67% are adenocarcinomas
- It is suspected that malignant change in an adenoma gives rise to most carcinomas, and adenomas may contain focus of adenocarcinoma

CLINICAL FINDINGS

SYMPTOMS AND SIGNS

- Jaundice
- GI bleeding from ampullary tumor
- Weight loss
- Abdominal pain

LABORATORY FINDINGS

- Elevated serum bilirubin
- Anemia

IMAGING FINDINGS

- **CT scan:** Dilation of the biliary tree and pancreatic duct; also for staging
- **Abdominal US:** Dilated biliary tree and pancreatic duct
- **ERCP:** Dilation of the biliary and pancreatic ducts
- In 75% of cases, the tumor is visible as an exophytic papillary lesion, an ulcerated tumor, or an infiltrating mass
- In 25% of cases, there is no intraduodenal growth, and endoscopic sphincterotomy is necessary to display the tumor
- An adequate biopsy specimen can usually be obtained from these lesions

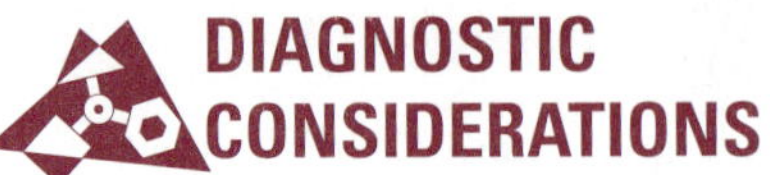

DIAGNOSTIC CONSIDERATIONS

- If a tumor of the ampulla of Vater is suspected but not visualized on duodenoscopy, a sphincterotomy should be performed to inspect the intraluminal surface of the ampulla
- A biopsy specimen of the tumor should be obtained to confirm an ampullary neoplasm and differentiate adenoma from adenocarcinoma

RULE OUT

- Benign causes of biliary obstruction
- Cholangiocarcinoma
- Pancreatic adenocarcinoma
- Duodenal adenoma or adenocarcinoma

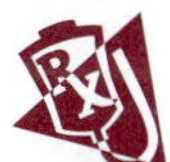

WORK-UP

- Abdominal US to identify biliary and pancreatic duct dilatation
- ERCP to identify lesion and perform biopsy
- CT scan for staging

WHEN TO ADMIT

- Symptomatic, high-grade biliary obstruction not amenable to endoscopic treatment
- Actively bleeding tumors

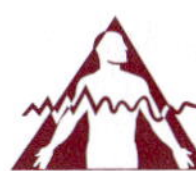

TREATMENT AND MANAGEMENT

- **Adenomas:** Local excision or pancreaticoduodenectomy; if invasive cancer found after excision, pancreaticoduodenectomy
- **Adenocarcinoma:** Pancreaticoduodenectomy

SURGERY

Indications

- All ampullary adenomas and adenocarcinomas
- Metastases to resectible peripancreatic lymph nodes is not a contraindication

Contraindications

- Distant metastases (hepatic): Endoscopic biliary drainage only

COMPLICATIONS

- Biliary and pancreatic duct obstruction

PROGNOSIS

- < 1 year survival without resection
- 5-year survival after resection of adenocarcinoma is 50%

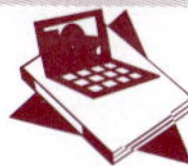

RESOURCES

REFERENCES

- Roberts RH et al. Pancreaticoduodenectomy of ampullary carcinoma. *Am Surg.* 1999;65:1043.
- Howe JR et al. Factors predictive of survival in ampullary carcinoma. *Ann Surg.* 1998;228:87.

PRACTICE GUIDELINES

- The National Comprehensive Cancer Network http://www.nccn.org/

CANCER STAGING

- See Ampulla of Vater Staging Table on page 744.

STAGE GROUPING

Stage 0	Tis	N0	M0
Stage IA	T1	N0	M0
Stage IB	T2	N0	M0
Stage IIA	T3	N0	M0
Stage IIB	T1	N1	M0
	T2	N1	M0
	T3	N1	M0
Stage III	T4	Any N	M0
Stage IV	Any T	Any N	M1

Anal Canal Cancer

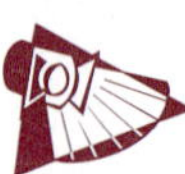

ESSENTIAL FEATURES

- Account for 1.5% of GI tract cancers
- Usually long history of perianal complaints
- Disease may be quite extensive at presentation
- Associated with chronic anal infection (human papillomavirus)
- Tumors anatomically found from the upper to lower border of the internal anal sphincter, 6–12 mm above dentate line
- Referred to as epidermoid carcinoma

EPIDEMIOLOGY

- Women are at increased risk
- Homosexual males at greatly increased risk
- 7/106 men; 9/106 women
- Increased incidence in males and females practicing anal sex
- Increased risk with history of anogenital warts; STD; > 10 sexual partners; cervical, vulvar, or vaginal cancer
- Increased incidence in persons who smoke or who are immunosuppressed (HIV infection and transplantation)

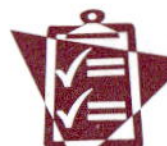

CLINICAL FINDINGS

SYMPTOMS AND SIGNS

- Perianal irritation, may be long-standing
- Palpable mass, may be indurated
- Bleeding
- Itching
- Tenesmus

LABORATORY FINDINGS

- No specific abnormalities

IMAGING FINDINGS

- **CT/MRI:** Reveal anal mass
- **Endorectal US:** Reveals size and depth of invasion and perianal nodes

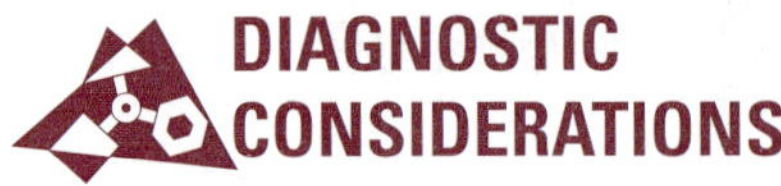

DIAGNOSTIC CONSIDERATIONS

- Tumor of anal margin
- Hemorrhoids
- Anal melanoma
- Perianal/perirectal abscess/fistula
- Low rectal cancer

RULE OUT

- Extension of low rectal adenocarcinoma
- Anal melanoma

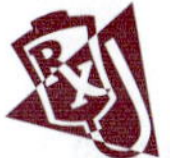

WORK-UP

- Physical exam with digital rectal exam
- Assessment for lymphadenopathy (groins)
- Exam under anesthesia, anoscopy with biopsy
- Endorectal US to assess size and depth of invasion
- Chest film, CT to assess for metastatic disease

WHEN TO ADMIT

- Severe bleeding with hemodynamic compromise
- Intractable symptoms: itching, pain

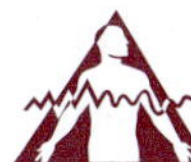

TREATMENT AND MANAGEMENT

- Chemoradiation is mainstay of therapy
- Role of surgery limited
- Overall reported recurrence rates with local excision high

SURGERY

Indications

- Local excision for small, well-differentiated, mobile lesions confined to the submucosa
- Surgery is largely used as salvage procedure or for recurrent/persistent disease (abdominal perineal resection)

Contraindications

- Nigro protocol of chemoradiation is first-line therapy

MEDICATIONS

- Radiation therapy (XRT): 30 Gray to primary tumor and pelvic and inguinal nodes
- Mitomycin is given on day 1 of XRT
- Two 4-day infusions of 5-fluorouracil (5-FU) given on day 1 and day 28 of chemoradiation therapy
- Cisplatin may be used in place of mitomycin

TREATMENT MONITORING

- Follow-up rectal and node exam

COMPLICATIONS

- Recurrence of disease
- Metastatic disease

PROGNOSIS

- Tumor size is best predictor
- Mobile lesions < 2 cm have cure rates of 80%
- Tumors > 5 cm associated with 50% mortality
- Metastatic disease more likely to be present with increasing depth of invasion, size, and histologic grade
- Lymph node disease at presentation is poor prognostic indicator
- 40% of patients die of disease outside the pelvis
- If surgery required for salvage (abdominoperineal resection [APR]), 5-year survival about 50%
- T1–T3 node negative, 5-year survival 88%; T1–T3 node positive, 5-year survival 52%

RESOURCES

REFERENCES

- Allal AS et al. Effectiveness of surgical salvage therapy for patients with locally uncontrolled anal carcinoma after sphincter-conserving treatment. *Cancer.* 1999;86:405.
- Epidermoid and cancer: results from the UKCCCR randomized trial of radiotherapy, 5-fluorouracil, and mitomycin. UKCCCR Anal Cancer Trial Working Party. UK Coordinating Committee on Cancer Research. *Lancet.* 1996;348:1049.
- Ryan DP et al. Carcinoma of the anal canal: treatment with chemotherapy and low-dose radiation therapy. *Radiology.* 1994;191:569.

PRACTICE GUIDELINES

- The National Comprehensive Cancer Network http://www.nccn.org/

CANCER STAGING

- See Anal Canal Staging Table on page 744.

STAGE GROUPING

Stage 0	Tis	N0	M0
Stage I	T1	N0	M0
Stage II	T2	N0	M0
	T3	N0	M0
Stage IIIA	T1	N1	M0
	T2	N1	M0
	T3	N1	M0
	T4	N0	M0
Stage IIIB	T4	N1	M0
	Any T	N2	M0
	Any T	N3	M0
Stage IV	Any T	Any N	M1

Anal Fissure & Ulcer

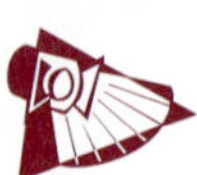

ESSENTIAL FEATURES

- **Fissure:** Split in the anoderm
- **Ulcer:** Chronic fissure
- Associated with skin tag (sentinel pile) once matured
- Located in midline, distal to dentate line
- Most commonly located posteriorly (90%)
- Caused by forceful dilatation of anal canal, usually from defecation, leading to sphincter spasm and local anoderm ischemia

EPIDEMIOLOGY

- Predisposing factors: previous anorectal surgery (hemorrhoidectomy, fistulotomy)
- Classically, initial insult is a firm, hard bowel movement
  - Pain resulting from the initial bowel movement may be great, leading to tendency to resist urge to defecate
  - This leads to the formation of harder stool

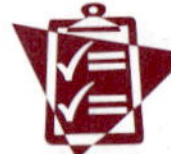

CLINICAL FINDINGS

SYMPTOMS AND SIGNS

- Pain and bleeding with defecation
- Pain may be tearing or burning, worst during defecation, may last for hours
- Blood may be noted on tissue or on stool but not mixed in
- Constipation may develop secondary to fear of recurrent pain
- May present as painless, nonhealing wounds that occasionally bleed
- Physical exam reveals disruption of anoderm in the midline at the mucocutaneous junction
- Sentinel skin tag or pile may be present at the inferior margin
- Digital exam may reveal sphincter spasm

LABORATORY FINDINGS

- No specific findings
- Anal manometry may demonstrate increased sphincter tone

IMAGING FINDINGS

- No specific findings

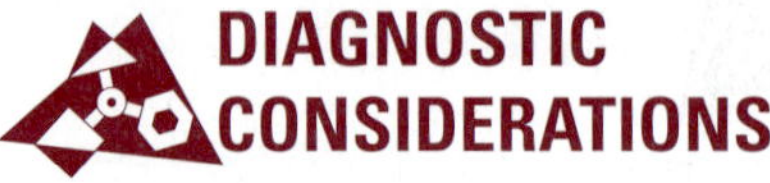

DIAGNOSTIC CONSIDERATIONS

- Crohn disease
- Anal tuberculosis
- Anal malignancy
- Abscess
- Fistula
- Cytomegalovirus
- Herpes
- Chlamydiosis
- Syphilis
- AIDS

RULE OUT

- Anal malignancy

WORK-UP

- History (including previous anorectal surgery) and physical exam
- Following diagnosis, patients should undergo anoscopy and sigmoidoscopy to evaluate for anorectal malignancy or inflammatory bowel disease
- Nonhealing ulcers should be biopsied

WHEN TO ADMIT

- Rarely, except for severe pain or bleeding leading to hemodynamic compromise, or both

TREATMENT AND MANAGEMENT

- Initial treatment is conservative with stool softeners, bulking agents, sitz baths

SURGERY

Indications

- Failure of conservative measures
- Perform lateral internal anal sphincterotomy

MEDICATIONS

- 0.2% nitroglycerin ointment
- Botulinum toxin infiltration into internal sphincters may aid healing
- Stool softeners
- Bulking agents

TREATMENT MONITORING

- Follow-up physical exam

COMPLICATIONS

- Sphincterotomy may result in fecal incontinence
- Recurrence

PROGNOSIS

- Conservative measures will result in healing in 90% cases
- A second episode has a 70% chance of healing with conservative treatment
- Lateral internal anal sphincterotomy is over 90% successful
- Recurrence rate is less than 10% after sphincterotomy

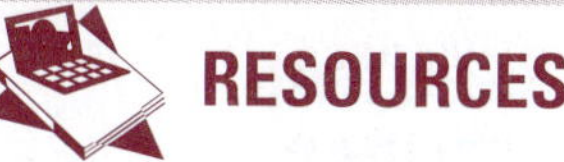

RESOURCES

REFERENCES

- Nelson RL. Meta-analysis of operative techniques for fissure-in-ano. *Dis Colon Rectum.* 1999;42:1424; discussion 1428.
- Brisinda G et al. A comparison of injections of botulinum toxin and topical nitroglycerin ointment for the treatment of chronic anal fissure. *N Engl J Med.* 1999;341:65.

Anal Margin Cancer

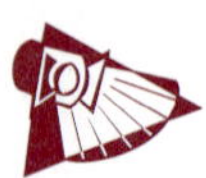

ESSENTIAL FEATURES

- Located at or outside the anal verge
- Usually well-differentiated, keratinizing tumors
- Behave similarly to squamous cell carcinomas of skin
- Lesions may be present for long periods before symptoms develop
- 4 types
  - Squamous cell
  - Basal cell
  - Bowen disease
  - Paget disease

EPIDEMIOLOGY

- Squamous, basal cell carcinoma, and Bowen disease more common in men
- Paget disease more common in women
- 50% patients with Paget disease have coexistent GI malignancy

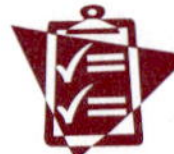

CLINICAL FINDINGS

SYMPTOMS AND SIGNS

- Mass
- Bleeding
- Pain
- Discharge
- Itching
- Tenesmus
- Lesions may be quite large with central ulceration
- **Paget disease:** Erythematous, eczematoid rash
- **Basal cell:** Raised edges with central ulcer
- **Bowen disease:** Scaly, erythematous, sometimes pigmented; often associated with condylomas in younger patients

LABORATORY FINDINGS

- Pap smear screening may be useful to detect dysplasia in immunocompromised patients

IMAGING FINDINGS

- **CT/MRI:** Reveal anal mass
- **Endorectal US:** Reveals size and depth of invasion and perianal nodes

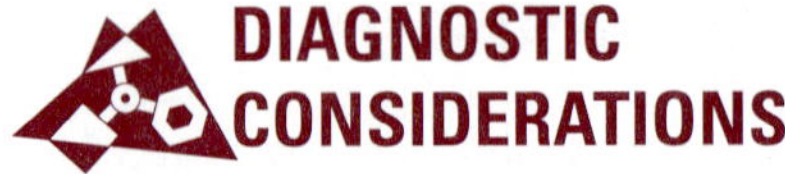

DIAGNOSTIC CONSIDERATIONS

- Chronic or nonhealing perineal ulcer
- Anal canal cancer
- Perianal abscess

RULE OUT

- Biopsy all chronic or nonhealing perineal ulcers

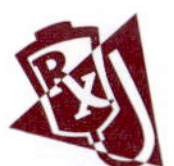

WORK-UP

- Physical exam with digital rectal exam
- Assessment for lymph adenopathy (groins)
- Exam under anesthesia, anoscopy with biopsy
- Endorectal US to assess size and depth of invasion
- Chest film, CT to assess for metastatic disease

WHEN TO ADMIT

- Intractable symptoms: Pain
- Severe bleeding with hemodynamic compromise

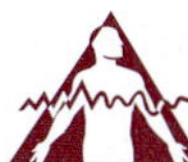

TREATMENT AND MANAGEMENT

- Mainstay of treatment is surgical (wide excision)
- Chemoradiation useful for aggressive lesions

SURGERY

Indications

- Small, well-differentiated lesions (< 4 cm) may be treated with wide excision
- Large, deep lesions involving sphincters require abdominoperineal resection (APR)
- Grossly involved lymph nodes should be resected
- Recurrences may be treated with reexcision or APR
- **For Bowen disease:** Wide local excision and 4-quadrant biopsy
- **For Paget disease:** Wide local excision and multiple perianal biopsies

MEDICATIONS

- Chemoradiation may have a role in advanced disease

TREATMENT MONITORING

- Surveillance physical exam with rectal exam and lymph node exam

COMPLICATIONS

- Infection/perianal sepsis
- Fistula

PROGNOSIS

- **Squamous cell carcinoma:** T stage determines survival; 5-year survival T1 (100%), T2 (60%)
- **Basal cell carcinoma:** Metastasis is rare; local recurrence is 30%
- **Bowen disease:** invasive squamous cell carcinoma develops in fewer than 10% of cases

RESOURCES

REFERENCES

- Marchesa P et al. Long-term outcome of patients with perianal Paget's disease. *Ann Surg Oncol.* 1997;4:475.
- Marchesa P et al. Perianal Bowen's disease: a clinicopathologic study of 47 patients. *Dis Colon Rectum.* 1997;40:1286.
- Peiffert D et al. Conservative treatment by irradiation of epidermoid carcinomas of the anal margin. *Int J Radiat Oncol Biol Phys.* 1997;39:57.

PRACTICE GUIDELINES

- The National Cancer Network web site http://www.nccn.org/

CANCER STAGING

- See Anal Canal Staging Table on page 744.

STAGE GROUPING

Stage 0	Tis	N0	M0
Stage I	T1	N0	M0
Stage II	T2	N0	M0
	T3	N0	M0
Stage IIIA	T1	N1	M0
	T2	N1	M0
	T3	N1	M0
	T4	N0	M0
Stage IIIB	T4	N1	M0
	Any T	N2	M0
	Any T	N3	M0
Stage IV	Any T	Any N	M1

Aneurysms, Peripheral

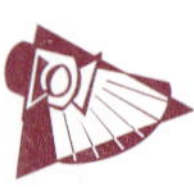

ESSENTIAL FEATURES

- **True aneurysms:** Involves all 3 layers of vessel wall
- **False aneurysm (pseudoaneurysm):** Disruption of artery causing contained hematoma confined by fibrous capsule

Lower Extremity

- 70% of peripheral aneurysms are of popliteal artery; femoral artery next most common site
- Persistence of sciatic artery
  - Rare anomaly
  - Large embryonic sciatic artery (originates from internal iliac artery) communicates directly with popliteal artery;
  - Propensity for aneurismal degeneration

Upper Extremity

- Subclavian artery aneurysms: Rare
  - Several causes: Pseudoaneurysms from drug addict injections increasing, poststenotic dilation from patient with cervical rib or thoracic outlet syndrome, congenital variant with aberrant artery arising from proximal descending thoracic aorta (Kommerell's diverticulum)
- Radial artery pseudoaneurysms: Increased as a result of increased radial artery catheters, occasionally infected

EPIDEMIOLOGY

- 0.5–6% incidence of pseudoaneurysm of femoral artery after puncture
- Popliteal aneurysms bilateral in 50%
- 33% of patients with popliteal aneurysm have AAA

CLINICAL FINDINGS

SYMPTOMS AND SIGNS

- Usually minimal until progressive thrombosis, stenosis occurs
- **Femoral:** Throbbing mass in groin often present
- **Popliteal:** Usually asymptomatic
  - First symptom often acute ischemia
  - Thrombosis, peripheral embolization cause acute ischemia
  - Occlusion may occur from fragmentation of mural thrombus
  - Thrombus may occlude lumen of aneurysm or embolize
  - Can progress rapidly to gangrene
  - Recurrent embolization presents with sudden ischemia of toe or foot with gradual resolution
  - Popliteal aneurysms rarely cause symptoms from compression of vein or tibial nerve
  - Palpation suggests diagnosis
- **Persistent sciatic artery aneurysms:** Painful, pulsatile buttock mass
- **Subclavian:** Emboli to fingers, dysphagia lusoria (difficulty swallowing)

IMAGING FINDINGS

- US confirms size, diagnosis, flow
- Arteriography advised before operation

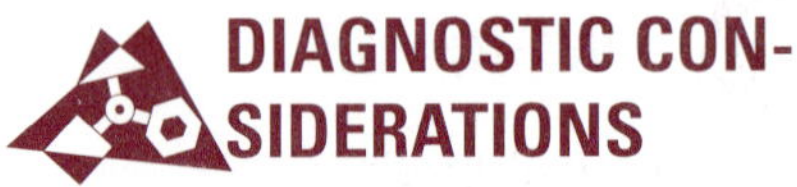

DIAGNOSTIC CONSIDERATIONS

- Evaluate for multiple sites of aneurysm
- Evaluate for distal ischemia or embolus

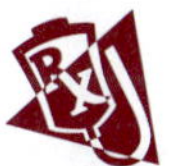

WORK-UP

- US confirms diagnosis
- Arteriography may not demonstrate aneurysm but is advised before operative repair to define distal arteries

TREATMENT AND MANAGEMENT

- Immediate operation or thrombolytic therapy indicated when pregangrenous
- Femoral pseudoaneurysm treated with US-guided compression

SURGERY

- **Femoral artery:** Replace diseased segment
- **Popliteal artery:** Exclude and bypass with saphenous vein
- **Sciatic nerve:** Exclude aneurysm and bypass with saphenous vein
- **Subclavian:** Resect first rib or cervical rib, divide scalenus anterior, replace aneurysm with graft
- **Radial pseudoaneurysm**
  - Normal Allen test, excise and ligate
  - Abnormal Allen test, reconstruct artery

Indications

- Pregangreneous ischemia
- Recurrent peripheral embolization
- Symptomatic aneurysm
- Asymptomatic aneurysm 3 × normal diameter

MEDICATIONS

- Thrombolytics for occluded popliteal aneurysms should be considered

PROGNOSIS

- Depends on outflow tract
- Late graft failures less common than operations done for peripheral vascular occlusive disease

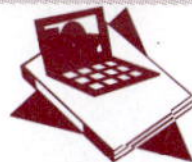

RESOURCES

REFERENCES

- Diwan A et al. Incidence of femoral and popliteal aneurysms in patients with abdominal aortic aneurysms. *J Vasc Surg.* 2000;31:863.
- Henry M et al. Percutaneous endovascular treatment of peripheral aneurysms. *J Cardiovasc Surg.* 2000;41:871.

Annular Pancreas

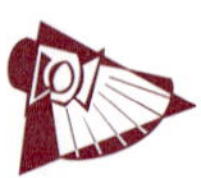

ESSENTIAL FEATURES

- Ring of pancreatic tissue from the head of the pancreas surrounds the descending duodenum, leading to obstruction, presenting either in infancy or adulthood
- Vomitus is bilious if obstruction is distal to the ampulla of Vater
- Air in the stomach and duodenum proximal to the obstruction on abdominal x-ray (double bubble sign)

EPIDEMIOLOGY

- Rare congenital condition in which a ring of pancreatic tissue from the head of the pancreas surrounds the descending duodenum
- The abnormality usually presents in infancy as duodenal obstruction with postprandial vomiting
- There is bile in the vomitus if the constriction is distal to the entrance of the common bile duct
- Occasionally, annular pancreas will present in adults with similar symptoms

CLINICAL FINDINGS

SYMPTOMS AND SIGNS

- Upper GI obstruction
- Vomiting
- Upper GI bleeding
- Epigastric pain

LABORATORY FINDINGS

- Hypochloremic metabolic alkalosis
- Hypokalemia

IMAGING FINDINGS

- **Abdominal x-ray**: Dilated stomach and proximal duodenum (double bubble sign) and little or no air in the rest of the small bowel
- **Upper GI contrast radiography:** Narrowing of the duodenum where it is encircled by the pancreatic head, with proximal dilation
- **ERCP:** Pancreatic duct in head of pancreas encircling duodenum

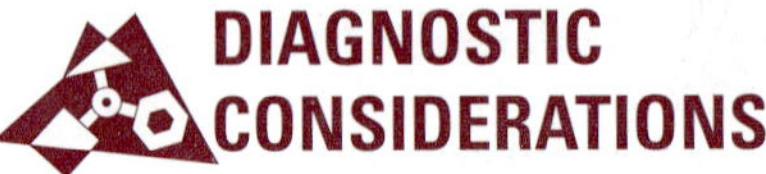

DIAGNOSTIC CONSIDERATIONS

- Signs and symptoms of upper GI obstruction should prompt radiographic imaging, which may suggest duodenal obstruction
- Always consider annular pancreas as a cause of duodenal obstruction
- May cause peptic ulcer disease or chronic pancreatitis in an adult

RULE OUT

- Other causes of duodenal obstruction

–Duodenal tumors
–Pancreatic head masses
–Duodenal atresia (infant)

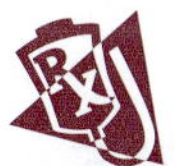

WORK-UP

- Abdominal x-ray
- Upper GI contrast radiography
- ERCP confirms the diagnosis but is not necessary

WHEN TO ADMIT

- All symptomatic cases

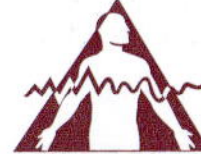

TREATMENT AND MANAGEMENT

- Correction of fluids and electrolytes
- The obstructed segment should be bypassed by a duodenojejunostomy
- The obstructing pancreas should not be resected; high risk for pancreatic fistula

SURGERY

Indications

- All cases in children
- All symptomatic cases in adults

COMPLICATIONS

- Chronic pancreatitis
- Peptic ulcer disease
- Obstruction
- Bleeding

PROGNOSIS

- Excellent after surgical bypass of obstruction

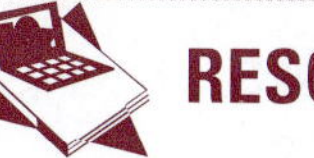

RESOURCES

REFERENCES

- Chen YC et al. Symptomatic adult annular pancreas. *J Clin Gastroenterol.* 2003;36:446.
- McCollum MO et al. Annular pancreas and duodenal stenosis. *J Pediatr Surg.* 2002;37:1776.

Anorectal Abscess & Fistula

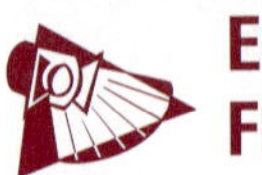

ESSENTIAL FEATURES

- Result from occlusion of anal glands and crypts at the dentate line
- Occlusion may follow impaction of vegetable matter or edema from trauma
- Abscesses are classified according to space they invade
  - Supralevator
  - Ischiorectal
  - Superficial
  - Intersphincteric
  - Transphincteric
- May also develop as a result of inflammatory bowel disease (Crohn)
- Fistula-in-ano from the anus to the perianal skin develops when abscess cavity maintains persistent communication with the crypt
- **Goodsall rule:** Used to identify direction of fistula tract
  - Anterior external opening: Tract extends in a radial direction to the dentate line
  - Posterior external opening: Fistula tract curves to the posterior midline

EPIDEMIOLOGY

- 10% of patients with Crohn disease have anorectal abscess fistulous disease with no prior history of inflammatory bowel disease

CLINICAL FINDINGS

SYMPTOMS AND SIGNS

- Severe anal/perianal pain, usually continuous and throbbing
- Pain may worsen with movement and straining
- Swelling and discharge may be noted
- Patients may have fever, urinary retention
- Severe, life-threatening perineal sepsis may develop
- Patients with fistula-in-ano may have pain and bloody discharge
- Exam findings may include tender perianal or rectal mass
- **Fistula:** Internal and external openings with mucopurulent drainage
- Fistulous tract is often palpable and firm

LABORATORY FINDINGS

- May have elevated WBC count, especially with perineal sepsis
- Drainage may have white blood cells, bacteria

IMAGING FINDINGS

- Imaging studies are unnecessary in uncomplicated cases
- Sinogram may reveal fistulous tract and branches
- Transrectal US may reveal extent of sphincter involvement
- CT scan may be helpful in identifying supralevator abscesses

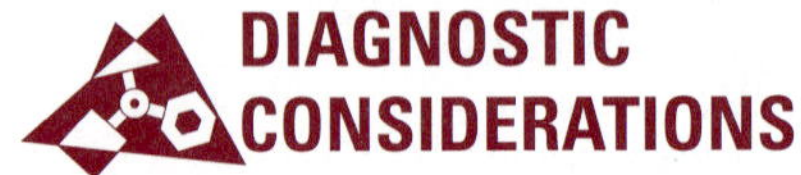

DIAGNOSTIC CONSIDERATIONS

- Inflammatory bowel disease (Crohn disease)
- Pilonidal disease
- Hidradenitis suppurativa
- Anal tuberculosis
- Actinomycosis
- Trauma
- Anal fissure
- Anal malignancy
- Radiation injury
- Chlamydiosis
- Diverticulitis
- Retrorectal tumors

RULE OUT

- Crohn disease
- Anorectal malignancy

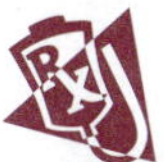

WORK-UP

- History and physical exam
  - Is there history of diabetes or immunocompromised conditions, including medications (steroids, chemotherapy)?
- Imaging studies are not indicated for uncomplicated cases

WHEN TO ADMIT

- Abscesses should be drained; admission will depend on extent of abscess drainage required
- Signs of perineal sepsis or complicated abscess
- Fistula-in-ano by itself is not a surgical emergency

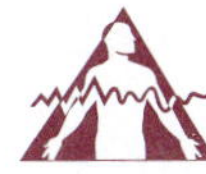

TREATMENT AND MANAGEMENT

- Treatment for abscess is surgical drainage
- Intersphincteric abscesses are treated with internal sphincterotomy
- Perianal and ischiorectal abscesses are drained through the perianal skin
- **Fistula-in-ano:** Fistulotomy, currette tract and granulation tissue, heal by secondary intention
- **Fistula-in-ano:** Involving external sphincter may be treated with seton placement or drainage with delayed repair with an endorectal advancement flap

SURGERY

Indications

- Anorectal abscesses require surgical drainage
- Patients with diabetes or immunocompromised require urgent attention since these patients are prone to necrotizing anorectal infections and sepsis

Contraindications

- Fistulotomy may be delayed until abscess is drained and inflammation subsides to allow identification of internal opening

MEDICATIONS

- Antibiotics are not necessary unless patient is immunocompromised, diabetic, has extensive cellulitis, or has valvular heart disease

COMPLICATIONS

- Recurrence
- Incomplete drainage
- Sphincter injury/fecal incontinence

PROGNOSIS

- Once the source for infection is identified and adequately drained, prognosis is good
- 50% of patients are cured with drainage alone
- Chronic fistula develops in 50% of patients
- Seton placement for fistula has 17% incontinence rate

RESOURCES

REFERENCES

- Garcia-Aguilar J et al. Anal fistula surgery. Factors associated with recurrence and incontinence. *Dis Colon Rectum.* 1996;39:723.
- Jun SH et al. Anocutaneous advancement flap closure of high and fistulas. *Br J Surg.* 1999;86:490.
- Knoefel WT et al. The initial approach to anorectal abscesses: fistulotomy is safe and reduces the chance of recurrences. *Dig Surg.* 2000;17:274.
- Practice parameters for treatment of fistula-in-ano—supporting documentation. The Standards Practice Task Force. The American Society of Colon and Rectal Surgeons. *Dis Colon Rectum.* 1996;39:1363.

Aortic Coarctation & Interrupted Aortic Arch, Congenital

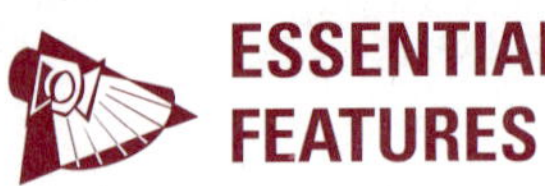

ESSENTIAL FEATURES

- Congenital obstructive lesions

Aortic Coarctation

- 98% are located near aortic isthmus (proximal to ductus arteriosus)
- Occurs in 3 contexts
  - Isolated
  - Associated with ventricular septal defect (VSD)
  - Associated with severe intracardiac anomalies and extensive arch involvement
- Associated anomalies (occur in 70% of neonates, 15% of older children): patent foramen ovale (PFO), ductus arteriosus, VSD, bicuspid aortic valve (40%), and Shone syndrome
- Obstruction leads to systolic and diastolic hypertension in upper extremities
- Collaterals eventually develop
- Patent ductus arteriosus maintains distal flow

Interrupted Aortic Arch

- **Type A (35%):** Absence of arch distal to left subclavian artery
- **Type B (60%):** Between left carotid and left subclavian artery
- **Type C (5%):** Between innominate and left carotid artery
- Ductus arteriosus maintains distal flow
- Almost always has associated VSD, truncus arteriosus, aortopulmonary window, subaortic stenosis, or transposition of great vessels
- Type B associated with aberrant right subclavian artery

EPIDEMIOLOGY

Aortic Coarctation

- Occurs in 0.2–0.6 per 1000 live births
- 5–8% of congenital cardiovascular anomalies
- 2–5 times more common in males
- 15–30% of patients with Turner syndrome have aortic coarctation

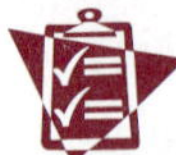

CLINICAL FINDINGS

SYMPTOMS AND SIGNS

Aortic Coarctation

- 2 distinct presentations
  - Early infancy: Severe congestive heart failure, sudden cardiovascular collapse with duct closure
  - Older children: Many asymptomatic; headache; pain in calves when running; frequent nose bleeds; hypertension of upper extremities; LV hypertrophy; classically, notched ribs (from enlarged intercostals vessels) seen in children older than 4 years

Interrupted Aortic Arch

- Symptomatic in first few days of life

IMAGING FINDINGS

Aortic Coarctation

- **Chest film:** Reversed “3” sign
- **Echocardiography:** Diagnostic
- **MRI:** Diagnostic

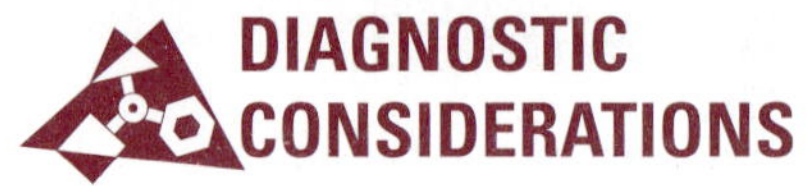

DIAGNOSTIC CONSIDERATIONS

- Evaluate for other cardiac or extracardiac anomalies

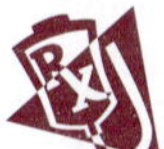

WORK-UP

- Echocardiography is usually sufficient to make diagnosis
- Arteriography occasionally useful

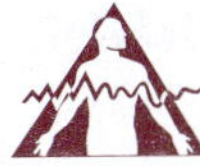

TREATMENT AND MANAGEMENT

Aortic Coarctation

- In neonate, alprostadil (PGE_1) to maintain ductus patency, mechanical ventilation, and HCO_3
- **Surgical options:** Resect with end-to-end anastomosis, subclavian flap aortoplasty ± resection, patch aortoplasty, interposition graft, percutaneous balloon
- Repair performed via left thoracotomy
- Median sternotomy if concomitant intracardiac anomaly repair
- **Neonate:** Primary repair or subclavian flap preferred
- **Child:** Primary repair or interposition graft preferred
- Recoarctation (gradient > 20 mm Hg), consider balloon or patch aortoplasty

Interrupted Aortic Arch

- PGE_1 maintains hemodynamics

SURGERY

Indications

- Once diagnosis of aortic coarctation is made, correct when stabilized
- Repair interrupted aortic arch early

COMPLICATIONS

- Operative: Hemorrhage, damage to recurrent laryngeal nerve, Horner syndrome, chylothorax, paraplegia
- Postoperative mesenteric vasculitis can be minimized with good blood pressure control

PROGNOSIS

Aortic Coarctation

- If untreated, mortality is 50% by age 30
- 5-year survival 95% but can be low (40%) if intracardiac anomaly
- Postoperative hypertension usually resolves in several days but should be treated aggressively

RESOURCES

REFERENCES

- Conte S et al. Surgical management of neonatal coarctation. *J Thorac Cardiovasc Surg.* 1995;109:663.

Aortic Stenosis

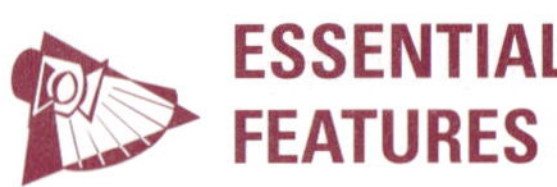

ESSENTIAL FEATURES

Aortic Valve (AV)

- Usually tricuspid, composed of fibrous skeleton, 3 cusps, and sinuses of Valsalva
- Free edge of each cusp is concave and thicker, with fibrous node at midpoint
- Eddy currents in sinuses of Valsalva prevent occlusion of coronary ostia during systole
- Cusps fall closed and coapt, supports ejected column of blood during diastole
- Coronary arteries arise from 2 of 3 sinuses of Valsalva

Aortic Stenosis (AS)

- Can be subvalvular, valvular, or supravalvular
- **Etiology in adult:** Congenital unicuspid, bicuspid valve; congenital subvalvular or supravalvular stenosis; rheumatic heart disease; or degenerative fibrosis and calcification (most common)
- LV outflow obstruction leads to concentric LV hypertrophy: decreased diastolic compliance, maintained ejection fraction (EF)
- Atrial systole important for LV filling
- Atrial fibrillation may precipitate congestive heart failure (CHF)
- LV hypertrophy leads to increased myocardial oxygen consumption, coronary artery disease (present in 25–50%), more myocardium at jeopardy

EPIDEMIOLOGY

- **Causes of valve disease**
  - Rheumatic carditis (most common)
  - Valve collagen degeneration
  - Infection
  - Less common causes include collagen-vascular disease, tumors, carcinoid, and Marfan syndrome
- Valvular heart disease: 89,000 hospital discharges in 1998

AS

- Likely congenital if patient is < 30 years old
- Likely bicuspid valve if patient is 30–65 years old
- Likely degenerative if patient is > 65 years old

CLINICAL FINDINGS

SYMPTOMS AND SIGNS

- Most asymptomatic for many years
- **Triad:** Angina, syncope, CHF
- Aortic valve gradient > 50 mm Hg, or valve area < 1 cm^2 usually symptomatic
- Angina from inadequate oxygen delivery
- Syncope usually exertional
- CHF is late finding and ominous sign
- Narrowed pulse pressure
- Decreased systolic pressure (parvus et tardus)
- Harsh midsystolic murmur: second intercostal space along left sternal border, radiating to carotids, not axilla or apex
- 25–50% also have aortic regurgitation murmur

LABORATORY FINDINGS

- **ECG:** LV hypertrophy

IMAGING FINDINGS

- **Chest film:** Heart usually normal size (may be dilated if CHF present), poststenotic aortic dilation, calcified aortic valve
- **Transesophageal echocardiography (TEE):** Evaluate for calcification, valve mobility, bicuspid anatomy, LV hypertrophy, EF, valvular gradients, aortic regurgitation
- **Cardiac catheterization:** Coronary anatomy, cardiac output, transvalvular pressure gradients, LV function, coexisting valvular lesions

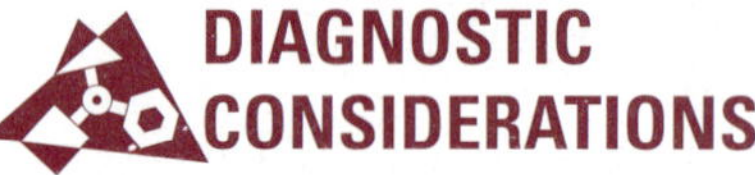

DIAGNOSTIC CONSIDERATIONS

- **TEE:** Evaluate for calcification, valve mobility, bicuspid anatomy, LV hypertrophy, EF, valvular gradients, aortic regurgitation
- **Cardiac catheterization:** Coronary anatomy, cardiac output, transvalvular pressure gradients, LV function, coexisting valvular lesions

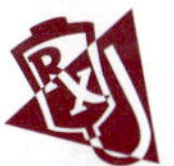

WORK-UP

- **Mild AS:** Aortic valve area > 1.5 cm^2
- **Moderate AS:** 1–1.5 cm^2
- **Severe AS:** ≤ 1 cm^2

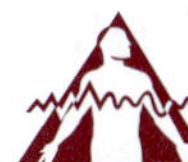

TREATMENT AND MANAGEMENT

- **Balloon valvotomy:** Limited role due to high restenosis rate within 6 mos; may be option if patient is decompensated with severe heart failure as a "bridge"
- **Valve replacement:** Mechanical or porcine

SURGERY

Indications

- Symptomatic AS with life expectancy of 1–3 years without intervention
- Asymptomatic with AV gradient > 50 mm Hg, or area ≤ 1 cm^2
- Presence of LV dysfunction or coexisting coronary disease is relative indication

PROGNOSIS

- Operative mortality < 5%
- LV dysfunction, advanced age, acute presentation increases surgical risk
- LV hypertrophy may regress for 10 years
- 5-year survival, > 85%
- 50% of late deaths noncardiac

RESOURCES

REFERENCES

- Knott-Craig CJ et al. Aortic valve replacement: comparison of late survival between autografts and homografts. *Ann Thorac Surg.* 2000;69:1327.
- Smedira NG et al. Balloon aortic valvuloplasty as a bridge to aortic valve replacement in critically ill patients. *Ann Thorac Surg.* 1993;55:914.

Aortic Valve Regurgitation

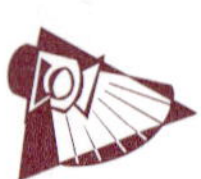

ESSENTIAL FEATURES

- **Aortic valve (AV):** Usually tricuspid, composed of fibrous skeleton, 3 cusps, and sinuses of Valsalva
- Free edge of each cusp is concave and thicker, with fibrous node at midpoint
- **During systole:** Eddy currents in sinuses of Valsalva prevent occlusion of coronary ostia
- **During diastole:** Cusps fall closed and coapt, supports ejected column of blood
- Coronary arteries arise from 2 of 3 sinuses of Valsalva
- Aortic regurgitation (AR) is caused by abnormal coaptation of valve leaflets, allowing blood to return from aorta to ventricle during diastole
- Etiology of chronic AR:
  - Rheumatic dilation
  - Annuloaortic ectasia
  - Cystic medial necrosis
  - Atherosclerosis
  - Syphilis
  - Arthritic inflammatory disease
  - Congenital bicuspid valve
- Etiology of acute AR:
  - Endocarditis
  - Acute aortic dissection
  - Trauma
- LV becomes eccentrically hypertrophied and dilated

EPIDEMIOLOGY

- Causes of valve disease: rheumatic carditis (most common), valve collagen degeneration, infection
- Less common causes: Collagen-vascular disease, tumors, carcinoid, and Marfan syndrome
- Valvular heart disease: 89,000 hospital discharges in 1998

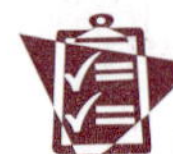

CLINICAL FINDINGS

SYMPTOMS AND SIGNS

- Acute AR:
  - Poorly tolerated
  - Severe pulmonary edema, congestive heart failure (CHF)
  - If diastolic murmur absent, indicates complete valve incompetence
- Chronic AR:
  - Patients with early disease are asymptomatic
  - Orthopnea, paroxysmal dyspnea, and CHF develops later
- Wide pulse pressure, diastolic pressure low (Corrigan pulse)
- Apical impulse: Sustained and lateral and inferiorly displaced
- Blowing high-pitched diastolic murmur heard at left lower sternal border at full expiration
- Third heart sound may be present
- Austin-Flint murmur: Diastolic rumbling—secondary mitral valve obstruction

LABORATORY FINDINGS

- ECG: LV hypertrophy with left axis deviation

IMAGING FINDINGS

- **Chest film**
  - Usually normal cardiac size
  - If chronic AR, LV enlargement, pulmonary congestion
- **Echocardiography:** Demonstrates LV function, chamber size, degree of regurgitation
- **Catheterization:** Define degree of AR and coronary artery, aortic root anatomy

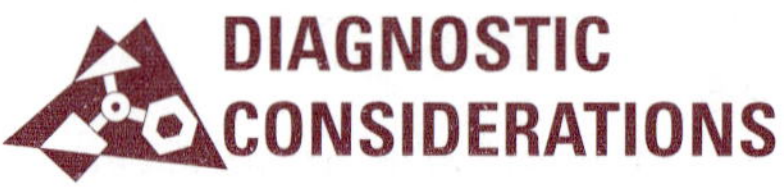

DIAGNOSTIC CONSIDERATIONS

- Evaluate for other valvular disease and secondary LV dysfunction

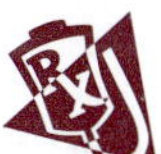

WORK-UP

- Echocardiographic measurement of LV dimensions: Significant ventricular dilation = LV end-diastolic dimension > 70 mm, or end-systolic > 50 mm

TREATMENT AND MANAGEMENT

- Vasodilator therapy
  - Useful in asymptomatic patients
  - Will not prevent need for future surgery
- AV replacement is standard
- Select patients can have valve repair with subcommissural annuloplasty if the lesion is simple annular dilation

SURGERY

Indications

- Replace valve before onset of irreversible LV dilation (see Work-up)

PROGNOSIS

- Medical therapy: 5- and 10-year mortality in severe AR is 25% and 50%, respectively
- 5-year survival postoperatively with normal ventricular function is 85%
- Abnormal LV function affects long-term survival

RESOURCES

REFERENCES

- Dujardin KS et al. Mortality and morbidity of aortic regurgitation in clinical practice. A long-term follow-up study. *Circulation.* 1999;99:1851.
- Knott-Craig CJ et al. Aortic valve replacement: comparison of late survival between autografts and homografts. *Ann Thorac Surg.* 2000;69:1327.

Appendiceal Neoplasms

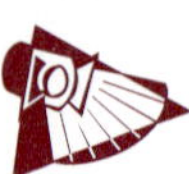

ESSENTIAL FEATURES

- Most diagnosed during appendectomy for acute appendicitis
- Some discovered as incidental findings during other abdominal procedures
- Mucin secretion from peritoneal cystadenocarcinoma implants is the cause of pseudomyxoma peritonei

EPIDEMIOLOGY

- 4.6% incidence of benign tumors in appendectomy specimens
- 1.4% incidence of malignant tumors in appendectomy specimens
- Benign lesions include small carcinoid and mucocele
- Malignant tumors include carcinoid, mucinous cystadenocarcinoma, and adenocarcinoma
- Appendix most common location of GI carcinoids
- Most carcinoids are < 2 cm and are located at the tip of the appendix
- Carcinoids > 1.5 cm may exhibit malignant behavior
- Widespread metastases are present in 10–50% of patients with appendiceal adenocarcinoma

CLINICAL FINDINGS

SYMPTOMS AND SIGNS

- Diagnosis virtually never made preoperatively
- Clinical presentation in most patients is either acute appendicitis or lack of symptoms
- Clinical presentation in small portion of patients is the carcinoid syndrome or evidence of widespread metastases
- Rarely is a palpable mass present
- Ascites may be present in patients with a ruptured or metastatic mucin-secreting tumor

LABORATORY FINDINGS

- Findings consistent with acute appendicitis
- Patients with carcinoid syndrome may have elevations of 5-hydroxyindoleacetic acid (HIAA)

IMAGING FINDINGS

- Most common radiographic findings are those consistent with acute appendicitis (enlarged appendix with peri-appendiceal fat stranding on CT)
- Up to 15% of patients have formed peri-appendiceal abscesses
- Tumors > 1–2 cm may be detected as an appendiceal mass on CT scan, although tumors usually obscured by surrounding bowel

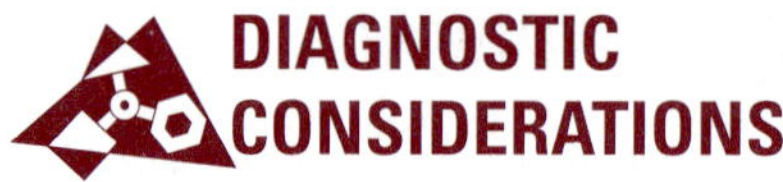

DIAGNOSTIC CONSIDERATIONS

- Acute appendicitis
- Appendiceal abscess
- Carcinoid
- Mucinous cystadenoma
- Mucinous cystadenocarcinoma
- Adenocarcinoma
- Adenocarcinoid
- Lymphoma
- Metastasis to the appendix

RULE OUT

- Synchronous carcinoid neoplasms
- Metastatic disease

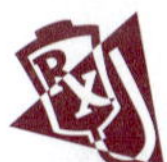

WORK-UP

- Most diagnoses depend on pathologic evaluation of the appendiceal specimen
- Abdominal/pelvic CT scan to evaluate for metastatic disease
- Somatostatin receptor scintigraphy can be helpful with carcinoid tumors
- Up to 35% of patients with adenocarcinoma have a second GI malignancy

WHEN TO REFER

- Patients with evidence of lymph node involvement or metastatic disease

TREATMENT AND MANAGEMENT

- Following recovery from initial surgical procedure, further resection should be considered

SURGERY

Indications

- Carcinoids < 2 cm are treated with appendectomy alone
- Carcinoids > 2 cm or with mucinous elements, or invasion of the mesoappendix or cecum, should have right hemicolectomy
- All (nonmetastatic) adenocarcinoma should be treated with right hemicolectomy
- Localized hepatic masses should be resected
- Debulking of cystadenocarcinoma mucin-secreting peritoneal implants provides symptomatic relief

Contraindications

- Unresectable metastatic disease

PROGNOSIS

- Very good for benign lesions and small carcinoids
- Adenocarcinoma 5-year survival 60% after right hemicolectomy
- Prolonged survival with metastatic carcinoid and mucinous cystadenocarcinoma is common

RESOURCES

REFERENCES

- Way L. Appendix. In: Way L, Doherty G (editors). *Current Surgical Diagnosis & Treatment,* 11e. McGraw-Hill; New York: 2003:672–673.

Appendicitis, Acute

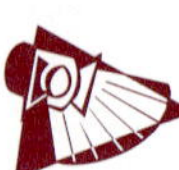

ESSENTIAL FEATURES

- Abdominal pain
- Anorexia, nausea, and vomiting
- Localized right lower quadrant pain
- Low-grade fever
- Leukocytosis

EPIDEMIOLOGY

- 7% of people in Western countries have appendicitis at some time in their lives
- 200,000 appendectomies for acute appendicitis are performed each year in the United States
- Incidence in developing countries has been increasing in proportion to economic gains and changes in lifestyle
- **Major causes:** Obstruction of the proximal lumen by fibrous bands, lymphoid hyperplasia, fecaliths, calculi, or parasites
- Evidence of temporal and geographic clustering of cases has suggested a primary infectious etiology
- Diagnosis is most difficult in the very young or old
- Highest incidence of false-positives occur in women between the ages of 20 and 40, attributable to pelvic inflammatory disease (PID) and other gynecologic conditions

CLINICAL FINDINGS

SYMPTOMS AND SIGNS

- Classically, abdominal pain develops prior to nausea and vomiting
- Peri-umbilical abdominal pain initially, then localizes to the right lower quadrant
- Right lower quadrant rebound or percussion tenderness (localized "peritoneal irritation")
- Constipation and indigestion are frequent complaints
- Patients complain of discomfort with movement, walking, or coughing
- Low-grade fever (99 °F–101 °F) unless perforation has occurred

LABORATORY FINDINGS

- Mild leukocytosis (10,000–15,000) with left shift
- Mild elevations in amylase
- UA frequently will show a few WBC and RBCs on microscopic exam
- Elevated C-reactive protein and ESR levels

IMAGING FINDINGS

- Plain films may show evidence of localized air fluid levels or localized ileus or increased soft-tissue density in the right lower quadrant
  - Less common findings include an appendiceal calculus, altered right psoas stripe, or an abnormal right flank stripe
- US may demonstrate a dilated tubular structure in the right lower quadrant although this technique is user- and institutional-dependant and is less sensitive in adults than in children
- Spiral CT (either abdominal/pelvic or a dedicated "appendiceal protocol") is the most sensitive and specific diagnostic radiographic test
  - An enlarged appendix with peri-appendiceal fat stranding is demonstrated in 90–95% of cases
  - CT scans are of greatest value in patients with atypical clinical presentation or laboratory findings

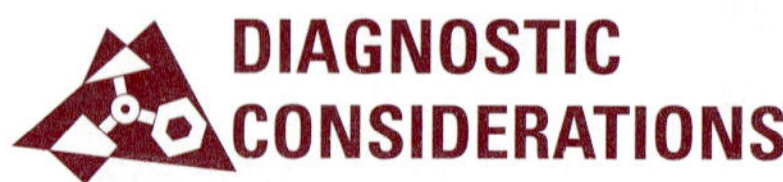

DIAGNOSTIC CONSIDERATIONS

- Acute salpingitis
- PID
- Regional enteritis/complicated Crohn disease
- Viral gastroenterologic infection
- Mesenteric adenitis
- Dysmenorrhea
- Ovarian lesions
- Urinary tract infections
- Small bowel obstruction
- Cecal volvulus
- Incarcerated hernia
- Mesenteric ischemia
- Acute cholecystitis
- Right-sided diverticulitis (true cecal or a redundant sigmoid that flops over into the right lower quadrant)
- Complicated peptic ulcer disease (with enteric contents collecting in the right paracolic gutter)
- Infarcted epiploic appendage

RULE OUT

- Nonsurgical etiology of right lower quadrant abdominal pain
  - Acute salpingitis
  - Dysmenorrhea
  - Urinary tract infections
  - Viral gastroenterologic infection
  - Mesenteric adenitis
  - Others
- Complicated appendicitis manifested by right lower quadrant abscess formation

WORK-UP

- Thorough history and physical exam (including rectal and pelvic in all females)
- CBC count
- Basic chemistries and liver profile
- Amylase and lipase
- UA
- Chest and abdominal films
- Obtain CT scans when clinical presentation or laboratory findings are atypical

WHEN TO ADMIT

- All patients with acute appendicitis or complicated appendicitis for definitive treatment
- In equivocal clinical presentations, 24-hour admission for serial abdominal exams is helpful in making the diagnosis of acute appendicitis
- Reliable patients that live close to the hospital may be sent home and asked to return to the emergency department if their pain worsens

WHEN TO REFER

- Referral to gynecology, gastroenterology, etc as clinically indicated
- Patients who present in a delayed fashion with a formed right lower quadrant abscess may be best managed by percutaneous drainage via interventional radiology

TREATMENT AND MANAGEMENT

- CT scan or 24-hour admission for serial abdominal exams or diagnostic laparoscopy for "nonclassic" presentation
- Appendectomy mainstay of treatment for uncomplicated acute appendicitis
- Appendectomy can be performed open or laparoscopically
- Patients with complicated appendicitis can be treated operatively with appendectomy and drainage or with percutaneous drainage followed by delayed appendectomy
- Abdominal drainage only for established abscesses
- Culturing abdominal fluid has no practical value as organisms are the usual fecal flora
- If a patient with appendicitis cannot be taken to a surgical facility for care, treatment should consist of antibiotics alone

SURGERY

Indications

- Uncomplicated acute appendicitis
- Diagnostic laparoscopy, especially in young women
- Interval appendectomy for patients with right lower quadrant abscess formation and who were treated initially with percutaneous drainage

MEDICATIONS

- Prophylactic antibiotics are indicated preoperatively only
- Single-drug regimen, usually a cephalosporin, is as effective as multidrug combinations

TREATMENT MONITORING

- Clinical improvement in symptoms
- Resolution of fever
- Normalization of WBC

COMPLICATIONS

- Wound complications
- Right lower quadrant abscess formation (up 30% in perforated appendicitis)
- Tubal infertility in complicated appendicitis

PROGNOSIS

- Mortality 0.1% for uncomplicated appendicitis
- Mortality 5% for perforated appendicitis

RESOURCES

REFERENCES

- Andersson RE et al. Repeated clinical and laboratory examinations in patients with an equivocal diagnosis of appendicitis. *World J Surg.* 2000;24:479.
- Stroman DL et al. The role of computed tomography in the diagnosis of acute appendicitis? *Am J Surg.* 1999;178:485.

Arterial Injuries

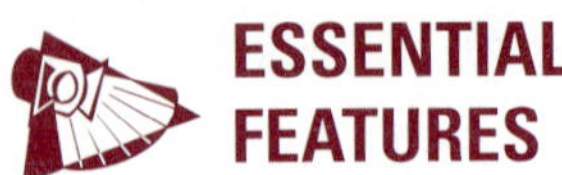

ESSENTIAL FEATURES

Penetrating Injuries

- Local and regional effects of are determined by mechanism of vessel injury
- Stab wounds, low-velocity (< 2000 ft/s) bullet wounds, iatrogenic injuries, and inadvertent intra-arterial injection of drugs produce less soft-tissue injury and less disruption of collateral circulation
- High-velocity missiles produce more extensive vascular injuries, which involve massive destruction and contamination of surrounding tissues
- Cavitational effect of high-velocity injury causes additional injury and may produce arterial thrombosis due to disrupted intima even when vessel not directly traumatized
- Shotgun blasts produce widespread damage and have higher likelihood of infection

Blunt Injuries

- Motor vehicle accidents are a major cause of blunt arterial injuries
- Most arterial injuries are indirect due to fractures
- Especially likely near joints where vessels are relatively fixed and vulnerable to shear forces
- Contusions or crush injuries may result in complete or partial disruption of arteries

EPIDEMIOLOGY

- Peripheral vascular trauma typically occurs in young men between the ages of 20 and 40 years
- Blunt trauma is the principal cause of over 8000 cases of thoracic aortic injuries per year in United States
- About 10–15% of deaths from MVA involve thoracic aortic rupture
- Most aortic ruptures occur in patients aged 20–30 years, with a 9:1 male to female predominance
- 10–20% of patients with acute thoracic disruption survive the initial trauma
  - Of these, 30% will die within 6 hours, 40% with 24 hours, 72% in first week, and 90% within 10 weeks without treatment
- Aortic disruption generally occurs at aortic isthmus (between left subclavian and ligamentum arteriosum)

CLINICAL FINDINGS

SYMPTOMS AND SIGNS

Hemorrhage

- When pulsatile external hemorrhage is present, diagnosis of arterial injury is obvious
- When blood accumulates in deep tissues the only manifestation may be shock
- Thrombus may form at ends of severed vessels making diagnosis difficult
- Presence of pulses distal to injury DO NOT preclude arterial injury (as many as 20% of injuries will be associated with preserved distal pulses)

Ischemia

- Must be diagnosed promptly to prevent tissue loss
- Must be suspected when patient has 1 or more of the "5 Ps": pain, pallor, paralysis, paresthesias, pulselessness

False Aneurysm

- Wall is primarily composed of fibrous tissue derived from nearby tissue (not arterial tissue)
- May rupture at any time
- Continue to expand due to absence of elastic fibers
- Spontaneous resolution is unlikely if > 3 cm
- Symptoms gradually appear with compression of surrounding nerves or collateral vessels from rupture or thrombosis

Arteriovenous Fistula (AVF)

- With simultaneous injury of adjacent artery and vein, a fistula may form that allows blood from the artery to enter the vein
- Long-standing AVF can lead to cardiac failure

IMAGING FINDINGS

- Fractures or dislocations near joints or the known course of arteries should prompt careful consideration of possible arterial injury
- Angiographic findings of injury (extravasation, thrombosis, intimal flaps, etc)
- Duplex Doppler findings of injury (hematoma, thrombosis, intimal flaps, etc)

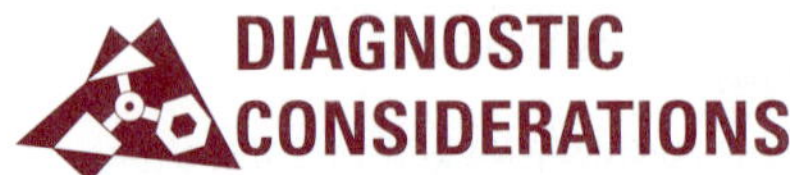

DIAGNOSTIC CONSIDERATIONS

- Arterial injury must be considered in any injured patient
- Patients in shock following penetrating or blunt trauma should be assumed to have vascular injury until proved otherwise
- Diagnosis is usually based on physical examination
- Look for "5 Ps" and listen for bruit, feel for a thrill, and look for an expanding hematoma
- Check ankle-brachial index (ABIs) (< 0.9 has sensitivity of 95% and specificity of 97% and negative predictive value of 99%)
- Only patients with "soft" signs (history of bleeding, diminished pulses, proximity injury, neurapraxia) and ABI < 0.9 require arteriography

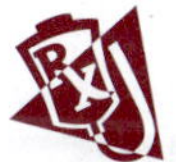

WORK-UP

- Physical examination ("5 Ps," bruit, thrill, expanding hematoma)
- ABIs
- Arteriography (most accurate)
- Duplex Doppler (noninvasive)

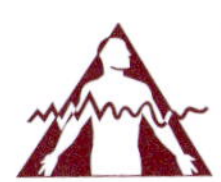

TREATMENT AND MANAGEMENT

Initial

- Repair within 12 hrs makes amputation unlikely
- Depending on the degree of ischemia, delay in repair will lead to lasting neuromuscular damage after only 4–6 hrs
- Restoration of blood volume and control of hemorrhage are done simultaneously
- Exsanguinating hemorrhage requires rapid move to operating room
- External bleeding is best controlled by direct pressure or packing
- Probes or fingers should not be inserted into the wound
- Atraumatic vascular clamps may be applied to visible vessels but should never be used in a blind fashion

Nonoperative

- May be appropriate for compliant patients who have
  - No active hemorrhage
  - Low-velocity injuries
  - Minimal arterial wall disruptions (< 5 mm)
  - Small (< 5 mm) intimal defects
  - Intact distal circulation
- Follow-up must include frequent physical exam and carefully performed noninvasive studies
- Antiplatelet agents may improve patency
- Endovascular management is an option with ever-expanding indications

Operative

- At least 1 uninjured extremity should be prepared for surgery to provide vein if necessary
- Intraoperative angiography should be available
- Incisions should be generous and parallel to the involved vessel
- Preservation of all arterial branches is desirable to preserve collateral flow
- Proximal and distal control should be achieved early when possible
- If large hematoma or multiple injuries make dissection difficult, use of a proximal orthopedic tourniquet is indicated
- Care must be taken to accurately delineate full extent of injury
- Resect only the grossly injured portion of the vessel
- Method of reconstruction depends on degree of damage
- End-to-end anastomosis is occasionally possible
- Interposition graft is performed if tension-free end-to-end repair not possible
- Autogenous vein is preferable to prosthetic graft in contaminated wounds
- Patch angioplasty is performed for closure of partially transected vessels when primary repair would cause narrowing
- Fogarty catheter should be used to clear thrombus both proximal and distal (good back-bleeding does NOT rule out thrombus)
- Completion arteriography is always indicated (even with palpable distal pulses)
- Current recommendations call for repair or shunting of vascular injury before stabilization of associated fracture
- Repaired vessels must be covered with healthy tissue (skin alone is inadequate)
- Fasciotomy is an important adjunctive treatment indicated when
  - Combined arterial and venous injury
  - Massive soft-tissue damage
  - Delay between injury and repair (4–6 hrs)
  - Prolonged hypotension
  - Excessive swelling or high tissue pressure
- Normal intracompartmental pressure is < 10 mm Hg; pressures > 30 mm Hg generally require fasciotomy

SURGERY

Indications

- Any significant arterial injury

Contraindications

- Injury in otherwise unsalvageable limb
- Nonoperative management is an option in certain well-defined instances

TREATMENT MONITORING

- Frequent neurovascular exams

COMPLICATIONS

- Tissue loss
- Nervous injury
- Venous insufficiency

PROGNOSIS

- Depends on extent of injury and delay to repair

PREVENTION

- Firearm regulation

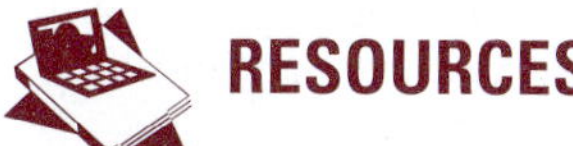

RESOURCES

REFERENCES

- Asensio JA et al. Operative management and outcome of 302 abdominal vascular injuries. *Am J Surg.* 2000;180:528.
- Biffl WL et al. The unrecognized epidemic of blunt carotid arterial injuries: early diagnosis improves neurologic outcome. *Ann Surg.* 1998;228:462.
- Sparks SR et al. Arterial injury in uncomplicated upper extremity dislocations. *Ann Vasc Surg.* 2000;14:110.
- Fujikama T et al. Endovascular stent grafting for the treatment of blunt thoracic aortic injury. *J Trauma.* 2001;50:223.
- Martinez D et al. Popliteal artery injury associated with knee dislocations. *Am Surg.* 2001;67:165.

Arterial Occlusion, Acute

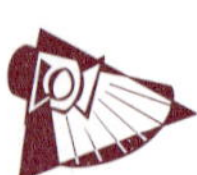

ESSENTIAL FEATURES

- Sudden occlusion of previously patent artery supplying an extremity
- Abrupt onset of ischemia: pain, coldness, numbness, motor weakness, absent pulses
- Tissue viability determined by collaterals and surgical intervention
- Line of demarcation occurs between viable and nonviable tissue
- Caused by embolus, thrombosis, trauma, or dissection

Embolus

- Heart source of embolus in 85%; higher risk in patients with atrial fibrillation, LV thrombus, mechanical valves; septic emboli from infective endocarditis
- Aneurysms in aortofemoral or popliteal arteries can be the source of emboli
- Cardiac tumors and paradoxic emboli (through patent foramen ovale) rarely source
- Source is unknown in 5–10% of cases (cryptogenic)

Thrombosis

- Sudden thrombosis in hypercoagulable states, patients with malignancy, or atherosclerotic vessel
- May be difficult to distinguish thrombotic from embolic event

Trauma

- Arterial damage by bone fracture or dislocation, penetrating injury, complication of catheterization or percutaneous transluminal angioplasty (PTA)

Dissection

- Most common in thoracic aorta and propogates distally
- May cause limb ischemia with iliofemoral involvement

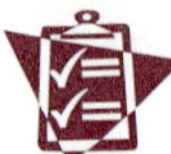

CLINICAL FINDINGS

SYMPTOMS AND SIGNS

- 5 Ps: pain, pallor, pulselessness, paresthesias, paralysis
- Sudden pain present in 80% indicates time of occlusion, may be absent with prompt onset of paresthesia/paralysis
- Pallor followed by mottled cyanosis
- Hyperesthesia followed by anesthesia; light touch lost, pressure, pain, and temperature often more preserved
- Motor paralysis: impending gangrene
- Symptoms > 12 h, unlikely salvageable
- Tense swelling and acute tenderness of gastrocnemius denotes irreversible infarction
- 4–6 hrs nerves and muscles ischemic; skin more resistant to ischemia
- Level of demarcation varies with site of occlusion
- Collateral flow may result in return of warmth and color of skin, lessening of sensory deficit with symptoms of chronic occlusion of artery

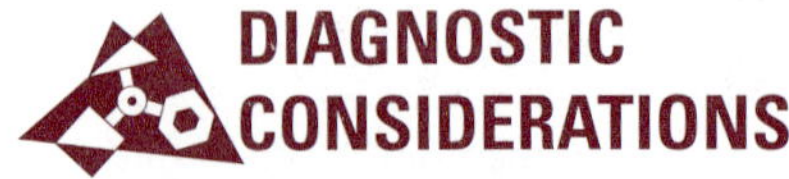

DIAGNOSTIC CONSIDERATIONS

- Consider both thrombosis and embolic events
- Must evaluate for secondary tissue loss or compartment syndrome

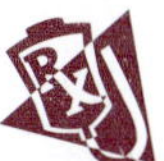

WORK-UP

- Immediate administration of heparin
- Arteriography may help differentiate thrombosis from embolus

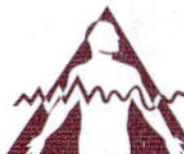

TREATMENT AND MANAGEMENT

Embolisms/Thrombosis

- Immediate administration of heparin
- Arteriography can help if no delay in treatment

Traumatic

- Repair arterial injury in addition to other injuries

SURGERY

Indications

- Advanced, reversible ischemia
- Fasciotomy often required with long ischemia time
- Thrombolysis, surgical embolectomy (least delay in reestablishing flow)
- Arterial reconstruction in thrombotic event with atherosclerosis (alternative to thrombolytic therapy)

Contraindications

- Irreversible ischemia

MEDICATIONS

- Heparin
- Thrombolytics

COMPLICATIONS

- **With reperfusion:** Myoglobinuria, renal failure, hyperkalemia

PROGNOSIS

- Good if reestablish blood flow within 6 hours

RESOURCES

REFERENCES

- Campbell WB et al. Current management of acute leg ischaemia: results of an audit by the Vascular Surgical Society of Great Britain and Ireland. *Br J Surg.* 1998;85:1498.
- Ouriel K et al. Acute lower limb ischemia: determinants of outcome. *Surgery.* 1998;124:336.

Arterial Trauma, Iatrogenic

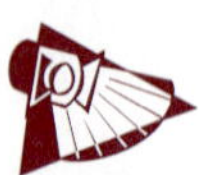

ESSENTIAL FEATURES

Traumatic Pseudoaneurysms

- Arterial access for catheter procedures has risk of pseudoaneurysm formation
- Pseudoaneurysms are arterial disruptions contained by fibrotic tissue
- Most resolve spontaneously

Intra-arterial Injections

- Seen among injecting drug abusers
- Brachial and femoral most common
- Vessel vasoconstriction results in thrombosis and distal ischemia

EPIDEMIOLOGY

- Percutaneous catheter-based procedures and anticoagulation: Increased frequency of pseudoaneurysms

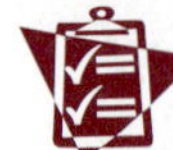

CLINICAL FINDINGS

SYMPTOMS AND SIGNS

Pseudoaneurysm

- Mass, may be pulsating
- Bleeding
- Pain

Intra-arterial Injection

- Burning pain of limb
- Gangrene of digits

IMAGING FINDINGS

- Duplex US can identify ongoing leak, patency of vessel

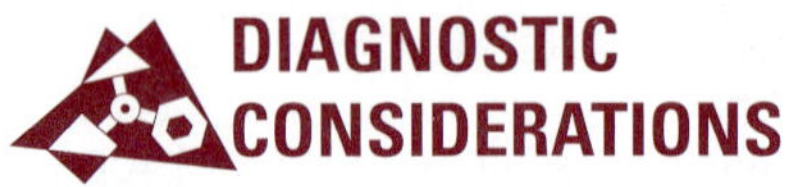

DIAGNOSTIC CONSIDERATIONS

- Evaluate for distal ischemia or embolus

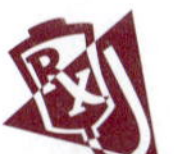

WORK-UP

- Physical exam
- Duplex US
- Arteriography (rarely)

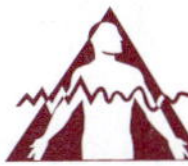

TREATMENT AND MANAGEMENT

Pseudoaneurysms

- Most resolve spontaneously
- US-guided compression can be very useful
- Operative therapy, if indicated, includes primary repair of artery versus interposition graft

Intra-arterial Injection

- If needle is still in place, irrigate with heparinized saline
- Intra-arterial vasodilators to reduce spasm
- Late complications, such as infection, treated by excision and ligation

SURGERY

Indications

- Distal ischemia
- Severe infection of pseudoaneurysm
- Ongoing hemorrhage
- Local integumentary/neurologic compromise

COMPLICATIONS

- Infection, pseudoaneurysm formation, chemical endarteritis late complications of intra-arterial injection

RESOURCES

REFERENCES

- Hye RJ. Compression therapy for acute iatrogenic femoral pseudoaneurysms. *Semin Vasc Surg.* 2000;13:58.
- Nehler MR et al. Iatrogenic vascular trauma. *Semin Vasc Surg.* 1998;11:283.

Arteriovenous Fistulas

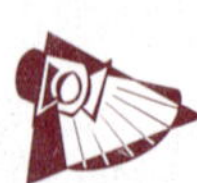

ESSENTIAL FEATURES

- Congenital or acquired
- Abnormal connection between artery and vein; located anywhere in body

Congenital

- Systemic effect minimal
- Noted in infancy or childhood
- Limb involvement leads to hypertrophied, longer extremity
- Frequently involve brain, viscera, lungs
- **Osler-Weber-Rendu syndrome (autosomal dominant):** Hemorrhages in form of epistaxis, GI bleeding, polycythemia, cyanosis, clubbing

Acquired

- Enlarge rapidly
- Can cause heart failure
- Generally, result from trauma or disease
- **Venous malformations:** Rarely cause hemodynamic effects

EPIDEMIOLOGY

Acquired

- Most commonly a result of traumatic injury
- Iatrogenic injury after angiography or angioplasty common
- Connective tissue disorders (Ehlers-Danlos), erosion of mycotic aneurysm, communication with prosthetic graft, neoplastic invasion can cause false aneurysm and arteriovenous fistula
- Rare cause is injury to aorta and inferior vena cava after excision of herniated disk

CLINICAL FINDINGS

SYMPTOMS AND SIGNS

- Determine time of onset and presence of associated disease
- Continuous murmur may be heard
- Palpable thrill and increased skin temperature
- Proximal vein dilatation, distal pulse diminished, distal coolness
- **Tachycardia:** Increased cardiac output
- **Branham sign:** Compression of fistula results in slowed heart rate
- **Venous malformations:** Mass; may be tender; no hemodynamic effects

IMAGING FINDINGS

- MRI study of choice for peripheral AV malformations
- Angiograms give precise delineation of AV fistulas

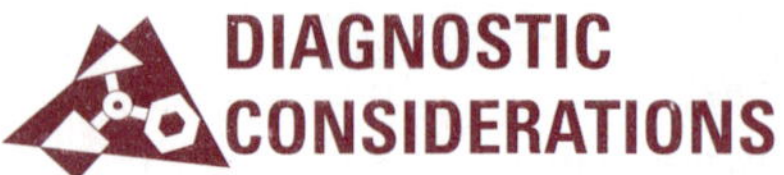

DIAGNOSTIC CONSIDERATIONS

- Evaluate for signs of systemic or distant intravascular infection

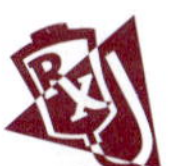

WORK-UP

- Physical exam
- Duplex US or MRI for most peripheral lesions
- Occasionally, use angiography to delineate further

TREATMENT AND MANAGEMENT

- Not all require treatment

Venous fistulas

- Compression garments when possible
- Injection of sclerosing agents possible

AV fistulas

- Monitor small peripheral fistulas
- Most managed with radiographic embolization; head and neck, pelvis best
- **Surgical:** Ligate all feeding vessels; amputate extremity; repair of fistula, oversewing defects (avoid for congenital fistulas)

Congenital

- En bloc resection of all tissue involved in fistula

SURGERY

Indications

- Hemorrhage
- Expanding false aneurysm
- Severe venous or arterial insufficiency
- Cosmesis
- Heart failure

Contraindications

- Congenital fistula (relative)

PROGNOSIS

- Vary according to extent, location, and type
- Traumatic type has better prognosis
- Congenital has worse prognosis because of high recurrence

RESOURCES

REFERENCES

- Jacobowitz GR et al. Transcatheter embolization of complex pelvic vascular malformations: results and long-term follow-up. *J Vasc Surg.* 2001;33:51.
- White RI Jr et al. Long-term outcome of embolotherapy and surgery for high-flow extremity arteriovenous maformations. *J Vasc Interv Radiol.* 2000;11:1285.

Ascites

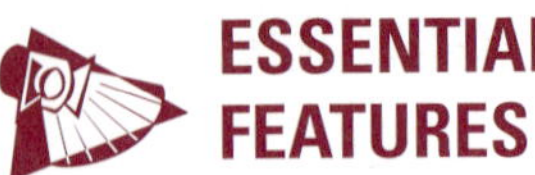

ESSENTIAL FEATURES

- Pathologic accumulation of free fluid within the abdominal cavity
- Ascites develops from
  - Decreased plasma oncotic pressure (liver disease, malnutrition)
  - Increased lymph/peritoneal fluid production (liver disease, malignant ascites)
  - Blockage or disruption of abdominal lymphatic drainage (chylous ascites, congenital)
- Patients typically complain of abdominal distention or vague constitutional symptoms

EPIDEMIOLOGY

- Over 80% of patients with ascites have portal hypertension secondary to chronic liver diseases
- Less common causes are chylous, malignant, or pancreatic ascites
- Chylous ascites is most commonly due to occult tumor obstructing the lymphatic ducts (lymphoma or adenocarcinoma), external trauma, operative disruption, or congenital anomalies
- Malignant ascites occurs secondary to peritoneal implants stimulating ascitic fluid production or if there is advanced venous or lymphatic obstruction

CLINICAL FINDINGS

SYMPTOMS AND SIGNS

- Vague, diffuse, constant abdominal discomfort associated with distention
- Ascites from cirrhosis associated with systemic signs of liver disease including palmar erythema, spider angiomas, gynecomastia, evidence of portosystemic shunting, and encephalopathy
- Malignant ascites associated with weight loss, a history of cancer, or symptoms related to the neoplasm (eg, fever, night sweats, and weight loss in cases of lymphoma)
- Chylous ascites often relatively asymptomatic with vague abdominal discomfort and mild abdominal distention

LABORATORY FINDINGS

Liver Failure

- Systemic
  - Hypoalbuminemia
  - Increased bilirubin
  - Increased prothrombin time/international normalized ratio (PT/INR)
- Paracentesis
  - Serum-ascites albumin
  - Gradient > 1.1

Chylous Ascites

- Systemic
  - Hypoalbuminemia
  - Lymphocytopenia
  - Anemia
- Paracentesis
  - Grossly milky appearance
  - Serum-ascites albumin gradient (SAAG) < 1.1
  - Triglyceride level > 200 mg/dL
  - Leukocyte count > 1000/mL

Malignant Ascites

- Systemic
  - Positive tumor markers
  - Evidence of malnutrition
- Paracentesis
  - Positive cytologic diagnosis
  - Aneuploidy (flow cytometry)
  - High lactic dehydrogenase (LDH) (> 500 IU/L)
  - High carcinoembryonic antigen (CEA)

IMAGING FINDINGS

- Abdominal US verifies the presence of ascites, suggests the presence of liver disease, and guides diagnostic/therapeutic paracentesis
- Abdominal/pelvic CT scans are useful in documenting ascites; suggesting liver disease; detecting lymphadenopathy and masses of the mesentery as well as of solid organs, such as the liver, ovaries, and pancreas

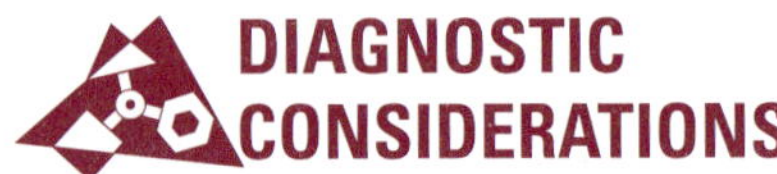

DIAGNOSTIC CONSIDERATIONS

- Portal hypertension
- Chylous ascites
- Malignant ascites
- Normal postoperative intra-abdominal fluid
- Sterile fluid collection
- Intra-abdominal abscess
- Hematoma
- Biloma
- Urinoma
- Soft-tissue neoplasm
- Chronic inflammatory peritonitis

RULE OUT

- Spontaneous bacterial peritonitis (SBP)
- Underlying malignancy

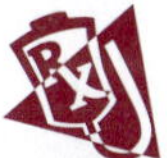

WORK-UP

- **Diagnostic paracentesis:** LDH level, albumin, amylase, triglyceride level, WBC count, cytologic studies, Gram stain, and culture
- **Abdominal/pelvic CT scan:**
  - Plus a full colonoscopy to search for primary neoplasm in malignant ascites
  - Used to search for underlying neoplasm in cases of chylous ascites occurring in adults with constitutional symptoms

WHEN TO ADMIT

- Cirrhotic patients with an exacerbation of ascites should be admitted to rule out SBP, and initiate or adjust medical management
- Most patients with symptomatic chylous or malignant ascites also will require hospitalization for diagnosis and medical management

WHEN TO REFER

- Advanced liver disease; consult with gastroenterologists and hepatologists
- Chylous and malignant ascites usually managed medically, often in conjunction with medical oncology

TREATMENT AND MANAGEMENT

- Diagnostic paracentesis
- Search for underlying malignancy
- Medical management with diuretics, therapeutic paracentesis, and chemotherapy when indicated
- Surgery to assist in diagnosis or treat medically refractory cases

SURGERY

Indications

- Diagnostic laparotomy to assess peritoneum for carcinomatosis or tumor/lymph node biopsy
- Portovenous decompression in patients with good liver synthetic function (Childs class A) and complicated portosystemic shunting
- Peritoneal-jugular shunt for refractory malignant ascites in select patients (ineffective for chylous ascites)

Contraindications

- Surgery is diagnostic or palliative only, thus should only be performed on patients with good preoperative function
- Childs class C cirrhosis

MEDICATIONS

- Spironolactone with or without furosemide
- Albumin in conjunction with therapeutic paracentesis

TREATMENT MONITORING

- Resolution or medical control of ascites

COMPLICATIONS

- Refractory ascites
- Clogging of peritoneal jugular shunt

PROGNOSIS

- Prognosis in liver failure correlates with Child class
- Life expectancy in malignant ascites is 2–6 months
- Chylous ascites due to external trauma, operative lymphatic disruption, or congenital anomalies has a favorable prognosis with regard to gradual resolution

PREVENTION

- Salt and water restriction
- Medical compliance

RESOURCES

REFERENCES

- Uriz J et al. Pathophysiology, diagnosis and treatment of ascites in cirrhosis. *Baillieres Best Pract Res Clin Gastroenterol.* 2000;14:927.
- Heneghan MA et al. Pathogenesis of ascites in cirrhosis and portal hypertension. *Med Sci Monit.* 2000;6:807.

Aspiration

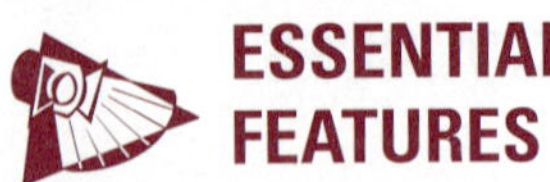

ESSENTIAL FEATURES

- Aspiration of gastric contents
- Hypoxemia

EPIDEMIOLOGY

- Occurs in patients unable to protect airway
- Post trauma
- Anesthetized patient
- Obtunded patient

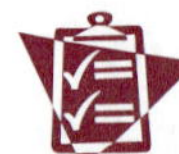

CLINICAL FINDINGS

SYMPTOMS AND SIGNS

- Vomiting
- Shortness of breath
- Gastric contents in airway on bronchoscopy

LABORATORY FINDINGS

- Hypoxemia

IMAGING FINDINGS

- Localized infiltrate on chest film

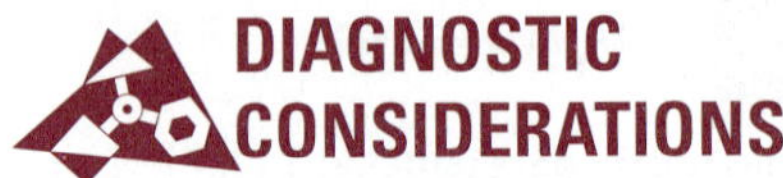

DIAGNOSTIC CONSIDERATIONS

- May occur in settings with other potential causes of hypoxemia (acute respiratory distress syndrome, sepsis, trauma)
- Patient often with altered level of consciousness

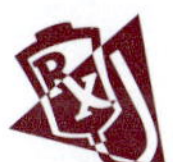

WORK-UP

- ABG measurements
- Chest film
- Bronchoscopy

TREATMENT AND MANAGEMENT

- Pulmonary hygiene
- Supplemental oxygen
- Intubation and mechanical ventilation
- Bronchoscopy

COMPLICATIONS

- Pneumonitis
- Pneumonia

PROGNOSIS

- Determined by patient's overall health

PREVENTION

- Aspiration precautions
- Avoid oversedation

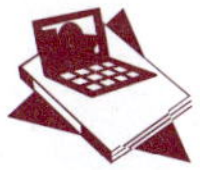

RESOURCES

REFERENCES

- Bulger EM et al. Current clinical options for the treatment and management of acute respiratory distress syndrome. *J Trauma.* 2000;48:562.

Atelectasis

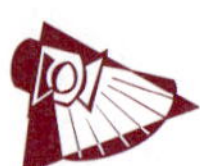

ESSENTIAL FEATURES

- Localized collapse of alveoli
- Hypoxemia

EPIDEMIOLOGY

- Prolonged immobilization
- Splinting
- Prolonged shallow respirations

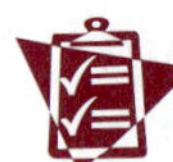

CLINICAL FINDINGS

SYMPTOMS AND SIGNS

- Hypoxemia
- Bronchial breath sounds over dependent portions of lungs

LABORATORY FINDINGS

- Hypoxemia

IMAGING FINDINGS

- Parenchymal collapse on chest film
- Small lung volumes on chest film

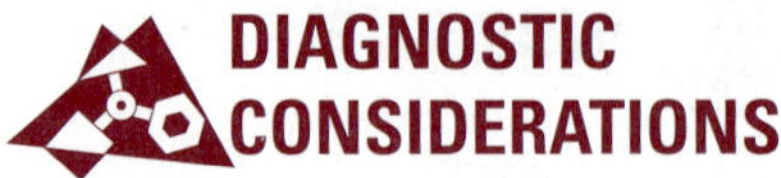

DIAGNOSTIC CONSIDERATIONS

- Frequently occurs postoperatively within 48 hours
- Fever often unaccompanied by other findings

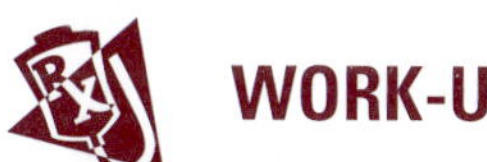

WORK-UP

- ABG measurements
- Chest film

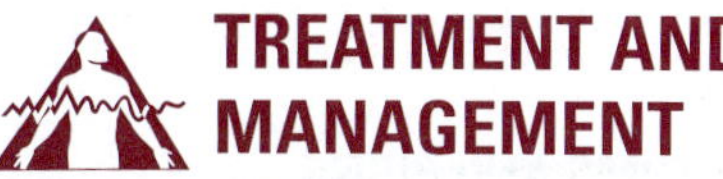

TREATMENT AND MANAGEMENT

- Encourage deep breathing
- Ambulation
- Encourage coughing
- Bronchoscopy
- Mechanical ventilation
- Diuresis if appropriate

MEDICATIONS

- Diuretics if appropriate
- Adequate pain relief

COMPLICATIONS

- Pneumonia

PROGNOSIS

- Excellent

PREVENTION

- Incentive spirometry

RESOURCES

REFERENCES

- Celi BR et al. A controlled trial of intermittent positive pressure breathing, incentive spirometry, and deep breathing exercises in preventing pulmonary complications after abdominal surgery. *Am Rev Respir Dis.* 1984;130:12.

Atrial Septal Defect (ASD)

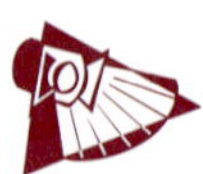

ESSENTIAL FEATURES

- A congenital heart lesion that increases pulmonary artery (PA) blood flow
- Causes left to right shunt, results in lung infection, pulmonary vascular congestion, PA hypertension, right heart failure, pulmonary vasoconstriction, pulmonary vascular obstructive disease
- **Eisenmenger syndrome:** Increased pulmonary hypertension to such extent that left to right shunt ceases and shunt becomes right to left, requiring heart-lung transplant
- Inhaled nitric oxide, oxygen, or IV tolazoline reverses PA vasoconstriction
- PA band is palliative and can reduce PA flow to alleviate RV failure and progression of pulmonary hypertension

EPIDEMIOLOGY

- **Ostium secundum type:** Most common and largest of ASDs
- Defects high in atrial septum, associated with partial anomalous pulmonary venous return, termed "sinus venosus defects"
- Reduced life expectancy because of RV failure, arrhythmias, pulmonary vascular disease
- Pulmonary vascular disease rare

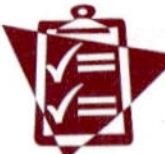

CLINICAL FINDINGS

SYMPTOMS AND SIGNS

- Acyanotic, asymptomatic often
- RV lift
- S_2 widely split and fixed
- Pulmonary systolic ejection murmur
- Diastolic flow murmur at left lower sternal border
- Heart failure may occur in kids, rare in adults
- Atrial dysrhythmias increase with age

IMAGING FINDINGS

- Echocardiography: Diagnostic

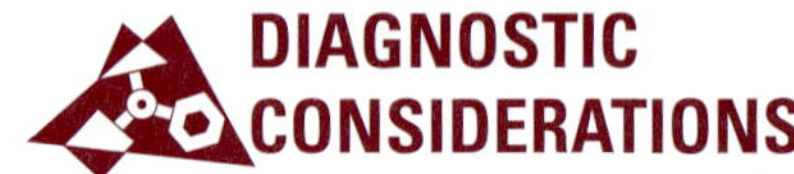

DIAGNOSTIC CONSIDERATIONS

- Evaluate for other associated cardiac or extracardiac anomalies

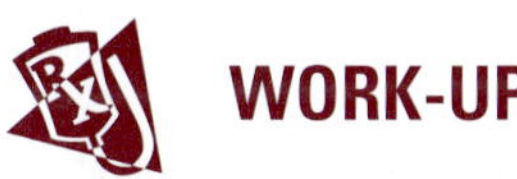

WORK-UP

- Echocardiography

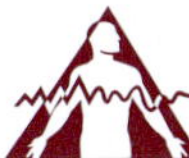

TREATMENT AND MANAGEMENT

- Most should be closed
- Optimal time debated
- Paradoxic embolism and endocarditis associated with delaying repair
- Open surgery is performed to close if patient is 1 or 2 years old
- Many now are closed percutaneously (patient must be 10 kg)

SURGERY

Indications

- Presence of ASD in low- to moderate-risBk patient

PROGNOSIS

- Excellent

RESOURCES

REFERENCES

- Berger F et al. Comparison of results and complications of surgical and Amplatzer device closure of atrial septal defects. *J Thorac Cardiovasc Surg.* 1999;118:674.

Atrioventricular Canal Defect

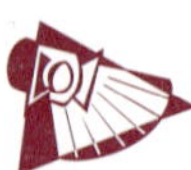

ESSENTIAL FEATURES

- A congenital heart lesion that increases pulmonary artery (PA) blood flow
- Causes left to right shunt, results in lung infection, pulmonary vascular congestion, PA hypertension, right heart failure, pulmonary vasoconstriction, pulmonary vascular obstructive disease
- **Eisenmenger syndrome:** Increased pulmonary hypertension to such extent that left to right shunt ceases and shunt becomes right to left, requiring heart-lung transplant
- Inhaled nitric oxide, oxygen, or IV tolazoline reverses PA vasoconstriction
- PA band is palliative and can reduce PA flow to alleviate RV failure and progression of pulmonary hypertension
- Deficiency of tissue in central region of heart (lower atrial septum-septum primum, mitral valve, tricuspid valve)
- Defect in endocardial and conal tissue development
- Range of defects possible
- **Partial AV canal defect:** Septum primum atrial septal defect (ASD), deficient lower atrial septum only
- **Transitional AV canal defect:** Intermediate form with ASD and minor deficiency in upper ventricular system
- **Complete AV canal defect:** ASD and severe valve anomalies
- Associated with left superior vena cava (SVC), additional ventricular septal defect (VSD), anomalous pulmonary venous connection, patent ductus arteriosus (PDA), tetralogy of Fallot

EPIDEMIOLOGY

- Can occur in patients with trisomy 21 (Down syndrome) who are more prone to pulmonary vascular obstructive disease

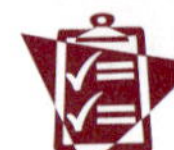

CLINICAL FINDINGS

SYMPTOMS AND SIGNS

- Heart failure common in infancy
- Cardiomegaly present
- Blowing pansystolic murmur (varies)
- Loud S_2, fixed split
- Left to right shunt modified by mitral regurgitation
- Severity depends on structural defects
- Partial defect may be asymptomatic
- Pulmonary hypertension and mitral regurgitation natural history

LABORATORY FINDINGS

- **ECG:** Left axis deviation and counterclockwise frontal QRS vector loop

IMAGING FINDINGS

- Echocardiography best for diagnosis
- Catheterization for patients older than 6 mos if pulmonary hypertension is a concern

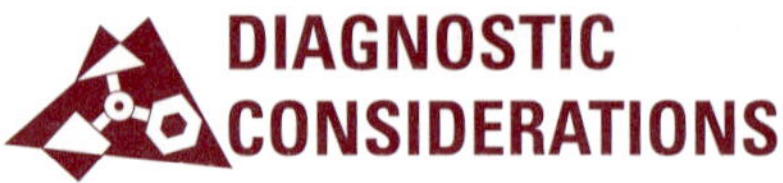

DIAGNOSTIC CONSIDERATIONS

- Must define extent of canal defect to plan correction

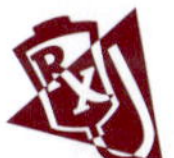

WORK-UP

- Echocardiography
- Cardiac catheterization if patient is older than 6 months

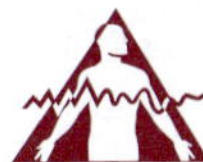

TREATMENT AND MANAGEMENT

- Timing of correction indicated by degree of anomaly and symptoms
- **Partial defect:** Patch closure
- **Complete defect:** Patch closure of septal defects and reconstruction of valves (suture closure of valve with or without annuloplasty)

SURGERY

Indications

- Defect warrants repair
- **Complete defect:** Repair by 6 months of age
  - Repair by 1 year of age in other less severe types
- **Mitral regurgitation:** Repair regardless of age

COMPLICATIONS

- **Postoperative mitral regurgitation:** 10–40%, 10% require reoperation
- Many patients will require additional mitral valve work in adulthood

PROGNOSIS

- Mortality varies with defect and age
- **Partial defect:** 10-year survival is 98%
- **Complete defect:**
  - Operative mortality is 3–5%
  - 10-year survival is 90%
  - < 1 year life expectancy from congestive heart failure

RESOURCES

REFERENCES

- Anderson RH et al. The diagnostic features of atrioventricular septal defect with common atrioventricular junction. *Cardiol Young*. 1998;8:33.

Barrett Esophagus

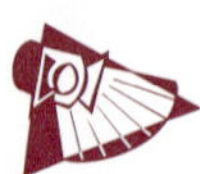

ESSENTIAL FEATURES

- Gastroesophageal reflux disease (GERD)
- Metaplastic changes from squamous to intestinal-type columnar epithelium in the distal esophagus
- Metaplasia may contain varying degrees of dysplasia, which is associated with increasing risk of developing esophageal adenocarcinoma
- Neither medical nor surgical treatment consistently causes regression of metaplastic changes but may prevent progression

EPIDEMIOLOGY

- Acquired intestinal-type metaplasia of any length that replaces the normal squamous epithelium of the distal esophagus; induced by chronic gastroesophageal reflux
- Found in 10–20% of patients with gastroesophageal reflux
- Male:female incidence of 2:1; increasing incidence with increased age
- Conveys a 2-fold increased risk of developing adenocarcinoma
- Adenocarcinoma is found in 10% of patients with Barrett epithelium at the time of first endoscopic exam
- Lower esophageal sphincter pressure averages 5 mm Hg; 24-hour pH monitoring reveals increased esophageal acid exposure and impaired clearing
- Reflux of bile acids may contribute to the development of Barrett esophagus along with acid and pepsin

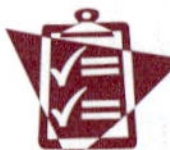

CLINICAL FINDINGS

SYMPTOMS AND SIGNS

- Heartburn, milder than in the absence of Barrett changes because the metaplastic epithelium is less sensitive than squamous epithelium
- Regurgitation
- Dysphagia

IMAGING FINDINGS

- **Esophagoscopy**: Pink epithelium in the lower esophagus instead of the shiny gray-pink squamous mucosa; must be verified by biopsy
- **Contrast radiography**: Hiatal hernia, esophageal stricture, or ulcer

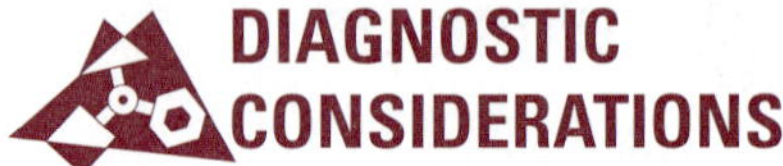

DIAGNOSTIC CONSIDERATIONS

- Patients with moderate to severe GERD should undergo endoscopy and biopsy to assess distal esophagus for metaplastic changes
- Only biopsy proven intestinal-type metaplasia is associated with increased risk of adenocarcinoma

RULE OUT

- High-grade dysplasia
- Adenocarcinoma

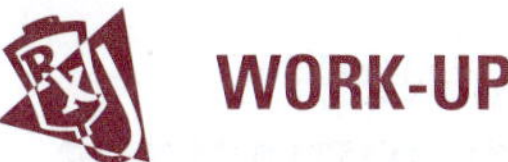

WORK-UP

- Esophagoscopy and biopsy

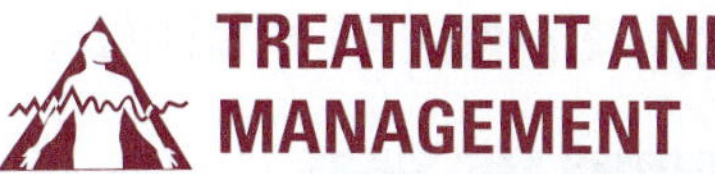

TREATMENT AND MANAGEMENT

- Treatment is the same as for GERD
- Surgical treatment is fundoplication
- Metaplastic epithelium rarely regresses after medical or surgical therapy

SURGERY

Indications

- Severe GERD refractory to medical treatment
- Esophageal strictures and ulcers
- Esophagectomy for high-grade dysplasia

MEDICATIONS

- H_2-blocking agents
- Proton pump inhibitors
- Antacids

TREATMENT MONITORING

- Routine endoscopy and biopsy should be performed every 6–12 months to assess degree of dysplasia

COMPLICATIONS

- Esophageal ulcer
- Esophageal stricture
- Esophageal adenocarcinoma

PROGNOSIS

- Estimated incidence of adenocarcinoma in patients with Barrett esophagus of 1:100 patient years of follow-up

PREVENTION

- Aggressive treatment of GERD

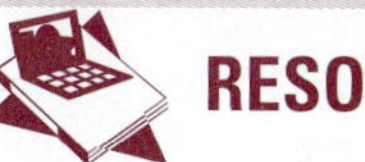

RESOURCES

REFERENCES

- Spechler SJ et al. Long-term outcome of medical and surgical therapies for gastroesophageal reflux disease: follow-up of a randomized controlled trial. *JAMA.* 2001;285:2331.

Biliary Atresia

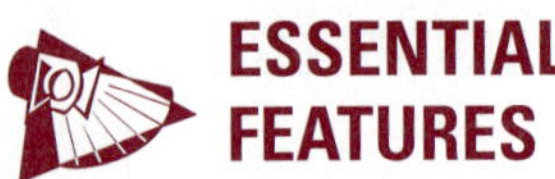

ESSENTIAL FEATURES

- Presents within first few weeks of life
- 67% of patients ultimately require liver transplantation

CLINICAL FINDINGS

SYMPTOMS AND SIGNS

- Progressive jaundice in newborns 2–4 weeks old
- Mild hepatomegaly
- Failure to feed well
- Growth failure

LABORATORY FINDINGS

- Hyperbilirubinemia
- Elevated alkaline phosphatase
- Elevated transaminases (occasionally)

IMAGING FINDINGS

- **^{99m}Tc-IDA scan:** Normal uptake into liver but failure to empty through bile duct into duodenum (100% sensitive, 94% specific)
- **US:** Diminutive or absence of gallbladder, absence of choledochocele

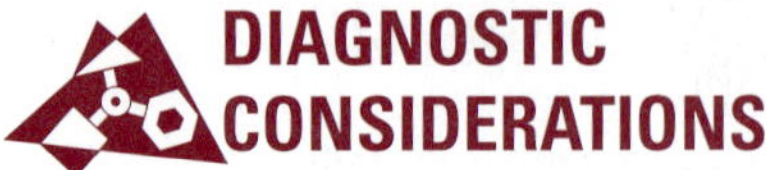

DIAGNOSTIC CONSIDERATIONS

- Age of patient at time of diagnosis will affect eventual success of treatment

RULE OUT

- Biliary hypoplasia or Alagille syndrome
- Other causes of neonatal jaundice
- α_1-Antitrypsin deficiency

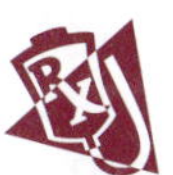

WORK-UP

- History and physical
- Liver function tests
- α_1-Antitrypsin level
- ^{99m}Tc-IDA scan
- US
- Possible liver biopsy to evaluate for other nonoperative causes of neonatal jaundice

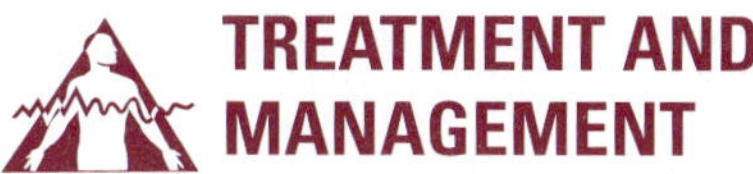

TREATMENT AND MANAGEMENT

SURGERY

- Portoenterostomy (Kasai)
- Liver transplantation

Indications

- Portoenterostomy when proximal bile ducts of adequate caliber are located (150 μm diameter most ideal)
- Liver transplantation if > 1 year of age and presence of liver failure or growth retardation following portoenterostomy

MEDICATIONS

- Phenobarbital to facilitate hepatocyte processing of bile preoperatively and postoperatively
- Ursodeoxycholic acid to facilitate bile flow postoperatively

TREATMENT MONITORING

- Bilirubin
- Temperature
- Growth rate

COMPLICATIONS

- Cholangitis (40–50%)
- Progressive liver failure
- Continued bile obstruction

PROGNOSIS

- 66–75% with bile flow after portoenterostomy if done before 60 days of age (90–95% if 150 μm ducts found)
- Bile flow unlikely if portenterostomy performed after 120 days of life
- 30–50% 5-year survival after portoenterostomy (25–35% 10-year)
- 66% ultimately require transplantation with ~ 80% 5-year survival

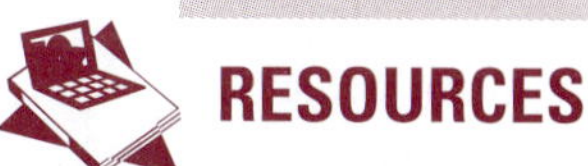

RESOURCES

REFERENCES

- Narkowicz MR: Biliary atresia: an update on our understanding of this disorder. *Curr Opin Pediatr.* 2001;13:435.

Biliary Neoplasms, Benign

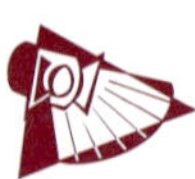

ESSENTIAL FEATURES

- **Gallbladder adenoma**
  - Rare
  - Considered premalignant lesion
  - Minimal to no risk if < 1 cm
- **Papillomatosis:** Multiple gallbladder adenomas
- **Adenomyomatosis:** Gallbladder wall hyperplasia that can be diffuse, possibly premalignant
- Leiomyomas, lipomas, hemangiomas, and heterotopic GI tissue are all other possible benign biliary neoplasms
- Approximately 67% of benign biliary neoplasms are polyps, adenomatous papillomas, or bile duct adenomas; not known to have malignant potential
- 47% of benign biliary neoplasms found in periampullary region and 27% found in common bile duct

EPIDEMIOLOGY

- 5% incidence of gallbladder polyps of which 50% are cholesterol polyps
- < 1% incidence of benign biliary tumors

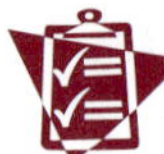

CLINICAL FINDINGS

SYMPTOMS AND SIGNS

- Asymptomatic
- Biliary colic or cholecystitis
- Jaundice
- Anorexia
- Fever
- Nausea

LABORATORY FINDINGS

- Leukocytosis if cholecystitis or cholangitis is present
- Hyperbilirubinemia
- Elevated alkaline phosphatase level

IMAGING FINDINGS

- Right upper quadrant US
  - Shows thickened gallbladder wall for adenomyomatosis
  - Shows submuscular hyperechoic areas in cholesterol polyps
  - Shows hyperechoic polypoid structures without shadowing for gallbladder adenomas
  - Shows biliary dilatation and possible stricture for benign biliary neoplasms
- ERCP and percutaneous transhepatic cholangiogram (PTC) reveal stricture and proximal biliary dilatation, suggesting benign biliary neoplasms

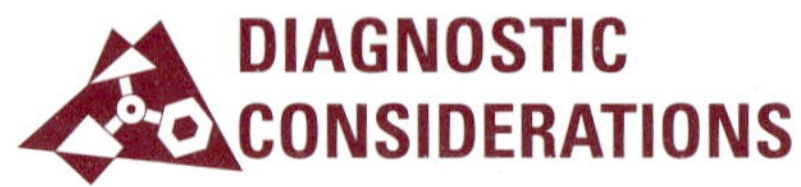

DIAGNOSTIC CONSIDERATIONS

RULE OUT

- Possible malignancy making resection often necessary to verify diagnosis

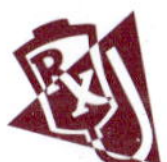

WORK-UP

- History and physical exam
- CBC count
- Liver function tests
- Carcinoembryonic antigen (CEA) and CA 19-9
- Right upper quadrant US
- PTC or ERCP

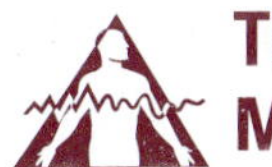

TREATMENT AND MANAGEMENT

SURGERY

- Cholecystectomy for gallbladder adenomatous polyps > 1 cm
- Resection of biliary stricture and bilioenteric reconstruction for benign biliary neoplasms causing jaundice or cholangitis

COMPLICATIONS

- Biliary leak or stricture

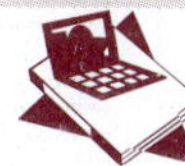

RESOURCES

REFERENCES

- Doherty GM, Way LW. Biliary Tract. In: Way LW, Doherty GM (editors). *Current Surgical Diagnosis & Treatment,* 11e. New York: McGraw-Hill; 2003:619.

Biliary Obstruction, Benign

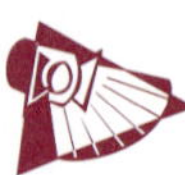

ESSENTIAL FEATURES

- Etiologies include:
  - Postoperative
  - Trauma
  - Chronic pancreatitis
  - Cholelithiasis or choledocholithiasis
  - Primary sclerosing cholangitis
  - Sphincter of Oddi stenosis
  - Duodenal ulcer
  - Crohn disease
  - Viral infection
  - Drug toxins
- 80% of cases occur post-cholecystectomy
- 10% of postoperative cases are recognized in first week, whereas 70% are recognized after 6 months
- Chronic pancreatitis < 10% of cases (3–29% of patients with chronic pancreatitis)

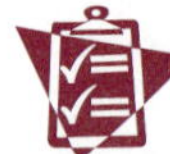

CLINICAL FINDINGS

SYMPTOMS AND SIGNS

- Fever
- Abdominal pain
- Jaundice

LABORATORY FINDINGS

- Hyperbilirubinemia
- Elevated alkaline phosphatase level
- Leukocytosis

IMAGING FINDINGS

- **Right upper quadrant US:** Associated biloma with postoperative stricture, biliary dilatation, atrophic/calcified pancreas
- **CT:** Shows associated biloma with postoperative ductal injury, biliary dilatation, atrophic/calcified pancreas
- **Magnetic resonance cholangiopancreatography (MRCP) or percutaneous transhepatic cholangiogram (PTC)**
  - Reveals long tapered stricture in intrapancreatic bile duct when stricture is caused by chronic pancreatitis
  - Long stricture when associated with postoperative or trauma

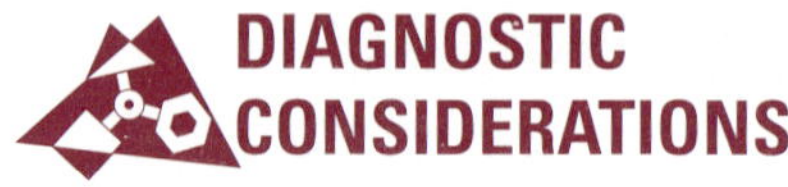

DIAGNOSTIC CONSIDERATIONS

- Recent operation
- History of pancreatitis
- History of choledocholithiasis

RULE OUT

- Biliary, pancreatic, or ampullary malignancy

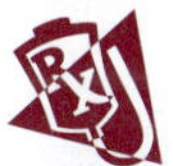

WORK-UP

- History and physical exam
- CBC count
- Liver function tests
- Right upper quadrant US
- CT
- MRCP
- PTC
- Endoscopic US if question of pancreatic head mass

WHEN TO ADMIT

- Cholangitis
- Infected biloma or bile peritonitis

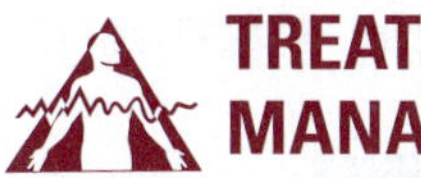

TREATMENT AND MANAGEMENT

SURGERY

Indications

- Hepaticojejunostomy for most postoperative or traumatic strictures
- Choledochoduodenostomy or choledochojejunostomy for chronic, pancreatitis-induced strictures
- Balloon dilatation indicated for some anastomotic biliary strictures post-repair

Contraindications

- If pancreatic malignancy is suspected, pancreaticoduodenectomy should be done

COMPLICATIONS

- Recurrent stricture/biliary leak
- Cholangitis

PROGNOSIS

- Excellent in 70–90% following surgical reconstruction
- Poor for balloon dilatation as primary therapy for strictures except as treatment for early post-repair stricture

RESOURCES

REFERENCES

- Nealon WH, Urrutia F. Long-term follow-up after bilioenteric anastomosis for benign bile duct stricture. *Ann Surg.* 1996;223:639.

Bites, Arthropod

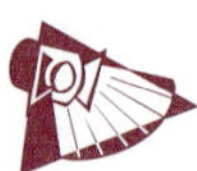

ESSENTIAL FEATURES

- Some arthropod bites can result in death by direct toxicity or by causing hypersensitivity reactions
- Venom of bees and wasps contains histamine, basic protein components of high molecular weight, free amino acids, hyaluronidase, and acetylcholine
- Only a few spider venoms are harmful to humans

Latrodectism

- Bite of the *Latrodectus* species of spiders, including the black widow (*Latrodectus mactans*) and the red-backed spider (*Latrodectus hasseltii*), has primarily systemic neurotoxic effects
- Female black widow spider can be identified by its characteristic black body with a red hourglass-like pattern on the abdomen (male of the species does not bite and is smaller)
  - Black widow venom: Neuromuscular toxic effects occur by presynaptic motor end plate neurotransmitter release, with release of norepinephrine and acetylcholine causing excessive stimulation and eventual fatigue of the motor end plate and muscle
- The brown recluse spider *(Loxosceles reclusa)* is dark tan and has a violin-shaped mark on the back of the main body

Loxoscelism

- Envenomation can have significant and prolonged local dermonecrotic effects, with development of deep necrotic wounds at the bite site that are very slow to heal

EPIDEMIOLOGY

- Because of their prevalence and numbers, bees and wasps kill more people than any other venomous animal, including snakes
- Very young, the elderly, and patients with comorbid medical conditions are at greatest risk for adverse outcomes

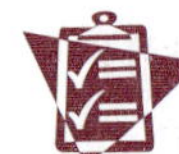

CLINICAL FINDINGS

SYMPTOMS AND SIGNS

Wasp and Bee Stings

- Symptoms may vary from minimal erythema to a marked local reaction of severe systemic toxicity
- Moderately severe reactions will present as generalized syncope or urticarial reactions

Latrodectism

- Symptoms of envenomation begin with pain at the bite location followed by later development of abdominal wall muscle rigidity, abdominal pain and cramping, respiratory difficulty with potential paralysis, and lower extremity weakness
- Massive hemolysis, severe hypotension, and cardiovascular collapse can occur
- Local skin changes are often minimal and can make identification of the bite difficult

Loxoscelism

- Bite may have local signs of erythema and edema but usually minimal associated pain
- Hemorrhagic bullae surrounded by localized ischemia develop over the next 24–48 hours
- Lesion usually progresses to a very slowly healing ulcer
- Symptoms may include fever, urticaria, lymphangitis, nausea

LABORATORY FINDINGS

- Hemolysis and disseminated intravascular coagulation are rare

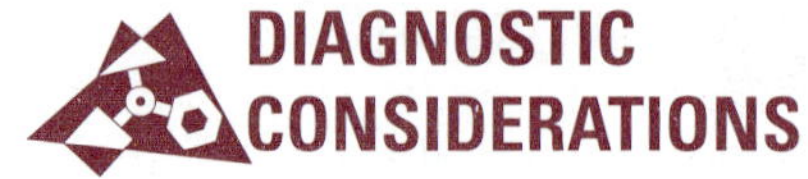

DIAGNOSTIC CONSIDERATIONS

RULE OUT

- Concomitant animal/insect bite
- Multiples bites or stings from multiple different animals or insects
- Associated injuries

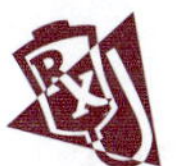

WORK-UP

- Determine type of insect bite or sting
- Physical exam to determine number of bites or stings
- Determine tetanus prophylaxis status

WHEN TO ADMIT

- Systemic signs or complications from bites or stings

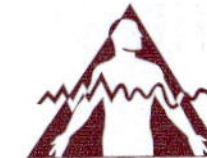

TREATMENT AND MANAGEMENT

- After being stung by a bee, the exuded poison sac should be scraped with a sharp knife; any attempt to pull the poison apparatus out will simply cause more venom to be squeezed into the tissue
- Early application of ice packs to reduce swelling
- Elevation of the extremity is useful

Loxoscelism

- Managed by supportive measures (cleansing of the bite, rest, elevation of the affected area)
- Prophylactic antibiotic therapy (eg, erythromycin) is appropriate

SURGERY

Indications

- Infected bites may require operative debridement

Contraindications

- **Bites from brown recluse spider:** Early excision of lesions associated with poor wound healing

MEDICATIONS

Bee and Wasp Stings

- Oral antihistamines may be of some use in reducing urticaria
- If infection occurs, treatment consists of local debridement and antibiotics
- If an anaphylactic reaction or severe reaction is present, aqueous epinephrine (0.5–1 mL of 1:1000 solution) should be given IM
- A repeat dose may be given in 5–10 minutes followed by 5–20 mg of diphenhydramine slowly IV
- Oxygen administration, plasma expanders, and pressor agents may be required in case of shock

Latrodectism

- IV administration of calcium gluconate may relieve muscle pain and spasm
- A horse antivenin is available but may cause allergic reactions
- Antivenin may be indicated in severely symptomatic patients to speed recovery and perhaps to prevent development of long-term symptoms related to neurologic dysfunction

Loxoscelism

- Corticosteroids or dapsone (50–100 mg/d) may be indicated if ulcers develop or if there is rapid progression of the local reaction

COMPLICATIONS

- Infection
- Generalized allergic reaction that resembles serum sickness
- Anaphylaxis/shock
- Systemic loxoscelism with intravascular coagulation and renal failure has been seen but is uncommon

PROGNOSIS

Latrodectism

- Most symptoms are self-limited and resolve within 48 hours with appropriate supportive therapy but full recovery may take over a week

PREVENTION

- Previously sensitized patients should carry identifying tags and a kit for emergency IM injection of epinephrine
- It is possible to immunize persons against bee and wasp stings, but cost-benefit analyses indicate that this is rarely—if ever—indicated

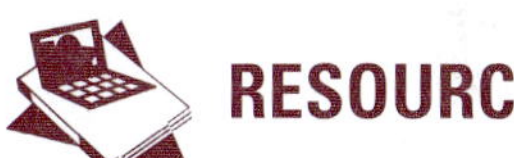

RESOURCES

REFERENCES

- Bond GR. Snake, spider, and scorpion envenomation in North America. *Pediatr Rev.* 1999;20:147.

Blast Injury

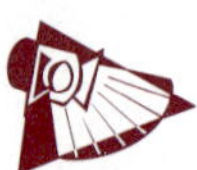

ESSENTIAL FEATURES

- Injuries occur from the effects of the blast itself, propelled foreign bodies, or falling objects
- Pathophysiology involves 2 mechanisms:
  1. Crush injury from rapid displacement of the body wall, leading to laceration and contusion of underlying structures
  2. Wave propagation transfers energy to internal sites

EPIDEMIOLOGY

- Fireworks, household explosions, industrial accidents
- Urban guerrilla warfare such as letter bombs, suitcase bombs, car bombs
- 10% of casualties have deep injuries to chest or abdomen

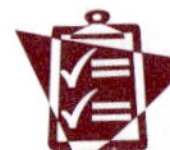

CLINICAL FINDINGS

SYMPTOMS AND SIGNS

- Depend on proximity to blast, space confinement, and detonation size
- Large explosion causes multiple foreign body impregnations, bruises, abrasions, and lacerations
- Blast-induced shock may be result of myocardial depression without compensatory circulatory vasoconstriction
- Lung damage from rupture of alveoli and hemorrhage
- Can cause pneumatic rupture of esophagus or bowel
- Letter bombs tend to injure eyes, hands, ears, and face

IMAGING FINDINGS

- **Chest film:** May be normal or show pneumothorax, pneumomediastinum, or infiltrates

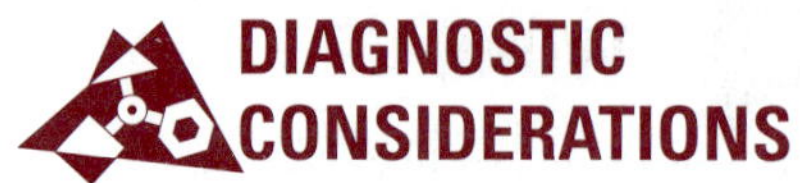

DIAGNOSTIC CONSIDERATIONS

- Must evaluate for associated penetrating trauma

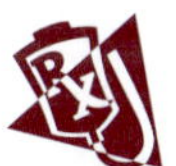

WORK-UP

- ABG of trauma evaluation
- Chest film, pelvic x-ray, and abdominal CT scans useful in stable patients

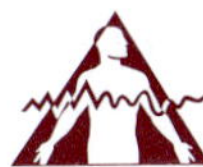

TREATMENT AND MANAGEMENT

- Severe injuries with shock from blood loss or hypoxia require resuscitative measures
- Usual criteria for exploring penetrating wounds of the thorax or abdomen
- High index of suspicion for hollow organ perforation (especially if victim was submerged at time of blast)

SURGERY

Indications

- Muscle devitalization
- Penetrating injury
- Cleansing of wounds
- Removal of foreign bodies

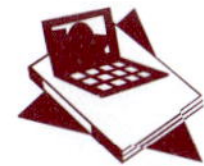

RESOURCES

REFERENCES

- Cernak I et al. Recognizing, scoring and predicting blast injuries. *World J Surg.* 1999;23:44.
- Guy RJ et al. Physiologic responses to primary blast. *J Trauma.* 1998;45:983.

Blind Loop Syndrome

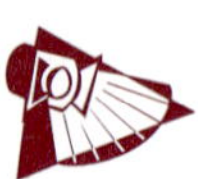

ESSENTIAL FEATURES

- Intestinal stasis and bacterial overgrowth related to disruption of propulsive forces or other factors that limit bacterial growth
- Proliferating bacteria deconjugate bile acids, making micellar formation inadequate resulting in increased colonic fatty acids and steatorrhea
- Megaloblastic anemia results from malabsorption of vitamin B_{12}.
- Treatment should be geared toward correcting the anatomic defect predisposing to bacterial overgrowth, or decreasing bacterial concentration through antibiotic treatment

EPIDEMIOLOGY

- Caused by the disruption of the mechanisms that limit bacterial growth
  - Peristalsis
  - Interdigestive migrating motor complex
  - Gastric acidity
  - Immunoglobulins
  - Prevention of reflux of colonic contents by the ileocecal valve
- Strictures, diverticula, fistulas, or poorly emptying segments of intestine cause stagnation and permit bacterial proliferation
- Stasis of intestinal contents may also result from a functional abnormality of motility (eg, scleroderma)

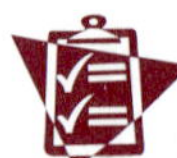

CLINICAL FINDINGS

SYMPTOMS AND SIGNS

- Steatorrhea
- Diarrhea
- Malnutrition

LABORATORY FINDINGS

- Megaloblastic anemia
- Hypocalcemia
- Impaired absorption of orally administered vitamin B_{12}
- Quantitative culture of upper intestinal aspirates (> 10^5/mL are abnormal)
- **^{14}C-D-xylose breath test:** Anaerobic bacteria in the small bowel metabolize xylose, releasing $^{14}CO_2$, which is detected in the breath

IMAGING FINDINGS

- **Upper GI contrast radiographic study or CT scan:** May reveal blind intestinal loop, intestinal stricture, or fistula

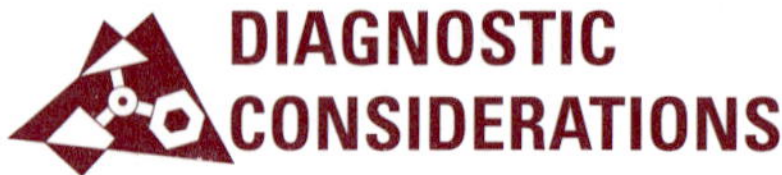

DIAGNOSTIC CONSIDERATIONS

- Steatorrhea is the consequence of bacterial deconjugation and dehydroxylation of bile salts in the proximal small bowel, resulting in micelle formation that is inadequate to solubilize ingested fat
- Hypocalcemia occurs because calcium is bound to unabsorbed fatty acids in the intestinal lumen
- Macrocytic anemia is due to malabsorption of vitamin B_{12}, largely because of binding of the vitamin by anaerobic bacteria

RULE OUT

- Other causes of malabsorption (short bowel syndrome, small intestinal lymphoma, pancreatic exocrine insufficiency, inflammatory bowel disease)

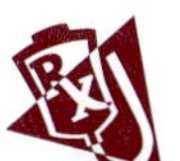

WORK-UP

- CBC count
- Peripheral blood smear
- Serum calcium
- Upper GI aspirate with culture
- ^{14}C-D-xylose breath test
- GI contrast radiography or CT scan for defining anatomic defects

WHEN TO ADMIT

- Severe malnutrition

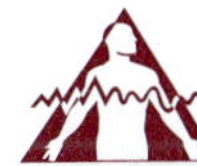

TREATMENT AND MANAGEMENT

- Surgical treatment of underlying fistula, blind loop, diverticula, or other lesion
- In others, treatment consists of broad-spectrum antibiotics and drugs to control diarrhea

SURGERY

Indications

- **Anatomic defects amenable to treatment:** Fistula, diverticulum, blind loop

MEDICATIONS

- Antibiotics
- Antidiarrheal agents

TREATMENT MONITORING

- CBC count
- Symptomatic control (diarrhea, steatorrhea, malnutrition)

PROGNOSIS

- Good if anatomic defect can be identified and corrected

RESOURCES

REFERENCES

- Rubesin SE et al. Small bowel malabsorption: clinical and radiologic perspectives. How we see it. *Radiology.* 1992;184:297.

Breast Cancer, Female

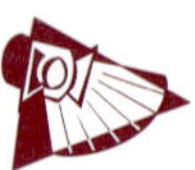

ESSENTIAL FEATURES

- Higher incidence in women who have delayed childbearing, those with family history of breast cancer, and those with a personal history of breast cancer or some types of mammary dysplasia

Early Findings

- Single, nontender, firm-to-hard mass with ill-defined margins
- Mammographic abnormalities
- No palpable mass

Later Findings

- Skin or nipple retraction
- Axillary lymphadenopathy
- Breast enlargement, redness, edema, pain
- Fixation of mass to skin or chest wall

Late Findings

- Ulceration
- Supraclavicular lymphadenopathy
- Edema of arm
- Bone, lung, liver, brain, or other distant metastases

EPIDEMIOLOGY

- Most common site of cancer in women
- Second to lung cancer as a cause of death from cancer in women
- Mean and median age for breast cancer is between 60 and 61 years
- About 182,000 new cases per year
- About 42,000 deaths per year
- Lifetime risk is between 1 in 8 and 9
- 90% of patients have no family history
- About 50% of patients will have involved axillary nodes at presentation
- 35–50% of breast cancers are found on mammogram alone
- 33% of abnormalities seen on mammogram are found to be malignant
- **Distribution of cancers by quadrant:** 45% in upper outer, 15% in upper inner, 5% in lower inner, 10% in lower outer, 25% in subareolar
- 1–3% of persons with ductal carcinoma in situ have an associated invasive carcinoma; untreated, invasive ductal carcinoma will eventually develop in the ipsilateral breast in 40–60% of women with DCIS
- An invasive malignancy develops (in either breast) in 20% of persons with lobular carcinoma in situ
- 1–2% of breast cancers occur during pregnancy or lactation
- Malignant pleural effusions develop in nearly 50% of patients with metastatic disease

CLINICAL FINDINGS

SYMPTOMS AND SIGNS

- Palpable mass (90% detected first by patient)
- Pain (less common for malignant disease than benign disease)
- Nipple discharge, especially bloody
- Nipple erosion
- Breast erythema or edema
- Skin or nipple retraction/dimpling
- Thickening in a portion of the breast
- **Adenopathy:** Axillary or supraclavicular

LABORATORY FINDINGS

- Pathologic analysis of tissue sample taken via fine-needle aspiration, core needle biopsy, stereotactic core needle biopsy, or open excision biopsy
- Serum markers for advanced breast cancer or metastatic disease include elevated ESR, elevated alkaline phosphatase, hypercalcemia, carcinoembryonic antigen, CA 15-3, CA 27-29

IMAGING FINDINGS

- Mammographic abnormality of increased density with microcalcifications and irregular border
- US demonstration of solid mass (versus cyst—usually benign)
- Chest film may show pulmonary metastases
- CT scan of the liver or brain may demonstrate metastases
- Bone scan may show increased uptake reflecting disease metastatic to bone

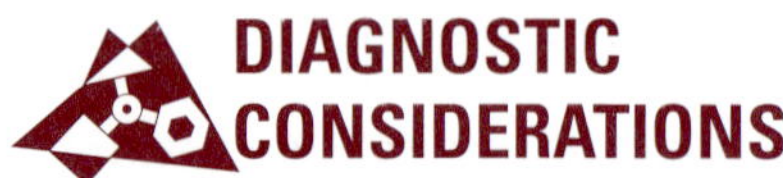

DIAGNOSTIC CONSIDERATIONS

- Risk factors include:
  - Family history of breast cancer (especially premenopausal or bilateral cancers)
  - Nulliparity
  - First full-term pregnancy after age 35
  - Early menarche (under age 12)
  - Late menopause (after age 50)
  - Mammary dysplasia with proliferative changes
  - Personal history of contralateral breast cancer
  - Personal history of uterine cancer

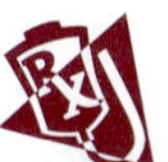

WORK-UP

- Complete history (including family and reproductive) and physical exam
- Bilateral mammograms
- Tissue diagnosis

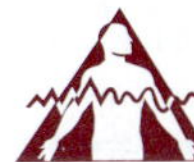

TREATMENT AND MANAGEMENT

- Early detection via routine self breast exams and screening is the key to improved survival; this includes recognition of high-risk patients
- Adjuvant hormonal therapy depends on receptor status (ER, PR, Her2/Neu)
- Aim for curative therapy but often only palliative with stages III and IV

SURGERY

Indications

- Stage I–III disease (extent of operation still controversial—lumpectomy, axillary interrogation, and postoperative radiation vs modified radical mastectomy)

Contraindications

- **Stage IV disease:** Generally treated with radiotherapy and hormonal therapy; may require mastectomy for local symptom control

MEDICATIONS

- Breast radiation often used in adjuvant setting
- Adjuvant hormonal therapy (tamoxifen) or combination chemotherapy often used depending on nodal involvement and estrogen receptor status
- Generally agreed that all women, regardless of age and menopausal status, whose tumors are estrogen receptor positive, should receive adjuvant tamoxifen

TREATMENT MONITORING

- Self breast exams
- Semiannual clinical breast exams
- Annual bilateral mammograms

COMPLICATIONS

- Edema of the arm
- Metastatic disease
- Malignant pleural effusions

PROGNOSIS

- Stage is best indicator
- Cancer localized to just breast has 75–90% cure rate
- With spread to axilla, 5-year survival is 40–50%, and 10-year survival is 25%

RESOURCES

REFERENCES

- Alberg AJ et al. Epidemiology, prevention, and early detection of breast cancer. *Curr Opin Oncol.* 1997;9:505.
- Krag D et al. The sentinel node in breast cancer—a multicenter validation study. *N Engl J Med.* 1998;339:941.
- Fish EB et al. Assessment of treatment for patients with primary ductal carcinoma in situ in the breast. *Ann Surg Oncol.* 1998;5:724.
- Margolese RG. Surgical considerations for invasive breast cancer. *Surg Clin North Am.* 1999;79:1031.
- Clarke M. Tamoxifen for early breast cancer: an overview of the randomized trials. *Lancet.* 1998;351:1451.

PRACTICE GUIDELINES

- The National Comprehensive Cancer Network http://www.nccn.org/

CANCER STAGING

- See Breast Staging Table on page 744.

STAGE GROUPING

Stage 0	Tis	N0	M0
Stage I	T1*	N0	M0
Stage IIA	T0	N1	M0
	T1*	N1	M0
	T2	N0	M0
Stage IIB	T2	N1	M0
	T3	N0	M0
Stage IIIA	T0	N2	M0
	T1*	N2	M0
	T2	N2	M0
	T3	N1	M0
	T3	N2	M0
Stage IIIB	T4	N0	M0
	T4	N1	M0
	T4	N2	M0
Stage IIIC	Any T	N3	M0
Stage IV	Any T	Any N	M1

*T1 includes T1mic

Note: Stage designation may be changed if post-surgical imaging studies reveal the presence of distant metastases, provided that the studies are carried out within 4 months of diagnosis in the absence of disease progression and provided that the patient has not received neoadjuvant therapy.

Breast Cancer, Male

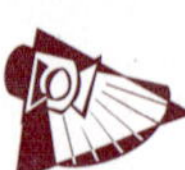

ESSENTIAL FEATURES

- Painless lump beneath the areola in a man who is usually over the age of 50
- Nipple discharge, retraction, or ulceration may be present

EPIDEMIOLOGY

- Rare disease, with an incidence only about 1% of that for carcinoma of the female breast
- Average age of occurrence is about 60 years
- 75% of males with nipple discharge have a breast carcinoma

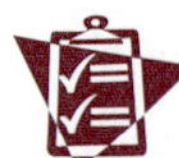

CLINICAL FINDINGS

SYMPTOMS AND SIGNS

- Hard, painless breast lump, often beneath the areola
- Nipple discharge, retraction, erosion, or ulceration
- May have accompanying gynecomastia

IMAGING FINDINGS

- Mass on mammography

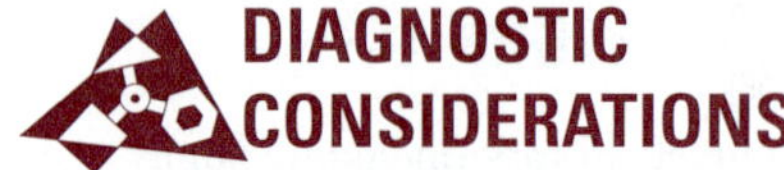

DIAGNOSTIC CONSIDERATIONS

- Blood-borne metastases often present at initial presentation, although may be latent

RULE OUT

- Gynecomastia
- Metastatic cancer from another site

WORK-UP

- History and physical exam
- Mammography
- Needle biopsy

TREATMENT AND MANAGEMENT

- Modified radical mastectomy is first-line therapy for surgical candidates
- Surgical candidates chosen by the same criteria as women
- Irradiation is the first step in treating localized metastases to skin, lymph nodes, or bone that are causing symptoms
- Tumor hormone receptor status may be of benefit in determining role of adjuvant biochemotherapy
- Castration is possible palliative measure for advanced metastatic disease

MEDICATIONS

- Tamoxifen for metastatic disease
- Potential role of aminoglutethimide to suppress adrenal androgen production (has replaced adrenalectomy)

PROGNOSIS

- Worse prognosis, stage for stage, than female breast carcinoma
- 5- and 10-year survival for stage I cancer is 58% and 38%, respectively
- 5- and 10-year survival for stage II cancer is 38% and 10%, respectively
- 5- and 10-year survival rates for all stages combined are 36% and 17%, respectively

RESOURCES

REFERENCES

- Joshi MG et al. Male breast carcinoma: an evaluation of prognostic factors contributing to a poor outcome. *Cancer.* 1996;77:490.
- Memon MA et al. Male breast cancer. *Br J Surg.* 1997;84:433.
- Winchester DJ. Male breast cancer. *Semin Surg Oncol.* 1996;12:364.

PRACTICE GUIDELINES

- The National Comprehensive Cancer Network http://www.nccn.org/

CANCER STAGING

- See Breast Staging Table on page 744.

STAGE GROUPING

Stage 0	Tis	N0	M0
Stage I	T1*	N0	M0
Stage IIA	T0	N1	M0
	T1*	N1	M0
	T2	N0	M0
Stage IIB	T2	N1	M0
	T3	N0	M0
Stage IIIA	T0	N2	M0
	T1*	N2	M0
	T2	N2	M0
	T3	N1	M0
	T3	N2	M0
Stage IIIB	T4	N0	M0
	T4	N1	M0
	T4	N2	M0
Stage IIIC	Any T	N3	M0
Stage IV	Any T	Any N	M1

*T1 includes T1mic

Note: Stage designation may be changed if post-surgical imaging studies reveal the presence of distant metastases, provided that the studies are carried out within 4 months of diagnosis in the absence of disease progression and provided that the patient has not received neoadjuvant therapy.

Breast Lesions, Benign

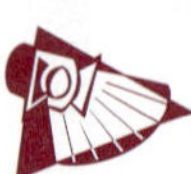

ESSENTIAL FEATURES

- Types of lesions include:
  - Mammary dysplasia (fibrocystic disease)
  - Fibroadenoma of the breast
  - Intraductal papilloma
  - Fat necrosis and mastitis
  - Breast abscess

EPIDEMIOLOGY

- Fibrocystic disease is most frequent lesion of the breast; common from 30 to 50 years of age but rare after menopause
- Fibroadenoma occurs more frequently in blacks than whites
- Only 50% of patients with fat necrosis report antecedent trauma
- Subareolar abscess can develop spontaneously in young or middle-aged women who are not lactating

CLINICAL FINDINGS

SYMPTOMS AND SIGNS

Fibrocystic Disease

- Painful, multiple, bilateral masses
- Rapid fluctuation in mass size
- Symptoms increase during premenstrual phase of cycle

Fibroadenoma

- Round, firm, discrete, mobile mass

Intraductal Papilloma

- Unilateral bloody nipple discharge

Fat Necrosis

- Mass with associated skin or nipple retraction; tenderness and ecchymosis occasionally seen

Mastitis/Breast Abscess

- Area of erythema, tenderness, and induration
- Localized mass

IMAGING FINDINGS

- Mammography often unreliable due to dense breast parenchyma in this age group
- US can distinguish solid from cyctic mass

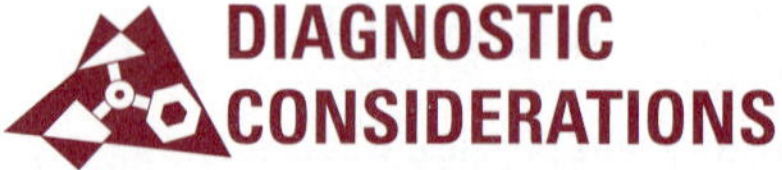

DIAGNOSTIC CONSIDERATIONS

- Nursing can continue with mastitis but should be discontinued with breast abscess
- Most common causative pathogen in mastitis and breast abscesses is *Staphylococcus*

RULE OUT

- Breast carcinoma
- Inflammatory breast carcinoma (when signs of breast abscess in the nonlactating breast)

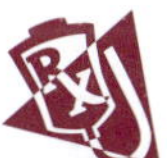

WORK-UP

- Complete history (including family and reproductive) and physical exam
- Mammography or US
- Biopsy if any possibility of cancer

TREATMENT AND MANAGEMENT

SURGERY

Indications

- Persistent dominant mass; mass after cyst aspiration
- Suspicious cytologic studies or biopsy results
- Fibroadenoma (excisional biopsy)
- Intraductal papilloma (total excision through circumareolar incision)
- Fat necrosis
- Subareolar abscess in the nonlactating breast

MEDICATIONS

- **Danazol:** Synthetic androgen; can reduce pain
- Symptomatic relief with vitamin E and with discontinuation of caffeine
- Antibiotics for mastitis/abscess

TREATMENT MONITORING

- Self breast exams
- Annual clinical breast exams
- Annual bilateral mammogram

PROGNOSIS

- Excellent

RESOURCES

REFERENCES

- Marchant DJ. Controversies in benign breast disease. *Surg Oncol Clin North Am.* 1998;7:285.
- Alle KM et al. Conservative management of fibroadenoma of the breast. *Br J Surg.* 1996;83:1798.
- Schein M. Subareolar breast abscess. *Surgery.* 1996;120:902.

Bronchial Adenomas & Carcinoid Tumors of Lung

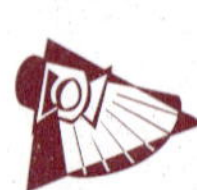

ESSENTIAL FEATURES

- Bronchial gland adenomas constitute 5% of all lung cancer
  - Misnomer since vast majority actually malignant
- Carcinoid lung tumors constitute 85% of bronchial adenomas
  - Classified as typical or atypical
  - Derived from Kulchitsky cells
  - Located in central, proximal airways
  - Slow growing, can metastasize widely, rarely cause carcinoid syndrome
- Adenoid cystic carcinoma (cylindromas)
  - Locally aggressive, metastasis involve lung
  - Slow growing, amenable to resection
- Mucoepidermoid cancer
  - Rare tumors; mucus secreting cells and squamous cells present
  - Less aggressive
- Mucous gland adenoma: Truly benign

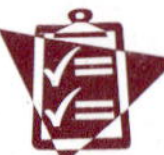

CLINICAL FINDINGS

IMAGING FINDINGS

- Chest film
- Chest CT scan

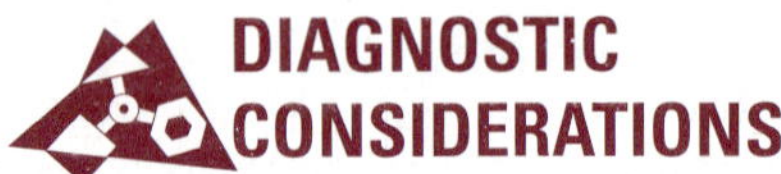

DIAGNOSTIC CONSIDERATIONS

- May present as a solitary pulmonary nodule, and require work-up as such
- Carcinoid syndrome rare with pulmonary tumors

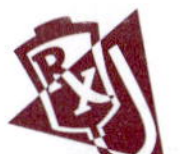

WORK-UP

- Chest film
- Chest CT
- **Bronchoscopy:** Biopsy for tissue diagnosis; beware of bleeding

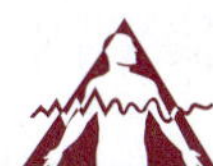

TREATMENT AND MANAGEMENT

SURGERY

- **Surgery primary treatment:** Lobectomy or sleeve
- **Adenoid cystic carcinomas:** Requires generous margins and frozen section exam at surgery
- Up to 8 cm of trachea can be removed with primary anastomosis

MEDICATIONS

- Chemotherapy indicated only for atypical carcinoid

PROGNOSIS

- Very good, in general
- Lymph node and distant metastasis portend poor prognosis

RESOURCES

REFERENCES

- Gould MK et al. Accuracy of positron emission tomography for diagnosis of pulmonary nodules and mass lesions: a meta-analysis. *JAMA.* 2001;285:914.
- Swanson SJ et al. Management of the solitary pulmonary nodule: role of thoracoscopy in diagnosis and therapy. *Chest.* 1999;116(6 Suppl):523S.

Bronchiectasis

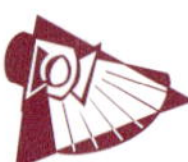

ESSENTIAL FEATURES

- Defined as abnormal dilation of bronchi
- Denotes clinical syndrome marked by:
  - Chronic dilation of bronchi
  - Paroxysmal cough producing mucopurulent sputum
  - Recurrent pulmonary infections
- 2 main types
  - Saccular: Follows most infections and bronchial obstruction
  - Cylindric: Associated with post-TB bronchiectasis
- Mixed or varicose: Third type; alternates saccular and cylindrical areas
- Involves second to fourth order branches
- Congenital often bilateral bronchiectasis
- TB/granulomatous disease more often unilateral, or bilateral but limited to upper lobes
- Pyogenic/pneumonias result in bronchiectasis of lower lobes, lingula

EPIDEMIOLOGY

- Congenital disease can cause bronchiectasis
  - Kartagener syndrome
  - Cystic fibrosis, Williams-Campbell syndrome
  - Mounier-Kuhn syndrome, immunoglobulin deficiency
  - α_1-Antitrypsin deficiency
- Most cases are not congenital but caused by infection and bronchial obstruction
  - Pertussis
  - Measles
  - Influenza
  - TB
  - Bronchopneumonia
- Repeated bouts or single severe pneumonia can causes bronchiectasis
- Foreign bodies, endobronchial neoplasms, hilar lymphadenopathy can lead to bronchiectasis
- **Common pathogens:** *H influenza, S aureus, K pneumoniae, E coli*

CLINICAL FINDINGS

SYMPTOMS AND SIGNS

- Recurrent febrile episodes
- Chronic or intermittent cough producing foul-smelling sputum (up to 500 mL/d)
- Hemoptysis (about 50% of patients)
- Advanced disease indicated by increased sputum production, fever, dyspnea, anorexia, fatigue, and weight loss
- History of sinus problems, infertility, or family history may indicate inherited disease

IMAGING FINDINGS

- **High-resolution chest CT:** Documents bronchial dilation

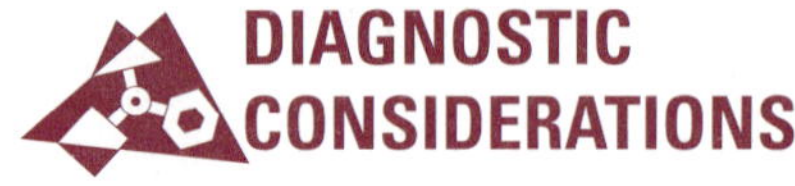

DIAGNOSTIC CONSIDERATIONS

RULE OUT

- Obstruction from neoplasm or foreign body

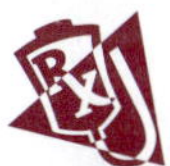

WORK-UP

- Culture for common pathogens *(E coli, Klebsiella, Staph, H influenza)*
- Culture for mycobacteria, fungi, *Legionella*
- **Chest CT scan:** Required preoperatively
- Bronchoscopy with bronchoalveolar lavage (BAL) for culture
- Bronchogram may be needed prior to operation

TREATMENT AND MANAGEMENT

- In most cases, conservative, medical treatment is sufficient
- Broad-spectrum antibiotics, bronchodilators, humidification, expectorants, mucolytics, and postural drainage
- **Continued infection:** Bronchoscopy with BAL for culture
- Influenza and pneumococcal vaccines may be needed
- Inhaled antibiotics (gentamicin or tobramycin) may help control infection

SURGERY

- **Goals:** Remove all active disease, preserve functioning lung as much as possible
- Maintain clear airway devoid of mucopurulent secretions or blood

Indications

- Criteria for failure of medical therapy include:
  - Localized disease and completely resectable
  - Adequate pulmonary reserve
  - Irreversible process
  - Significant symptoms despite medical treatment

COMPLICATIONS

- Hemoptysis, lung, and brain abscess; empyema; respiratory failure; death
- All complications decreased since anti-TB medications emerged

PROGNOSIS

- **Local disease:** 80% success with surgery
- **Diffuse disease:** 36% surgical success
- **Prognostic factors:** Unilateral disease in basal segments, young age, absence of sinusitis or rhinitis, history of pneumonia, no airway obstruction
- **Morbidity:** 3–5%; mortality < 1%

PREVENTION

- Long-term antibiotic therapy may be needed for prophylaxis (sulfamethoxazole-trimethoprim, ciprofloxacin, etc)

RESOURCES

REFERENCES

- Ip M et al. Multivariate analysis of factors affecting pulmonary function in bronchiectasis. *Respiration.* 1993;60:45.
- Trucksis M, Swartz MN. Bronchiectasis: a current view. *Curr Clin Top Infect Dis.* 1991;11:170.

Broncholithiasis

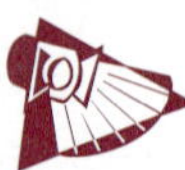

ESSENTIAL FEATURES

- Presence of broncholiths (calculi) in tracheobronchial tree
- Causes include:
  - Calcified parabronchial lymph node eroding into bronchial wall lumen (most common)
  - Severely inspissated mucus may calcify
- Broncholiths may remain attached to bronchial wall, lodge in bronchus, or be expectorated (lithoptysis)

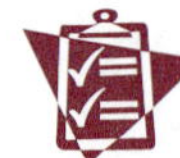

CLINICAL FINDINGS

SYMPTOMS AND SIGNS

- Hemoptysis
- Lithoptysis (30%)
- Cough, sputum production, pleuritic chest pain
- Fever, chills
- Wheezing
- Pneumonia may occur from obstructive broncholith

IMAGING FINDINGS

- **Chest film:** Hilar calcification, segmental atelectasis, pneumonia

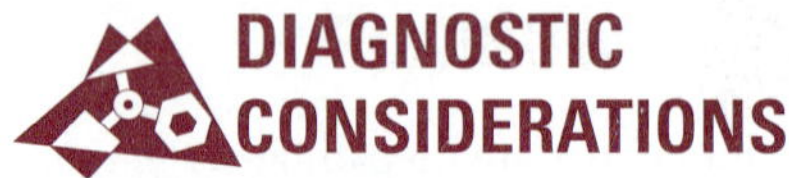

DIAGNOSTIC CONSIDERATIONS

- Diagnosis is confirmed with lithoptysis or presence of broncholith

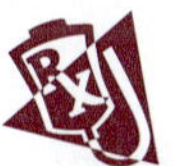

WORK-UP

- Chest film
- Bronchoscopy to identify stone

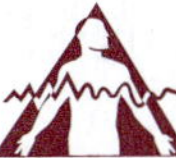

TREATMENT AND MANAGEMENT

- Treat underlying pulmonary disease
- Treatment directed at removal of stone

SURGERY

- Bronchoscopy successful 20% of time to remove stone
  - Risk is massive
  - Hemorrhage if attached to wall or use excessive force to remove
- **80% require surgery:** Bronchotomy and stone extraction or segmentectomy/ lobectomy

Indications

- Unable to remove via bronchoscopy (80% of cases)
- **Tracheoesophageal fistulas:** Repair with intercostals muscle flap between airway and esophagus to prevent recurrence

COMPLICATIONS

- Hemoptysis, may be massive
- Midesophageal traction diverticular
- Tracheoesophageal fistula

PROGNOSIS

- Excellent after surgery

RESOURCES

REFERENCES

- Galdermans D et al. Broncholithiasis: present clinical spectrum. *Respir Med.* 1990;84:155.
- Conces DJ Jr et al. Broncholithiasis: CT features in 15 patients. *AJR Am Roentgenol.* 1991;157:249.

Buerger Disease

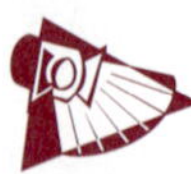

ESSENTIAL FEATURES

- Also known as thromboangiitis obliterans
  - Characterized as multiple segmental small arteries occlusions in distal extremities
- Involves all 3 layers of arterial wall with infiltration of round cells
- Healing of lesion results in fibrous obliteration of lumen in segmental fashion
- Upper and lower extremities affected
- Many patients have specific cellular immunity against arterial antigens and elevated immune complexes

EPIDEMIOLOGY

- Young cigarette-smoking men

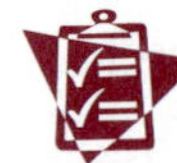

CLINICAL FINDINGS

SYMPTOMS AND SIGNS

- Migratory phlebitis
- Symptoms range from digital pain to coolness and cyanosis, to necrosis and gangrene
- Foot claudication may be first symptom
- On exam, patients often have irregular pattern of ischemia
- Allen test demonstrates delayed filling of affected digital arteries

IMAGING FINDINGS

- Angiography findings distinctive but not pathognomonic; tapering of proximal vessel, artery is smooth, not irregular, multiple wispy collateral present

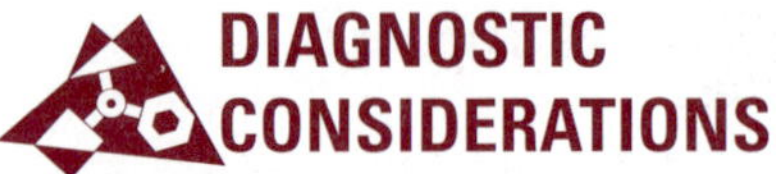

DIAGNOSTIC CONSIDERATIONS

- Precise diagnosis only made by microscopic evaluation

WORK-UP

- HLA typing may distinguish patients with Buerger disease from those with atherosclerosis
- Microscopic diagnosis necessary
  –Shows lymphocytic infiltration into all layers of vessel wall
- Arteriographic findings distinctive but not pathognomonic

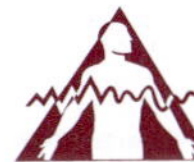

TREATMENT AND MANAGEMENT

- Cessation of smoking essential to avoid disease progression and may even become dormant
- Sympathectomy decreases arterial spasm in some patients
- Amputation for pain/gangrene

SURGERY

Indications

- Severe symptoms
- Necrosis/gangrene

RESOURCES

REFERENCES

- Eichorn J et al. Antiendothelial cell antibodies in thromboangiitis obliterans. *Am J Med.* 1998;315:17.

Burns

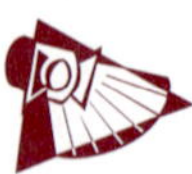

ESSENTIAL FEATURES

- Severe thermal injury is 1 of the most devastating physical and psychological injuries a person can suffer
- Skin is the largest organ of the body, ranging from 0.25 m^2 in infants to 1.8 m^2 in adults
- Skin has 2 layers: epidermis and dermis
  - The outermost cells of the epidermis are dead cornified cells that act as a tough protective barrier
  - The dermis is chiefly composed of fibrous connective tissue and contains the blood vessels and nerves to the skin and epithelial appendages of specialized function
  - The dermis prevents loss of body fluids and loss of excess body heat
- Nerve endings that mediate pain are found only in the corium
  - Partial-thickness injuries may be extremely painful
  - Full-thickness burns are usually painless
- **Second-degree** (or **partial-thickness**) burns are deeper, involving all of the epidermis and some of the dermis
  - The systemic severity and quality of subsequent healing are related to the amount of undamaged dermis
- Complications are rare from superficial partial-thickness burns and usually heal in 10–14 days
- **Deep partial-thickness** burns heal over 25–35 days with a fragile epithelial covering that arises from residual uninjured epithelium of the deep dermal sweat glands and hair follicles
  - Severe hypertrophic scarring occurs when such an injury heals
  - Evaporative losses remain high
  - Conversion to **full-thickness** by bacteria is common
- Skin grafting, when feasible, improves the physiologic quality and appearance of the skin cover

EPIDEMIOLOGY

- Over 2 million burn injuries require medical attention each year in United States
- Over 14,000 deaths per year in United States
- House fires responsible for 5% of fires but 50% of deaths, most from smoke inhalation
- 75,000 patients require hospitalization and 25,000 for more than 2 months

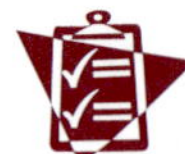

CLINICAL FINDINGS

SYMPTOMS AND SIGNS

- **First-degree burn:**
  - Involves only the epidermis
  - Characterized by erythema and minor microscopic changes
  - Tissue damage is minimal
  - Pain, the chief symptom, usually resolves in 48–72 hours and healing takes place uneventfully
- **Superficial partial-thickness burns:**
  - Characterized by blistering while deeper partial-thickness burns have a reddish appearance or a layer of whitish nonviable dermis adherent to the remaining viable tissue
- **Full-thickness (third-degree) burns:**
  - Have a characteristic white, waxy appearance
  - May appear to the untrained eye as unburned skin
  - The diagnostic findings are lack of sensation in the burned skin, lack of capillary refill, and a leathery texture that is unlike normal skin
- All epithelial elements are destroyed, leaving no potential for reepithelialization

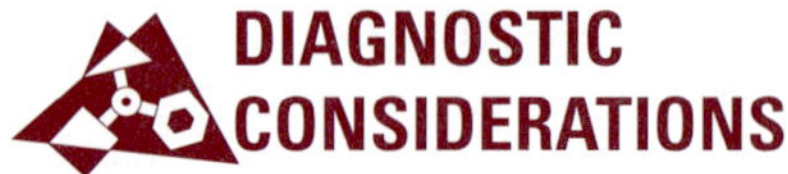

DIAGNOSTIC CONSIDERATIONS

RULE OUT

- Must evaluate for associated injuries, such as blunt trauma (falls)

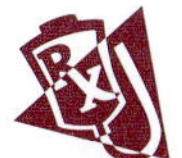

WORK-UP

- Burn victim should be assessed and treated like any patient with major trauma
- If smoke inhalation is possibility, ABG measurements, oxygen saturation, and carboxyhemoglobin levels should be obtained

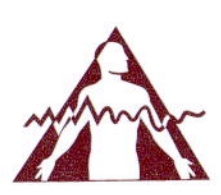

TREATMENT AND MANAGEMENT

Acute Care

- Oxygen should be administered
- Endotracheal intubation is indicated if patient is semicomatose, has deep burns to the face and neck, or is otherwise critically injured
- Intubation should be done early, as edema will make it more difficult later
- If burns > 20%, then a Foley catheter should be placed to monitor urinary output
- Large-bore IV access obtained, preferably in peripheral vein since central access is associated with infection in burn patients
- Isotonic crystalloid fluid is infused to counterbalance the loss of plasma volume into the extravascular space and the loss of extracellular fluid to the intracellular space
- Fluid should be administered to keep pulse < 120 beats per minute and urinary output > 0.5 mL/kg/h
- Rough estimate of fluid requirement is calculated as 4 mL/%TBSA/kg with 50% given over first 8 hours and remaining over the next 16 hours
- Colloids should not be given until capillary leak subsides (usually 4–8 hrs after injury)
- Wounds should be debrided of all dirt and loose skin, taking care to avoid hypothermia
- Tetanus toxoid, 0.5 mL, should be administered to all patients with significant burn injury

After 24 Hours

- IV fluid therapy during the second 24 hour period should consist of glucose in hypotonic salt solution to replace evaporative losses
- Pain, hypothermia, and anxiety all need to be aggressively controlled
- Nutritional support should begin as early as possible to maximize wound healing and minimize immune deficiency
- Broad-spectrum antibiotics should NOT be given
- Vitamin A, E, and C, and zinc should be given until the burn wound is closed

SURGERY

Indications

- Debridement of dirt and loose skin
- Rapid closure of burn wounds decreases the rate of sepsis and, in full-thickness burn injuries in excess of 60% of body surface, significantly decreases the death rate
- Approach to operative debridement varies from an extensive burn excision and grafting within several days of injury to a more moderate approach of limited debridements
- Excision should be to viable tissue, referred to as tangential excision
  - Advantageous because it provides a vascular base for grafting while preserving remaining viable tissue

MEDICATIONS

- Tetanus toxoid
- Narcotics (IV)
- Silver sulfadiazine is effective against a wide spectrum of gram-negative organisms and is moderately effective in penetrating the burn eschar; a transient leucopenia secondary to bone marrow depression is usually self-limiting and the agent does not have to be discontinued
- Mafenide penetrates the burn eschar and is a more potent antibiotic, but there are more complications with its use
  - Causes considerable pain in 50% of patients
  - Metabolic acidosis can occur with its use in large burns
  - It is chiefly used on burns that do not respond to silver sulfadiazine
- Porcine xenografts are a biologic dressing that can be applied to clean partial-thickness wounds and to cover primarily excised areas when grafting must be delayed
- Homografts (human skin), and a number of synthetic skin substitutes are also available; all these agents are particularly effective on second-degree burns

TREATMENT MONITORING

- Monitor blood pressure, pulse, urinary output
- Infection (*S aureus, P aeruginosa, C albicans)*
- Acute gastroduodenal (Curling) ulcers
- Circumferential burns
- Seizures (children)
- Acute gastric dilation

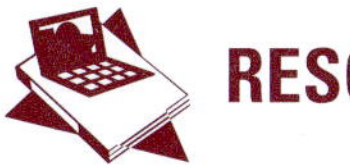

RESOURCES

REFERENCES

- Nguyen T et al. Current treatment of severely burned patients. *Ann Surg.* 1996;223:14.
- Kaups KL et al. Base deficit as an indicator of resuscitation needs in patients with burn injuries. *J Burn Care Rehabil.* 1998;19:346.
- Forjuoh SN. The mechanisms, intensity of treatment and outcomes of hospitalized burns: issues for prevention. *J Burn Care Rehabil.* 1998;19:456.

Burns, Respiratory Injury

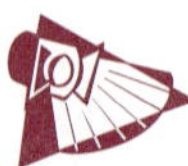

ESSENTIAL FEATURES

- Major cause of death after burns is respiratory tract injury or complications in the respiratory tract
- **Problems include:**
  - Inhalation injury
  - Aspiration
  - Bacterial pneumonia
  - Pulmonary edema
  - Pulmonary embolism
  - Post-traumatic pulmonary insufficiency
- Direct inhalation injuries are divided into 3 categories
  1. Heat injury to the airway
  2. Carbon monoxide poisoning
  3. Inhalation of noxious gases
- **Heat injury** is a rare cause of injury below the vocal cords because the upper airway effectively cools the inspired gases and reflexive closure of the cords halts full inhalation
  - Acute edema of the upper tract may cause airway obstruction and asphyxiation without lung damage
  - Treatment is primarily supportive with pulmonary toilet, mechanical ventilation (as needed), and antibiotics
- **Carbon monoxide** poisoning must be considered in every patient in whom inhalation injury is suspected
  - ABG and carboxyhemoglobin levels must be measured
  - COHgb levels > 5% in nonsmokers and > 10% in smokers indicates carbon monoxide poisoning
  - **Mild** carbon monoxide poisoning (< 20% COHgb) is manifested by headache, slight dyspnea, mild confusion, and diminished visual acuity
  - **Moderate** carbon monoxide poisoning (20–40% COHgb) leads to irritability, impairment of judgement, dim vision, nausea, and fatigability
  - **Severe** carbon monoxide poisoning (40–60% COHgb) produces hallucinations, confusion, ataxia, collapse, and coma
  - Levels in excess of 60% COHgb are usually fatal
- **Toxic inhalation** of different chemicals produces specific respiratory injuries
  - Inhalation injury causes severe mucosal edema followed soon by sloughing of the mucosa
  - The destroyed mucosa in the larger airways is replaced by a mucopurulent membrane
  - Edema fluid enters the airway and, when mixed with the pus, may form casts and plugs in the smaller bronchioles
- Less common causes of respiratory failure are pulmonary embolus and overload pulmonary edema
- **Pulmonary emboli** usually occur later in the course of treatment after prolonged bed rest and should be suspected if respiratory function suddenly deteriorates
- **Pulmonary edema** usually occurs only in patients with preexisting heart disease
- Probably the most common cause of respiratory failure is **bacterial pneumonia** due to either inhalation injury, contamination of the lungs through a tracheostomy or endotracheal tube, airborne infection, or hematogenous spread of bacteria from the burn wound
- Alteration of oropharyngeal normal flora with colonization by pathogens and subsequent **aspiration** of infected secretion is the most common cause of the lung infections
- **Pulmonary insufficiency** is associated with systemic sepsis; differentiating acute respiratory distress syndrome (ARDS) from bacterial pneumonia may be difficult

CLINICAL FINDINGS

SYMPTOMS AND SIGNS

- Airway erythema
- Airway edema
- Stridor
- Dyspnea
- Carbonaceous sputum

LABORATORY FINDINGS

- Hypoxemia
- Carboxyhemoglobinemia
- Bacterial cultures

IMAGING FINDINGS

- **Chest film:** Edema, pneumonia, ARDS, etc.

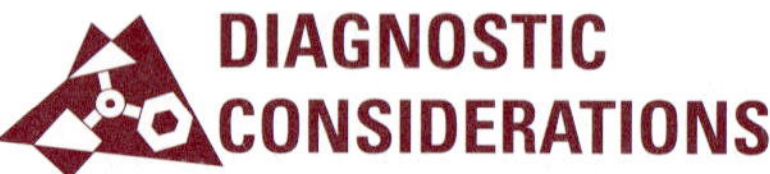

DIAGNOSTIC CONSIDERATIONS

- Must also evaluate for skin burns and blunt trauma (falls)

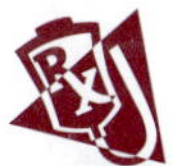

WORK-UP

- ABG measurement
- Carboxyhemoglobin measurement
- Direct laryngoscopy is probably as helpful as fiberoptic laryngoscopy
- Fiberoptic laryngoscopy can detect injury but is not quantitative
- Daily sputum examination to follow for development of bacterial infection
- Frequent evaluation of the lungs throughout the hospital stay

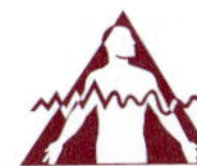

TREATMENT AND MANAGEMENT

- All patients who initially have evidence of smoke inhalation should receive humidified oxygen in high concentration
- If carbon monoxide poisoning has occurred, 100% oxygen should be given until the carboxyhemoglobin returns to normal levels and symptoms resolve
- Corticosteroids are **contraindicated**
- Bronchodilators and chest physical therapy with postural drainage
- Intubation and mechanical ventilation as indicated
- Tracheostomy is indicated in the first several days for patients who are expected to require ventilatory support for a few weeks or more
- Heparin is indicated in patients with pulmonary embolism

MEDICATIONS

- Corticosteroids are **contraindicated**

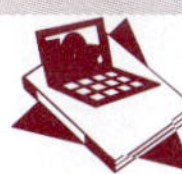

RESOURCES

REFERENCES

- Nguyen T et al. Current treatment of severely burned patients. *Ann Surg.* 1996;223:14.
- Kaups KL et al. Base deficit as an indicator of resuscitation needs in patients with burn injuries. *J Burn Care Rehabil.* 1998;19:346.
- Forjuoh SN. The mechanisms, intensity of treatment and outcomes of hospitalized burns: issues for prevention. *J Burn Care Rehabil.* 1998;19:456.

Carcinoma, Inflammatory

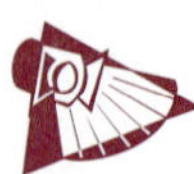

ESSENTIAL FEATURES

- Rapidly growing, painful mass of the breast
- No distinct mass as tumor infiltrates breast diffusely
- Name refers to clinical appearance not specific histologic subtype of mammary carcinoma

EPIDEMIOLOGY

- 3% of all breast cancer cases
- Average age of diagnosis is 55
- Rarely seen in men or children
- No predisposition conferred by pregnancy or lactation

CLINICAL FINDINGS

SYMPTOMS AND SIGNS

- Breast mass
- Erythematous, edematous, warm skin on breast
- Failure to respond to antibiotics (if initially diagnosed as breast cellulitis) within 1–2 weeks
- Peau d'orange changes, most notable over dependent portions of the breast

LABORATORY FINDINGS

- Biopsy shows invasion of subdermal lymphatics

IMAGING FINDINGS

- Mammography can demonstrate a mass, stromal coarsening, increased parenchymal density, or skin thickening

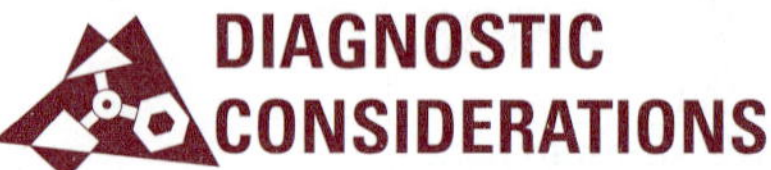

DIAGNOSTIC CONSIDERATIONS

- Metastases tend to occur early and widely
- Skin changes may precede palpable breast mass
- Tumors are more likely to be estrogen receptor negative compared with tumors that do not have an inflammatory component

RULE OUT

- Mastitis/breast abscess

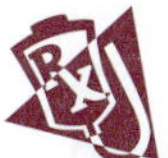

WORK-UP

- Complete history (including family and reproductive) and physical exam
- Bilateral mammography
- Breast biopsy

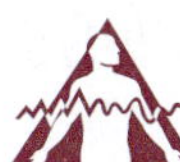

TREATMENT AND MANAGEMENT

- Rarely curable
- Mastectomy rarely indicated alone
- Multimodal therapy with radiation, chemotherapy, and hormonal therapy

SURGERY

Indications

- Mastectomy for local control of disease

MEDICATIONS

- Anthracycline-based combination chemotherapy
- External beam radiation

TREATMENT MONITORING

- Self breast exams
- Semiannual clinical breast exam
- Annual bilateral mammogram

COMPLICATIONS

- Edema of the arm
- Metastatic spread
- Local chest wall involvement

PROGNOSIS

- Rarely curable as metastases occur early and widely
- 5-year survival about 50%

RESOURCES

REFERENCES

- Gradishar WJ. Inflammatory breast cancer: the evolution of multimodality treatment strategies. *Semin Surg Oncol.* 1996;12:352.
- Moore MP et al. Inflammatory breast cancer. *Arch Surg.* 1991;126:304.

PRACTICE GUIDELINES

- The National Comprehensive Cancer Network http://www.nccn.org/

CANCER STAGING

- See Breast Staging Table on page 744.

STAGE GROUPING

Stage 0	Tis	N0	M0
Stage I	T1*	N0	M0
Stage IIA	T0	N1	M0
	T1*	N1	M0
	T2	N0	M0
Stage IIB	T2	N1	M0
	T3	N0	M0
Stage IIIA	T0	N2	M0
	T1*	N2	M0
	T2	N2	M0
	T3	N1	M0
	T3	N2	M0
Stage IIIB	T4	N0	M0
	T4	N1	M0
	T4	N2	M0
Stage IIIC	Any T	N3	M0
Stage IV	Any T	Any N	M1

*T1 includes T1mic

Note: Stage designation may be changed if post-surgical imaging studies reveal the presence of distant metastases, provided that the studies are carried out within 4 months of diagnosis in the absence of disease progression and provided that the patient has not received neoadjuvant therapy.

Cardiac Compressive Shock

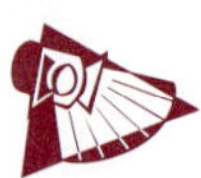

ESSENTIAL FEATURES

- Inadequate perfusion
- Compression of the heart or great veins

EPIDEMIOLOGY

- Pericardial tamponade
- Tension pneumothorax
- Abdominal compartment syndrome
- Diaphragmatic rupture with abdominal viscera in chest

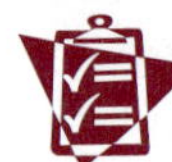

CLINICAL FINDINGS

SYMPTOMS AND SIGNS

- Distended neck veins
- Postural hypotension
- Oliguria
- Sweating
- Mental status changes
- **Kussmaul sign:** Distention of neck veins with deep inspiration is pathognomonic of pericardial tamponade
- **Paradoxic pulse:** A fall of > 10 mm Hg with inspiration supports diagnosis
- Equalization of heart chamber pressures with pulmonary artery catheter placement

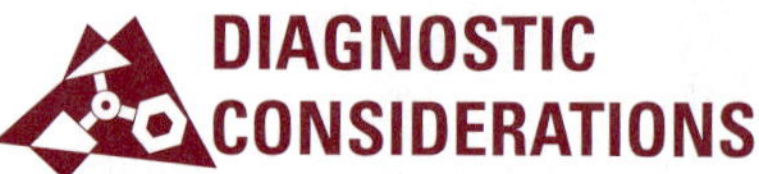

DIAGNOSTIC CONSIDERATIONS

- Mechanism of injury often raises suspicion
- Decision must sometimes be made for intervention without full confirmation of diagnosis, eg, thrombectomy or aspiration for penetrating chest injuries and loss of signs of life

WORK-UP

- Physical exam/trauma work-up

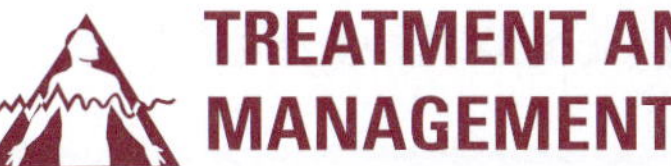

TREATMENT AND MANAGEMENT

- Fluid infusion can bring transient improvement
- Definitive treatment must correct mechanical abnormality
- See Thoracic Injuries and Abdominal Injuries
- See Small Intestine, Obstruction

SURGERY

Indications

- See section on particular etiology

TREATMENT MONITORING

- Blood pressure
- ECG

PROGNOSIS

- Varies with etiology and severity

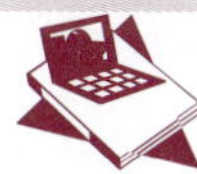

RESOURCES

REFERENCES

- Asensio JA et al. Penetrating cardiac injuries: a prospective study of variables predicting outcomes. *J Am Coll Surg.* 1998;186:24.

Cardiac Tumors

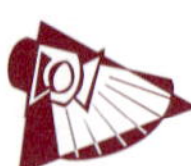

ESSENTIAL FEATURES

- Most common cardiac neoplasm is a metastatic lesion (carcinoma of lung or breast, sarcoma, melanoma)
- 75% of primary cardiac neoplasms are benign (myxoma, rhabdomyoma)

Myxoma

- 75% of benign primary cardiac tumors
- Appearance ranges from smooth, round, firm encapsulated mass to loose conglomeration of gelatinous material
- Most attached to fossa ovalis of left atrial septum; some may occur in right atrium or ventricles
- Histologically, contains various mesenchymal cells
  - Abnormal DNA ploidy may correlate with recurrence
- Papillary fronds attached to aortic valve associated with cerebral and coronary embolization
- Fibromas occur in pediatric patients, slowly invading conduction system
  - Can cause sudden death from arrhythmias

EPIDEMIOLOGY

- Primary tumors of heart are rare
  - 0.002–0.3% of autopsies
- Occur in any age

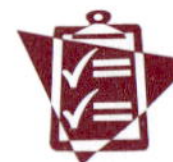

CLINICAL FINDINGS

SYMPTOMS AND SIGNS

- Presentation depends on type and location of tumor
- **Malignant tumors:** Rapidly progressive congestive heart failure from valvular or myocardial infiltration
- **Myxoma:** Fever, weight loss, anemia, systemic embolization
- Mitral stenosis can occur from tumor causing characteristic early diastolic sound "tumor plop"
- Fibromas can cause sudden death from arrhythmias

LABORATORY FINDINGS

- **Myxoma:** Abnormal ESR, gamma globulin, liver aminotransferases
- Anemia, thrombocytopenia common in many tumors
- **Transesophageal echocardiography:** Procedure of choice
- MRI and CT may be helpful in infiltrative lesions

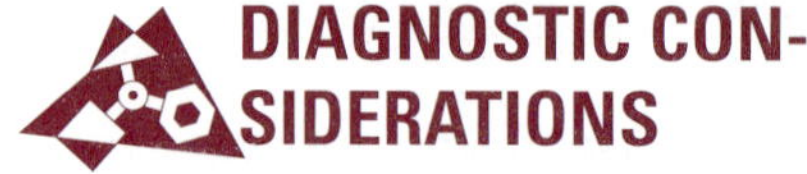

DIAGNOSTIC CONSIDERATIONS

- Evaluate for other sites of tumor

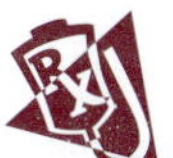

WORK-UP

- Physical exam
- Echocardiography, possibly trans-esophageal
- MRI for invasive lesions

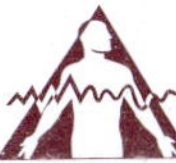

TREATMENT AND MANAGEMENT

- **Most benign lesions:** Resectable/curable
- **Myxomas**
  - Cardiopulmonary bypass required
  - Resect tumor and rim of normal tissue around attachment stalk
- Surgery for cardiac sarcomas and metastatic lesions is usually for diagnosis; occasionally palliative
- Orthotopic heart transplantation (rarely)

SURGERY

Indications

- Suspected myxoma, consider repair

COMPLICATIONS

- Embolization during tumor manipulation

PROGNOSIS

- Operative mortality < 1%
- Long-term survival for malignant cardiac lesions remains poor

PREVENTION

- Resect rim of normal tissue around attachment stalk to prevent recurrence of myxomas

RESOURCES

REFERENCES

- Araoz PA et al. CT and MR imaging of primary cardiac malignancies. *Radiographics.* 1999;19:1421.
- Lobo A et al. Intracardiac masses detected by echocardiography: case presentation and review of the literature. *Clin Cardiol.* 2000;23:702.
- Shapiro LM. Cardiac tumours: diagnosis and management. *Heart.* 2001;85:218.

Cardiogenic Shock

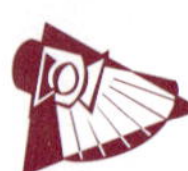

ESSENTIAL FEATURES

- Inadequate tissue perfusion due to heart pump failure

EPIDEMIOLOGY

- Arrhythmia
- Bradycardia (< 50 bpm) or tachycardia (> (230 – age)×0.8)
- Ischemia-induced myocardial failure
- Valvular or septal defects
- Systemic or pulmonary hypertension
- Myocarditis
- Myocardiopathies

CLINICAL FINDINGS

- Elevated right heart/central venous and jugular venous pressure
- Decreased cardiac output
- Peripheral hypoperfusion
- Peripheral edema/pulmonary edema

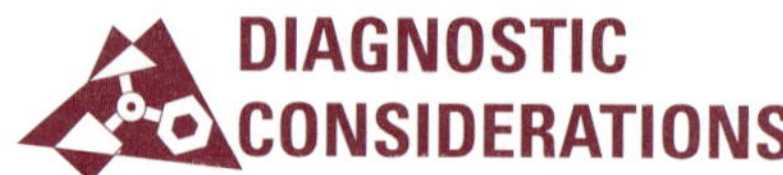

DIAGNOSTIC CONSIDERATIONS

- Intrinsic cardiac dysfunction
- Myocardial ischemia
- Arrhythmia

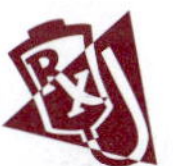

WORK-UP

- Physical exam
- ECG
- Echocardiogram

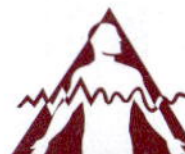

TREATMENT AND MANAGEMENT

- Aimed at underlying medical condition and optimizing cardiac output
- **Opioids** relieve pain, provide sedation, block adrenergic discharge, decrease right ventricular filling, and lessen stress on heart
- **Diuretics** decrease vascular volume, decrease right and left atrial pressures, and alleviate peripheral and pulmonary edema
- **Chronotropes** rarely indicated, should be used to raise heart rate only to tolerable levels
- **Inotropes** increase blood flow in the cardiovascular system
- **Vasodilators** in patients with elevated systemic vascular resistance
- **β-Blockers** in those with ischemia and a rapid heart rate
- **Vasoconstrictors** are occasionally useful to increase coronary perfusion pressure
- Transaortic balloon pump is effective in resuscitating selected patients with severe reversible LV dysfunction

RESOURCES

REFERENCES

- Feliciano DV et al. Advances in the diagnosis and treatment of thoracic trauma. *Surg Clin North Am.* 1999;79:1417.

Cardiomyopathy, Idiopathic

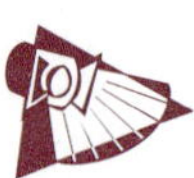

ESSENTIAL FEATURES

- 2 most common causes: dilated (idiopathic) and ischemic
- **Idiopathic**
  - Unknown etiology
  - Often multifactorial resulting in large, dilated heart with poor ventricular function
- **Ischemic**
  - Coronary artery disease causing severe ventricular dysfunction
  - See Cardiomyopathy, Ischemic

EPIDEMIOLOGY

- 60% of patients with NYHA Class IV disease will die within 1 year
- Medical therapy for cardiomyopathy carries dismal prognosis

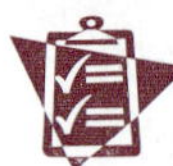

CLINICAL FINDINGS

SYMPTOMS AND SIGNS

- Heart failure symptoms

LABORATORY FINDINGS

- **ECG:** Q waves, widened QRS, conduction defects

IMAGING FINDINGS

- **Chest film:** Pulmonary congestion, enlarged heart

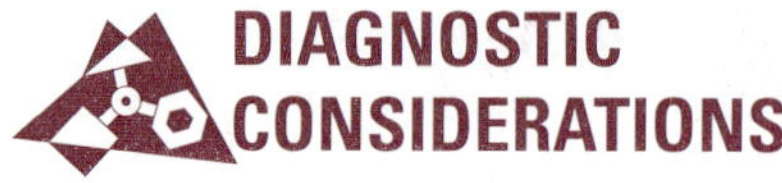

DIAGNOSTIC CONSIDERATIONS

- Echocardiography
- Catheterization

RULE OUT

- Other causes of heart failure

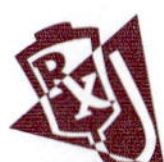

WORK-UP

- Physical exam
- ECG
- Echocardiography

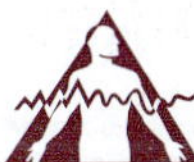

TREATMENT AND MANAGEMENT

- **Idiopathic**
  - Cardiac transplantation may have best long-term results
  - Mitral valve annuloplasty if enlarged annular size from LV enlargement
  - **Batista procedure:** ventricular reduction; limited use
  - **Biventricular pacing:** Restores normal depolarization to ventricles, increasing ejection fraction significantly
- **Ischemic**
  - Consider coronary artery bypass grafting (CABG) if suitable target vessels and evidence of "hibernating" myocardium

SURGERY

Indications

- **CABG:** If suitable target vessels, hibernating myocardium on PET scan or stress thallium
- **Idiopathic:** Cardiac transplantation in suitable candidates

PROGNOSIS

- Batista procedure: Limited survival, high mortality
- Medical therapy carries dismal prognosis
- See Cardiomyopathy, Ischemic

RESOURCES

REFERENCES

- Braile DM et al. Dynamic cardiomyoplasty: long-term clinical results in patients with dilated cardiomyopathy. *Ann Thorac Surg.* 2000;69:1445.
- Starling RC, McCarthy PM. Partial left ventriculectomy: sunrise or sunset? *Eur J Heart Fail.* 1999;1:313.

Cardiomyopathy, Ischemic

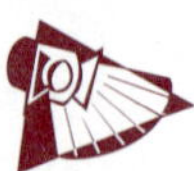

ESSENTIAL FEATURES

- Normal coronary blood flow: 1 mL per gram of myocardium per minute
- Oxygen extraction from coronary bed: 75% at rest, 100% during stress
- Coronary flow primarily during diastole
- Mean coronary resistance is 3–6 times the totally vasodilated value, implying extreme vasodilator reserve
- **Atherosclerosis progression:** Intimal incorporation of lipids → expanding plaque with fibrosis and calcification → finally rupture of plaque causing thrombosis → acute infarction
- Subtotal occlusions important in pathogenesis of unstable angina
- **Usual pattern**
  - Short, proximal stenoses of left coronary artery
  - In right coronary artery, disease more diffuse, involving proximal and middle portions of artery
  - Patients with type 1 diabetes mellitus have diffuse disease
- Blood flow may be adequate at rest; exercise and stress may produce ischemia
- **Acute coronary insufficiency (angina pectoris):** Immediate decrease in myocardial work
- After only 15 minutes of reversible ischemia, may take 24–48 hrs for complete recovery

EPIDEMIOLOGY

- Coronary artery disease responsible for 20% deaths
- Cardiovascular disease accounts for > 40% of all deaths
- Atherosclerosis identified in up to 50% of autopsies of patients in second decade of life
- **Risk factors**
  - Smoking (secondhand increases death rate from coronary disease by 30%; smoking cessation decreases coronary risk by 50% after 1 year of abstinence)
  - Hypercholesterolemia
  - Male
  - Diabetes mellitus
  - Hypertension
  - Family history
  - Obesity
  - Inactivity
- Coronary mortality rate directly proportional to number of vessels affected and LV function

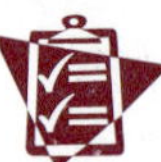

CLINICAL FINDINGS

SYMPTOMS AND SIGNS

- Retrosternal chest pain
  - Pressure
  - Choking
  - Tightness
  - Frequently radiates down left arm, left neck, occasionally right arm, mandible, ear
- Exercise, cold exposure, eating can precipitate symptoms
- Stable, progressive, or unstable angina
- Pulmonary edema from ischemia (poor prognosis)
- Some have no symptoms (silent myocardial ischemia)

LABORATORY FINDINGS

- **ECG**
  - Normal in 50% of patients
  - May have inverted T waves, ST segment abnormalities, or Q waves at rest

IMAGING FINDINGS

- **Coronary angiography:** Highest sensitivity and specificity of any test available (10% of patients underestimated)
- **Screening**
  - Stress ECG
  - Stress echocardiography
  - Dobutamine echocardiography
  - Stress thallium may identify viability

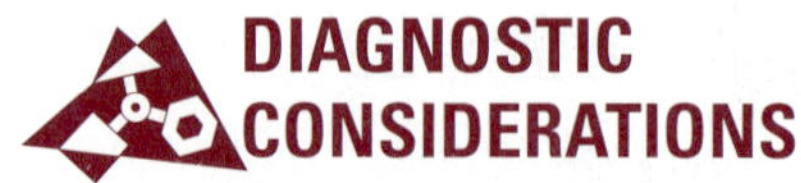

DIAGNOSTIC CONSIDERATIONS

- Consider other causes of chest pain, including gastroesophageal reflux disease, aneurysms, aortic dissection

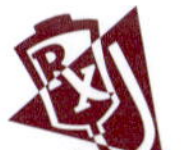

WORK-UP

- Screening test
- If high suspicion, proceed to angiography

TREATMENT AND MANAGEMENT

- **Risk reduction:** Smoking cessation, hypertension control, lipid reduction
- Percutaneous transluminal coronary angioplasty (> 90% successful but repeat interventions common)
- **Operative therapy:** Complete revascularization associated with improved outcome
- Evaluate carotid bruits, renal function, respiratory status, coagulation studies

Conventional Coronary Artery Bypass Grafting (CABG)

- Internal mammary (preferred), saphenous vein, or radial artery used to bypass on average 3–4 coronary vessels
- Graft patency affected by smoking, low-density lipoprotein

Minimally Invasive

- Off-pump coronary artery bypass (OPCAB)
  - Performed without cardiopulmonary bypass
  - Best for left anterior descending, diagonal, proximal right coronary arteries
- Transmyocardial laser revascularization (TMR)
  - For inoperable coronary disease, > 70% have symptomatic improvement, without change in survival

SURGERY

Indications

- Severe or progressive angina on medical therapy
- Refractory unstable angina
- Significant left main coronary disease
- Multivessel coronary disease in persons with diabetes
- Ventricular impairment with reduced ejection fraction

MEDICATIONS

- Nitroglycerin, β-blockers, calcium channel blockers, aspirin
- Heparin effective in preventing infarction in setting of unstable angina
- Glycoprotein IIB/IIIA inhibitors (abciximab, tirofiban) for unstable angina
- **Postinfarction patients:** ACE inhibitors improve remodeling

COMPLICATIONS

- **Graft closure**
  - < 30 days, technical error, poor graft quality, poor runoff
  - 1 month to 3 years, intimal hyperplasia
  - > 3 years, graft atherosclerosis

PROGNOSIS

- **CABG**
  - 5-year and 10-year survival: 92% and 81%
  - Angina free at 5 years and 10 years: 83% and 63%
  - Poor with continued smoking, diabetes, advanced age, reduced ejection fraction, nonuse of internal mammary artery
- < 1% require repeat revascularization within 4 years
- Operative mortality = 2.8%
- **Surgery:** 39% and 17% reduction in mortality at 5 and 10 years
- Minimal angina (stable) easily tolerated
- Worsening angina or unstable angina has poor prognosis

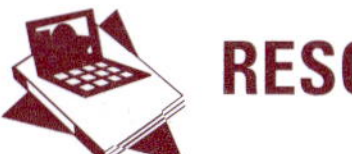

RESOURCES

REFERENCES

- Eagle KA et al. ACC/AHA Guidelines for Coronary Artery Bypass Graft Surgery: a Report of the American College of Cardiology/American Heart Association Task Force on Practice Guidelines (Committee to Revise the 1991 Guidelines for Coronary Artery Bypass Graft Surgery). American College of Cardiology/American Heart Association. *J Am Coll Cardiol.* 1999;34:1262.
- Hannan EL et al. A comparison of three-year survival after coronary artery bypass graft surgery and percutaneous transluminal coronary angioplasty. *J Am Coll Cardiol.* 1999;33:63.
- Myers WO et al. CASS Registry long term surgical survival. Coronary Artery Surgery Study. *J Am Coll Cardiol.* 1999;33:488.

Carotid Aneurysms, Extracranial

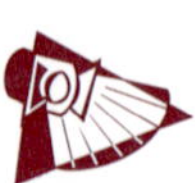

ESSENTIAL FEATURES

- Rare
- May occur anywhere along extracranial portion

EPIDEMIOLOGY

True Aneurysms

- Caused by
  - Atherosclerosis
  - Occasionally by cystic medial necrosis, Marfan syndrome, or fibromuscular dysplasia

False Aneurysms

- Occur rarely after carotid endarterectomy
- Occur as result of trauma, or infection (pharyngeal abscess)

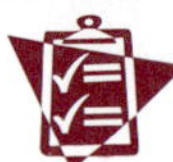

CLINICAL FINDINGS

SYMPTOMS AND SIGNS

- Pulsatile neck mass
- Dysphagia can occur from protrusion into oropharynx
- Neck pain, radiating to jaw
- 30% present with transient ischemic attacks
- Rupture (more common with false aneurysms) into oropharynx, ear canal, soft tissues of neck

IMAGING FINDINGS

- **Duplex US:** Initial test
- Arteriography necessary to plan surgery

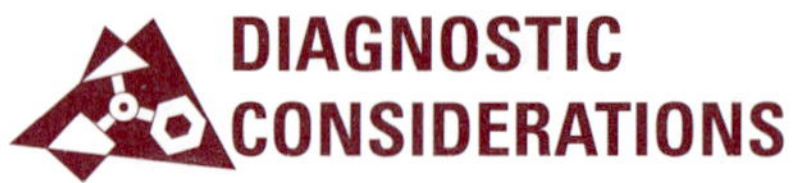

DIAGNOSTIC CONSIDERATIONS

- Duplex US will differentiate redundant carotid artery from aneurismal and identify occlusive disease

RULE OUT

- Coiled or redundant carotid artery, subclavian artery (can present as pulsatile neck mass)

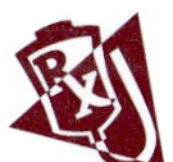

WORK-UP

- Duplex US
- Angiography prior to surgery
- Consider CT if infection or traumatic

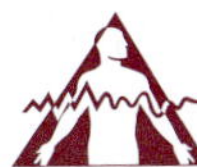

TREATMENT AND MANAGEMENT

- If accessible, resect and replace aneurysm with graft or vein
- Endovascular stenting may be an option
- False aneurysms should be repaired
- Can ligate extensive aneurysm if back pressure > 65 mm Hg
  - Can identify potential candidates with awake arteriography and balloon occlusion

SURGERY

Indications

- True or false aneurysm

PROGNOSIS

- Good if repairable

RESOURCES

PREFERENCES

- El-Sabrout R et al. Extracranial carotid artery aneurysms: Texas Heart Institute experience. *J Vasc Surg.* 2000;31:702.
- Rosset E et al. Surgical treatment of extracranial internal carotid artery aneurysms. *J Vasc Surg.* 2000;31:713.

Carotid Body Tumor

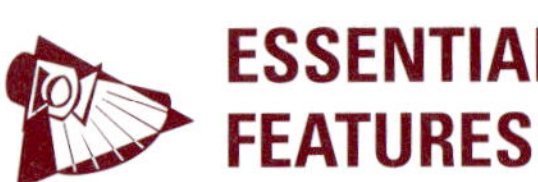

ESSENTIAL FEATURES

Carotid Body

- Normal carotid body 3–6 mm
- Nest of chemoreceptor cells of neuroectodermal origin
- Responds to decrease in PO_2, increase in PCO_2, decrease in pH, or blood temperature increase
- Results in increase in blood pressure, heart rate, depth and rate of respiration

Carotid Sinus

- In contrast, carotid sinus is baroreceptor
- Stimulation causes reflex bradycardia and hypotension
- **Tumors of carotid body**
  - Cervical chemodectomas
  - Paragangliomas
  - Glomus tumors
  - Nonchromaffin paragangliomas
- 10% metastatic
- Histologically, tumors resemble normal carotid body
- Often extends to local structures

EPIDEMIOLOGY

- Incidence equal in genders
- Bilaterality is common when tumor is familial
- Incidence increased in hypoxic persons (cyanotic heart disease, high altitude)

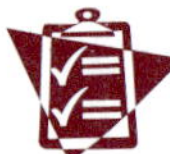

CLINICAL FINDINGS

SYMPTOMS AND SIGNS

- Slow enlargement of asymptomatic cervical mass
- Rarely, hypertension secondary to release of catecholamines
- Rarely, cranial nerve dysfunction from tumor extension
- Solitary midlateral pulsatile neck mass that is firm and rubbery
- Mass mobile in horizontal plane not vertical plan
- 50% bruits

IMAGING FINDINGS

- Duplex scanning is often diagnostic
- **Angiography:** Characteristic tumor blush at carotid bifurcation, with wide separation of internal and external carotid arteries

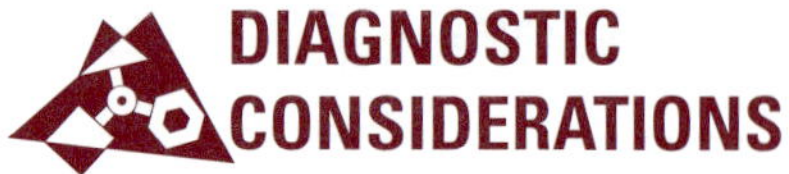

DIAGNOSTIC CONSIDERATIONS

- Duplex scanning often diagnostic
- Angiography shows characteristic tumor blush at carotid bifurcation, with wide separation of internal and external carotid arteries
- Percutaneous needle or incisional biopsy is dangerous

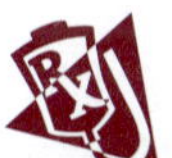

WORK-UP

- Physical exam
- Cervical US
- CT scan or MRI

TREATMENT AND MANAGEMENT

- **Preferred treatment:** Complete excision and possible arterial reconstruction
- Radiation therapy and chemotherapy not helpful
- Preoperative embolization carries risk of stroke and generally not performed

COMPLICATIONS

- > 40% incidence of cranial nerve dysfunction after resection

RESOURCES

REFERENCES

- Westerband A et al. Current trends in the detection and management of carotid body tumors. *J Vasc Surg.* 1998;28:84.

Cellulitis

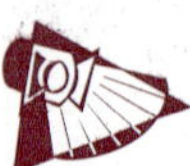

ESSENTIAL FEATURES

- Common invasive nonsuppurative infection of connective tissue
- Diffuse inflammation in the absence of findings indicating necrotizing infection
- Usually appears on an extremity
- A surgical wound, puncture, skin ulcer, or patch of dermatitis is usually identifiable as a portal of entry
- Most often caused by group A streptococci and *S aureus*

EPIDEMIOLOGY

- Often occurs in susceptible patients, eg, alcoholics with postphlebitic leg ulcers
- Cellulitis due to gram-negative bacterial infection (*Proteus mirabilis* and *Klebsiella*) may develop in immunocompromised patients

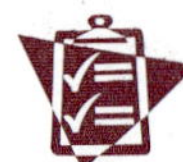

CLINICAL FINDINGS

SYMPTOMS AND SIGNS

- Brawny red or reddish-brown area of edematous skin
- Advances rapidly from its starting point, and the advancing edge may be vague or sharply defined
- Moderate or high fever is almost always present
- Warm, erythematous, edematous area
- Painful spreading inflammation of the skin
- Nonelevatated, poorly defined, advancing margins
- Lymphangitis arising from cellulitis produces red, warm, tender streaks 3–4 mm wide leading from the infection along lymphatic vessels

LABORATORY FINDINGS

- Most cases are caused by streptococci or staphylococci, but other bacteria have been involved
- Bacteria are difficult to obtain for culture
- Blood cultures positive only 2% of the time
- Needle aspiration yields positive cultures only 20–40% of the time
- Leukocytosis

IMAGING FINDINGS

- Radiographs may reveal nonspecific edematous soft tissue

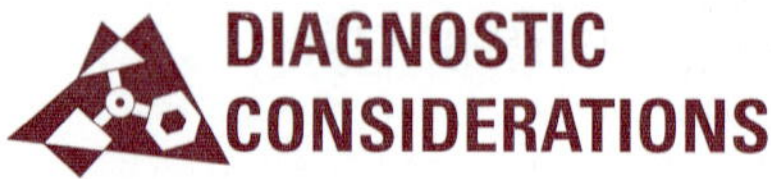

DIAGNOSTIC CONSIDERATIONS

- Thrombophlebitis
- Contact dermatitis
- Chemical inflammation due to drug injection
- Hemorrhagic bullae and skin necrosis suggests necrotizing fasciitis

RULE OUT

- Must be distinguished from necrotizing infection

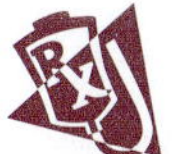

WORK-UP

- Complete history and physical exam
- History of open wound, break in skin, puncture
- Swab may be taken from lesion for culture

WHEN TO ADMIT

- High fever, spreading inflammation, failure of oral antibiotic regimen
- Cellulitis of the face, hand, orbits, periorbital region

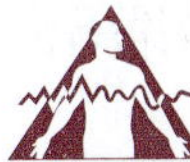

TREATMENT AND MANAGEMENT

- Therapy should consist of rest, elevation, warm packs, and a PO or IV antibiotic
- Warm packs may be used to elevate subcutaneous tissue temperature
- Treatment is predominantly nonoperative

SURGERY

Indications

- If there is progression to necrotizing infection
- Abscesses require drainage

MEDICATIONS

- Penicillins or first-generation cephalosporins given IV

TREATMENT MONITORING

- If a clear response has not occurred in 12–24 hours, an abscess should be suspected or consider the possibility that the causative agent is a gram-negative rod or resistant organism
- Patient must be examined once daily or more often to detect a hidden abscess masquerading within or under an area of cellulitis

COMPLICATIONS

- Sepsis

RESOURCES

REFERENCES

- Cobb JP et al. Inflammation, Infection, & Antibiotics. In: Way LW, Doherty GM (editors). *Current Surgical Diagnosis & Treatment,* 11e. New York: McGraw-Hill; 2003:123.

Cerebrovascular Disease, Atherosclerotic

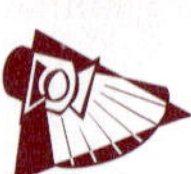

ESSENTIAL FEATURES

- Symptoms more often result from emboli than hypoperfusion
- 80% of patients with occlusive cerebrovascular disease have accessible arterial lesion in neck/chest
- When blood supply decreases below critical level, cellular death occurs in minutes
- Embolization most common mechanism of stroke from carotid lesions
- Most strokes due to lesions of internal carotid but can be from innominate/aorta
- Low wall shear stress, flow separation, loss of unidirectional flow may lead to atherosclerosis in carotid bulb
- Neurologic dysfunction without infarction can be produced in 2 ways:
  1. Cerebral embolization by microembolic fragments
  2. Transient reduction in cerebral perfusion
- Antiplatelet therapy decreases stroke rates by 5%

EPIDEMIOLOGY

- 33% of patients who have had transient ischemic attacks (TIAs) eventually suffer stroke
- 20% of patients with amaurosis fugax will suffer stroke
- Stroke risk after TIA correlates with severity of internal carotid stenosis
- Mortality from initial stroke is 20–30%
- Subclavian stenosis more common in left artery than in right

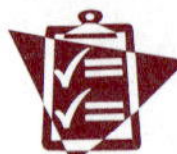

CLINICAL FINDINGS

SYMPTOMS

- **Asymptomatic disease**
  - Bruit may be heard
- **TIA**
  - Short-lived paresis or numbness of contralateral arm or leg that lasts < 24 h
  - Symptoms depend on location and size of embolus, which determines rate of dissolution
- **Amaurosis fugax**
  - Microembolus to ophthalmic artery produces temporary mononuclear vision loss (lamp shade), Hollenhorst plaques (emboli visible in retina)
- **Acute unstable neurologic defect**
  - Patients may have crescendo TIA, stroke in evolution, waxing and waning deficits
  - Treat urgently or may progress to stroke
- **Completed stroke**
  - 50% will suffer another stroke
- **Vertebrobasilar disease**
  - Emboli or hypoperfusion of posterior system causes drop attacks, clumsiness, vertigo, diplopia, dysphagia, dysequilibrium

SIGNS

- **Palpation**
  - Only the pulse of common carotid can be felt directly
  - Thus, internal carotid may be occluded even when neck pulse is normal
- **Bruits**
  - High in lateral neck indicates common carotid bifurcation stenosis
  - Of lower trapezius indicates vertebral stenosis
  - Along full length of right common carotid and subclavian indicates innominate stenosis
- **Brachial blood pressure discrepancy**
  - Indicates arterial stenosis (greater in left subclavian artery than in right)
- **Subclavian steal syndrome**
  - Neurologic symptoms upon exercise of upper extremity due to reversal of vertebral artery flow (collateral to arm)
  - Arm effort fatigue with proximal stenosis

IMAGING FINDINGS

- **Carotid duplex US:** Screening for stenosis
- **Cerebral arteriography:** Provide extracranial and intracranial anatomy of carotid and vertebral arteries

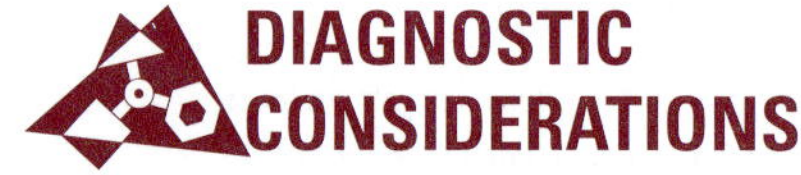

DIAGNOSTIC CONSIDERATIONS

- Carotid duplex US useful to demonstrate plaque morphology and degree of stenosis rapidly and accurately
- Carotid duplex US velocity criteria indicates degree of luminal narrowing—increases with increased stenosis

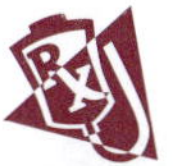

WORK-UP

- Duplex US is initial test
- Arteriogram should be only done selectively
- **NASCET trial:** Reported in 2 major parts
  - Symptomatic patients with 70–99% stenosis randomized to receive aspirin alone or aspirin plus carotid endarterectomy
  - 2-year stroke rate was 26% for aspirin alone vs 9% for aspirin plus carotid endarterectomy
  - In patients with moderate stenosis (50-69%), 2-year stroke rate was 22% for aspirin alone versus 16% for aspirin plus carotid endarterectomy
- **ACAS trial**
  - Patients with asymptomatic stenosis of 60% or more were randomized to medical therapy or carotid endarterectomy
  - 5-year stroke risk was 11% in aspirin group and 5% in aspirin plus carotid endarterectomy group

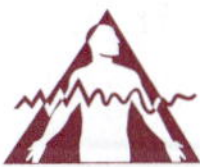

TREATMENT AND MANAGEMENT

- Objective to prevent TIAs and strokes
- Aspirin plus risk factor reduction
- Endarterectomy preferred for lesions of internal carotid, right vertebral, and right subclavian arteries
- Left vertebral artery best to transplant onto adjacent common carotid artery
- **Left proximal carotid stenosis:** Left carotid-subclavian bypass
- Carotid stenting may be more common in future

SURGERY

Indications

- (A)symptomatic 80–99% on duplex US
- Subclavian steal syndrome (carotid-subclavian bypass)

Contraindications

- Recent stroke (relative)

MEDICATIONS

- Aspirin (clopidogrel may be slightly more effective to decrease risk of stroke)
- Low-density lipoprotein lowering agents
- Hypertension treatment
- Smoking cessation
- Anticoagulation has no effect on risk of future stroke

COMPLICATIONS

- Stroke (ranges from 1% to 5% depending on if symptomatic and contralateral supply to brain)
- Death
- Permanent nerve injury < 5% (CN XII injury most common)

PROGNOSIS

- Excellent if no stroke perioperatively

RESOURCES

REFERENCES

- Endarterectomy for asymptomatic carotid artery stenosis. Executive Committee for the Asymptomatic Carotid Atherosclerosis Study (ACAS). *JAMA.* 1995;273:1421.
- Ferguson GG et al. The North American Symptomatic Carotid Endarterectomy Trial: surgical results in 1415 patients. *Stroke.* 1999;30:1751.
- Roubin GS et al. Immediate and late clinical outcomes of carotid artery stenting in patients with symptomatic and asymptomatic carotid artery stenosis: a 5-year prospective analysis. *Circulation.* 2001;103:532.

Cerebrovascular Disease, Nonatherosclerotic

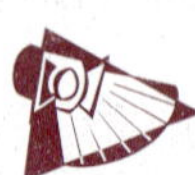

ESSENTIAL FEATURES

- Primary disease of extracranial arteries other than atherosclerosis is rare

Takayasu Arteritis

- Obliterative arteriopathy involving aortic arch vessels
- Abdominal aorta and pulmonary arteries can be affected

Internal Carotid Dissection

- Originates in internal carotid artery
- Acute event that narrows or obliterates lumen
- Primary lesion is intimal tear at distal end of carotid bulb
- May develop spontaneously

Fibromuscular Dysplasia

- Nonatherosclerotic angiopathy, unknown cause affects specific arteries
- Usually bilateral disease, involves middle third of internal carotid
- Irregular zones of overgrowing media, causing concentric rings
- 20% already had stroke at presentation

EPIDEMIOLOGY

Takayasu Arteritis

- More common in women

Internal Carotid Dissection

- Due to trauma or hypertension
- Most frequent in young adults

Fibromuscular Dysplasia

- Primarily young women affected

CLINICAL FINDINGS

SYMPTOMS AND SIGNS

Internal Carotid Dissection

- Ipsilateral cerebral ischemic symptoms
- Acute neck pain, cervical tenderness at the angle of mandible

Fibromuscular Dysplasia

- 20% already had stroke

IMAGING FINDINGS

Internal Carotid Dissection

- **Duplex US:** Indicates narrowing
- **Arteriography:** Characteristic tapered narrowing; if lumen persists, it resumes normal caliber beyond bony foramen

Fibromuscular Dysplasia

- **Arteriography:** Characteristic "string of beads" appearance

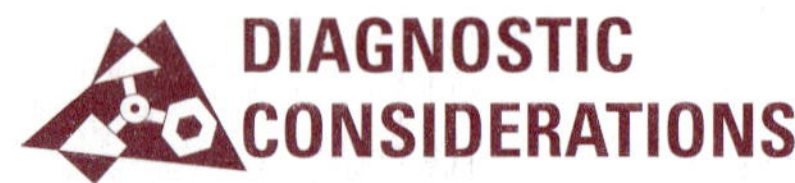

DIAGNOSTIC CONSIDERATIONS

RULE OUT

- Atherosclerotic cerebral disease
- Takayasu arteritis
- Dissecting aortic aneurysm
- Internal carotid dissection
- Fibromuscular dysplasia

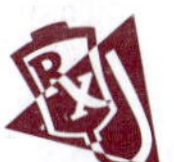

WORK-UP

- Duplex US
- Arteriography

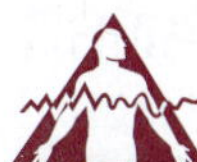

TREATMENT AND MANAGEMENT

Takayasu Arteritis

- Corticosteroids and cyclophosphamide are effective
- Operative treatment avoided unless active arteritis

Internal Carotid Dissection

- Anticoagulation treatment of choice
  - In most cases, intramural clot is resorbed restoring normal lumen
- Operation only for recurrent transient ischemic attacks (TIAs)
  - If dissection only proximal, replace segment with graft,
  - If stump pressure > 65 mm Hg, consider proximal ligation
  - Extracranial-intracranial bypass possible

Fibromuscular Dysplasia

- High incidence of neurologic disability
  - Correct surgically—intraoperative graduated balloon dilation

SURGERY

Indications

- Recurrent TIAs

RESOURCES

REFERENCES

- Diwan A et al. Incidence of femoral and popliteal aneurysms in patients with abdominal aortic aneurysms. *J Vasc Surg.* 2000;31:863.

Chest Wall Osteomyelitis

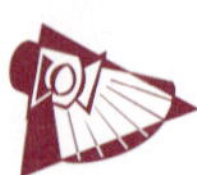

ESSENTIAL FEATURES

- Can occur in ribs or sternum
- In past, caused by typhoid or TB
- Sternal infections common after median sternotomy
  - Increased risk among diabetics in whom bilateral internal mammary arteries have been used for coronary artery bypass grafting
- In children, caused by hematogenous infection

EPIDEMIOLOGY

- **Ribs:** Due to hematogenous osteomyelitis, which is rare except in children
- **Sternum:** Occurs in 1–2% after sternotomy
- Often gram-positive, but occasionally due to TB

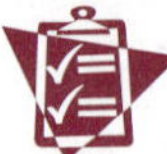

CLINICAL FINDINGS

SYMPTOMS AND SIGNS

- **Sternum:** Postoperative wound infection or medistinitis
- Serous drainage increases suspicion
- Sternal click signifies nonunion of bone and may be due to infection
- Erythema
- Fever
- Fluctuance

LABORATORY FINDINGS

- Elevated WBC count

IMAGING FINDINGS

- **Chest film:** Substernal air may be deep infection
- CT scan can confirm
- PET scan
- Gallium scan

DIAGNOSTIC CONSIDERATIONS

- Differentiate superficial from deep infection using imaging studies and clinical suspicion

RULE OUT

- Costal cartilage infection
- Bone tumor
- Cartilage tumor
- Tietze syndrome
- Chest wall metastasis
- Eroding aortic aneurysm
- Bronchocutaneous fistula

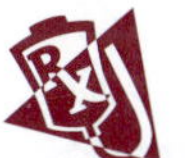

WORK-UP

- Physical exam
- Chest film
- CT scan
- Gallium or PET scan if questionable

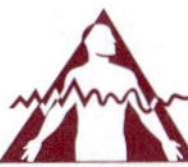

TREATMENT AND MANAGEMENT

- Differentiate superficial from deep infection
  - Topical antibiotics, wound packing, IV antibiotics for superficial infection
  - Surgery for deep infection

SURGERY

Indications

- **Deep infection:** Aggressive debridement with cultures and muscle flap closure
- Debridement and closed drainage system is alternate method of treatment
- Continue IV antibiotics

MEDICATIONS

- IV antibiotics

TREATMENT MONITORING

- Temperature, continued drainage, healing of bone, and pain
- Can be difficult to clear infection

RESOURCES

REFERENCES

- Mansour KA et al. Sternal resection and reconstruction. *Ann Thorac Surg.* 1993;55:838.
- Siegman-Igra Y et al. Serious infectious complications of midsternotomy: a review of bacteriology and antimicrobial therapy. *Scand J Infect Dis.* 1990;22:633.

Chest Wall Tumors, Benign Skeletal

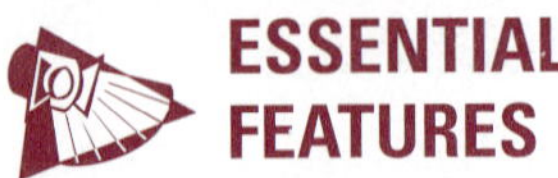

ESSENTIAL FEATURES

Fibrous Dysplasia

- Accounts for 33% of benign skeletal tumors
- Involves ribs 50% of time
- Not associated with hyperparathyroidism
- Usually single tumor, associated with trauma

Chondromas, Osteochondromas, Myxochomdromas

- Combined equal 30–45% of benign skeletal tumors

Eosinophilic Granuloma

- Occurs in clavicle and scapula usually; rarely in sternum
- Lung infiltrates are common
- Benign form of Litterer-Siwe disease or Hand-Schuller-Christian disease

Hemangioma

- Cavernous hemangioma of ribs
  - Painful mass during childhood
- Multiple radiolucent areas or single trabeculated cyst seen on radiograph

EPIDEMIOLOGY

Chondroma

- Occurs equally among males and females, between childhood and fourth decade

CLINICAL FINDINGS

SYMPTOMS AND SIGNS

- Most often painless
- Swelling and tenderness may occur with fibrous dysplasia
- Chondromas occur along anterior costal margin
- Lung infiltrates—consider eosinophilic granuloma
- Fever, malaise, leukocytosis—consider eosinophilic granuloma
- Bone pain—consider eosinophilic granuloma

IMAGING FINDINGS

- X-ray often diagnostic
- Lung infiltrates—consider eosinophilic granuloma

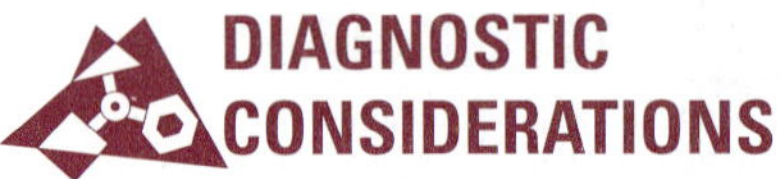

DIAGNOSTIC CONSIDERATIONS

- Can be difficult to distinguish from malignant lesions

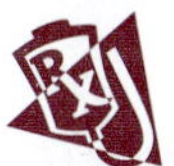

WORK-UP

- Physical exam to assess skin involvement
- CT scan of thorax including bone windows
- Bone scan
- Incisional biopsy for large mass (> 4 cm)
- Excisional biopsy if small and amenable

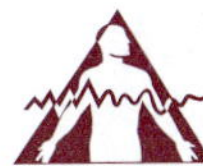

TREATMENT AND MANAGEMENT

- Wide local excision often necessary for cure

RESOURCES

REFERENCES

- Burt M et al. Primary bony and cartilaginous sarcomas of chest wall: results of therapy. *Ann Thorac Surg.* 1992;54:226.
- Brodsky JT et al. Desmoid tumors of the chest wall: a locally recurrent problem. *J Thorac Surg.* 1992;104:900.

Chest Wall Tumors, Benign Soft Tissue

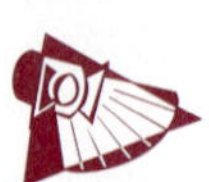

ESSENTIAL FEATURES

- **Lipomas**
  - Most common benign tumors
  - Small potential for malignancy
  - Dumbbell-shaped
- **Neurogenic tumors**
  - Arise from intercostal nerves
  - Solitary neurofibromas most common
- **Cavernous hemangiomas**
  - Usually painful
  - Occur in children
  - If involves lung, consider Rendu-Osler-Weber syndrome
- **Lymphangiomas**
  - Rare lesion seen in kids
  - Poorly defined borders

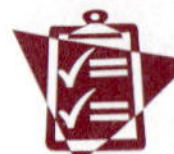

CLINICAL FINDINGS

SYMPTOMS AND SIGNS

- Mostly asymptomatic
- Cavernous hemangiomas can be painful

IMAGING FINDINGS

- US and CT may be helpful

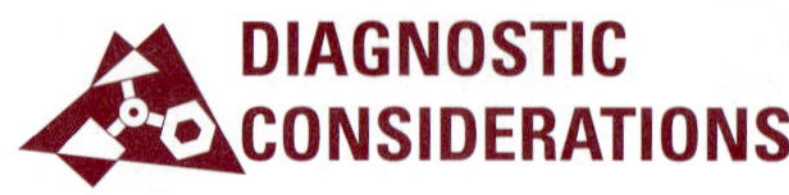

DIAGNOSTIC CONSIDERATIONS

RULE OUT

- Neoplasm

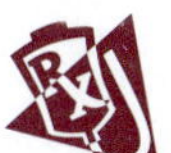

WORK-UP

- Physical exam
- If tumor not solely subcutaneous, CT scan
- Excisional biopsy for small, amenable lesions, otherwise incisional biopsy

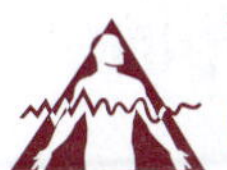

TREATMENT AND MANAGEMENT

SURGERY

Indications

- Growing tumors should be excised
- If large (> 5 cm), consider incisional biopsy to rule out malignancy

RESOURCES

REFERENCES

- Kim JY et al. Atypical benign lipomatous tumors in the soft tissue. *J Comp Assist Tomog.* 2002;26:1063.

Chest Wall Tumors, Malignant Skeletal

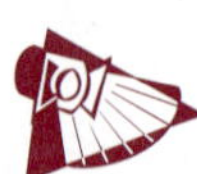

ESSENTIAL FEATURES

- Chondrosarcomas, osteosarcomas, myelomas, Ewing sarcoma, lymphoma, and metastatic cancer

Chondrosarcoma

- Most common primary malignancy of chest wall (30%)
- Commonly develop at costochondral junction
- First 4 ribs commonly affected; spreads locally

Osteosarcoma

- More malignant than chondrosarcoma
- Propensity to metastasize to lung or bone
- < 5% arise in chest wall
- Majority present on extremity

Myeloma

- Rare lesions, causing 5–20% of chest wall tumors
- 75% of the time solitary chest wall plasmacytomas are harbingers of diffuse disease

Ewing Sarcoma

- 10–15% of primary chest wall tumors
- < 15% present in chest

Metastatic

- Kidney, thyroid, lung, breast, prostate, stomach, uterus, or colon
- Renal and thyroid high propensity to metastasize to sternum
- Direct extension occurs with breast and lung cancers

EPIDEMIOLOGY

Chondrosarcomas

- Patients are 20- to 40-years-old

Osteosarcoma

- Patients are 20- to 40-years-old
- 60% of cases occur in men;40% in women

Myeloma

- Patients are 40- to 60-years-old
- More common in men

Ewing Sarcoma

- Disease of childhood/adolescence

CLINICAL FINDINGS

SYMPTOMS AND SIGNS

- Pain is rare
- Mass
- Ewing sarcoma
  - Large, warm, painful, soft-tissue mass
  - Systemic symptoms common, including fever, malaise, weight loss
- Metastatic disease may present as pulsatile mass due to vascularity

IMAGING FINDINGS

Chondrosarcoma

- **Radiography**
  - Destruction of cortical bone with ossification
  - Tumor border indistinct

Osteosarcoma

- **Radiography**
  - Bone destruction and recalcification at right angles causing characteristic "sunburst" appearance

Myeloma

- **Radiography**
  - Classic "punched-out" lytic lesion without new bone formation

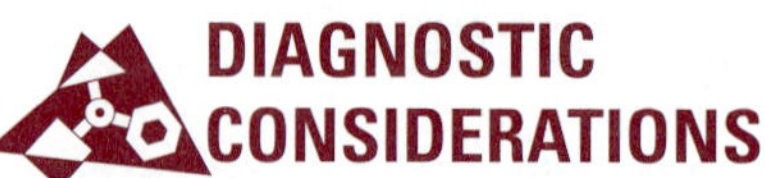

DIAGNOSTIC CONSIDERATIONS

- **Ewing sarcoma**
  - Fine-needle aspiration cytology or incisional biopsy to diagnose
  - Histology reveals broad sheets of small polyhedral cells with pale cytoplasm staining periodic acid-Schiff-positive

RULE OUT

- Aortic aneurysm before obtaining biopsy specimen of any lesion, especially if pulsatile

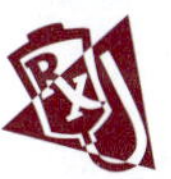

WORK-UP

- Physical exam
- Chest film
- Chest CT scan
- Incisional or excisional biopsy depending on size and configuration

TREATMENT AND MANAGEMENT

- Wide excision, en bloc
- Negative margins is goal
- Postoperative chemotherapy for osteosarcoma

SURGERY

Indications

- Large tumors (> 20 cm) can be cured surgically
- Important in diagnosis of myeloma

MEDICATIONS

- Radiation therapy is useful in myeloma to control pain
- Chemotherapy is primary treatment for myeloma
- Chemotherapy followed by radiation therapy or surgery for Ewing sarcoma

TREATMENT MONITORING

- Local recurrence portends future metastatic disease

PROGNOSIS

Chondrosarcoma

- Positive margins much worse prognosis
- Histologic grade clear predictor
  - Low grade: 5-year, 60-80%
  - High grade: 5-year, 25%

Osteosarcoma

- 5-year survival, 15%
- Metastases will develop in 60–70% of resected cancers

Myeloma

- 5-year survival, 35–40%; 10-year survival, 15–20%

Ewing Sarcoma

- Most important: Distant metastasis
- 5-year survival, 15–48%

RESOURCES

REFERENCES

- Burt M. Primary malignant tumors of the chest wall. The Memorial Sloan-Kettering Cancer Center experience. *Chest Surg Clin North Am.* 1994;4:137.
- Burt M et al. Primary bony and cartilaginous sarcomas of chest wall: results of therapy. *Ann Thorac Surg.* 1992;54:226.

PRACTICE GUIDELINES

- The National Comprehensive Cancer Network http://www.nccn.org/

Chest Wall Tumors, Malignant Soft Tissue

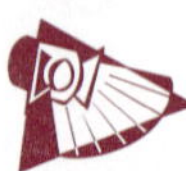

ESSENTIAL FEATURES

- Up to 50% of all malignant chest wall masses
- Only 5% of all malignant soft-tissue sarcomas located in chest wall
- Prognosis determined by histologic grade, completeness of resection, and metastatic disease
- Metastasize commonly to lungs (75%)
- Types of tumors:
  - Desmoids: Low grade
  - Fibrosarcoma: Most common in this location, especially in young adults
  - Liposarcoma: 33% of all primary cancers of chest wall, especially in men
  - Neurofibrosarcomas: 2 × more common in this location than any other, often in Recklinghausen disease, originating from intercostals nerves

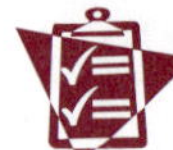

CLINICAL FINDINGS

IMAGING FINDINGS

- US, CT, and MRI can be useful

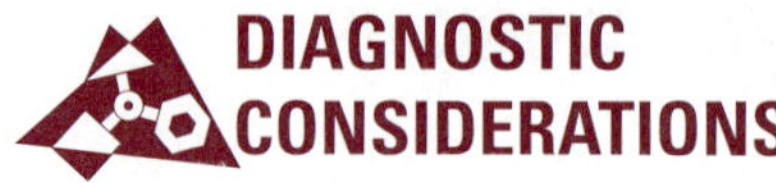

DIAGNOSTIC CONSIDERATIONS

- Most often metastasize to lungs

RULE OUT

- Metastatic disease with chest CT

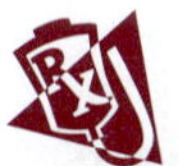

WORK-UP

- Physical exam
- Chest film
- Chest CT scan
- Incisional or excisional biopsy depending on size and configuration

TREATMENT AND MANAGEMENT

- Goal to achieve negative margins (1–2 cm)
- Marlex mesh/methyl methacrylate to correct chest wall deformity
- Soft-tissue flaps for coverage
- **Positive margins:** Radiation therapy
- Adjuvant chemotherapy if high grade

SURGERY

Indications

- Resectable lesion
- Localized metatstatic disease to lungs if amenable to negative margins

PROGNOSIS

- Depends on histologic grade
  - Low grade: 5-year survival, 90%
  - High grade: 5-year survival, 30–50%
- Completeness of surgical resection helps determine
- Metastases greatly decrease survival

RESOURCES

REFERENCES

- Burt M. Primary malignant tumors of the chest wall. The Memorial Sloan-Kettering Cancer Center experience. *Chest Surg Clin North Am.* 1994;4:137.

PRACTICE GUIDELINES

- The National Comprehensive Cancer Network http://www.nccn.org/

Cholangiocarcinoma

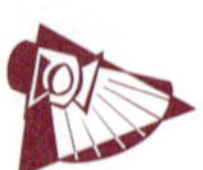

ESSENTIAL FEATURES

- Arises from biliary epithelium
- Risk factors
  - Primary sclerosing cholangitis
  - Choledochal cysts
  - *Clonorchis* infection

EPIDEMIOLOGY

- < 4500 patients per year
- Average age, 50–70 years
- Evenly distributed among men and women

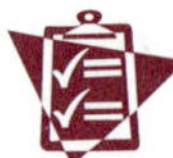

CLINICAL FINDINGS

SYMPTOMS AND SIGNS

- Painless jaundice
- Right upper quadrant pain
- Pruritus
- Anorexia
- Malaise
- Weight loss
- Cholangitis
- Asymptomatic

LABORATORY FINDINGS

- Hyperbilirubinemia
- Elevated alkaline phosphatase
- Elevated CA 19-9

IMAGING FINDINGS

- US showing dilated extrahepatic and intrahepatic biliary ducts (depending on level of tumor)
- CT or MRI with biliary dilatation and occasional visible hepatic tumor
- Percutaneous transhepatic cholangiography (PTC) or magnetic resonance cholangiopancreatography (MRCP) visualizing proximal and distal extent of tumor
  - PTC provides opportunity for brushings for cytologic studies of tumor
- Mesenteric angiography for question of portal vasculature involvement

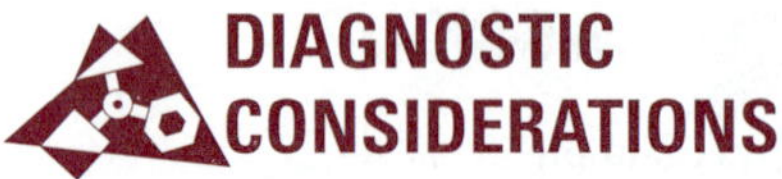

DIAGNOSTIC CONSIDERATIONS

- History of pancreatitis (possible benign stricture)
- History of ulcerative colitis (possible primary sclerosing cholangitis)
- Choledocholithiasis

RULE OUT

- Extrahepatic disease or bilobar involvement
- Choledocholithiasis

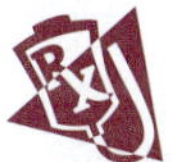

WORK-UP

- History and physical exam
- Liver function tests
- CA 19-9
- US to screen for anatomic causes of hyperbilirubinemia
- Abdominal CT
- PTC or MRCP (PTC if brushings needed)
- Angiography if portal vessel involvement suspected

TREATMENT AND MANAGEMENT

SURGERY

- Biliary resection followed by biliary-enteric resection
- Extended right or left lobectomy if proximal disease noted (isolated to 1 side) above secondary radicals or if unilateral portal vein or hepatic artery involvement
- Pancreaticoduodenectomy (Whipple) for distal common bile duct (CBD) tumors
- Biliary-enteric bypass for PTC-placed wall stent for palliation

Indications

- Resectable cholangiocarcinoma or diagnosis of benign stricture can be difficult to distinguish
- Presence of choledochal cyst

Contraindications

- Bilobar involvement or second order biliary radicals bilaterally
- Extrahepatic disease
- Main portal vein, bilateral portal vein, or bilateral hepatic artery involvement

COMPLICATIONS

- Anastomotic leak or stricture
- Cholangitis
- Recurrent disease
- Liver failure
- Hemorrhage

PROGNOSIS

- 10–30% 5-year survival with curative resection of proximal biliary tumor
- 30–50% 5-year survival with distal CBD tumor

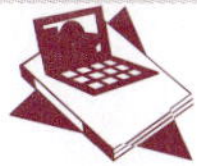

RESOURCES

REFERENCES

- Ahrendt SA et al. Cholangiocarcinoma. *Clin Liver Dis.* 2001;5:191.
- Jarnagin WR. Cholangiocarcinoma of the extrahepatic bile ducts. *Semin Surg Oncol.* 2000;19:156.

PRACTICE GUIDELINES

- The National Comprehensive Cancer Network http://www.nccn.org/

CANCER STAGING

- See Extrahepatic Bile Ducts Staging Table on page 748.

STAGE GROUPING			
Stage 0	Tis	N0	M0
Stage IA	T1	N0	M0
Stage IB	T2	N0	M0
Stage IIA	T3	N0	M0
Stage IIB	T1	N1	M0
	T2	N1	M0
	T3	N1	M0
Stage III	T4	Any N	M0
Stage IV	Any T	Any N	M1

- See Liver (Including Intrahepatic Bile Ducts) Staging Table on page 750.

STAGE GROUPING			
Stage I	T1	N0	M0
Stage II	T2	N0	M0
Stage IIIA	T3	N0	M0
IIIB	T4	N0	M0
IIIC	Any T	N1	M0
Stage IV	Any T	Any N	M1

Cholangitis, Primary Sclerosing

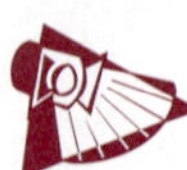

ESSENTIAL FEATURES

- Associated with ulcerative colitis 40–60%, pancreatitis 12–25%, diabetes mellitus 5–10%, and rarely other autoimmune disorders
- Onset during fourth or fifth decade of life
- Increased risk for cholangiocarcinoma

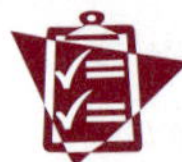

CLINICAL FINDINGS

SYMPTOMS AND SIGNS

- Intermittent jaundice
- Fever
- Right upper quadrant pain
- Pruritus

LABORATORY FINDINGS

- Elevated alkaline phosphatase
- Hyperbilirubinemia
- Leukocytosis

IMAGING FINDINGS

- Right upper quadrant US, ERCP, and magnetic resonance cholangiopancreatography (MRCP) may show multiple dilatations and strictures of extrahepatic biliary ducts

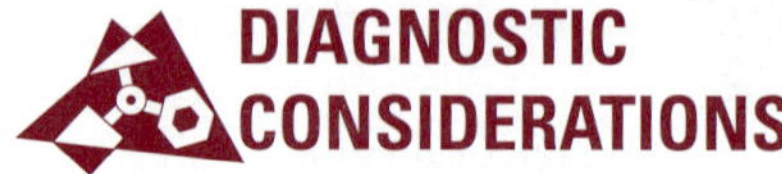

DIAGNOSTIC CONSIDERATIONS

- Cholangiocarcinoma
- Presence of cirrhosis

RULE OUT

- Cholangiocarcinoma

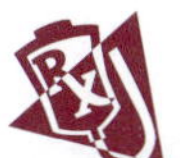

WORK-UP

- History and physical exam
- Liver function tests
- Abdominal US
- ERCP
- Liver biopsy if question of cirrhosis
- Brushings by percutaneous transhepatic cholangiography (PTC) or ERCP if question of malignancy

WHEN TO ADMIT

- Cholangitis

TREATMENT AND MANAGEMENT

SURGERY

- Balloon dilatation of multiple strictures
- Resection of dominant stricture followed by biliary reconstruction
- Liver transplantation (preferably before onset of cirrhosis)

Contraindications

- Cirrhosis

MEDICATIONS

- Ursodiol (improves liver function and histology but no difference in 5-year clinical outcome)

TREATMENT MONITORING

- Alkaline phosphatase levels

COMPLICATIONS

- Cholangitis
- Recurrent strictures
- Primary nonfunction
- Allograft rejection
- Recurrent stricture post-transplant

PROGNOSIS

- 85% survival rate 5 years post transplant
- 71% actuarial survival at 5 years for resection of dominant stricture (only 20% if cirrhosis present)
- 43% long-term success with balloon therapy for multiple strictures

RESOURCES

REFERENCES

- Kim WR et al. A revised natural history model for primary sclerosing cholangitis. *Mayo Clin Proc.* 2000;75:688.
- van Hoogstraten HJ et al. Ursodeoxycholic acid therapy for primary sclerosing cholangitis: results of a 2-year randomized controlled trial to evaluate single versus multiple daily doses. *J Hepatol.* 1998;29:417.

Cholecystitis (Acute & Chronic)

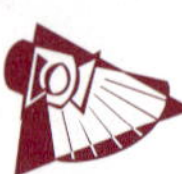

ESSENTIAL FEATURES

- Cholesterol stones form in 20% of women and 10% of men by age 60
- Cholesterol stone risk factors include:
  - Female gender
  - Age
  - Obesity
  - Estrogen exposure
  - Fatty diet
  - Rapid weight loss

EPIDEMIOLOGY

- Symptoms develop in about 3% of asymptomatic patients each year (20–30% over 20 years)
- Acalculous cholecystitis affecting patients with acute, severe systemic illness

CLINICAL FINDINGS

SYMPTOMS AND SIGNS

- Biliary colic but becoming unremitting and steady in epigastrium or right upper quadrant
- Fever
- Nausea
- Vomiting
- Right upper quadrant pain to palpation with peritoneal signs
- Murphy sign
- Anorexia

LABORATORY FINDINGS

- Leukocytosis

IMAGING FINDINGS

- Right upper quadrant US showing gallstones, gallbladder wall thickening (> 4 mm), or pericholecystic fluid (no stones if acalculous cholecystitis)
- HIDA scan showing failure of filling of gallbladder (> 95% sensitive)
- CT showing gallbladder wall thickening (> 4 mm), pericholecystic fluid (for patients with suspected acalculous cholecystitis) as sensitive as US

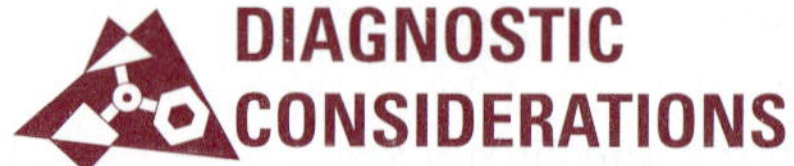

DIAGNOSTIC CONSIDERATIONS

- Other causes of acute abdominal pain

RULE OUT

- Choledocholithiasis
- Pancreatitis

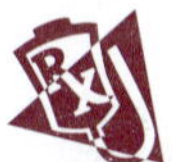

WORK-UP

- History and physical exam
- CBC count
- Amylase and lipase
- Liver function tests
- Right upper quadrant US
- HIDA scan for difficult cases
- CT if abdominal US not technically possible (patients with suspected acalculous cholecystitis, large wounds etc)

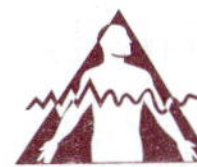

TREATMENT AND MANAGEMENT

MEDICAL

- All patients require IV fluids and antibiotics
- Management then can include either early cholecystectomy (generally preferred) or cholecystectomy after about 6 weeks

SURGERY

- Laparoscopic cholecystectomy
- Open cholecystectomy
- Cholecystostomy tube (if cholecystectomy too hazardous)

Indications

- Suspected acute cholecystitis
- Suspected acalculous cholecystitis
- Failure to resolve cholecystitis on antibiotics

COMPLICATIONS

- Bile duct injury or leak
- Empyema
  - Suppurative cholecystitis occurs with frank pus in the gallbladder, high fever, chills and systemic toxicity
  - Percutaneous drainage or cholecystectomy is necessary
- Pericholecystic abscess
  - Localized perforation at the gallbladder can result in a pericholecystic abscess
  - Treatment requires drainage with or without initial cholecystectomy
- Free perforation
  - Rare but causes generalized peritonitis
  - This occurs when a gangrenous portion of the wall necroses prior to local adhesion formation
  - The diagnosis is rarely made before urgent laparotomy
  - Treatment is cholecystectomy
- Cholecystoenteric fistula
  - Perforation at the gallbladder into an adjacent viscous generally resolves the acute episode
  - Symptomatic fistula and/or patients with continued gallstone symptoms should have cholecystectomy and closure at the fistula

RESOURCES

REFERENCES

- Berber E et al. Selective use of tube cholecystostomy with interval laparoscopic cholecystectomy in acute cholecystitis. *Arch Surg.* 2000;135:341.
- Svanvik J. Laparoscopic cholecystectomy for acute cholecystitis. *Eur J Surg.* 2000;(Suppl 585):16.

Choledochal Cyst

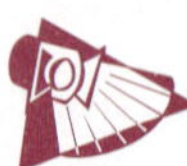

ESSENTIAL FEATURES

- Type I cysts (fusiform dilation of common bile duct [CBD]) account for 85–90%
- Type II (true diverticula of CBD) 1–2% of cases
- Type III (choledochocele—dilation of distal/intramural portion of CBD) < 2% of cases
- Type IV (multiple cysts involving intrahepatic and extrahepatic ducts) as high as 15% of cases in some series
- Type V (cystic malformation of intrahepatic ducts) rare
- 3–5% incidence of carcinoma

EPIDEMIOLOGY

- Onset of symptoms usually in infancy or childhood

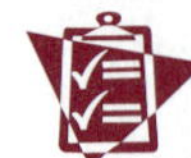

CLINICAL FINDINGS

SYMPTOMS AND SIGNS

- Jaundice
- Fever
- Pain
- Palpable right upper quadrant mass
- Hepatomegaly
- Bleeding varices
- Asymptomatic

LABORATORY FINDINGS

- Hyperbilirubinemia
- Elevated alkaline phosphatase
- Leukocytosis
- Elevated amylase and lipase

IMAGING FINDINGS

- US showing characteristic cystic dilation of biliary tree corresponding to type as well as proximal dilation in presence of obstruction
- ERCP or magnetic resonance cholangiopancreatography (MRCP) showing cystic dilation corresponding to type and proximal obstruction in presence of obstruction

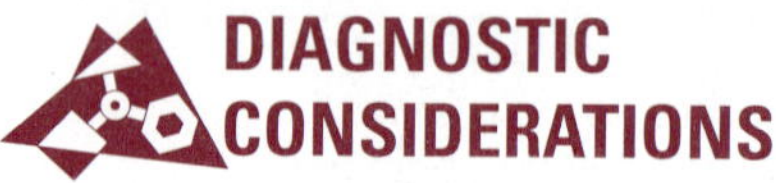

DIAGNOSTIC CONSIDERATIONS

- Type of choledochal cyst

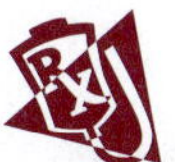

WORK-UP

- History and physical exam
- Liver function tests
- CBC count
- Amylase and lipase
- Abdominal US
- ERCP or MRCP (adults)
- HIDA scan or MRCP (children)

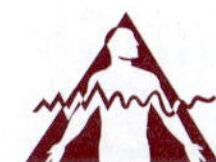

TREATMENT AND MANAGEMENT

SURGERY

- Cyst excision and biliary reconstruction (types I–III)
- Types IV and V individualized and may require partial hepatectomy if unilobar involvement

TREATMENT MONITORING

- Surveillance for carcinoma since patients still at increased risk for remainder of biliary tree

COMPLICATIONS

- Biliary stricture or leak
- Cholangitis

RESOURCES

REFERENCES

- Vercruysse R, Van den Bossche MR. Choledochal cyst in adults. *Acta Chir Belg.* 1998;98:220.

Choledocholithiasis & Gallstone Pancreatitis

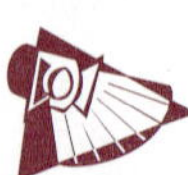

ESSENTIAL FEATURES

- Cholesterol stone risk factors include:
  - Female gender
  - Age
  - Obesity
  - Estrogen exposure
  - Fatty diet
  - Rapid weight loss
- Complicated gallstone disease affects < 0.5% annually of patients who are asymptomatic

EPIDEMIOLOGY

- Average age generally 10 years older than those affected by cholelithiasis (eg, 40–50 years of age)

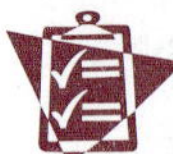

CLINICAL FINDINGS

SYMPTOMS AND SIGNS

- Right upper quadrant pain
- Painless jaundice
- Both pain and jaundice
- Fever
- Asymptomatic
- Nausea
- Vomiting
- Anorexia

LABORATORY FINDINGS

- Conjugated hyperbilirubinemia (for choledocholithiasis)
- Elevated alkaline phosphatase (for choledocholithiasis)
- Leukocytosis (for pancreatitis or cholangitis)

IMAGING FINDINGS

- Right upper quadrant US showing presence of gallstones, dilated common bile duct (CBD) (> 6 mm) and CBD stone in only 20–30% of patients with choledocholithiasis
- ERCP showing dilated CBD and presence of single or multiple CBD stones in patients with choledocholithiasis
- ERCP showing impacted ampullary gallstone in < 10 % of patients with gallstone pancreatitis

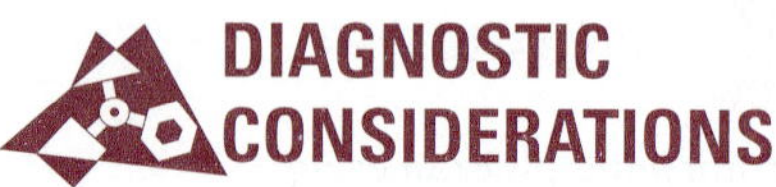

DIAGNOSTIC CONSIDERATIONS

- Presence of signs or symptoms suggestive of cholangitis

RULE OUT

- Biliary stricture

Choledocholithiasis & Gallstone Pancreatitis

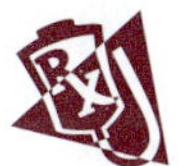

WORK-UP

- History and physical exam
- CBC count
- Liver function tests
- Amylase and lipase
- Right upper quadrant US
- ERCP or laparoscopic cholangiogram

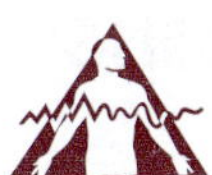

TREATMENT AND MANAGEMENT

SURGERY

- ERCP with sphincterotomy and stone extraction followed by laparoscopic cholecystectomy (preferred when cholangitis present or if pancreatitis does not resolve)
- Laparoscopic cholecystectomy with CBD exploration
- Laparoscopic cholecystectomy and cholangiogram followed by ERCP and stone extraction (preferred stone extraction technique is center specific for stones noted on screening cholangiogram following resolution of gallstone pancreatitis)
- Percutaneous transhepatic cholangiography and stone extraction if ERCP unsuccessful and cholangitis present

Indications

- Choledocholithiasis noted to be symptomatic or asymptomatic
- Gallstone pancreatitis

MEDICATIONS

- Antibiotics to cover GI flora for cases of cholangitis

COMPLICATIONS

- Pancreatitis (for ERCP)
- Bile duct injury or leak

PROGNOSIS

- Gallstone pancreatitis resolves in > 90% of cases

PREVENTION

- Treatment of symptomatic cholelithiasis

RESOURCES

REFERENCES

- Binmoeller KF, Schafer TW. Endoscopic management of bile duct stones. *J Clin Gastroenterol.* 2001;32:106.
- Rosenthal RJ et al. Options and strategies for the management of choledocholithiasis. *World J Surg.* 1998;22:1125.

Cholelithiasis

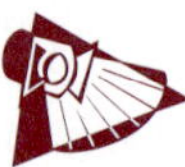

ESSENTIAL FEATURES

- Divided into symptomatic and asymptomatic
- Caused by cholesterol (most common), black pigment, or brown pigment stones
- Cholesterol stones form in 20% of women and 10% of men by age 60
- Cholesterol stone risk factors include:
  - Female gender
  - Age
  - Obesity
  - Estrogen exposure
  - Fatty diet
  - Rapid weight loss
- Black pigment stone risk factors include:
  - Hemolytic disorders
  - Living in Asia
- Brown pigment stone risk factors include:
  - Biliary stasis
  - Biliary infections

EPIDEMIOLOGY

- 20 million affected in United States
- Symptoms develop in about 3% of asymptomatic patients each year (20–30% over 20 years)
- Each year, complicated gallstone disease affects 3–5% of patients who are symptomatic
- Each year, complicated gallstone disease affects < .5% of patients who are asymptomatic

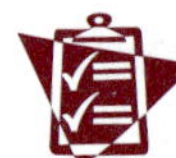

CLINICAL FINDINGS

SYMPTOMS AND SIGNS

- Asymptomatic
- Biliary colic
  - Right upper quadrant or epigastric
  - Episodic, often after meals or at night, lasting as long as 2–4 hours
- Nausea
- Vomiting
- Diarrhea
- Mild right upper quadrant tenderness to palpation

LABORATORY FINDINGS

- Normal liver function tests, normal amylase and lipase, normal WBC count

IMAGING FINDINGS

- Right upper quadrant US showing acoustically dense stones in gallbladder with acoustic shadowing without evidence of gallbladder wall thickening or pericholecystic fluid (> 90% sensitive for gallstones)

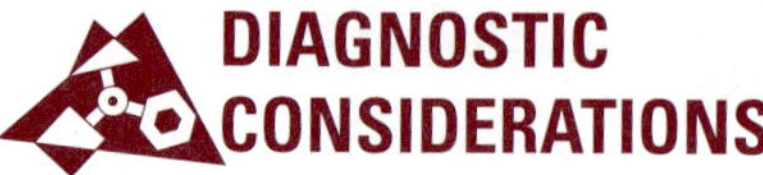

DIAGNOSTIC CONSIDERATIONS

- Other causes of abdominal pain

RULE OUT

- Cholecystitis
- Choledocholithiasis
- Pancreatitis

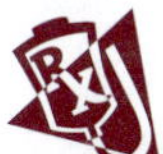

WORK-UP

- History and physical exam
- CBC count
- Liver function tests
- Amylase and lipase
- Right upper quadrant US

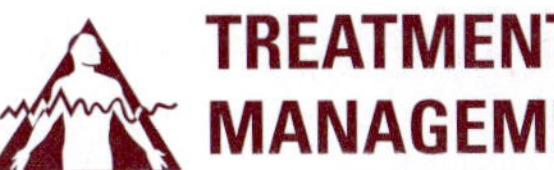

TREATMENT AND MANAGEMENT

SURGERY

- Laparoscopic cholecystectomy
- Open cholecystectomy

Indications

- Symptomatic cholelithiasis
- Porcelain gallbladder (25% risk of carcinoma)

Contraindications

- First or third trimester of pregnancy (relative)
- Previous upper abdominal surgeries (laparoscopic)

COMPLICATIONS

- Bile duct injury or leak

RESOURCES

REFERENCES

- Fletcher DR et al. Complications of cholecystectomy: risks of the laparoscopic approach and protective effects of operative cholangiography: a population-based study. *Ann Surg.* 1999;229:449.
- Montori A et al. Endoscopic and surgical integration in the approach to biliary tract disease. *J Clin Gastroenterol.* 1999;28:198.

Cholelithiasis, Rare Complications

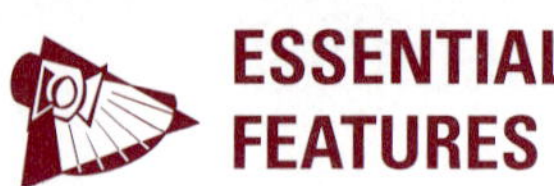

ESSENTIAL FEATURES

Gallstone Ileus

- Small bowel obstruction secondary to 1 or more large gallstones entering via cholecystoduodenal fistula

Mirizzi Syndrome

- Biliary stricture secondary to direct compression by chronically impacted cystic duct gallstone or chronic inflammation secondary to chronically inflamed gallbladder

EPIDEMIOLOGY

- Both gallstone ileus and Mirizzi syndrome are rare complications mainly affecting patients older than 60 years

CLINICAL FINDINGS

SYMPTOMS AND SIGNS

Gallstone Ileus

- Signs and symptoms of small bowel obstruction and possible antecedent history of biliary colic

Mirizzi Syndrome

- Chronic or history of right upper quadrant pain along with jaundice

LABORATORY FINDINGS

Gallstone Ileus

- Hypokalemia
- Prerenal azotemia
- Hypernatremia
- Leukocytosis

Mirizzi Syndrome

- Hyperbilirubinemia
- Elevated alkaline phosphatase

IMAGING FINDINGS

Gallstone Ileus

- **Abdominal x-ray**
  - Air-fluid levels
  - Dilated loops of small bowel
  - Possible pneumobilia
- **US**
  - Cholelithiasis and pneumobilia
- **Hypaque swallow**
  - Fistula between duodenum and gallbladder

Mirizzi Syndrome

- **US**
  - Biliary dilatation (> 6 mm)
  - Cholelithiasis
  - Possible thickened wall of gallbladder
- **ERCP or percutaneous transhepatic cholangiogram (PTC)**
  - Stricture of common bile duct

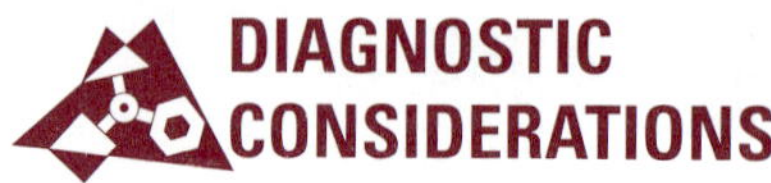

DIAGNOSTIC CONSIDERATIONS

Gallstone Ileus

- Overall clinical status of patient

Mirizzi Syndrome

- Evaluate for malignant causes of stricture

Cholelithiasis, Rare Complications

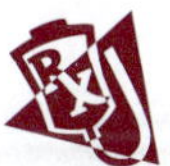

WORK-UP

Gallstone Ileus

- History and physical exam
- CBC count
- Electrolytes
- Blood urea nitrogen, creatinine
- Plain abdominal x-ray
- Right upper quadrant US
- Small bowel contrast study if partial small bowel obstruction

Mirizzi Syndrome

- History and physical exam
- CBC count
- Liver function tests
- Right upper quadrant US

TREATMENT AND MANAGEMENT

SURGERY

Gallstone Ileus

- Removal of retained small bowel gallstone(s) via enterostomy or partial resection if bowel ischemic
- Cholecystectomy and resection of fistula and duodenal closure at same operation or as staged procedure

Mirizzi Syndrome

- Cholecystectomy and resection and/or bypass of stricture via hepaticojejunostomy

Contraindications

- Clinical status of patient during laparotomy for gallstone ileus

COMPLICATIONS

Gallstone Ileus

- Missed enteral gallstone and recurrent obstruction
- Duodenal leak
- Bile duct injury or leak

Mirizzi Syndrome

- Anastomotic leak or stricture
- Cholangitis

RESOURCES

REFERENCES

- Doherty GM, Way LW. Biliary Tract. In: Way LW, Doherty GM (editors). *Current Surgical Diagnosis & Treatment,* 11e. New York: McGraw-Hill; 2003:611–612.

Cirrhosis

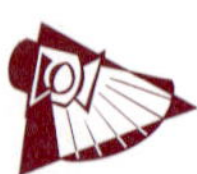

ESSENTIAL FEATURES

- Develops in 15% of alcoholics
- Alcoholism most common cause
- Other causes include:
  - Idiopathic
  - Viral hepatitis
  - Hemochromatosis
  - Wilson disease
  - Primary biliary cirrhosis
  - Primary sclerosing cholangitis
  - Budd-Chiari syndrome
  - Tricuspid regurgitation or stenosis
- Chronic allograft rejection in patients with liver transplant

EPIDEMIOLOGY

- Increasing incidence in United States
- Males affected more than females
- Third leading cause of death among men during the fifth decade
- 10–30% of patients with chronic hepatitis B and C have cirrhosis
- 30% mortality rate at 1 year after diagnosis
- Variceal bleeding, 50%
- Variceal bleed mortality, 50%
- Viral hepatitis most common worldwide

CLINICAL FINDINGS

SYMPTOMS AND SIGNS

- Jaundice
- Ascites
- Bleeding varices
- Edema
- Spider angiomas
- Dark urine
- Light-colored stools
- Encephalopathy
- Splenomegaly
- Hepatomegaly (early)
- Palmar erythema
- Gynecomastia
- Dupuytren contractures
- Dyspnea

LABORATORY FINDINGS

- Hyperbilirubinemia
- Hypoalbuminemia
- Prolonged prothrombin time
- Elevated creatinine
- Occasional elevated transaminases

IMAGING FINDINGS

- Ascites on CT or US
- Hepatic fibrosis and nodularity on CT or US
- Hepatofugal portal vein flow on duplex or thrombosis
- Splenomegaly on CT
- Dilated venous collaterals on CT

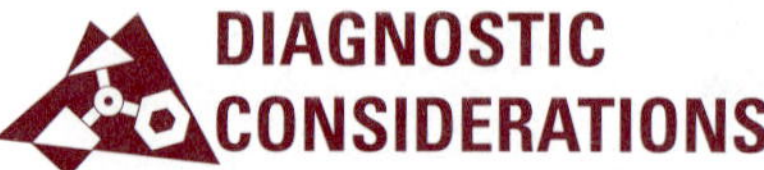

DIAGNOSTIC CONSIDERATIONS

- Etiology (alcohol, viral, hemochromatosis, Wilson disease)
- Liver biopsy
- Hepatoma
- GI bleeding
- Infection
- Model for End-Stage Liver Disease (MELD) criteria:
  - Bilirubin
  - International normalized ratio (INR)
  - Creatinine (Cr)
  - Etiology
- MELD change over time

Child-Pugh classification of functional status in liver diseases.

	Class: A Risk: Low	B Moderate	C High
Ascites	Absent	Slight to moderate	Tense
Encephalopathy	None	Grades I–II	Grades III–IV
Serum albumin (g/dL)	> 3.5	3.0–3.5	< 3.0
Serum bilirubin (mg/dL)	< 2.0	2.0–3.0	> 3.0
Prothrombin time (seconds above control)	< 4.0	4.0–6.0	> 6.0

RULE OUT

- GI bleeding, hepatoma, and infection all could cause cirrhotic decompensation or first presentation of cirrhosis

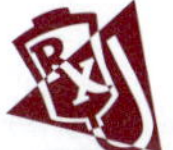

WORK-UP

- History and physical exam
- Liver function tests
- Cr
- Hepatitis serologies
- Liver biopsy (for unclear cases)
- Urine sodium and Cr for hepatorenal syndrome
- Esophagoscopy with or without sclerotherapy for varices

WHEN TO ADMIT

- Decompensated cirrhosis

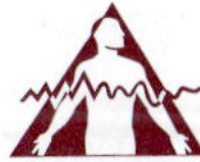

TREATMENT AND MANAGEMENT

SURGERY

- Liver transplantation
- Resection for selected hepatomas
- Radiofrequency ablation for selected hepatomas
- Transjugular intrahepatic portasystemic shunt (TIPS) vs surgical shunt for portal hypertension

Indications

- Relative MELD score for liver transplantaion
- Residual liver function for resection vs radiofrequency ablation for hepatoma
- Bleeding varices for shunt

Contraindications

- To liver transplantation
  - Continued alcoholism
  - Medical comorbidities

MEDICATIONS

- Aldactone
- Lactulose
- β-Blockers
- Low protein, low salt diet
- Change or increase immunosuppression for chronic allograft rejection following transplantation

TREATMENT MONITORING

- MELD criteria: Bilirubin, INR, Cr
- Esophagoscopy

COMPLICATIONS

- Of liver transplantation
  - Primary nonfunction
  - Rejection
  - Biliary leak or stricture
  - Hemorrhage
  - Hepatic artery thrombosis

PROGNOSIS

- 30% mortality rate at 1 year after diagnosis
- Variceal bleeding, 50%
- Variceal bleed mortality, 50%
- 60–70% 5-year survival following liver transplant

PREVENTION

- Prevention of viral hepatitis
- Alcohol cessation
- Monitoring of immunosuppressive drug trough levels following transplantation

RESOURCES

REFERENCES

- Menon KV et al. Pathogenesis, diagnosis, and treatment of alcoholic liver disease. *Mayo Clin Proc.* 2001;76:1021.
- Menon KV, Kamath PS. Managing the complications of cirrhosis. *Mayo Clin Proc.* 2000;75:501.
- Kamath PS et al. A model to predict survival in patients with end-stage liver disease. *Hepatology.* 2001;33:464.

Cirrhosis, Primary Biliary

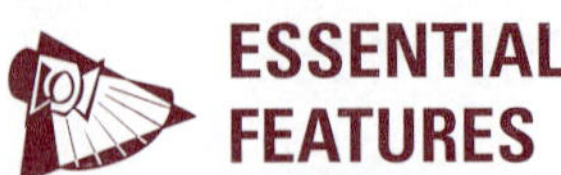

ESSENTIAL FEATURES

• Autoimmune disease characterized by portal tract inflammation

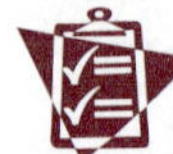

CLINICAL FINDINGS

SYMPTOMS AND SIGNS

• Gradual increasing fatigue and pruritus

LABORATORY FINDINGS

• Gradual hyperbilirubinemia often evolving over 20 years

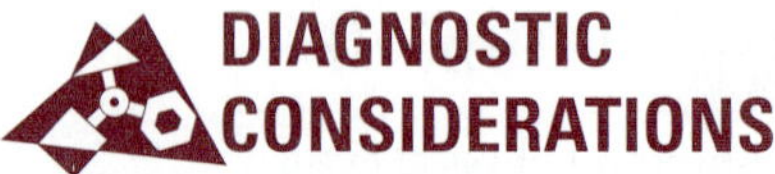

DIAGNOSTIC CONSIDERATIONS

RULE OUT

• Biliary obstruction secondary to anatomic lesion

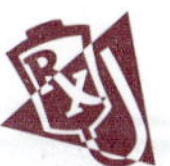

WORK-UP

- History and physical exam
- CT abdomen
- ERCP
- Liver function tests
- C-reactive protein levels
- Anti-smooth muscle cell antibody
- Anti-mitochondrial antibody
- Liver biopsy

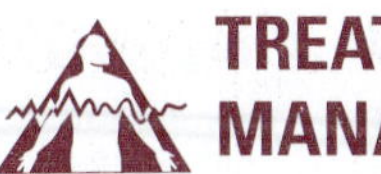

TREATMENT AND MANAGEMENT

SURGERY

- Liver transplantation

Indications

- Bilirubin > 10

Contraindications

- Medical comorbidity, active malignancy

TREATMENT MONITORING

- Bilirubin level

COMPLICATIONS

- Primary nonfunction
- Rejection
- Biliary leak or stricture
- Hemorrhage
- Hepatic artery thrombosis

PROGNOSIS

- 60–70% 5-year survival following liver transplant

RESOURCES

REFERENCES

- Talwalkar JA, Lindor KD. Primary biliary cirrhosis. *Lancet.* 2003;362:53.

Colitis, Antibiotic-Associated

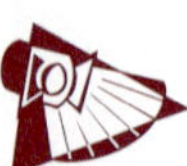

ESSENTIAL FEATURES

- Results from antibiotic therapy or alteration in colonic flora
- Diarrhea with or without gross mucosal abnormalities
- Caused by *Clostridium difficile* toxins A and B
- Also referred to as pseudomembranous colitis
- Clindamycin, ampicillin, cephalosporins are common inciting antibiotics
- May progress to toxic megacolon, perforation
- Symptoms may develop up to 6 weeks following antibiotic treatment

EPIDEMIOLOGY

- Transmitted in hospital or closed environments
- Epidemics noted on surgical wards
- Can be transmitted by health care personnel, making wearing gloves and washing hands essential
- Infection can be especially severe in immunocompromised patients

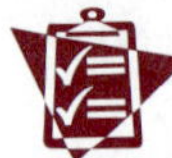

CLINICAL FINDINGS

SYMPTOMS AND SIGNS

- Watery, green diarrhea, sometimes bloody
- Crampy abdominal pain, cramping
- Vomiting
- Fever
- Complications including toxic megacolon or perforation may lead to peritoneal signs

LABORATORY FINDINGS

- Leukocytosis
- Positive tests for *C difficile* cytotoxin
- Positive stool culture

IMAGING FINDINGS

- **Endoscopy (sigmoidoscopy)**
  - Elevated plaques
  - Pseudomembranes
  - Erythematous, edematous mucosa
- **Biopsy**
  - Leukocytes
  - Necrotic epithelium
  - Fibrin

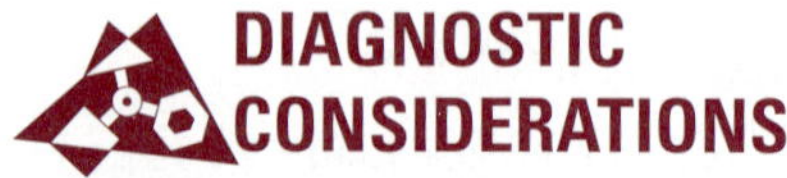

DIAGNOSTIC CONSIDERATIONS

- Malignancy
- Stricture
- Ischemic colitis
- Diverticulitis

RULE OUT

- Other causes of infectious colitis
  - Amebic
  - Actinomycosis
  - Cytomegalovirus (in immunocompromised patients)

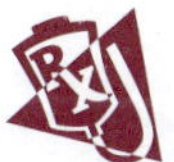

WORK-UP

- Sigmoidoscopy/colonoscopy with or without biopsy
- Stool culture, *C difficile* cytotoxin
- WBC count
- History of antibiotic therapy

WHEN TO ADMIT

- Dehydration
- Worsening abdominal pain/distention

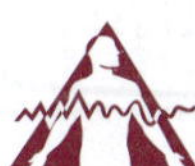

TREATMENT AND MANAGEMENT

- Discontinue inciting antibiotic
- Oral vancomycin for 7–10 days
- Oral metronidazole for 7–14 days
- Avoid antidiarrheal medications

SURGERY

Indications

- Failure of medical management with worsening clinical course/progression to toxic megacolon, peritonitis, perforation

MEDICATIONS

- Oral vancomycin
- Oral metronidazole

TREATMENT MONITORING

- Serial abdominal exams
- Serial WBC count

COMPLICATIONS

- Sepsis
- Colonic dilatation, perforation
- Hypovolemia/shock

PROGNOSIS

- Recurrence after treatment is 20%

PREVENTION

- Proper hand washing and protective barrier (gown and gloves) with infected patients
- Discontinue unnecessary antibiotics

RESOURCES

REFERENCES

- Marts BC et al. Patterns and prognosis of *Clostridium difficile* colitis. *Dis Colon Rectum.* 1994;37:837.
- Kelly CP et al. *Clostridium difficile* colitis. *N Engl J Med.* 1994;330:257.
- Fekety R, Shah AB. Diagnosis and treatment of *Clostridium difficile* colitis. *JAMA.* 1993;269:71.

Colitis, Ischemic

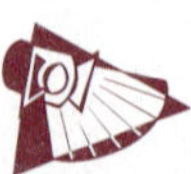

ESSENTIAL FEATURES

- Most common form of GI ischemia
- May occur following low-flow states: shock, myocardial infarction, abdominal aortic aneurysm (AAA) repair
- Reversible or irreversible
- Vascular compromise by occlusive or nonocclusive mechanisms
- May affect any portion of colon
- Watershed areas (splenic flexure, rectosigmoid junction) especially vulnerable
- No pathognomonic findings or signs; requires high index of suspicion

EPIDEMIOLOGY

- Ischemia of the right colon seen in patients with coronary artery disease (CAD), aortic stenosis
- Affects elderly most often (> 60 years)
- May occur in association with diabetes, lupus, sickle cell crisis, pancreatitis
- Left-sided ischemic colitis 1–2% following aortic reconstruction, higher incidence with ruptured AAA

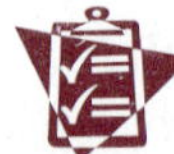

CLINICAL FINDINGS

SYMPTOMS AND SIGNS

- Abrupt onset of abdominal pain
- Diarrhea (may be bloody)
- Nausea
- Vomiting
- Tenesmus
- Fever
- Physical exam may be unremarkable
- Pain out of proportion to exam findings

LABORATORY FINDINGS

- Nonspecific, no pathognomonic abnormalities
- May have leukocytosis

IMAGING FINDINGS

- **Abdominal x-rays:** Nonspecific Abdominal catastrophe: free air, pneumatosis intestinalis, portal vein air
- **Barium enema:** May feature thumbprints
- **CT:** May show thicken bowel wall
- **Angiography:** May reveal major mesenteric vascular occlusion, stenosis, spasm
- **Colonoscopy**
  - May reveal edematous, hemorrhagic mucosa with or without ulcerations
  - Advanced ischemia appears as blue-black discoloration, patchy areas of black, nonviable mucosa
- Grayish membrane resembles pseudomembranous colitis

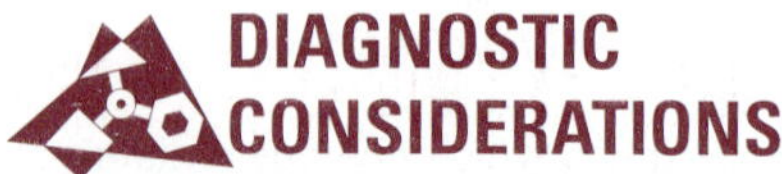

DIAGNOSTIC CONSIDERATIONS

- Colorectal cancer
- Diverticulitis
- Inflammatory bowel disease
- Pseudomembranous colitis
- Infectious colitis

RULE OUT

- Neoplasm
- Ulcerative colitis
- Diverticulitis

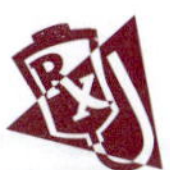

WORK-UP

- Comprehensive history and physical exam
- Is there recent history of low-flow state (AAA repair, cardiac event), pancreatitis
- Colonoscopy
- CT scan
- Diagnosis requires high index of suspicion
- Consider work-up for hypercoaguable state, embolic source (transesophageal echocardiography, aortography)

WHEN TO ADMIT

- Patients with suspicion of ischemic colitis should be admitted for work-up, hydration, IV antibiotics, and observation to be certain that the problem is reversible

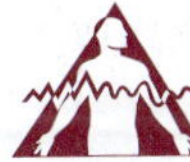

TREATMENT AND MANAGEMENT

- IV hydration
- Broad-spectrum antibiotics
- Inpatient hospitalization
- Bowel rest
- NG decompression

SURGERY

Indications

- Irreversible disease, failure of conservative measures (hydration, antibiotics, bowel rest) with persistence of symptoms
- Full thickness necrosis (gangrenous ischemic colitis)
- Development of stricture/obstruction
- Worsening clinical course (fever, tachycardia, leukocytosis, acidosis, hypotension)

MEDICATIONS

- IV broad-spectrum antibiotics

TREATMENT MONITORING

- Serial abdominal exam
- Serial WBC count
- Follow-up endoscopy

COMPLICATIONS

- Severe ischemic disease often associated with other medical comorbidities
- Overall mortality rate ~ 50%
- Ischemic stricture
- Peritonitis
- Perforation

PROGNOSIS

- In transient disease, 80–90% will completely heal
- Gangrenous ischemic colitis occurs 10–20%
- For gangrenous ischemic colitis, mortality approaches 60–90%
- Strictures develop in 2%
- Recurrence ~ 5%

RESOURCES

REFERENCES

- Balthazar EJ et al. Ischemic colitis: CT evaluation of 54 cases. *Radiology.* 1999;211:381.
- Hwang RF, Schwartz RW. Ischemic colitis: a brief review. *Curr Surg.* 2001;58:192.

WEB SITES

- http://www.postgradmed.com/issues/1999/04_99/alapati.htm

Colitis, Ulcerative

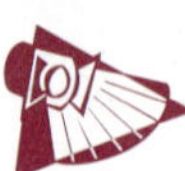

ESSENTIAL FEATURES

- Diffuse inflammatory disease confined to mucosa and submucosa
- Crypts of Lieberkühn abscesses
- Most commonly affects rectum
- May spread to involve entire colon and distal ileum (backwash ileitis)
- Diseased areas are contiguous
- Increase in colorectal cancer risk

EPIDEMIOLOGY

- Bimodal age distribution
  - 15–30 years
  - 60–80 years
- Females affected slightly more than males
- Incidence 5–12/100,000
- Etiology unknown

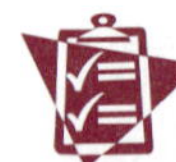

CLINICAL FINDINGS

SYMPTOMS AND SIGNS

- Rectal bleeding
- Diarrhea
- Tenesmus
- Rectal urgency
- Anal incontinence
- Crampy abdominal pain
- Fever
- Vomiting
- Weight loss
- Dehydration
- Extracolonic manifestations, including arthropathy, uveitis, iritis, pyoderma gangrenosum, and aphthous ulcers

LABORATORY FINDINGS

- Anemia
- Leukocytosis
- Elevated ESR
- Hypoalbuminemia
- Electrolyte depletion

IMAGING FINDINGS

- **Sigmoidoscopy**
  - Loss of normal vascular pattern
  - Friable
  - Hyperemic rectal mucosa
  - Mucosal granularity
  - Ulcers with bleeding and purulent exudates in advanced disease
- **Barium enema**
  - Diffuse reticulated pattern
  - "Collar button" ulcers
  - Disappearance of haustral markings ("lead pipe")
  - Shortening of colon
- **Abdominal x-ray**
  - Colonic dilation
  - Loss of haustral markings
- **CT scan of abdomen**
  - May be helpful in puzzling cases
  - Colonic dilation
  - Loss of haustral markings

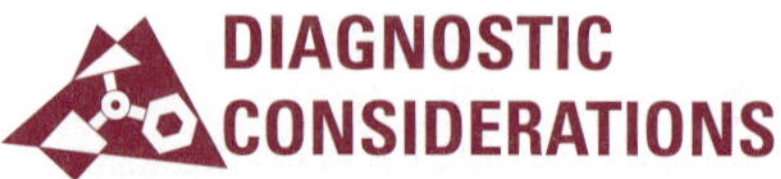

DIAGNOSTIC CONSIDERATIONS

- No radiographic, histologic, endoscopic findings pathognomonic
- Infectious colitis
- Mesenteric insufficiency
- Neoplasm
- Antibiotic-associated colitis
- Chagas disease

RULE OUT

- Infectious diarrhea (shigellosis, salmonellosis, *E coli,* amebiasis)
- Crohn disease
- Malignancy
- Diverticular disease
- *Clostridium difficile* colitis
- Toxic megacolon
- Infectious colitis and pseudomembranous colitis

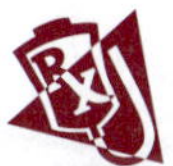

WORK-UP

- Flexible sigmoidoscopy and colonoscopy
- Contrast enema
- Obtain CBC count, metabolic panel, liver function panel

WHEN TO ADMIT

- Dehydration or malnutrition
- Severe rectal bleeding
- Abdominal pain
- Bowel obstruction
- Intractable diarrhea
- Severe, acute, or fulminant attack

WHEN TO REFER

- Unclear diagnosis
- Impending perforation
- Suspicion of toxic megacolon

TREATMENT AND MANAGEMENT

- Initially, medical unless complications arise
- Surgery potentially curative
- Treatment focus on containing and reducing inflammation

SURGERY

- Total colectomy, rectal mucosectomy, and ileoanal anastomosis
- Proctocolectomy with ileostomy or continent ileal pouch
- Subtotal colectomy with ileorectal anastomosis
- Emergent procedures should be tailored to fit the extent of the illness; typically total abdominal colectomy and ileostomy

Indications

- Emergency surgery for perforation
- Urgent surgery for
  - Medically refractory toxic megacolon
  - Massive hemorrhage
  - Fulminant acute flare unresponsive to medication
  - Acute obstruction
  - Suspicion or demonstration of colorectal cancer
- Medically refractory chronic disease resulting in malnutrition, complications from medical management, or inability to work or perform activities of daily living

MEDICATIONS

- Sulfasalazine
- Corticosteroids
- Mesalamine
- Cyclosporine for steroid-resistant colitis

TREATMENT MONITORING

- Endoscopy

COMPLICATIONS

- Increase colorectal cancer risk
- Chronic steroid use complications, including diabetes, osteoporosis, Cushing syndrome, and avascular necrosis

PROGNOSIS

- Mortality declining over last 2 decades
- 1–2 % per year colorectal cancer risk
- Emergent surgery increases risk of complications
- 10% of patients who present with proctitis develop colonic disease within 10 years of diagnosis
- Left-sided colitis and pancolitis have worse prognosis

RESOURCES

REFERENCES

- D'Haens G et al. Intravenous cyclosporine versus intravenous corticosteroids as single therapy for severe attacks of ulcerative colitis. *Gastroenterology.* 2001;120:1323.
- Eaden JA et al. The risk of colorectal cancer in ulcerative colitis: a meta-analysis. *Gut.* 2001;48:526.

WEB SITES

- http://www.ccfa.org
- http://www.niddk.nih.gov

INFORMATION FOR PATIENTS

- Crohn and Colitis Foundation of America
- National Institute of Diabetes & Digestive & Kidney Diseases (NIDDK)

Colorectal Adenocarcinoma

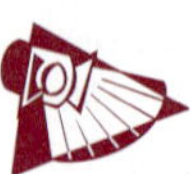

ESSENTIAL FEATURES

- Colorectal cancer second leading cause of cancer deaths (after lung)
- Adenocarcinoma accounts for 95% of malignant colorectal tumors
- Genetic predisposition in familial adenomatous polyposis and hereditary nonpolyposis colorectal cancer (HNPCC)
- Conditions predisposing to colorectal cancer
  - Ulcerative colitis
  - Crohn colitis
  - Schistosomal colitis
  - Exposure to radiation
  - Presence of ureterocolostomy
- Possible dietary influences
  - High caloric intake
  - High saturated fat intake
  - Decreased dietary calcium
  - Decreased fiber intake
- Carcinogenesis multi-step process involving dysfunction of tumor suppressor genes, including APC, DCC, P53
- Distribution of colorectal cancer
  - 25% right colon
  - 10% transverse colon
  - 15% left colon
  - 20–50% rectosigmoid colon
- Spreads through direct extension, hematogenously, lymph nodes, transperitoneal, intraluminal
- Synchronous lesions occur in 3–5%

EPIDEMIOLOGY

- 156,000 cases diagnosed per year
- 65,000 colorectal cancer deaths per year
- Incidence increases with age
- Colon cancer is more common in women than men
- Rectal cancer is more common in men than women
- Multiple synchronous colonic cancers found in 5% of patients
- 5% lifetime risk
- 6–8% occurs before age 40 years

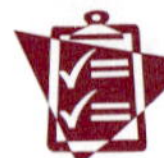

CLINICAL FINDINGS

SYMPTOMS AND SIGNS

- Symptoms depend on anatomic location and extent of lesion
- Right colon lesions may become large before symptoms develop
  - May cause occult bleeding, anemia
- Left colon lesions often cause crampy abdominal pain
- Large bowel obstruction ~ 10% cases
- Fatigue, weakness, vague abdominal pain, abdominal mass (< 10%), anemia
- Constipation alternating with increased frequency of defecation
- Dark or blood tinged stool
- Change in stool caliber
- Rectal cancers
  - Hematochezia
  - Tenesmus
- Physical exam findings may include abdominal mass, lymphadenopathy, rectal mass

LABORATORY FINDINGS

- Patients may have microcytic, hypochromic anemia
- Positive occult blood on guiac stool test
- Carcinoembryonic antigen (CEA) elevation (nonspecific, more useful for surveillance following resection), prompts additional imaging (CT scan)
- Elevation of biochemical markers (nonspecific): CA 19-9, CA 72-4, plasma prolactin

IMAGING FINDINGS

- Contrast enema-filling defect, "apple core lesion"; constricted area or intraluminal mass
- **Total colonoscopy:** Should be performed to evaluate lesion and presence of synchronous lesions

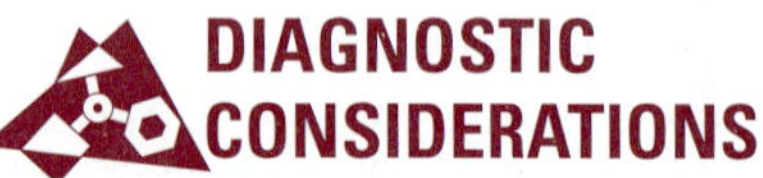

DIAGNOSTIC CONSIDERATIONS

- Ulcerative colitis
- Crohn colitis
- Ischemic colitis
- Parasite infection, amebiasis
- Diverticulitis
- Diverticulosis
- Appendicitis
- Peptic ulcer disease
- Other neoplasms of colon/rectum
  - Lymphoma
  - Carcinoid

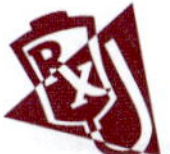

WORK-UP

- Complete history (including family) and physical exam
- Total colonoscopy with biopsy
- Obtain plain abdominal x-ray and water-soluble contrast enema in patients with bowel obstruction
- Once diagnosis is made, staging studies should be performed
  - Chest x-ray
  - CT scan: Helpful to assess extramural extension or metastatic lesions
  - Liver function tests
- **Endorectal US:** Helpful for determining depth of invasion in rectal lesions

WHEN TO ADMIT

- Bowel obstruction/perforation
- Hemodynamically significant lower GI bleeding

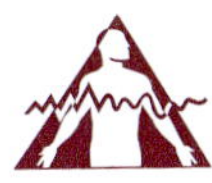

TREATMENT AND MANAGEMENT

- Mainstay of management is surgical with good mechanical bowel prep
- Lesion and regional lymphatic drainage basin need to be resected, adherent visceral structures resected en bloc
- Margins should be at least 2 cm
- Abdominal exploration carried out to search for other lesions (liver metastasis)
- Avoid spillage or unnecessary manipulation of lesion
- Multiple carcinomas or neoplastic polyps may require subtotal colectomy
- **Rectal cancer:** Type of operation (abdominoperineal resection vs low anterior resection) determined by distance from anal verge and ability to achieve adequate margins (at least 2 cm)
- **Right-sided lesions:** Resection includes distal ileum, ileocolic, right colic, and right branch of middle colic vessels
- **Transverse colon lesion:** Transverse or extended right colectomy
- **Left-sided lesions:** Takes inferior mesenteric artery (IMA) at its origin

SURGERY

Indications

- Primary tumor is resected even if distant metastases have occurred to prevent future obstruction, bleeding
- Rejection offers best chance at long-term survival
- In carefully selected patients, local excision of small, well-differentiated mobile, polypoid lesions may serve as surgical therapy
- Unresectable rectal cancer may be palliated by fulguration, photocoagulation, diverting colostomy for obstructing, unresectable tumors

Contraindications

- Severe medical comorbidity
- Metastatic lesions may be amenable to palliative procedures to bypass malignant obstruction

MEDICATIONS

- Preoperative radiotherapy increases 5-year survival and decreases local recurrence in rectal cancer
- Postoperative chemotherapy (5-fluorouracil) and radiation beneficial for stage II rectal cancer in terms of local control and survival
- Stage II colon cancer
  - Efficacy of chemotherapy unclear
  - Radiation generally not used for colon cancer
- Oral levamisole and IV 5-fluorouracil may be useful in stage III colon cancer

TREATMENT MONITORING

- Surveillance colonoscopy
- Follow serial CEA levels
- Fecal occult blood testing
- Rising CEA should prompt CT scan and liver function tests

COMPLICATIONS

- Recurrence
- Metastasis, extension to adjacent viscera
- Malignant bowel obstruction
- Perforation
- Hemorrhage

PROGNOSIS

- Results for surgical treatment better for colon cancer than for rectal cancer
- Low rectal cancers worse prognosis than high rectal cancer
- 5-year survival per Dukes stage: A (80%), B (60%), C (30%), D (5%)
- Diploid lesions may have better prognosis than aneuploid lesions
- Approximately 10% of lesions are not resectable at time of operation
  - 20% of patients have metastatic disease at operation
- Curative resection can be performed in about 70% of patients
- Operative mortality, 2–4%
- Overall survival (all stages), 35%
- Prognosis adversely influenced by complications
- Prognosis may be adversely affected by perioperative blood transfusion
- 90% recurrences occur with first 4 years after surgery

RESOURCES

PRACTICE GUIDELINES

- The National Comprehensive Cancer Network http://www.nccn.org/

WEB SITES

- http://www.cancer.gov/cancerinfo/types/colon-and-rectal

CANCER STAGING

- See Colon and Rectum Staging Table on page 746.

STAGE GROUPING

Stage	T	N	M	Dukes*	MAC*
0	Tis	N0	M0	-	-
I	T1	N0	M0	A	A
	T2	N0	M0	A	B1
IIA	T3	N0	M0	B	B2
IIB	T4	N0	M0	B	B3
IIIA	T1-T2	N1	M0	C	C1
IIIB	T3-T4	N1	M0	C	C2/C3
IIIC	Any T	N2	M0	C	C1/C2/C3
IV	Any T	Any N	M1	-	D

*Dukes B is a composite of better (T3 N0 M0) and worse (T4 N0 M0) prognostic groups, as is Dukes C (Any TN1 M0 and Any T N2 M0). MAC is the modified Astler-Coller classification.

Note: The y prefix is to be used for those cancers that are classified after pretreatment, whereas the r prefix is to be used for those cancers that have recurred.

Colorectal Cancer, Hereditary Nonpolyposis (HNPCC)

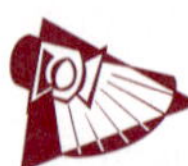

ESSENTIAL FEATURES

- Perhaps 6% of patients with cancer of the colon or rectum have HNPCC
- Most common form of hereditary colorectal cancer
- Gene responsible for this syndrome has been localized to chromosome 2p
- **Lynch syndrome II:**
  - Early onset (average age 44)
  - Proximal dominance
  - Synchronous and metachronous cancers and other associated extracolonic adenocarcinomas, especially endometrial carcinoma
- **Lynch syndrome I:** Hereditary site-specific colon cancer shows the same characteristics except that there are no extracolonic cancers
- Autosomal dominant inheritance
- Cancers arise in discrete adenomas but polyposis (ie, hundreds of polyps) does not occur
- **Diagnostic criteria (Amsterdam criteria)**
  - Families must have at least 3 relatives with colorectal cancer, 1 of whom is a first-degree relative of the other 2
  - Colorectal cancer must involve at least 2 generations, and at least 1 cancer case must occur before age of 50
- Adenomas and carcinomas in HNPCC arise at an early age
  - Adenomas may occur in patients in their 20s and 30s, with a mean age for carcinoma development of 40 to 45 years
  - Are often proximal in location and multiple
- Alterations in DNA mismatch repair genes that help maintain DNA fidelity during replication are characteristic of patients with HNPCC: (hMLH1, hPMS1 and hPMS2, and hMSH2, hMSH3, and hMSH6) may lead to the inability to repair base pair mismatches and result in DNA replication errors or microsatellite instability
- Accelerated carcinogenesis occurs in hereditary nonpolyposis colorectal cancer compared with sporadic cases

EPIDEMIOLOGY

- The frequency of HNPCC in the general population is yet to be determined, but HNPCC may account for as many as 6% of colorectal cancer cases
- Multiple generations are affected with colorectal cancer at an early age (mean, approximately 45 years) with a predominance of right-sided colorectal cancer (approximately 70% proximal to the splenic flexure)
- Excess of synchronous colorectal cancer and metachronous colorectal cancer
- Excess of extracolonic cancers—namely, carcinoma of the endometrium (second only to colorectal cancer in frequency), ovary, stomach (particularly in Asian countries such as Japan and Korea), small bowel, pancreas, hepatobiliary tract, brain, and upper uroepithelial tract
- As compared with sporadic colorectal cancer, tumors in HNPCC are more often poorly differentiated, with an excess of mucoid and signet-cell features

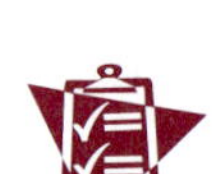

CLINICAL FINDINGS

SYMPTOMS AND SIGNS

- Most patients are asymptomatic
- Lower GI bleeding, although most bleeding is occult
- Vague abdominal pain

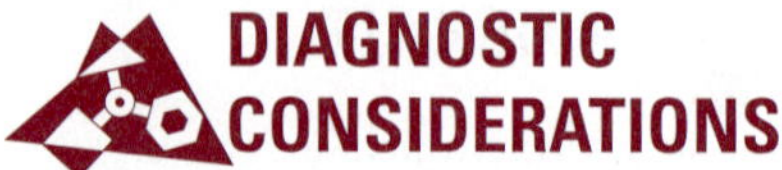

DIAGNOSTIC CONSIDERATIONS

- Must always evaluate for synchronous colon carcinoma

Colorectal Cancer, Hereditary Nonpolyposis (HNPCC)

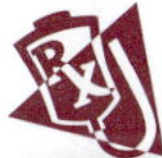

WORK-UP

- History and physical exam
- Digital rectal exam
- Colonoscopy
- Mainstay of the diagnosis of Lynch syndromes is a detailed family history
  - A nuclear pedigree should be obtained from any patient with suspected cancer, as well as a history of colonic polyps
  - When a pedigree is identified, genetic counseling should be provided to decide about testing for genetic markers

WHEN TO REFER

- Suspicion of familial component of colorectal malignancy

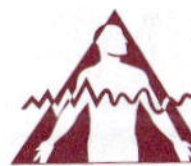

TREATMENT AND MANAGEMENT

- When colon cancer is detected, an abdominal colectomy and ileorectal anastomosis is the procedure of choice
- In the case of a woman with no further plans for childbearing, a prophylactic total abdominal hysterectomy and bilateral salpingo-oophorectomy is recommended

TREATMENT MONITORING

- Extracolonic screening
  - Particularly of the endometrium and ovary, the sites of the second and third most common cancers in this disorder
  - With respect to the endometrium, annual transvaginal US and endometrial aspiration for pathologic assessment should be begun at the age of 30 years and repeated annually
  - In the case of the ovary, the evaluation should include transvaginal ovarian US and CA-125 screening, also beginning at the age of 30

PREVENTION

- Patients with a family history of HNPCC should have colonoscopy every 1–2 years beginning at age 20–30, then annually after age 40
- The role of prophylactic colectomy for patients with HNPCC is still controversial, although most experts in the field now favor it

RESOURCES

REFERENCES

- Lynch HY, de la Chapelle A. Hereditary colorectal cancer. *N Engl J Med.* 2003;348:919.

PRACTICE GUIDELINES

- The National Comprehensive Cancer Network http://www.nccn.org/

CANCER STAGING

- See Colon and Rectum Staging Table on page 746.

STAGE GROUPING

Stage	T	N	M	Dukes*	MAC*
0	Tis	N0	M0	-	-
I	T1	N0	M0	A	A
	T2	N0	M0	A	B1
IIA	T3	N0	M0	B	B2
IIB	T4	N0	M0	B	B3
IIIA	T1-T2	N1	M0	C	C1
IIIB	T3-T4	N1	M0	C	C2/C3
IIIC	Any T	N2	M0	C	C1/C2/C3
IV	Any T	Any N	M1	-	D

*Dukes B is a composite of better (T3 N0 M0) and worse (T4 N0 M0) prognostic groups, as is Dukes C (Any TN1 M0 and Any T N2 M0). MAC is the modified Astler-Coller classification.

Note: The y prefix is to be used for those cancers that are classified after pretreatment, whereas the r prefix is to be used for those cancers that have recurred.

Colorectal Tumors, Uncommon

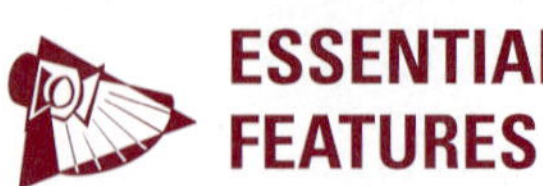

ESSENTIAL FEATURES

Carcinoids

- Uncommon in large bowel; most occur in the rectum
- Lesions < 2 cm in diameter usually are asymptomatic, behave benignly, and can be managed by local excision
- Larger tumors arising in the colon (mainly the right side) or rectum cause local symptoms, often metastasize, and require standard cancer surgeries
- Carcinoid syndrome appears in fewer than 5% of patients with metastatic carcinoid of the large bowel
- Derived from cells that are capable of synthesizing a wide variety of hormones
- 60% of rectal carcinoids present as asymptomatic submucosal nodules measuring < 2 cm in diameter

Lymphomas

- Rrare and account for < 0.5% of all colorectal malignancies
- The documentation of widespread dissemination of lymphoma in most cases underscores the concept that lymphoma of the GI tract is a systemic disease in which tumor cells are present in other organ sites

Sarcoma

- Extremely rare and account for < 0.1% of all large bowel malignancies
- Most common histologic subtype is leiomyosarcoma
- Most significant prognostic indicator is the tumor grade

EPIDEMIOLOGY

- **Carcinoids** of the colon are uncommon (2% of GI carcinoids) and most of them occur in the rectum (15% of GI carcinoids)
- **Lymphomas** are the most common noncarcinomatous malignant tumors of the large bowel; primary non-Hodgkin colonic lymphoma account for 10% of GI lymphomas
- **Sarcomas** represent < 1% of colonic tumors, with peak incidence in sixth decade of life

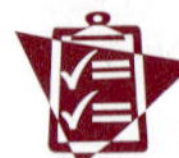

CLINICAL FINDINGS

SYMPTOMS AND SIGNS

- Abdominal pain
- Abdominal distention
- Obstipation, constipation
- Change in bowel habits
- Weight loss
- Hematochezia
- Abdominal mass

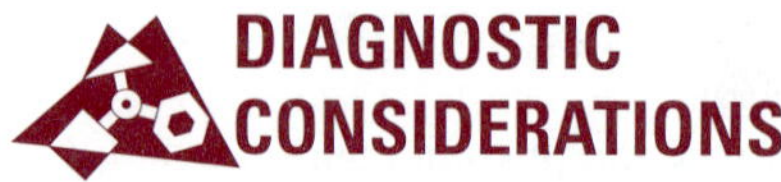

DIAGNOSTIC CONSIDERATIONS

- Adenocarcinoma
- Stricture: Inflammatory, radiation-induced
- Appendicitis
- Diverticular disease

RULE OUT

- Neoplasm

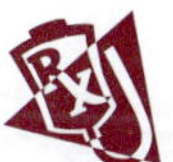

WORK-UP

- History and physical exam
- Colonoscopy with biopsy
- **Staging studies:** Chest film, abdominal CT scan, liver function tests
- **For lymphoma:** Bone marrow biopsy

WHEN TO ADMIT

- Bleeding
- Obstruction
- Perforation/peritonitis

TREATMENT AND MANAGEMENT

Lymphoma

- Because this disease is highly responsive to chemotherapy and radiation, surgery is not always the primary mode of therapy
- Usually, for localized, low-grade colorectal lymphomas, radiation is considered first-line therapy
- Intermediate- and high-grade lymphomas, chemotherapy combined with radiation therapy should be the primary treatment

Sarcoma

- If the tumors are clinically localized at initial presentation, a radical en bloc excision should be performed to obtain a margin of uninvolved normal tissue; nodal dissection indicated if gross nodal involvement

Carcinoid

- Surgery mainstay of therapy, degree of resection depends on size (lesions > 2 cm may require formal resection; < 2 cm may be amenable to local excision)

SURGERY

Indications

- **Rectal carcinoid:** Transanal local excision suffices for definitive therapy because small tumors rarely metastasize
- **Lymphoma:** Surgery has been primarily for diagnostic and staging purposes and for the management of treatment-related complications (ie, perforation or bleeding).
- **Sarcoma:** If tumors are clinically localized at initial presentation, a radical en bloc excision should be performed to obtain a margin of uninvolved normal tissue

PROGNOSIS

Carcinoid

- Size is an extremely important prognostic factor; malignant potential is seen almost exclusively in tumors larger than 2 cm
- Results of radical excisions for large rectal carcinoids are poor because these tumors tend to metastasize

Sarcoma

- Most significant prognostic indicator is the tumor grade and size
  - Patients with high-grade tumors do poorly
  - These tumors usually metastasize to the liver and peritoneal surfaces
- 5-year survival with tumor < 5 cm, 71%; > 5 cm, 25%
- Radiation and chemotherapy have not proved efficacious

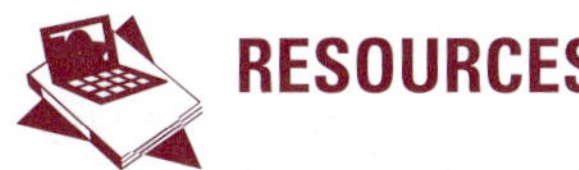

RESOURCES

REFERENCES

- Saclarides TJ et al. Neuroendocrine cancers of the colon and rectum: results of a ten-year experience. *Dis Colon Rectum.* 1994;37:635.
- Soga J. Carcinoids of the colon and ileocecal region: a statistical evaluation of 363 cases collected from the literature. *J Exp Clin Cancer Res.* 1998;17:139.

PRACTICE GUIDELINES

- The National Comprehensive Cancer Network http://www.nccn.org/

Colovesical Fistula

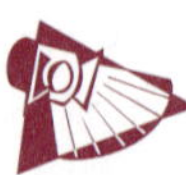

ESSENTIAL FEATURES

- **Fistula:** Communication between 2 epithelialized surfaces
- Classified by output
  - High output > 500 mL/d
  - Low output < 500 mL/d
- Most common causes include:
  - Prior abdominal operation, especially for inflammatory bowel disease
  - Malignancy
  - Extensive adhesions
  - Abscesses
  - Anastomotic leaks
  - Diverticular disease
  - Radiation
  - Trauma
  - Foreign body
- Malnutrition also major risk factor in fistula formation/failure to heal
- Colovesical fistula
  - Most common communication between bladder and GI tract
  - Diverticulitis is most common cause
  - Refractory, recurrent urinary tract infection (UTI) is common presentation

EPIDEMIOLOGY

- Affects more men than women (3:1)
- Complicates 2–4% cases of diverticulitis
- 67–80% fistulas follow abdominal surgery

CLINICAL FINDINGS

SYMPTOMS AND SIGNS

- **Colovesical fistula**
  - Patients may be asymptomatic
  - Patients may have chronic, refractory UTI and present with fecaluria, pneumaturia
  - Physical exam usually not revealing
  - Patient may show signs of dehydration
- **Colocutaneous fistula**
  - Draining sinus at the skin with enteric content or stool
  - Often located at wound or incision with surrounding erythema, excoriation, induration

LABORATORY FINDINGS

- No pathognomonic abnormalities
- UA may reveal fecaluria, infection
- Low serum albumin, prealbumin, transferring indicative of compromised nutritional status

IMAGING FINDINGS

- **Sigmoidoscopy** is usually unrevealing, though may disclose inflammation or mass at the fistula site
- **Cystoscopy** usually fails to visualize opening
- **CT** may detect small amounts of air in bladder
- **Contrast enema** may demonstrate large fistulas but commonly misses small openings
- **Fistulogram** if tract is mature
- **Pyelography** and **cystography** may be used to discern connection with urinary tract

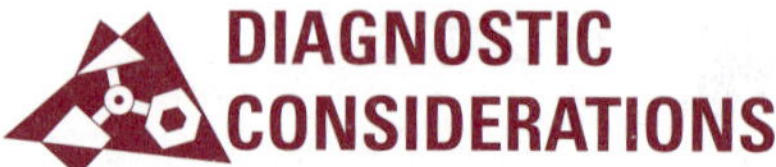

DIAGNOSTIC CONSIDERATIONS

- Consider etiology of fistula formation and reasons for failed closure (eg, foreign body, radiation injury, abscess, distal obstruction, neoplasm, inflammatory conditions, epithelialization)

RULE OUT

- GI malignancy or primary bladder malignancy as cause of fistula

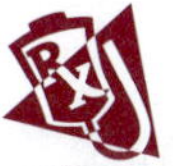

WORK-UP

- UA
- CT scan to evaluate for location of fistula, possible source (eg, sigmoid diverticulitis, mass, abscess)
- Obtain nutrition status markers
  - Serum albumin
  - Prealbumin
  - Transferrin
- Endoscopic evaluation of GI tract, bladder

WHEN TO ADMIT

- Severe nutritional depletion
- Septic complications
- Severe dehydration

TREATMENT AND MANAGEMENT

- Persistent fistulae require surgical intervention, although no need for urgent or emergent surgery
- Up to 50% of colovesical fistulas secondary to diverticulitis close spontaneously
- Treat volume loss with adequate fluid resuscitation
- Correct electrolyte abnormalities
- Improve nutritional status (low output, distal fistulas may be treated with enteral feeding); use total parenteral nutrition if high output or intolerance to enteral feeding
- Sepsis must be aggressively addressed early
- Drain abscesses
- IV antibiotics when infection present
- Open, debride, and pack infected wounds
- Control and measure fistula output
- Protect skin surrounding cutaneous fistula opening

SURGERY

Indications

- Recurrent UTI
- Failure to close spontaneously
- GI malignancy requires disk of involved bladder wall to be resected with primary specimen

Contraindications

- Prohibitive medical comorbidities

MEDICATIONS

- Antibiotic therapy for recurrent UTI

TREATMENT MONITORING

- Follow-up CT scan to evaluate abscess drainage
- Consider repeat endoscopy or contrast study (fistulogram) to document persistent communications or healing

COMPLICATIONS

- Sepsis
- Electrolyte abnormalities

PROGNOSIS

- **Mortality of all fistulas:** 5–20%
- Sepsis is major determinant of mortality and morbidity from fistulas
- Improvement of nutritional status may have profound impact on morbidity and mortality
- Colonic fistulas have high rate of spontaneous closure

PREVENTION

- Identification of high risk patients
- Meticulous operative technique
- Good mechanical bowel prep

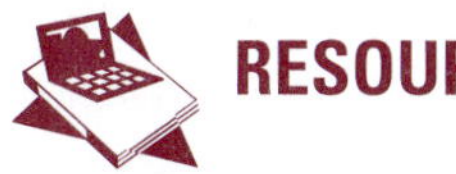

RESOURCES

REFERENCES

- Vasilevsky CA et al. Fistulas complicating diverticulitis. *Int J Colorectal Dis.* 1998;13:57.

Condylomata Acuminata

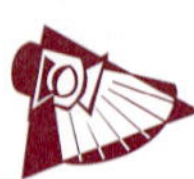

ESSENTIAL FEATURES

- Human papillomavirus (HPV) is the cause of condylomata acuminata
- Multiple types have been identified
  - Types HPV-6 and HPV-11 are associated with the common benign genital wart
  - HPV-16 and HPV-18 are associated with the development of high-grade anal dysplasia and anal cancer
- Most common sexually transmitted viral disease

EPIDEMIOLOGY

- 1 million new cases reported per year in the United States
- Most common anorectal infection of homosexual men and is particularly prevalent in HIV-positive patients
- Disease is not limited to men or women who practice anoreceptive intercourse
- In women, the virus may track down from the vagina, and in men it may pool and track from the base of the scrotum
- Immunosuppression, either from drugs after transplantation or from HIV, increases susceptibility to condylomatous disease with prevalence rates of 5% and 85%, respectively

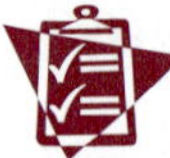

CLINICAL FINDINGS

SYMPTOMS AND SIGNS

- Complaint is that of a perianal growth
- Pruritus, discharge, bleeding, odor, and anal pain common complaints
- Classic cauliflower-like lesion, which may be isolated, clustered, or coalescent
- Warts tend to run in radial rows out from the anus

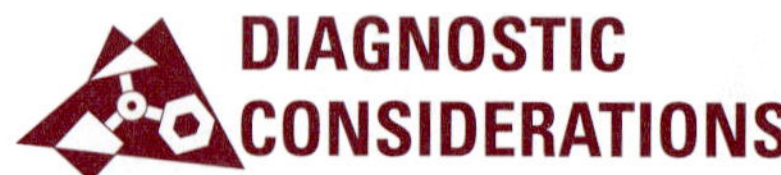

DIAGNOSTIC CONSIDERATIONS

- Condylomata lata lesions of secondary syphilis
- Anal squamous cell carcinoma

RULE OUT

- Malignancy

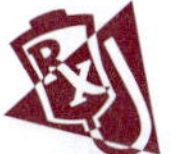

WORK-UP

- History and physical exam
- Anoscopy and proctosigmoidoscopy are essential because the disease extends internally in more than 75% of patients
- HPV-16 and HPV-18 are causally associated with squamous cell carcinomas of the anal canal
  - Representative biopsies of clinically apparent condylomas should be sent for pathologic study because unsuspected low-grade or high-grade dysplasia or squamous cell carcinoma of the anal canal may be found

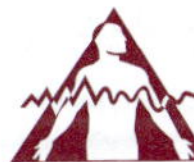

TREATMENT AND MANAGEMENT

- Extent of the disease and the risk of malignancy determine the treatment
- Minimal disease is treated in the office with topical agents
- Warts respond promptly to therapy
- More extensive disease may require an initial treatment session under anesthesia so that random lesions can be excised for pathologic evaluation to rule out dysplasia and the remainder coagulated
- Laser therapy is another method of condyloma destruction

SURGERY

Indications

- Extensive disease may require an initial treatment session under anesthesia so that random lesions can be excised for pathologic evaluation to rule out dysplasia

MEDICATIONS

- **Topical agents:** Bichloracetic acid or 25% podophyllum resin in tincture of benzoin

TREATMENT MONITORING

- Patients should be seen at regular intervals until resolution is complete
- Follow-up evaluation may reveal residual disease, but this is often easily treated with topical agents in the office

COMPLICATIONS

- Squamous cell carcinoma of the anal canal is the major complication

PROGNOSIS

- **Laser fulguration:** Recurrence rates are low
- Disease may respond to excision or destruction followed by intralesional interferon or autogenous vaccine created from excisional biopsies of the lesions

RESOURCES

REFERENCES

- Rompalo AM. Diagnosis and treatment of sexually acquired proctitis and proctocolitis: an update. *Clin Infect Dis.* 1999;28 (Suppl 1):S84.
- El-Attar SM et al. Anal warts, sexually transmitted diseases, and anorectal conditions associated with human immunodeficiency virus. *Prim Care.* 1999;26:81.

Crohn Disease

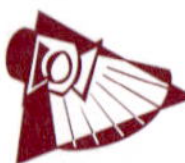

ESSENTIAL FEATURES

- Diarrhea
- Abdominal pain and palpable mass
- Low-grade fever, lassitude, weight loss
- Anemia
- Radiographic findings of thickened, stenotic bowel with ulceration and internal fistulas

EPIDEMIOLOGY

- A chronic progressive granulomatous inflammatory disorder affecting any part of the GI tract
- From 2 to 9 cases per 100,000 are detected annually in the United States
- There is geographic variation (more common in urban dwellers and Northern residents of the United States), and there is a relatively high incidence among Ashkenazi Jews
- The peak incidence occurs between the second and fourth decades
- The cause is unknown; appears to result from the interaction of genetic and environmental factors.
- The distal ileum is the most frequent site of involvement, eventually becoming diseased in 75% of cases
- Small bowel alone is involved in 15–30%, both the distal ileum and the colon in 40–60%, duodenum in 0.5–7%.

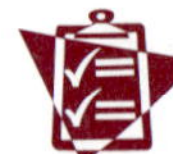

CLINICAL FINDINGS

SYMPTOMS AND SIGNS

- **Diarrhea:** Characteristically contains no blood if small bowel alone is diseased
- Acute and recurrent abdominal pain
- Malaise
- Weight loss
- Malnutrition
- Fever
- Palpable abdominal mass
- Abdominal tenderness
- **Anorectal lesions:** Chronic anal fissures, large ulcers, complex anal fistulas, or pararectal abscesses

LABORATORY FINDINGS

- Iron deficiency or macrocytic anemia due to vitamin B_{12} or folate deficiency
- Elevated ESR
- Hypoalbuminemia
- Abnormal D-xylose absorption suggests extensive disease or fistula formation, since carbohydrate is normally absorbed in the jejunum.

IMAGING FINDINGS

- Upper GI contrast radiography
  - Thickened bowel wall with stricture
  - Longitudinal ulceration
  - Deep transverse fissures and cobblestone formation
  - Fistulas and abscesses may also be detected
- Upper GI endoscopy
  - Mucosal lesions appear grossly as tiny hemorrhagic spots or shallow ulcers
  - Fissures serpiginous or linear ulcers surrounding islands of intact mucosa overlying edematous submucosa give a cobblestone appearance to the luminal surface
  - Stricture formation

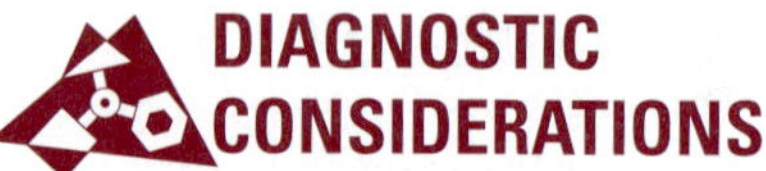

DIAGNOSTIC CONSIDERATIONS

- Systemic manifestations include:
  - Hepatobiliary disease
  - Uveitis
  - Arthritis
  - Ankylosing spondylitis
  - Aphthous ulcers
  - Erythema nodosum
  - Amyloidosis
  - Thromboembolism
  - Vascular disorders
  - Cutaneous ulcers with a granulomatous reaction
- About 70% of patients with Crohn disease undergo a definitive operation
- If multiple strictures are encountered, they can be treated by “strictureplasty,” in which the bowel is incised through the stricture and the wall is sutured or stapled so that the lumen is widened.

RULE OUT

- Ulcerative colitis
- Appendicitis
- TB
- Lymphoma
- Carcinoma
- Amebiasis
- Ischemia
- Eosinophilic gastroenteritis

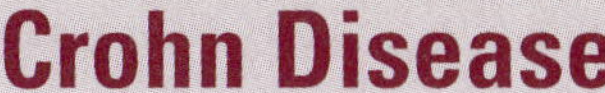

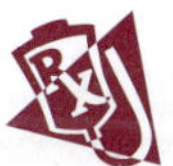

WORK-UP

- Upper GI contrast radiography
- Upper GI endoscopy

WHEN TO ADMIT

- Acute exacerbations
- Obstruction
- Perforation
- Abscess

WHEN TO REFER

- Most cases of Crohn disease of the small bowel should be managed in conjunction with a gastroenterologist

TREATMENT AND MANAGEMENT

- Surgery should be used to manage complications in coordination with medical therapy and is palliative, not curative

SURGERY

Indications

- Obstruction
- Perforation
- Internal or external fistulae
- Abscess
- Growth failure in children

Contraindications

- Extensive involvement of small bowel is unfavorable for curative resection
  - Resection is limited to the area responsible for complications.

MEDICATIONS

- Steroids, aminosalicylates, immunosuppressives, and metronidazole (perianal disease)
- Infliximab

COMPLICATIONS

- Obstruction
- Perforation
- Internal or external fistulae
- Abscess

PROGNOSIS

- **Symptomatic recurrence rates after resection:** 25–50% at 5 years, 35–80% at 10 years, 45–85% at 15 years.

RESOURCES

REFERENCES

- Ricart E et al. Infliximab for Crohn's disease in clinical practice at the Mayo Clinic: the first 100 patients. *Am J Gastroenterol.* 2001;96:722.
- Sutherland LR et al. Prevention of relapse of Crohn's disease. *Inflamm Bowel Dis.* 2000;6:321.

Cystic Disease of Lungs, Congenital

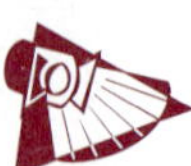

ESSENTIAL FEATURES

- Uncommon aberrations of respiratory tract development
  - Starts at 4th week of fetal life
  - Initial phase of airway branching until 16th wk
  - Canalicular phase: Capillaries develop (16th to 26th wk)
  - Alveolar phase: 26th wk on, alveolar air sacs form with type I, II pneumocytes
- **Tracheobronchial atresia (TA)**
  - Can occur at any level
  - May involve isolated or multiple areas
  - Diffuse disease is fatal
  - Isolated bronchial atresia results in bronchus with blind pouch leads to compression of surrounding lung and emphysematous changes
  - Anomalous tracheal or esophageal bronchi and diverticular are related diseases
- **Bronchogenic cysts (BC)**
  - Abnormal budding of foregut may result in formation of BC
  - Commonly occur in pulmonary hilum or mediastinum, occasionally pulmonary parenchyma
  - Usually single, lined by cuboidal respiratory epithelium, preferentially in lower lobes
  - Cysts generally thin walled, occasionally with cartilage
  - May communicate with tracheobronchial tree
  - Known to enlarge rapidly and rupture causing tension pneumothorax
- **Bronchopulmonary dysplasia (BPD):** Cluster of diseases includes pulmonary agenesis, aplasia, and primary and secondary hypoplasia
  - **Unilateral agenesis** occurs when 1 lung and vessels fail to develop
  - **Pulmonary aplasia:** Blind bronchial tumor stump exists and soils normal lung with secretions
  - **Pulmonary hypoplasia:** Low radial alvelolar count and low lung to body weight ratio without inciting cause
  - **Secondary pulmonary hypoplasia:** Occurs due to fetal or maternal abnormalities such as congenital diaphragmatic hernia, oligohydramnios, Potter syndrome, abnormal bone development
- **Pulmonary sequestration (PS)**
  - Abnormal budding of foregut leading to lung parenchyma without bronchial communication
  - Can be intralobar (85%) or extralobar
  - Often have systemic blood supply from abdominal aorta, 96% drain into pulmonary venous system
- **Cystic adenomatoid malformation (CAM)**
  - Overgrowth of terminal bronchiolar structures lined by respiratory epithelium with disorganized elastic connective tissue and smooth muscle
  - Solid structures interspersed with cysts resembling immature alveoli
- **Congenital Lobar Emphysema (LE)**
  - Hypoplastic bronchial cartilage in 25–75% of patients; increased alveoli number in 37% (polyalveoli)
  - Neonates with prolonged vent support may develop LE from catheter trauma and barotraumas, affecting right lower lobe (RLL)

EPIDEMIOLOGY

- **BPD:** 50% have associated cardiac anomalies
- **PS:** Left lung affected 58% of time
- **LE:** Left upper lobe (LUL) most commonly involved, then right middle lobe (RML)

CLINICAL FINDINGS

SYMPTOMS AND SIGNS

- Often presents early in life
- Some remain occult until adulthood
- **TA:** Neonates present with intractable cyanosis with normal larynx on intubation
- **Isolated bronchial atresia:** Wheezing, stridor, pulmonary infections due to mucocele formation and compression of normal lung
- **BC:** Mediastinal present with airway compression, parenchymal present with pulmonary infection
- **BPD (agenesis):** Neonates present with tachypnea and cyanosis
- **BPD:** Some patients present in childhood; dyspnea and wheezing and tracheal deviation toward side of agenesis
- **BPD (hypoplasia):** Presents in neonates with tachypnea and hypoxemia resistant to oxygen; persistent fetal circulation
- **PS:** Presentation ranges from asymptomatic lower lobe masses to recurrent lower lobe infections due to seeding from pores connected to normal lung, rarely hemoptysis, congestive heart failure due to left to right shunt
- **CAM:** 3 types
  - Solid lung masses: associated with anasarca, ascites, stillbirth and prematurity
  - Intermediate: Mixed solid and cystic present with respiratory distress
  - Cystic lesion: Presents later, occasionally in adulthood with recurrent pulmonary infections
- **LE**
  - Most present within 6 mos of life with respiratory distress
  - Almost all have tracheal deviation away from affected side
  - Hyperresonance
  - Decreased breath sounds on affected side

IMAGING FINDINGS

- **BC:** Discrete round densities often sharp and air-filled, or as pulmonary nodule
- **PS**
  - Chest film, CT scan diagnostic
  - Angiography indicated only if questions arise regarding diagnosis, arterial blood supply, or venous drainage
- **CAM:** Chest CT and abdominal x-ray helps make diagnosis and rule out diaphragmatic hernia
- **LE**
  - Chest film demonstrates hyperlucency of affected lobe with compression of normal lung
  - CT may be necessary to rule out other etiology

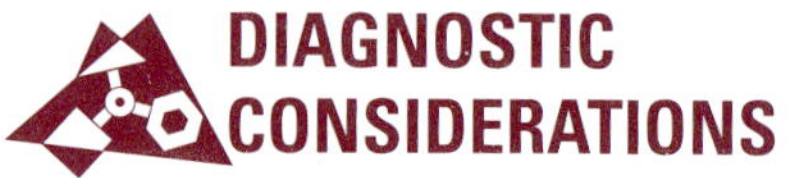

DIAGNOSTIC CONSIDERATIONS

- **BC:** May present as solitary pulmonary nodule or pulmonary abscess

RULE OUT

- **BPD:** Rule out total lung atelectasis from foreign body aspiration, total lung sequestration, esophageal bronchus
- **CAM:** Congenital diaphragmatic hernia, congenital lobar emphysema
- **LE:** Foreign body (bronchoscopy may be necessary)

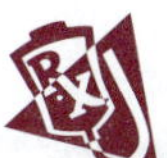

WORK-UP

- Chest film, esophagogram, chest CT may be required to exclude other diagnosis

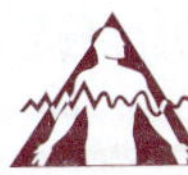

TREATMENT AND MANAGEMENT

- **TA:** Mask ventilation can palliate diffuse disease
- **PS:** Great care to identify systemic arterial and venous origins to avoid infarction of normal lung

SURGERY

Indications

- **TA:** Emergency tracheostomy lifesaving if isolated subglottic atresia
- **BC:** Simple or segmental resection, rarely lobectomy required
- **BPD (pulmonary aplasia):** Resect pulmonary stump
- **PS:** Segmental resection or lobectomy
- **CAM:** Surgical resection, may be required in neonates with acute respiratory distress
- **LE:** Lobectomy

PROGNOSIS

- **TA:** Diffuse disease is fatal
- **BC:** Good after resection
- **BPD (aplasia):** < 50% 5-year survival due to cardiac diseases
  - Hypoplasia, 75% mortality
- **PS:** Favorable after resection
- **CAM:** Good following resection for intermediate and cystic types
- **LE:** Good after resection

RESOURCES

REFERENCES

- Eber E, Zach MS. Long term sequelae of bronchopulmonary dysplasia (chronic lung disease of infancy). *Thorax.* 2001;56:317.
- Louie HW et al. Pulmonary sequestration: 17-year experience at UCLA. *Am Surg.* 1993;59:801.
- Stigers KB et al. The clinical and imaging spectrum of findings in patients with congenital lobar emphysema. *Pediatr Pulmonol.* 1992;14:160.

Cystic Fibrosis

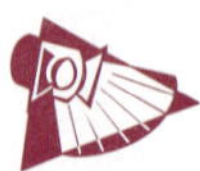

ESSENTIAL FEATURES

- Serious congenital disorder, autosomal recessive disorder
- Most common mutation is deletion of amino acid in position 508 (Phe)
- Defect in chloride transport, results in more NaCl absorption in the airway
- Defect occurs in apocrine sweat glands tracheobronchial tree, pancreas, GI tract
- Airway secretions are low in volume and high in viscosity
- Mucoid plugs form and are rubbery, semisolid, gray to greenish yellow in color resulting in impaction
- Often history of recurrent upper respiratory tract infection, fever, and chest pain

EPIDEMIOLOGY

- 1 in 25 whites heterozygous carrier
- 1 in 2000 homozygous
- Single most common mutation characterized

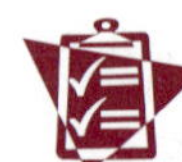

CLINICAL FINDINGS

SYMPTOMS AND SIGNS

- Recurrent respiratory infection
- Fever
- Chest pain
- Meconium ileus in newborn, meconium in terminal ileum causes obstruction

LABORATORY FINDINGS

- Positive sweat test (NaCl in sweat)

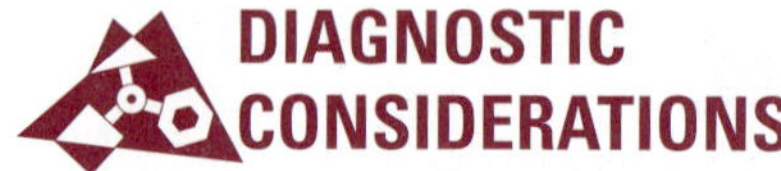

DIAGNOSTIC CONSIDERATIONS

RULE OUT

- Bronchogenic carcinoma
- Bronchiectasis
- Abscess
- Bacterial pneumonia
- Lipoid pneumonia
- Pulmonary eosinophilic granuloma
- Löffler syndrome

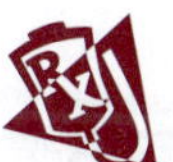

WORK-UP

- Chloride sweat test
- Pilocarpin iontophoresis (NaCl concentrations exceeding 60 mEq/L)

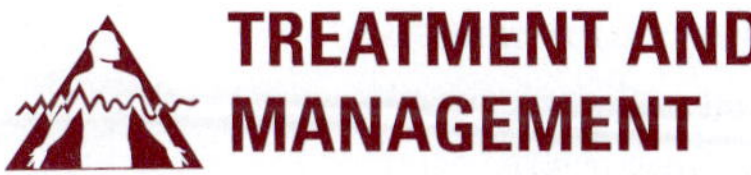

TREATMENT AND MANAGEMENT

SURGERY

- Double lung transplant

Indications

- End stage pulmonary disease

COMPLICATIONS

- Bronchitis, bronchiectasis
- Pulmonary fibrosis
- Emphysema
- Lung abscess
- **Complication of transplant:** Chronic bronchitis obliterans major obstacle and cause of eventual transplant failure

PROGNOSIS

- 1-year survival, 85%
- 5-year survival, 50%

RESOURCES

REFERENCES

- Fiel SB. Clinical management of pulmonary disease in cystic fibrosis. *Lancet.* 1993;341:1070.

Deep Venous Thrombosis (DVT)

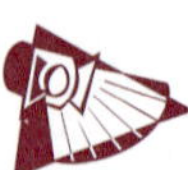

ESSENTIAL FEATURES

- **Virchow's triad:** Stasis, vascular injury, hypercoagulability
  - **Stasis:** Venous insufficiency, heart failure, prolonged bed rest/plane travel
  - **Endothelial injury:** Direct trauma, chemotherapy infusion, previous DVT, phlebitis, operative trauma all increase release of tissue factor increasing thrombin and decreasing fibrinolysis
  - **Hypercoagulability:** Malignancy, protein C or S deficiency, disseminated intravascular coagulation (DIC), liver failure, elevated homocysteine, factor V Leiden, prothrombin gene variant, paroxysmal nocturnal hemoglobinuria
- Important risk factors
  - Recent surgery
  - Trauma
  - Cancer
  - Prolonged immobilization
  - Oral contraceptive use
- Other risks
  - Advanced age
  - Type A blood group
  - Obesity
  - Prior DVT
  - Multiparity
  - Inflammatory bowel disease
  - Systemic lupus erythematosus
- Most common in calf veins, may arise in femoral or iliac
- 25% calf DVT progress proximally
- Proximal DVT (femoral or iliac)
  - Chronic venous insufficiency, 25%
  - Fatal pulmonary embolism (PE), 10%
- Phlegmasia cerulea dolens caused by iliofemoral venous thrombosis, which is characterized by cyanosis of limb from venous outflow obstruction; potentially limb-threatening
- In phlegmasia alba dolens, leg is pulseless, pale, cool; potentially limb-threatening

EPIDEMIOLOGY

- Affects 500,000 persons in United States each year
- Up to 21% mortality in elderly
- 20–30% of new DVT have occult malignancy (lung, pancreas, prostate, breast, ovary most common)
- Surgery increases risk 21-fold
- Complication rates
  - General surgery, 20%
  - Neurosurgery, 24%
  - Hip/knee arthroplasty, 50%

CLINICAL FINDINGS

SYMPTOMS AND SIGNS

- 50% are asymptomatic
- Thigh or calf pain with or without edema
- Extensive DVT
  - Massive edema
  - Cyanosis
  - Dilated superficial veins
- Low-grade fever, tachycardia
- 50% have positive Homans sign (calf pain with ankle dorsiflexion)
- Acute PE
- Phlegmasia

IMAGING FINDINGS

- **Duplex US**
  - Sensitivity/specificity > 95%
  - Evaluate vein for flow, dilation, and incompressibility (indicate clot present)
  - Acute clot anechogenic, chronic clot echogenic
  - Less accurate to detect calf thrombosis
- **Magnetic resonance venography (MRV)**
  - Sensitivity/specificity nearly 100%
  - Gadolinium MRV for thrombus age
- **D-dimer levels**
  - Too nonspecific

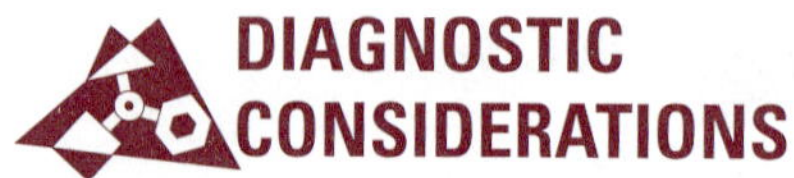

DIAGNOSTIC CONSIDERATIONS

RULE OUT

- Local muscle strain
- Achilles tendon rupture
- Cellulitis
- Lymphedema
- Baker cyst obstructing popliteal vein
- Retroperitoneal mass (obstructing iliac vein)
- Congestive heart failure (CHF), liver, kidney failure, inferior vena cava (IVC) obstruction (bilateral edema)

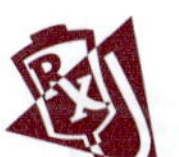

WORK-UP

- Duplex US
- Consider hypercoaguable work-up if idiopathic

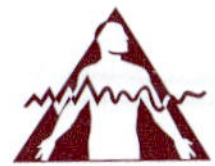

TREATMENT AND MANAGEMENT

- Goal is to reduce complications

Anticoagulation

- Primary treatment
- Decreases recurrence and PE risk by 80%
- Limits propagation of clot (no effect on clot lysis)
- Iliofemoral thrombosis
  - Thrombolytic therapy
  - Surgical thrombectomy
- IVC filter is contraindication to anticoagulation

SURGERY

Indications

- Calf compartment syndrome
- Massive extremity edema

MEDICATIONS

Heparin

- Potentiates antithrombin III, inhibits thrombin
- Partial thromboplastin time (PTT) goal of 2 times normal
- Effective heparinization within 24 hrs decreases risk of DVT recurrence
- Thrombocytopenia peaks at 5–10 days

Warfarin

- Initiated when PTT therapeutic
- First few days, may be hypercoaguable due to inhibition of anticoagulants proteins C and S
- For first episode of uncomplicated DVT, 3–6 months of therapy is recommended (international normalized ratio [INR]: 2.0–3.0)
- For second episode of DVT or hypercoaguable state, lifelong therapy is recommended

Low-Molecular-Weight Heparin (LMWH)

- Inhibits factor Xa activity
- Lower risk of bleeding
- No treatment monitoring; dose response is predicable
- May cause thrombus regression

Fibrinolytics/ Thrombolytics

- Faster clot lysis but no change in incidence of long-term sequelae
- Institute within 1 week of clot formation
- Treatment of acute iliofemoral thrombosis causing massive edema, cyanosis, calf compartment syndrome

TREATMENT MONITORING

- Heparin monitored with PTT
- Warfarin monitored with INR

COMPLICATIONS

- Varicose veins
- Chronic venous insufficiency
- Postphlebitic syndrome
- Recurrent DVT
- PE

PROGNOSIS

- Iliofemoral thrombectomy, 40–90% success; treatment failures due to residual thrombosis, stenosis of proximal vein

PREVENTION

- Surgical patients
  - Subcutaneous heparin
  - LMWH
  - Sequential compression devices
- Consider IVC filter in cases of prolonged immobility

RESOURCES

REFERENCES

- Hirsh J et al. Clinical trials that have influenced the treatment of venous thromboembolism: a historical perspective. *Ann Intern Med.* 2001;134:409.

Deep Venous Thrombosis (DVT), Upper Extremity

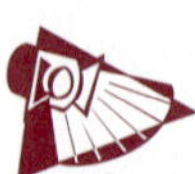

ESSENTIAL FEATURES

- Axillary-subclavian thrombosis: 3 etiologies
  1. Paget-Schroetter syndrome: Also called "effort thrombosis"
     - Results from intermittent obstruction of vein during repetitive arm/shoulder movements
     - Subclavian vein compressed between first rib, anterior scalene muscle, and clavicle
  2. Primary subclavian venous thrombosis occurs in patients with hypercoagulable states
  3. Secondary subclavian venous thrombosis results from venous injury (central lines, external trauma, pacemaker wires)

EPIDEMIOLOGY

- Thrombosis of axillary/subclavian vein < 5% of DVT; 12% result in PE
- Paget-Schroetter affects more men than women (4:1); 56% are hypercoaguable
  - Occurs in healthy young athletes and persons who perform manual labor

CLINICAL FINDINGS

SYMPTOMS AND SIGNS

Paget-Schroetter

- Repetitive arm activity and exercise
- Significant superficial venous distention in arm/shoulder
- Aching pain
- Cyanosis of chest wall, axilla, shoulder, and arm
- Other symptoms of thoracic outlet syndrome may be present (see Thoracic Outlet Syndrome)

Subclavian Venous Thrombosis

- Edematous, cyanotic arm, hand

IMAGING FINDINGS

- Duplex US of upper extremity
- Venography + thrombolysis considered if duplex US is abnormal (positional venography with arm abducted 120 degrees)
- **Chest film:** Exclude cervical rib

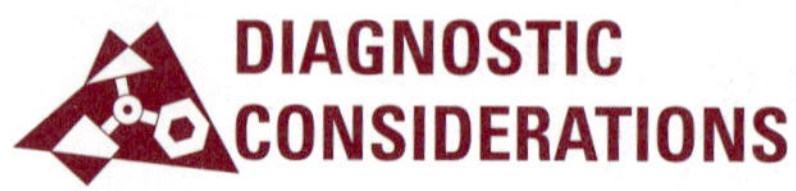

DIAGNOSTIC CONSIDERATIONS

- Evaluate for other evidence of hypercoagulability

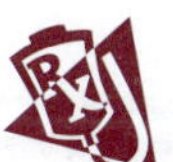

WORK-UP

- Duplex US
- Possible venogram

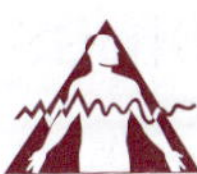

TREATMENT AND MANAGEMENT

- Remove indwelling central lines/ pacemakers
- Elevate arm, hydrate with IV fluid
- Thrombolysis
  - If vein stenotic, perform angioplasty on vein segment
- Vein compression with large collaterals suggests venous thoracic outlet syndrome and necessitates early operation
- Surgical thoracic outlet decompression
  - Resect anterior scalene muscle
  - First rib resection
  - Venoplasty

SURGERY

Indications

- Venous thoracic outlet syndrome

COMPLICATIONS

- Without surgery, venous thoracic outlet syndrome carries a 35–65% risk of rethrombosis

PROGNOSIS

- Excellent if treated early
- If thrombosis exists > 3 mos, it does not respond to therapy and may cause significant long-term disability

RESOURCES

- Urschel HC et al. Paget-Schroetter syndrome: what is the best management? *Ann Thorac Surg.* 2000;69:1663.

Dehydration (Volume & Electrolyte Depletion)

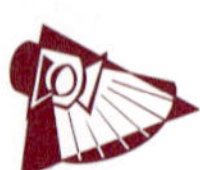

ESSENTIAL FEATURES

- Water deficit without solute deficit
- Rare in surgical patients
- Water deficit can be estimated from serum Na concentration
- Water deficit: ((140 – serum Na) × total body water))/140

EPIDEMIOLOGY

- Occurs in patients unable to regulate water intake
- Insensible water loss from fever
- Tube feedings with inadequate water content
- Diabetes insipidus

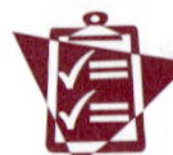

CLINICAL FINDINGS

SYMPTOMS AND SIGNS

- Concentrated urine
- CNS depression
- Lethargy
- Coma
- Muscle rigidity
- Tremors
- Spasticity
- Seizures

LABORATORY FINDINGS

- Hypernatremia
- Low urine Na despite hypernatremia

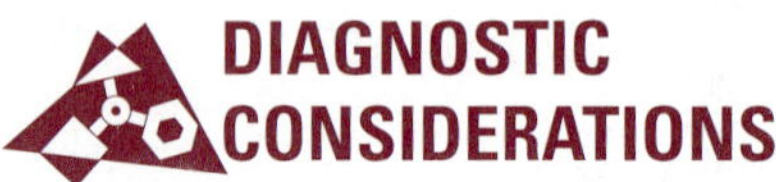

DIAGNOSTIC CONSIDERATIONS

- Water deficit usually accompanied by solute (Na^+) deficit

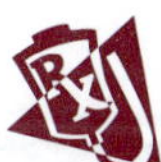

WORK-UP

- Physical exam
- Serial serum Na

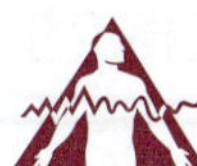

TREATMENT AND MANAGEMENT

- Replacement of enough water to return serum Na concentration to normal
- Treat patient with D5W unless hypotension has developed in which case hypotonic saline should be used

TREATMENT MONITORING

- Serum Na

PROGNOSIS

- Excellent

PREVENTION

- Adequate water intake

RESOURCES

REFERENCES

- Palevsky PM et al. Hypernatremia in hospitalized patients. *Ann Intern Med.* 1996;124:197.
- Body JJ. Current and future directions in medical therapy: hypercalcemia. *Cancer.* 2000;88(12 Suppl):3054.

Desmoid Tumor

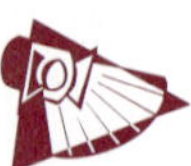

ESSENTIAL FEATURES

- Soft-tissue neoplasms that originate form aponeurotic tissues
- Referred to as "aggressive fibromatosis" and behave as low-grade malignant lesions
- Locally aggressive but virtually never metastasize
- Clinically, the lesions present as enlarging, often painless, soft-tissue mass
- Most often occur in abdominal wall scars, especially in a cesarean section incision
- Strongly associated with familial polyposis syndromes
- Intra-abdominal desmoids occur most commonly in the setting of familial adenomatous polyposis (FAP)

EPIDEMIOLOGY

- Strong female predominance, presentation 1–2 years after parturition, and reports of spontaneous degeneration after menopause all suggest a strong hormonal component to desmoid development
- Desmoids occur with increased frequency in patients with FAP, classically in the mesentery following total proctocolectomy

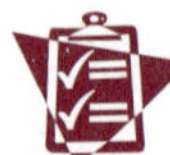

CLINICAL FINDINGS

SYMPTOMS AND SIGNS

- Enlarging, often painless, soft-tissue mass occurring in or near the vicinity of an incision with sporadic desmoid formation
- Abdominal mass formation or small bowel obstruction may occur secondary to mesenteric desmoid formation in patients with familial polyposis syndrome following total proctocolectomy

LABORATORY FINDINGS

- No specific abnormalities

IMAGING FINDINGS

- Plain films may demonstrate visceral displacement or obstruction
- US useful in characterizing abdominal wall desmoid extent
- Abdominal pelvic CT scan or MRI will demonstrate a soft-tissue mass that is radiographically indistinguishable from a soft-tissue sarcoma
  - Both methods will localize and characterize extent of the lesion

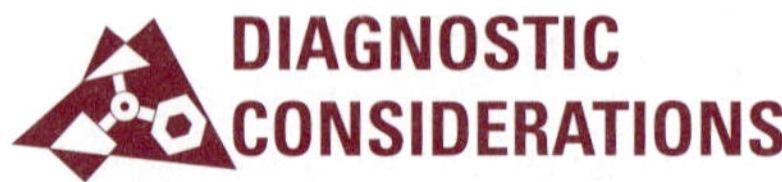

DIAGNOSTIC CONSIDERATIONS

- Soft-tissue sarcoma
- Rectus sheath hematoma
- Benign abdominal wall masses
  - Lipoma
  - Hemangioma
  - Fibroma
  - Endometrioma
- Abdominal wall metastasis
- Mesenteric metastasis
- Mesenteric cyst
- Interloop abscess
- Mesenteric hematoma

RULE OUT

- Soft-tissue sarcoma
- Abdominal wall metastases

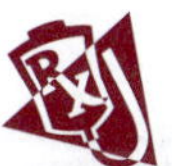

WORK-UP

- Complete history and physical exam
- Radiographic characterization of tumor extent
- Core needle biopsy or incisional biopsy to establish diagnosis

WHEN TO ADMIT

- Abdominal wall lesions usually can be managed on an outpatient basis

WHEN TO REFER

- Incompletely excised lesions with microscopically positive margins may benefit from postoperative radiation
- Most patients can be treated by the general surgeon

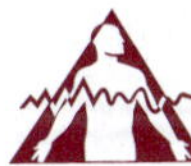

TREATMENT AND MANAGEMENT

- Resect desmoid tumor to a histologically negative margin
- Re-excision or radiation therapy for positive or close to positive margins
- Abdominal wall reconstruction with avoidance of alloplastic materials if possible
- Mesenteric desmoids associated with FAP are managed conservatively for as long as possible

SURGERY

Indications

- Resectable abdominal wall desmoid tumor
- Bowel obstruction secondary to desmoid that does not respond to conservative treatment

Contraindications

- Avoid resection of major neurovascular structures or adjacent organs unless absolutely necessary

MEDICATIONS

- Tamoxifen
- Sulindac
- Chemotherapy last resort

TREATMENT MONITORING

- Excision site recurrence

COMPLICATIONS

- Recurrence
- Compression of vital structures

PROGNOSIS

- Tumors virtually never metastasize but are locally invasive, thus location of the tumor predicts prognosis

RESOURCES

REFERENCES

- Soravia C et al. Desmoid disease in patients with familial adenomatous polyposis. *Dis Colon Rectrum.* 2000;43:363.

PRACTICE GUIDELINES

- The National Comprehensive Cancer Network http://www.nccn.org/

Diaphragmatic Hernia, Congenital

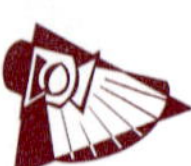

ESSENTIAL FEATURES

- 1/2000 and 1/5000 births
- 33% with associated congenital defects, including neural tube defects and cardiac defects
- 80% are left-sided; 20% are right-sided
- Right side, hepatic veins may drain ectopically into right atrium
- 10–20% present after first 24 hrs
- Associated with pulmonary hypoplasia on affected side

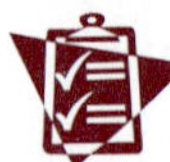

CLINICAL FINDINGS

SYMPTOMS AND SIGNS

- Dyspnea
- Chest retractions
- Decreased breath sounds on affected side
- Polyhydramnios prenatally (80%)
- Cyanosis
- Scaphoid abdomen

LABORATORY FINDINGS

- Respiratory acidosis

IMAGING FINDINGS

- **Prenatal US:** Accurate in 40–90% of cases showing herniation of abdominal contents in thorax
- **Chest film:** Herniation of abdominal contents into thorax and associated pulmonary hypoplasia with occasional compression of mediastinum away from affected side

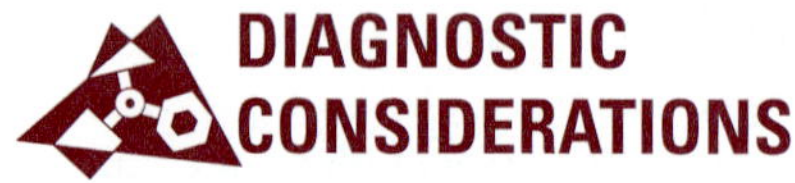

DIAGNOSTIC CONSIDERATIONS

- Cardiac and neural tube defects

RULE OUT

- Associated neural tube or cardiac defects

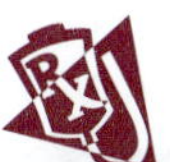

WORK-UP

- History and physical exam
- Chest film
- ABG measurements
- Echocardiogram
- US for neural tube defects

TREATMENT AND MANAGEMENT

SURGERY

Indications

- Primary repair or using mesh once respiratory status has been stabilized and optimized

MEDICATIONS

- Mechanical ventilation if necessary
- NG decompression
- High frequency oscillatory ventilation if necessary
- Extracorporeal membrane oxygenation (ECMO) if necessary

COMPLICATIONS

- Chronic lung disease
- Skeletal muscle abnormalities
- Acute respiratory failure postoperatively
- Developmental delay
- Growth delay

PROGNOSIS

- 39–95% survival

PREVENTION

- In utero repair efforts under investigation

RESOURCES

REFERENCES

- Harrison MR et al. Correction of congenital diaphragmatic hernia in utero IX: fetuses with poor prognosis (liver herniation and low lung-to-head ratio) can be saved by fetoscopic temporary tracheal occlusion. *J Pediatr Surg.* 1998;33:1017.
- Wilson JM et al. Congenital diaphragmatic hernia—a tale of two cities: the Boston experience. *J Pediatr Surg.* 1997;32:401.

Diaphragmatic Hernia, Traumatic

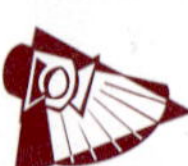

ESSENTIAL FEATURES

- May be acute or chronic following either penetrating or blunt trauma
  - Acute form associated with respiratory distress
  - Chronic form marked by pain and bowel obstruction
- Chest film showing NG tube, air fluid level, or abdominal vicera in the chest is diagnostic

EPIDEMIOLOGY

- Traumatic rupture of the diaphragm may occur as a result of penetrating wounds or severe blunt external trauma
- Lacerations usually occur in the tendinous portion of the diaphragm, most often on the left side
- Abdominal viscera may immediately herniate through the defect in the diaphragm into the pleural cavity (acute) or may gradually insinuate themselves into the thorax over a period of months or years (chronic)
- In the acute form, the patient has recently experienced blunt trauma or a penetrating wound to the chest, abdomen, or back
- In the chronic form, the diaphragmatic tear is unrecognized at the time of the original injury

CLINICAL FINDINGS

SYMPTOMS AND SIGNS

- Acute herniation
  - Symptoms from concomitant injuries
  - Respiratory insufficiency
- Chronic herniation
  - Pain
  - Bowel obstruction

IMAGING FINDINGS

- **Chest film**: A radiopaque area and occasionally an air fluid level if hollow viscera have herniated
- If the stomach has entered the chest, the abnormal path of an NG tube may be diagnostic
- **US, CT scan, and MRI**: Demonstrate the diaphragmatic rent

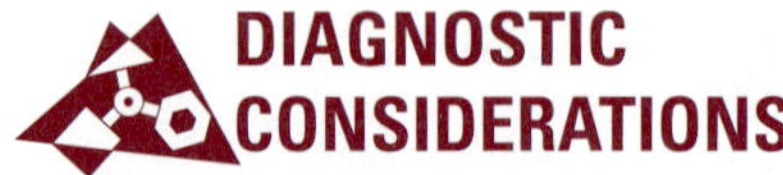

DIAGNOSTIC CONSIDERATIONS

- In an acute traumatic setting, focus attention on life-threatening injury
  - Diaphragmatic herniation may be considered as a possible source of respiratory distress
- In a patient with a history of abdominal trauma and a clinical picture of bowel obstruction, missed diaphragmatic hernia should be considered

RULE OUT

- Atelectasis
- Space-consuming tumors of the lower pleural space
- Pleural effusion
- Intestinal obstruction due to other causes

WORK-UP

- Chest film
- CT scan

WHEN TO ADMIT

- All acute cases
- Chronic cases with evidence of bowel obstruction, severe pain

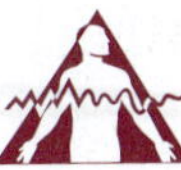

TREATMENT AND MANAGEMENT

- **Acute:** Repair after stabilized or at the same time as other injuries are treated if multiple injuries.
- **Chronic**
  - – Symptomatic, urgent repair
  - – Asymptomatic, elective repair

SURGERY

Indications

- All diaphragmatic hernias should be repaired

COMPLICATIONS

- Respiratory insufficiency
- Intestinal obstruction and perforation
- Intestinal bleeding

PROGNOSIS

- Excellent after surgical repair; very seldom recurrent

RESOURCES

REFERENCES

- Grover SB, Ratan SK. Simultaneous dual posttraumatic diaphragmatic and abdominal wall hernias. *J Trauma.* 2001;51:583.
- Meyer G et al. Laparoscopic repair of traumatic diaphragmatic hernias. *Surg Endosc.* 2000;14:1010.

Diverticulitis

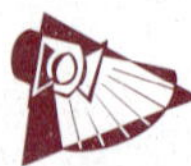

ESSENTIAL FEATURES

- Results from perforation and/or infection of colonic diverticulum
- Most common in sigmoid colon
- Becomes clinically significant when infection spreads through wall of colon, into pericolic tissue
- May lead to intra-abdominal abscess, peritonitis
- Believed to result from increased intraluminal pressure
- Cecal diverticulitis may resemble appendicitis clinically
- May be complicated by colonic fistulae (colovesical, coloenteric)
- Involvement of the entire colon in up to 10%
- **Noncomplicated:** Localized to colon, pericolic tissue
- **Complicated:** Abscess, fistula, obstruction, peritonitis

EPIDEMIOLOGY

- In western countries, diverticula develop in perhaps 50% of persons (10% by age 40; 65% by age 80)
- Dietary factors may contribute to formation of diverticula (low fiber)
- Natural history of patients with diverticula: 10–25% become symptomatic

CLINICAL FINDINGS

SYMPTOMS AND SIGNS

- May present with localized abdominal pain
- Constipation or increased frequency of defecation
- Dysuria with inflammatory process involving bladder
- Nausea, vomiting
- Fever
- Abdominal distention
- Pelvic or lower quadrant mass
- Localized to diffuse peritonitis if freely perforated
- May present as large bowel obstruction

LABORATORY FINDINGS

- Leukocytosis
- Stool may be guaiac positive

IMAGING FINDINGS

- **Abdominal x-ray:** May show free abdominal air if a diverticulum has freely perforated
- Radiographic picture of ileus or bowel obstruction
- **CT (oral and IV contrast)**
  - Effacement of pericolonic fat
  - Abscess
  - Fistula
  - Bowel wall thickening
- Abscesses found on CT may be concomitantly percutaneously drained
- Avoid colonoscopy (because of risk of perforation)
- **Water soluble contrast enema:** May reveal abscess, fistula, extrinsic compression by a paracolic mass

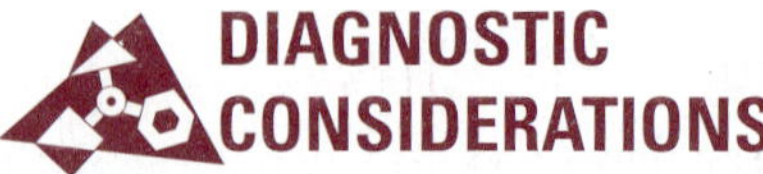

DIAGNOSTIC CONSIDERATIONS

- Colonic/visceral malignancy
- Appendicitis
- Renal colic
- Other causes of bowel obstruction
  - Stricture
  - Incarcerated hernia
  - Internal hernia
- Crohn disease
- Ulcerative colitis
- Ischemic colitis
- Antibiotic-associated colitis
- Irritable bowel syndrome

RULE OUT

- Colonic malignancy
- Perforated carcinoma
- Appendicitis

WORK-UP

- Plain x-ray to evaluate for free abdominal air
- Contrast CT scan with percutaneous catheter drainage if abscess identified and accessible
- Avoid colonoscopy or barium enema with acute presentation

WHEN TO ADMIT

- Signs of peritonitis or severe abdominal pain
- Mild attacks (noncomplicated) without signs of peritonitis or other indicators of perforation or obstruction may be managed as outpatient
- Signs of sepsis, obstruction, fistulas

TREATMENT AND MANAGEMENT

- Mild to moderate cases may be treated as outpatient with oral antibiotics
- NPO, IV hydration
- IV broad-spectrum antibiotics
- Percutaneous drainage if abscess found on CT
- NG decompression
- Avoid opioid pain medications
- May perform colonoscopy a week or so after acute process subsides

SURGERY

Indications

- **Emergency surgery**
  - Free perforation
  - Peritonitis
  - Massive bleeding
  - Complete obstruction
- **Urgent surgery**
  - Failure of medical therapy
  - Immediate recurrence following resolution
  - Partial colonic obstruction
- **Elective surgery**
  - Recurrent disease
  - Fistulas
  - Recurrent hemorrhage

MEDICATIONS

- Broad-spectrum antibiotics (IV for patients admitted to hospital)
- IV fluids

TREATMENT MONITORING

- Serial abdominal exams
- Serial blood counts
- Serial abdominal films
- Failure to improve, may obtain repeat CT scan

COMPLICATIONS

- Perforation
- Fistula formation
- Hemorrhage
- Colonic obstruction
- Abscess formation

RESOURCES

REFERENCES

- Baevsky R. Acute diverticulitis. *N Engl J Med.* 1998;339:1082.
- Gooszen AW et al. Operative treatment of acute complications of diverticular disease: primary or secondary anastomosis after sigmoid resection. *Eur J Surg.* 2001;167:35.
- Roberts P et al. Practice parameters for sigmoid diverticulitis. The Standards Task Force American Society of Colon and Rectal Surgeons. *Dis Colon Rectum.* 1995;38:125.
- Young-Fadok TM et al. Colonic diverticular disease. *Curr Probl Surg.* 2000;37:457.

WEB SITES

- http://www.niddk.nih.gov/health/digest/pubs/divert/divert.htm

Diverticulosis

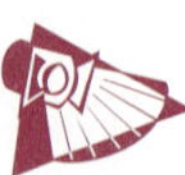

ESSENTIAL FEATURES

- Diverticula are more common in the colon than in any other portion of the GI tract
- Diverticulosis is the presence of multiple false diverticula
- Colonic diverticula are acquired and are classified as false because they consist of mucosa and submucosa that have herniated through the muscular coats
- Colonic diverticula are pulsion (rather than traction) diverticula because they are pushed out by intraluminal pressure
- They vary from a few millimeters to several centimeters in diameter; the necks may be narrow or wide; and some contain inspissated fecal matter
- Cultural factors, especially diet, play an important etiologic role
  - Chief among the dietary influences is the fiber content of foods.
- The pathogenesis of diverticula requires defects in the colonic wall and increased pressure in the lumen relative to the serosal surface

EPIDEMIOLOGY

- 95% of patients with diverticula have involvement of the sigmoid colon
- Descending > transverse > ascending
- Solitary cecal and multiple right colonic diverticula seen in Asian people
- In Western countries, diverticula develops in perhaps 50% of persons; 10% by age 40 and 65% by age 80
- Diverticular disease is more common in Western nations than in Japan or in developing countries of the tropics

CLINICAL FINDINGS

SYMPTOMS AND SIGNS

- Diverticulosis probably remains asymptomatic in about 80% of people and is detected incidentally on barium enema x-rays or endoscopy if it is discovered at all
- May present with lower GI bleeding
- Episodic pain, constipation, diarrhea
- Left lower quadrant tenderness
- Left colon is sometimes palpable as a firm tubular structure

LABORATORY FINDINGS

- Normal WBC count in uncomplicated cases
- Leukocytosis, anemia in complicated cases

IMAGING FINDINGS

- **Barium enema**
  - Diverticula
  - Segmental spasm
  - Muscular thickening that may narrow lumen
  - Saw-toothed appearance

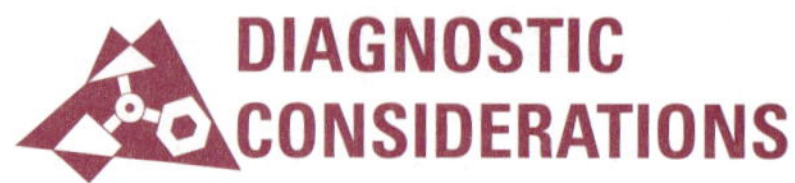

DIAGNOSTIC CONSIDERATIONS

- Diverticulitis
- Neoplasm (colonic, anal)
- AV malformation
- Hemorrhoids

RULE OUT

- Neoplasm

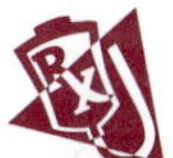

WORK-UP

- History and physical exam
- Digital rectal exam
- Lower endoscopy
  - Colonoscopy
  - Flexible sigmoidoscopy

WHEN TO ADMIT

- Abdominal pain
- GI bleeding
- Inability to distinguish diverticular disease from neoplasm

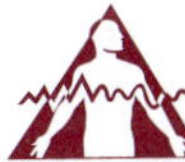

TREATMENT AND MANAGEMENT

- Asymptomatic persons with diverticulosis may be given a high-fiber diet
- Symptomatic patients also can be treated with a high-fiber diet
- Analgesics should be avoided, but if pain relief is necessary, nonopioid medications are preferred
- Education, reassurance, and a strong relationship between physician and patient are important to successful management

SURGERY

Indications

- Massive hemorrhage or to rule out carcinoma in some patients

Contraindications

- Colon resection for uncomplicated diverticular disease or irritable bowel syndrome is rarely necessary or advisable

MEDICATIONS

- Dietary fiber
- Bulking agents (psyllium seed or hemicellulose products)

COMPLICATIONS

- Diverticulitis
- Massive hemorrhage

PROGNOSIS

- Natural history of diverticulosis has not been defined
  - 10–20% of patients with diverticulosis develop diverticulitis or hemorrhage when monitored for many years
- 75% of complications of diverticular disease develop in patients with no prior colonic symptoms

RESOURCES

REFERENCES

- Young-Fadok TM et al. Colonic diverticular disease. *Curr Probl Surg.* 2000;37:457.
- Miura S et al. Recent trends in diverticulosis of the right colon in Japan: retrospective review in a regional hospital. *Dis Colon Rectum.* 2000;43:1383.

Double-Outlet Right Ventricle

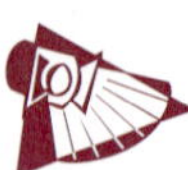

ESSENTIAL FEATURES

- A congenital heart lesion that decreases pulmonary arterial blood flow resulting in a right to left shunt
- Cyanosis and decreased oxygen delivery causes compensatory polycythemia (Hct > 70%) and spontaneous thrombosis
- Exercise, acidosis, pain worsens cyanosis and can cause hypoxic spells
- Squatting increases systemic resistance, causing increased pulmonary flow and blood oxygenation
- β-Blockers (decreases spasm), fluid intake, HCO_3 administration, norepinephrine (increases systemic resistance) may help decrease hypoxia
- Clubbing due to proliferation of capillaries and AV fistulas in extremities
- Bronchial and mediastinal arteries enlarge
- Ductus arteriosus maintains flow to lungs during fetal development
- Alprostadil early can allow time for optimization before definitive treatment
- Operative options to increase pulmonary flow:
  - Fontan procedure: Superior vena cava and inferior vena cava rerouted to pulmonary artery

Double-Outlet Right Ventricle (DORV)

- Both great arteries (50% of annulus of each valve) arise from right ventricle
- Uncommon and extremely complex
- Location of ventricular septal defect (VSD) (always present) determines classification
  - Subaortic
  - Subpulmonary
  - Noncomitted (proximal to valve annuli)
  - Double committed (adjacent to annuli and flow directed at both arteries)
- 33% of subaortic has subpulmonary obstruction and vice versa
- Great vessel and coronary artery anatomy can vary
- Subaortic VSD, rightward, posterior arrangement more common

Single Ventricle (SV)

- 1 ventricular chamber receiving blood from both tricuspid and mitral valves
- Associated with
  - Abnormal great vessel arrangements, 85%
  - Common AV valve, 30%
  - Stenosis or regurgitation of AV valve, 25%
  - Pulmonary stenosis or atresia, 50%
  - Aortic stenosis, 33%
  - Situs inversus, dextrocardia, and asplenia, 20%
- Clinical findings and prognosis related to relative pulmonary and systemic blood flow

EPIDEMIOLOGY

DORV

- Extremely rare

SV

- 3–5% of congenital heart defects
- 75% dominant left portion of ventricle

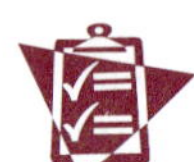

CLINICAL FINDINGS

SYMPTOMS AND SIGNS

DORV

- Symptoms depend on location of VSD and degree of outflow obstruction

SV

- Variable based on amount of pulmonary and systemic blood flow

IMAGING FINDINGS

- Echocardiography
- Catheterization

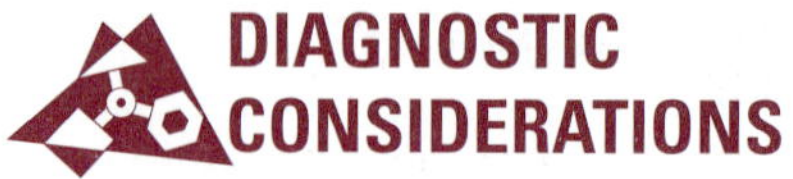

DIAGNOSTIC CONSIDERATIONS

- Echocardiography and catheterization for diagnosis

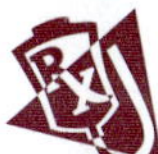

WORK-UP

- Echocardiography and catheterization for diagnosis

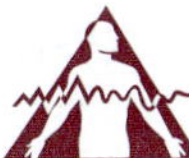

TREATMENT AND MANAGEMENT

DORV

- Surgical treatment depends on anatomy
- Creation of intraventricular baffle to direct LV flow to aorta, closing septal defect, avoiding subpulmonary obstruction
- Arterial switch is option

SV

- **Initial:** Shunt/pulmonary artery band, ventricular partitioning, then staged correction toward Fontan procedure

PROGNOSIS

DORV

- 10-year survival, 60–80%
- 33% require reintervention for outflow tract reobstruction

SV

- 1-year survival, 40–80%

RESOURCES

REFERENCES

- Planche C et al. Double-outlet right ventricle with non-committed ventricular septal defect. *Eur J Cardiothorac Surg.* 1999;15:747.
- Takeuchi K et al. Surgical outcome of double-outlet right ventricle with subpulmonary VSD. *Ann Thorac Surg.* 2001;71:49.
- Mayer JE et al. Factors associated with marked reduction in mortality for Fontan operations in patients with single ventricle. *J Thorac Cardiovasc Surg.* 1992;103:444.
- Mosca RS et al. Modified Norwood operation for single left ventricle and ventriculoarterial discordance: an improved surgical technique. *Ann Thorac Surg.* 1997;64:1126.

Drowning

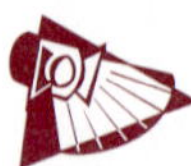

ESSENTIAL FEATURES

- Effects of drowning or near-drowning are due to hypoxemia and aspiration
- Physiologic effects of salt water aspiration are different than those of fresh water aspiration
  - Salt water aspiration produces hypovolemia, hemoconcentration, and hypertonicity but not hemolysis
  - Aspirated fresh water is quickly absorbed across the alveoli, leads to hypervolemia, hypotonicity, hemolysis, and electrolyte abnormalities

EPIDEMIOLOGY

- Major cause of accidental death in United States
- Particularly common among children
- 5500 deaths per year
- Up to 50 deaths per day in summer
- 25% of victims are teenagers; 20% are younger than 10 years
- 85% of victims are male
- Most cases in United States occur fresh water
- Alcohol plays a role in 40% of adult drownings

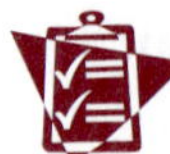

CLINICAL FINDINGS

SYMPTOMS AND SIGNS

- Hypoxemia
- Neurologic impairment/unconsciousness

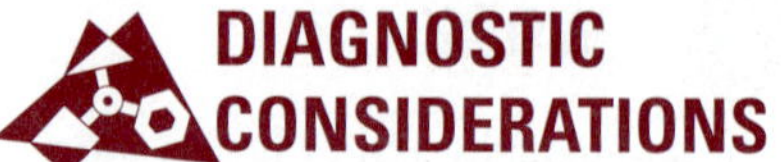

DIAGNOSTIC CONSIDERATIONS

- Evaluate for associated injuries (from a dive or fall) or toxic substances (drugs or alcohol)

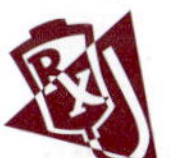

WORK-UP

- After restoring ventilation
  - Physical exam
  - Chest film
  - ABG measurements
  - Blood alcohol levels and drug screen

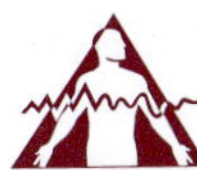

TREATMENT AND MANAGEMENT

- Immediate restoration of ventilation
- Do not waste time trying to empty lungs of aspirated water
- Correct residual hypoxemia, acidosis, and electrolyte abnormalities
- Endotracheal intubation and mechanical ventilation often necessary
- Aspiration at time of near-drowning is cause of late fatalities
- Prophylactic antibiotics and steroids have not shown benefit

COMPLICATIONS

- Aspiration-related late acute respiratory failure
- Red cell lysis (hypotonicity) can lead to hemoglobinuria and acute renal failure
- Neurologic injury related to hypoxia

RESOURCES

REFERENCES

- Cummings P et al. Trends in unintentional drowning: the role of alcohol and medical care. *JAMA.* 1999;281:2198.
- De Nicola LK et al. Submersion injuries in children and adults. *Crit Care Clin.* 1997;13:477.
- Graf WD et al. Outcome of children after near drowning. *Pediatrics.* 1998;101:160.

Duodenal Diverticula

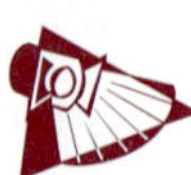

ESSENTIAL FEATURES

- Endoscopic or contrast radiographic evidence of diverticulum

EPIDEMIOLOGY

- Duodenal pulsion diverticula are acquired outpouchings of the mucosa and submucosa
- Found in 20% of autopsies and 5–10% of upper GI series
- 90% are on the medial aspect of the duodenum
- Most are solitary and within 2.5 cm of the ampulla of Vater
- Rare before age 40
- Symptoms are uncommon, and only 1% of cases found by x-ray warrant surgery
- Wind sock type of congenital intraluminal diverticulum is rare

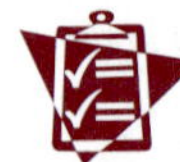

CLINICAL FINDINGS

SYMPTOMS AND SIGNS

- Most are asymptomatic
- A few patients have chronic postprandial abdominal pain or dyspepsia
- May present with symptoms from complications of diverticulum
  - Hemorrhage
  - Perforation
  - Pancreatitis
  - Biliary obstruction
- Wind sock type of intraluminal diverticulum usually presents with vague epigastric pain and postprandial fullness
  - Intestinal bleeding or pancreatitis is occasionally seen

LABORATORY FINDINGS

- Anemia

IMAGING FINDINGS

- Diverticulum visualized on upper GI contrast radiographic studies or upper GI endoscopy

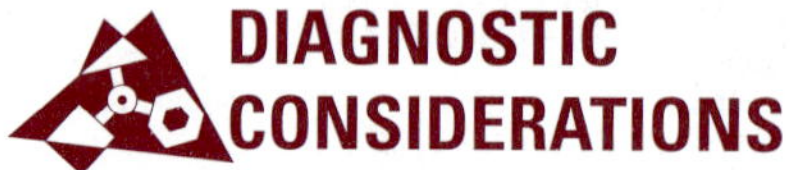

DIAGNOSTIC CONSIDERATIONS

- High level of suspicion is required for diagnosis
- Suspect duodenal diverticula in patients with upper GI bleeding, perforation or biliary obstruction in which no other source is evident

RULE OUT

- Other causes of upper GI perforation, bleeding, acute pancreatitis, or biliary obstruction

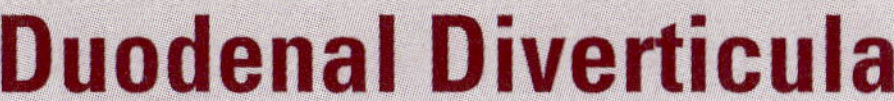

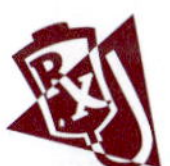

WORK-UP

- Signs and symptoms of duodenal diverticula or complications
- The diagnosis can be made by upper GI contrast radiographic studies or upper GI endoscopy

WHEN TO ADMIT

- Upper GI bleeding
- Perforation
- Biliary obstruction
- Pancreatitis
- Severe abdominal pain

TREATMENT AND MANAGEMENT

- Excision and a 2-layer closure
- Endoscopic sphincterotomy or stent placement may be preferable to treat biliary obstruction

SURGERY

Indications

- All complications
- Severe persistent postprandial abdominal pain or dyspepsia

Contraindications

- Asymptomatic patients

MEDICATIONS

- Antacids and anticholinergics

COMPLICATIONS

- Bleeding
- Perforation
- Acute pancreatitis
- Biliary obstruction

PROGNOSIS

- Good with expedient surgical treatment of complications

RESOURCES

REFERENCES

- Lobo DN et al. Periampullary diverticula and pancreaticobiliary disease. *Br J Surg.* 1999;86:588.

Duodenal Tumors, Benign

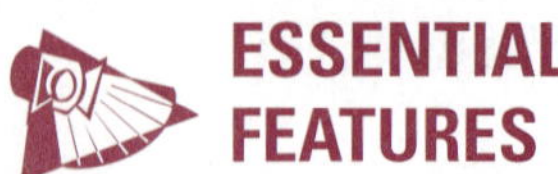

ESSENTIAL FEATURES

- Upper GI endoscopic or contrast radiographic evidence of duodenal tumor

EPIDEMIOLOGY

Adenomas

- Sessile or pedunculated
- May be associated with familial adenomatous polyposis
- **Tubular**: Low malignant potential
- **Villous**
  - High malignant risk
  - 30% of those > 3 cm with malignant focus
  - Often periampullary
- **Brunner gland**
  - Hyperplasia of exocrine glands
  - **Often asymptomatic**

Gastrointestinal stromal tumors (GIST)

- Difficult to distinguish benign from malignant on histologic studies

Carcinoid Tumors

- Often endocrinologically active

Hamartomas

- Associated with Peutz-Jeghers syndrome
- Rare malignant potential

Lipomas

- No malignant potential

CLINICAL FINDINGS

SYMPTOMS AND SIGNS

- Gastric outlet obstruction
- Biliary obstruction and jaundice
- Upper GI bleeding
- Carcinoid syndrome (flushing, diarrhea) if hepatic metastases are present

LABORATORY FINDINGS

- Carcinoid tumors: Elevated serotonin; 5-hydroxyindoleacetic acid (5-HIAA)
- Anemia

IMAGING FINDINGS

- Duodenal tumor evident on upper GI endoscopy or contrast radiography

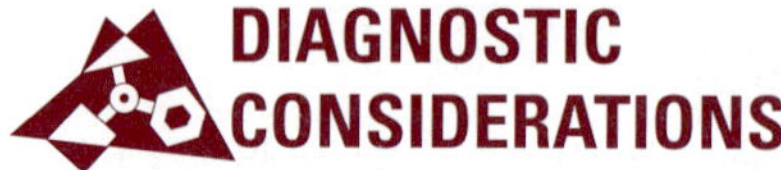

DIAGNOSTIC CONSIDERATIONS

- Duodenal mass
- Often asymptomatic
- CT scan may help differentiate tumor type

RULE OUT

- Malignant duodenal tumors or focus of malignancy in a benign tumor

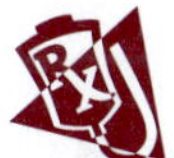

WORK-UP

- Symptoms and signs of duodenal mass
- Upper GI endoscopy or contrast radiography
- Endoscopic biopsy or polpectomy
- CT scan to distinguish tumor type and rule out metastases

WHEN TO ADMIT

- Severe gastric obstruction prohibiting eneteral intake
- GI bleeding
- Biliary obstruction

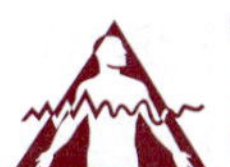

TREATMENT AND MANAGEMENT

- Endoscopic removal if possible

SURGERY

Indications

- Failure of endoscopic removal
- If malignancy found, pancreaticoduodenectomy usually indicated

MEDICATIONS

- GIST: Imatinib mesylate.
- Carcinoid syndrome: Octreotide.

TREATMENT MONITORING

- Repeated interval upper GI endoscopy or contrast radiography

COMPLICATIONS

- Bleeding
- Gastric outlet obstruction
- Biliary obstruction

PROGNOSIS

- If benign, most tumors cured by removal
- If malignancy found, 60% overall 5-year survival

RESOURCES

REFERENCES

- Demetri GD et al. Efficacy and safety of imatinib mesylate in advanced gastrointestinal stromal tumors. *N Engl J Med.* 2002;347:472.
- Blanchard DK et al. Tumors of the small intestine. *World J Surg.* 2000;24:421.

Duodenal Tumors, Malignant

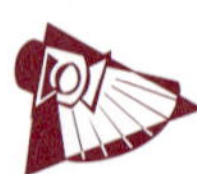

ESSENTIAL FEATURES

- Upper GI endoscopic or contrast radiographic evidence of duodenal tumor

EPIDEMIOLOGY

Adenocarcinoma

- 67% periampullary
- Risk factors
  - Crohn disease
  - Ulcerative colitis
  - Polyposis syndromes
  - Villous adenomas
  - Hereditary nonpolyposis colon cancer

Lymphoma

- Risk factors
  - Malabsorptive and inflammatory diseases
  - Immunosuppression

Gastrointestinal Stromal Tumor (GIST)

- 10–30% are malignant
- Difficult to distinguish benign from malignant on histologic studies

CLINICAL FINDINGS

SYMPTOMS AND SIGNS

- Abdominal pain
- GI or biliary obstruction
- GI bleeding (hematochezia or melena)
- Weight loss
- **Lymphoma:** Fever, night sweats
- Palpable abdominal mass

LABORATORY FINDINGS

- Anemia

IMAGING FINDINGS

- **Barium x-ray studies:** Duodenal tumors, particularly those in the third and fourth portions of the duodenum, may be missed
- **Endoscopy and biopsy:** Usually diagnostic

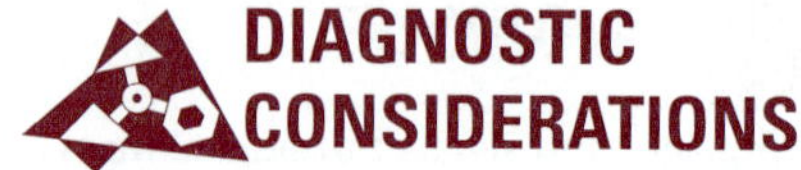

DIAGNOSTIC CONSIDERATIONS

- Symptoms should prompt upper GI contrast radiography or endoscopy and biopsy, which will be diagnostic

RULE OUT

- Benign duodenal tumors

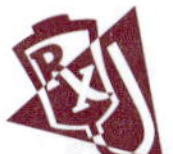

WORK-UP

- Signs and symptoms of duodenal tumor
- Upper GI endoscopy and biopsy will be diagnostic

WHEN TO ADMIT

- High grade obstruction
- Acute upper GI bleeding
- Severe abdominal pain
- Obstructive jaundice

TREATMENT AND MANAGEMENT

- Pancreaticoduodenectomy may be necessary for proximal duodenal malignancy

SURGERY

Indications

- Resect all adenocarcinoma and GIST
- Resect lymphoma if localized

Contraindications

- **Disseminated lymphoma:** Chemotherapy and radiation

MEDICATIONS

- **GIST:** Imatinib mesylate

TREATMENT MONITORING

- Endoscopic surveillance after resection

COMPLICATIONS

- GI and biliary obstruction
- GI bleeding

PROGNOSIS

- After curative resections, the overall 5-year survival rate is 30%
- **Adenocarcinoma:** 5-year survival stage I, 80%; Stage III, 10–15%.

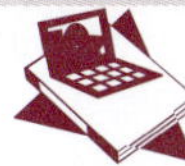

RESOURCES

REFERENCES

- Bakaeen FG et al. What prognostic factors are important in duodenal adenocarcinoma? *Arch Surg.* 2000;135:635.
- Isomoto H et al. Clinical and endoscopic features of adult T-cell leukemia/lymphoma with duodenal involvement. *J Clin Gastroenterol.* 2001;33:241.

PRACTICE GUIDELINES

- The National Comprehensive Cancer Network http://www.nccn.org/

Duodenal Ulcer

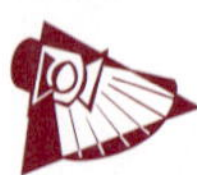

ESSENTIAL FEATURES

- Epigastric pain relieved by food or antacids
- Epigastric tenderness
- Normal or increased gastric acid secretion
- Signs of ulceration on upper GI studies
- *Helicobacter pylori* infection

EPIDEMIOLOGY

- More common in young and middle-aged patients (20–45 years old)
- Men affected more often than women
- 95% of ulcers occur within 2 cm of pylorus within the duodenal bulb
- *H pylori* infection is principal cause of duodenal ulcer, making the duodenum more vulnerable to acid and pepsin
- Prevalence of duodenal ulcer reflects prevalence of *H pylori* infection
- Majority of patients infected with *H pylori* do not develop ulcer disease
- Duodenal ulcers not associated with *H pylori* due mostly to NSAID use
- Gastric acid secretion is characteristically elevated compared with normal

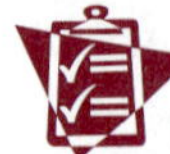

CLINICAL FINDINGS

SYMPTOMS AND SIGNS

- Epigastric pain temporarily relieved by food, milk, or antacids
- Nausea and vomiting may be present even in absence of obstruction
- Back pain may be present if ulcer perforates through posterior duodenal wall
- Localized epigastric tenderness may be present on physical exam
- Many patients have few vague abdominal symptoms

LABORATORY FINDINGS

- Increased basal acid output (male, 5.5 mEq/h; female, 3.0 mEq/h)
- Increased maximal acid output after stimulation by histamine or pentagastrin (male, 40 mEq/h; female, 30 mEq/h)
- Fasting serum gastrin > 200 pg/mL suggests gastrinoma
- Serum antibodies for *H pylori*
- Antral biopsy showing *H pylori* infection (histology, urease)

IMAGING FINDINGS

- Esophagogastroduodenoscopy showing duodenal ulceration
- Radiographic upper GI contrast study showing ulcer niche, duodenal deformity, and distortion of duodenal bulb

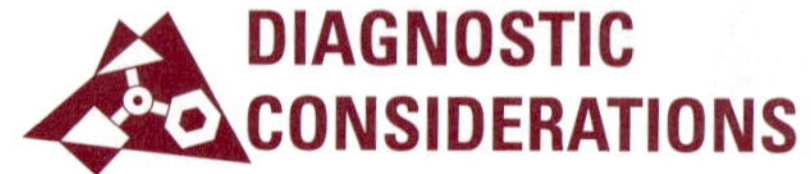

DIAGNOSTIC CONSIDERATIONS

RULE OUT

- Zollinger-Ellison syndrome (gastrinoma) in patients with severe or refractory duodenal ulcer

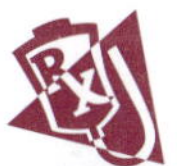

WORK-UP

- History and physical exam
- Endoscopic or radiographic evidence of duodenal ulceration
- Evaluate for *H pylori* infection by serum testing for screening or endoscopic biopsy testing
- Evaluate basal acid output and fasting serum gastrin in severe or refractory disease to exclude Zollinger-Ellison syndrome (gastrinoma)

WHEN TO ADMIT

- Free ulcer perforation
- Ulcer bleeding
- Severe duodenal obstruction

TREATMENT AND MANAGEMENT

- Goals are reduction of acid secretion and eradication of *H pylori* infection

SURGERY

- Parietal cell or truncal vagotomy with pyloroplasty
- Antrectomy and vagotomy

Indications

- Intractibility and failure of medical treatment
- Bleeding
- Perforation
- Duodenal obstruction

Contraindications

- Inadequate medical treatment

MEDICATIONS

- H_2 blockers
- Proton pump inhibitors
- Antacids
- Treatment of *H pylori* infection

TREATMENT MONITORING

- Endoscopy to confirm ulcer healing
- Resolution of symptoms

COMPLICATIONS

- Bleeding
- Perforation
- Obstruction

PROGNOSIS

- 80% heal within 6 weeks when treated with H_2 blockers
- 80% recurrence within 1 year if *H pylori* not eradicated

PREVENTION

- Avoidance of *H pylori* infection

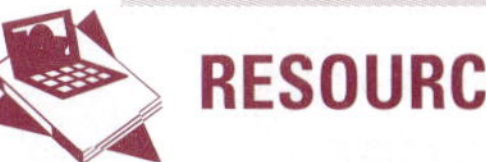

RESOURCES

REFERENCES

- Jamieson GG. Current indications for surgery in peptic ulcer disease. *World J Surg.* 2000;24:256.
- Zittel TT et al. Surgical management of peptic ulcer disease today—indication, technique and outcome. *Langenbecks Arch Surg.* 2000;385:84.

Echinococcosis

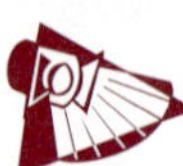

ESSENTIAL FEATURES

- Hydatid disease caused by the microscopic cestode parasites *Echinococcus granulosus* and *Echinococcus multilocularis*
- Form larval cysts in mammalian tissue
- Foxes, coyotes, dogs, and cats are the definitive hosts that harbor the adult tapeworms in their intestines
- Host animals are not harmed by the worms and are asymptomatic
- Ova are passed in the feces and are ingested by intermediate hosts such as cattle, humans, rodents, and particularly sheep
- Ova penetrate the intestine and pass via the portal vein to the liver (75%) and then to the lung (15%) or other tissues
- Ovum typically develops into a cyst filled with clear fluid
- Scoleces bud into the cyst lumen
- Cysts grow slowly; patients may be asymptomatic for several years
- Endocysts may cause secondary intraperitoneal cyst formation if spilled into the peritoneal cavity
- 80% of hydatid cysts are single and in the right lobe

EPIDEMIOLOGY

- Most common cystic lesions of liver outside of the United States

CLINICAL FINDINGS

SYMPTOMS AND SIGNS

- Abdominal pain (especially in right upper quadrant)
- Weight loss
- Hepatomegaly
- Jaundice
- Portal hypertension
- Hepatic mass

LABORATORY FINDINGS

- Eosinophilia is present in about 40% of patients
- Serologic tests (eg, indirect hemagglutination, complement fixation, dot immunobinding, and ELISA) are specific and sensitive, yielding positive results in 80% or more of cases of hepatic hydatid cyst
- Elevated liver function tests
- Casoni skin test

IMAGING FINDINGS

- **US and CT scanning:** Calcification and daughter cysts within the parent cyst
- **Nuclear medicine imaging:** Can also reveal uptake characteristic of hydatid cyst
- **Abdominal x-ray:** Can show calcific mass

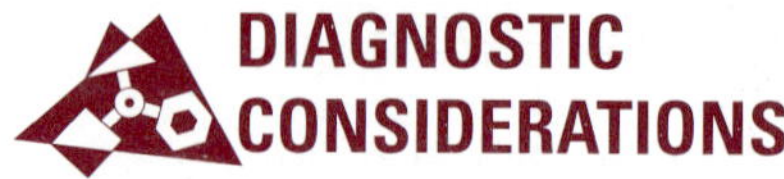

DIAGNOSTIC CONSIDERATIONS

- Nonparasitic cyst
- Cystic neoplasm
- Hepatic malignancy (primary or metastatic)
- Hepatitis
- Hemangioma
- Pyogenic abscess
- Amebic abscess
- Polycystic liver disease

RULE OUT

- Nonparasitic cysts
- Hepatic neoplasm

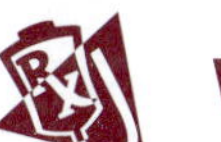

WORK-UP

- Complete history and physical exam
- History of animal contact
- Recent travel history

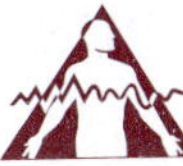

TREATMENT AND MANAGEMENT

- In some patients, the parasite dies, the cyst wall calcifies, and therapy is not required
- The surgical aim is to remove any cysts without disseminating the organism
- Excision of the intact cyst
- Scolicidal agent (hypertonic sodium chloride solution or sodium hypochlorite solution) can be placed into the cyst
- Care must be taken to avoid rupturing the cyst and spilling its contents into the peritoneal cavity because of the dangers of anaphylaxis or implantation
- Consider percutaneous drainage and albendazole

SURGERY

Indications

- Symptomatic and asymptomatic cysts, unless asymptomatic cysts completely circumferentially calcified
- Abdomen explored and cysts are isolated
- Superificial cysts may be excised
- Large cysts may be unroofed and contents removed piecemeal
- Pericystectomy is excision of the cyst between the host pericyst and liver tissue
- Rarely, hepatic lobectomy required for multiple cysts

Contraindications

- Disseminated echinococosis or systemic illness should be treated with antiparasitic agents first

MEDICATIONS

- Albendazole
- Praziquantel
- Mebendazole

COMPLICATIONS

- Cholangitis
- Biliary obstruction
- Rupture into the peritoneal cavity, anaphylaxis
- Perforation of the diaphragm, empyema, pulmonary cysts, biliary-bronchial fistulae, or pericardial collection

PROGNOSIS

- Overall death rate is about 15%, but it is only 4% in surgically treated cases

RESOURCES

REFERENCES

- Taylor BR et al. Current surgical management of hepatic cyst disease. *Adv Surg.* 1997;31:127.

Ectopic Pregnancy, Ruptured

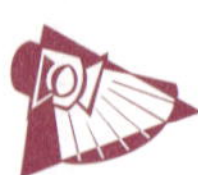

ESSENTIAL FEATURES

- Severe abdominal tenderness with guarding
- Hemodynamic instability
- Adnexal mass

EPIDEMIOLOGY

- Incidence has increased with the use of advanced reproductive technologies
- At least 2 in every 100 pregnancies are ectopic
- Mortality 0.3% in ectopic pregnancy
- 95% of ectopic pregnancies occur in the uterine tube, usually in the ampullary portion
- In vitro fertilization has increased the incidence of heterotopic pregnancy (intrauterine + ectopic)
- Risk factors include:
  - Prior ectopic pregnancy
  - History of pelvic inflammatory disease (PID)
  - Prior pelvic surgery
  - In vitro fertilization
  - Current intrauterine device use
  - Smoking
  - Diethylstilbestrol exposure
  - Increasing age

CLINICAL FINDINGS

SYMPTOMS AND SIGNS

- Sudden-onset lower abdominal pain with guarding
- Lower back discomfort
- Hemodynamic instability
- Adnexal mass
- Amenorrhea
- Current or recent history of vaginal spotting/bleeding

LABORATORY FINDINGS

- Positive β-hCG
- Lowered Hct
- Slight leukocytosis
- Lower values of quantitative β-hCG for gestational age of fetus
- Progesterone level < 5 ng/mL

IMAGING FINDINGS

- Transvaginal US is the radiographic procedure of choice
  - Free fluid in the cul-de-sac
  - Absence of intrauterine gestational sac —especially when β-hCG level is > 2000 mIU/mL (a threshold value above which an intrauterine gestational sac should be detected)
  - Presence of adnexal mass

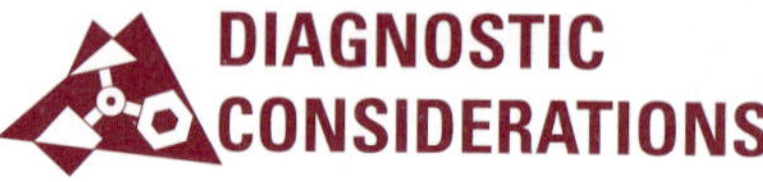

DIAGNOSTIC CONSIDERATIONS

- Threatened spontaneous abortion
- Missed abortion
- Acute appendicitis
- Acute PID
- Ruptured corpus luteum cyst
- Ureteral colic
- Hemorrhagic ovarian cysts or tumors
- Torsed ovarian cysts or tumor

RULE OUT

- Threatened abortion
- Missed abortion

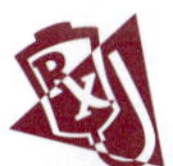

WORK-UP

- CBC count
- Basic chemistries
- β-hCG
- Serum progesterone
- Prothrombin time and partial thromboplastin time
- Transvaginal US

WHEN TO ADMIT

- Many uncomplicated ectopic pregnancies are diagnosed and managed in clinician's offices as an outpatient
- All patients with a ruptured ectopic pregnancy should be admitted for urgent surgical exploration

WHEN TO REFER

- All patients with suspected ectopic pregnancy should be managed by a gynecology-trained surgeon

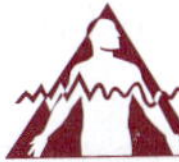

TREATMENT AND MANAGEMENT

- Treatment is surgical
- Goals are to control hemorrhage and preserve as much uterine tube as possible
- Serial Hct evaluation
- Cross-matched blood on reserve
- Determine Rh status

SURGERY

Indications

- All patients with ruptured ectopic pregnancy require immediate laparotomy
- Laparoscopic approaches to nonruptured ectopic pregnancies are gaining popularity

MEDICATIONS

- RH_0(D) immune globulin to patients who are Rh negative

TREATMENT MONITORING

- β-hCG levels should return to normal values
- Hct stabilization

COMPLICATIONS

- Infertility
- Repeat ectopic pregnancy

PROGNOSIS

- 0.3% mortality

RESOURCES

REFERENCES

- Lehner R et al. Ectopic pregnancy. *Arch Gynecol Obstet.* 2000;263:87.

Electrical Injury

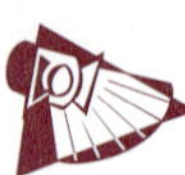

ESSENTIAL FEATURES

- 3 kinds of electrical injuries
  1. Current injury
  2. Electrothermal burns from arcing current
  3. Flame burns from ignited clothing
- Damage from electrical current is directly proportional to its intensity (Ohm's law): Amperage = Voltage/Resistance
- Voltages > 40 V are dangerous
- Current path through body depends on resistances: bone>fat>tendon>skin>muscle>blood>nerve
- Pathway of current determines survival
- Type of current also relates to severity of injury (AC>DC)
- Electrical injuries are often more than just burns (thrombosis, hemorrhage, fractures, dislocations, etc.)
- Deep destruction not initially evident
- Flame burns (clothing) often most significant injury

EPIDEMIOLOGY

- House current (AC) particularly dangerous (cardiac arrest common)

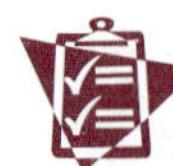

CLINICAL FINDINGS

SYMPTOMS AND SIGNS

- Skin burn usually depressed gray or yellow area of full-thickness burn with surrounding hyperemia
- Charring may be present if arc injury coexists
- Deep destruction not initially evident

LABORATORY FINDINGS

- Myoglobinuria
- Rapid drop in Hct (lysis)

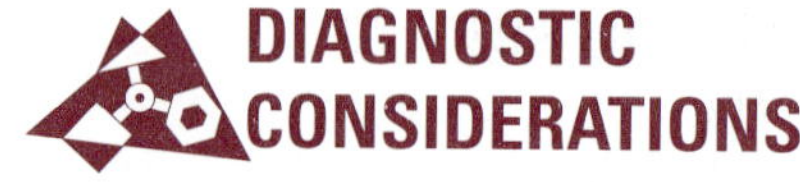

DIAGNOSTIC CONSIDERATIONS

RULE OUT

- Must evaluate for associated injuries, such as from blunt trauma (falls)

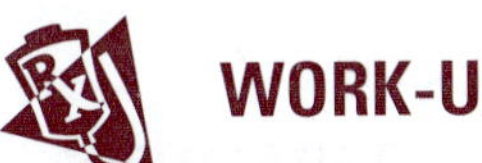

WORK-UP

WHEN TO REFER

- Always transfer significant electrical injuries to specialized centers after initial resuscitation

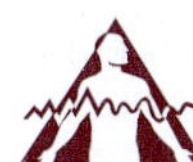

TREATMENT AND MANAGEMENT

- All dead and devitalized tissue must be debrided
- Second debridement often indicated 24–48 hrs after the injury
- Referral to specialized center after initial resuscitation
- Alkalinization of urine and osmotic diuresis if myoglobinuria present

SURGERY

Indications

- Dead or devitalized tissue

COMPLICATIONS

- Acute tubular necrosis

PROGNOSIS

- Related to voltage, path, type

PREVENTION

- Public education

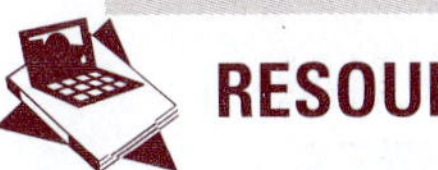

RESOURCES

REFERENCES

- Haberal M. An eleven year survey of electrical burn injuries. *J Burn Care Rehabil.* 1995;16:43.

Empyema

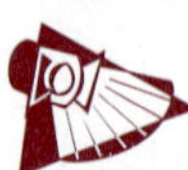

ESSENTIAL FEATURES

- **Pyothorax:** Pus within pleural cavity, usually thick, creamy, malodorous
- Etiology includes:
  - In setting of pneumonia, lung abscess, bronchiectasis, it is referred to as parapneumonic (60%)
  - Postsurgical (20%)
  - Post-traumatic (10%)
  - Less common causes include esophageal rupture and other chest wall or mediastinal infections
- 3 temporal phases:
  1. Acute exudative
  - Sterile low viscosity pleural fluid
  - Low WBC count and lactic dehydrogenase (LDH)
  - Normal glucose
  - Normal pH
  2. Transitional (fibrinopurulent)
  - Increase in turbidity, WBC, and LDH
  - Low glucose and pH
  - Fibrin deposited thereby fixing the lung
  3. Chronic organizing
  - Occurs 7–28 days after disease onset
  - Exudates thickens, causing further fixation of lung
  - pH < 7.0
  - Glucose < 40 mg/dL

EPIDEMIOLOGY

- Most organisms are anaerobic bacteria: bacteroides, fusobacterium, peptococcus
- *Staphylococcus* is cause in > 90% of children under 2 years; common cause in adults also
- *E coli, Pseudomonas* cause 66% of aerobic, gram-negative empyemas
- Rarely fungi and *Entamoeba histolytica* can cause empyemas
- Average number of bacterial species isolated: 3.2 per patient
- **Incidence of complications with *Staph* pneumonias in adults:**
  - Abscess (25%)
  - Empyema (15%)
  - Effusion (30%)
- **Incidence of complications with *Staph* pneumonias in kids:**
  - Abscess (50%)
  - Empyema (15%)
  - Pneumatocele (35%)
  - Effusion (55%)

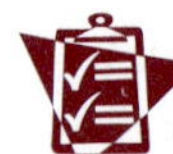

CLINICAL FINDINGS

SYMPTOMS AND SIGNS

- Rarely asymptomatic
- Fever, pleuritic chest pain, dyspnea, hemoptysis, cough
- Tachycardia, anemia, tachypnea, diminished breath sounds, clubbing

IMAGING FINDINGS

- **Chest film and chest CT:**
  - Pneumonia
  - Lung abscess
  - Pleural effusion
  - Mediastinal shift away if large empyema

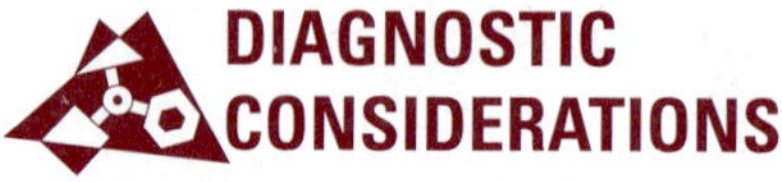

DIAGNOSTIC CONSIDERATIONS

- Thoracentesis is diagnostic
  - In early empyema, pleural fluid may not be purulent
  - pH < 7.0
  - Glucose < 40 mg/dL
  - LDH > 1000 U/L
  - Suggests evolving empyema despite negative Gram stain and culture
  - Frank pus usually develops later in empyema development

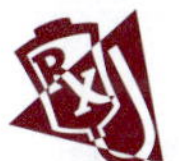

WORK-UP

- **Chest CT:** May be necessary if loculated
- **Bronchoscopy:** Performed to exclude presence of endobronchial obstruction
- **Thoracentesis:** Diagnostic

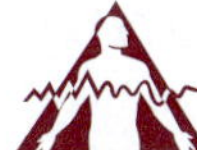

TREATMENT AND MANAGEMENT

- Goals:
  - Control infection
  - Remove purulent material with lung reexpansion
  - Eliminate underlying disease process
- Options:
  - Repeated thoracentesis
  - Chest tube drainage
  - Rib resection with open drainage
  - Decortication and empyemectomy
  - Thoracoplasty
  - Muscle flap closure

Treatment Algorithm: Empyema

- Clear thoracentesis
  - Check Gram stain and culture
  - If positive, thoracentesis/chest tube
  - If negative, check pH, glucose, LDH; chest tube if indicated
- Pus on thoracentesis
  - Place chest tube
  - Convert to open drainage
  - Perform sinogram: **No cavity**, then withdraw tube; **small cavity**, evaluate how well drained—if well drained, then slowly advance tube—if not well drained, then consider rib resection, thoracoscopy, or new chest tube; **large cavity,** if well drained, slowly advance tube—if no reexpansion, consider decortication—if not well drained, consider early decortication, rib resection, or Eloesser procedure
- Residual spaces, continued sepsis: Consider open drainage procedures 10–14 days after chest tube (allows time for pleural fusion
- Rib resection: Of short segments of 1–3 ribs in dependent portion
- Eloesser procedure: Simple rib resection and open flap drainage
- Creation of U-shape flap: Chest wall sewn to parietal pleura with rib resection
- Empyemectomy with decortication: Performed early in good-risk patients; best for post-traumatic empyema with normal underlying lung

Postlobectomy Empyema Algorithm

- Difficult to manage: Bronchopulmonary fistula often present
  - No space present: Chest tube or Eloesser procedure; if bronchopleural fistula, close fistula
  - Space present (with or without bronchopleural fistula): Chest tube if unstable Eloesser or thoracoplasty; if stable, myoplasty with muscle flap

Postpneumonectomy Empyema Algorithm

- Difficult problem since empty space
- Can attempt antibiotic irrigation with catheters in apex and base of pleural space: Successful in 20–88% if no fistula
  - No fistula: Chest tube, modified Clagett; if fails, complete flap
  - Fistula present: Chest tube if fistula closed, modified Clagett; if fistula open, Eloesser → complete flap
- Flaps typically used: Pectoralis major, lattissimus, serratus, rectus muscles ± omentum
- Modified Clagett: 2-stage procedure to remove infection and obliterate space

TREATMENT MONITORING

- Evaluate with chest CT after chest tube insertion to evaluate adequacy of drainage and lung reexpansion

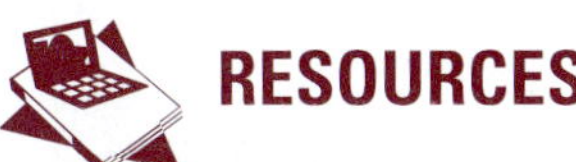

RESOURCES

REFERENCES

- Alfageme I et al. Empyema of the thorax in adults: etiology, microbiologic findings, and management. *Chest.* 1993;103:839.

Endocarditis

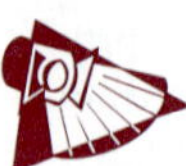

ESSENTIAL FEATURES

- Infection of any part of cardiac endothelium (usually bacterial)
- Valves most frequently involved
  - Vegetations may destroy leaflets or embolize
- Abscess formation can cause heart block or persistent sepsis
- **Subacute:** Symptoms for months, usually caused by hemolytic streptococci
- **Acute/fulminant:** Days to weeks; typically caused by *S aureus*
- Result in aortic regurgitation (AR), failure, sepsis, emboli

EPIDEMIOLOGY

- Patients at risk for endocarditis include those with congenital or preexisting valvular defects, indwelling cardiac catheters, or prosthetic heart valves
- Injection drug users and persons with prosthetic heart valves have highest incidence of gram-negative bacterial and fungal infections
- Fourth leading cause of life-threatening infections in United States

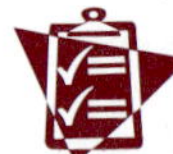

CLINICAL FINDINGS

SYMPTOMS AND SIGNS

- Fever, bacteremia, peripheral emboli
- Immunologic vascular phenomena:
  - Glomerulonephritis
  - Osler's nodes (painful, erythematous nodules on pulp of fingers)
  - Roth spots (retinal hemorrhages)
- Subungual splinter hemorrhages: Peripheral hemorrhages
- Janeway lesions: Flat, painless red spots on palms and soles of feet

LABORATORY FINDINGS

- 3 sets of blood cultures 1 hr apart: Positive
- Culture-negative endocarditis occurs in < 5% of cases (due to antibiotics, fastidious organism, fungal infection)
- ECG
  - Nonspecific usually
  - PR prolongation may be seen in cases of annular abscess and is ominous

IMAGING FINDINGS

- **Chest film:**
  - Signs of heart failure including interstitial pulmonary edema and cardiomegaly
  - Parenchymal nodules (septic emboli) seen in right-sided heart involvement
- **Echocardiography:** Document location and degree of valve involvement, vegetation size, presence of annular abscess
- **Catheterization:** Contraindicated if aortic valve vegetations or annulus abscess

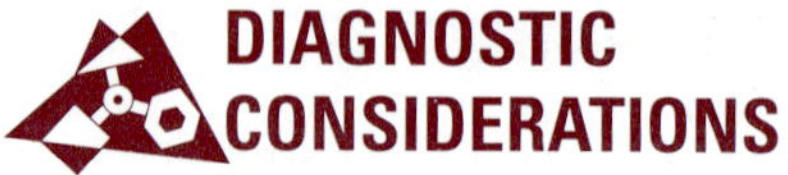

DIAGNOSTIC CONSIDERATIONS

- Evaluate for other sites of endovascular infection
- Evaluate for secondary effects on cardiac muscle function

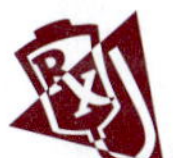

WORK-UP

- Vegetations > 1 cm (especially on mitral valve) have higher risk of embolization

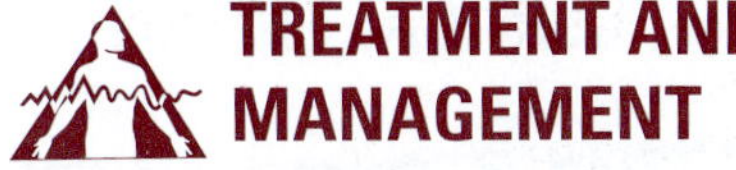

TREATMENT AND MANAGEMENT

- IV antibiotics
- Acute AR from endocarditis poorly tolerated
  - Pulmonary edema, congestive heart failure rapid
- AV replacement with allograft preferred due to high resistance to infection
- Mitral valve repair with debridement of vegetation and pericardial patch reconstruction is possible in a small fraction of patients

SURGERY

Indications

- Severe valvular regurgitation with heart failure
- Abscess of valve annulus
- Persistent bacteremia > 7 days with adequate antibiotic therapy
- Fungal or gram-negative bacterial infection
- Recurrent emboli
- Mobile vegetations > 1 cm

PROGNOSIS

- Untreated mortality is nearly 100%; parenteral antibiotics, 30–50% mortality
- Overall mortality with antibiotics and surgery is 10%
- Many injection drug users die of prosthetic valve infection or drug overdose after repair

RESOURCES

REFERENCES

- Bayer AS et al. Diagnosis and management of infective endocarditis and its complications. *Circulation.* 1998;98:2936.
- Moon MR et al. Treatment of endocarditis with valve replacement: the question of tissue versus mechanical prosthesis. *Ann Thorac Surg.* 2001;71:1164.
- Ferguson E et al. The surgical management of bacterial valvular endocarditis. *Curr Opin Cardiol.* 2000;15:82.

Endometriosis

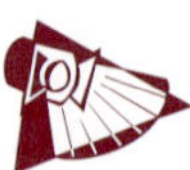

ESSENTIAL FEATURES

- Dysmenorrhea
- Constant aching lower abdominal pain, beginning 2–7 days before the onset of menses, and increasing in severity until menstrual flow subsides
- Clinical diagnosis is presumptive and must be confirmed in severe cases with laparoscopy or laparotomy

EPIDEMIOLOGY

- Prevalence in United States is 2% among fertile women and 3- to 4-fold greater in infertile women

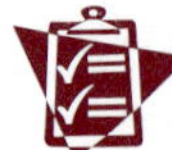

CLINICAL FINDINGS

SYMPTOMS AND SIGNS

- Lower abdominal pain
- Infertility
- Dyspareunia
- Rectal pain with or without hematochezia when ectopic endometrial implants involve the rectum
- Tender indurated nodules in the cul-de-sac (can appreciate best during menses)

LABORATORY FINDINGS

- β-hCG negative
- UA normal
- WBC count within normal range

IMAGING FINDINGS

- **US:** Findings will often reveal complex fluid-filled masses that cannot be distinguished from neoplasms
- **MRI:** More sensitive and specific in diagnosing adnexal masses
- **Barium enema:** May delineate colonic involvement

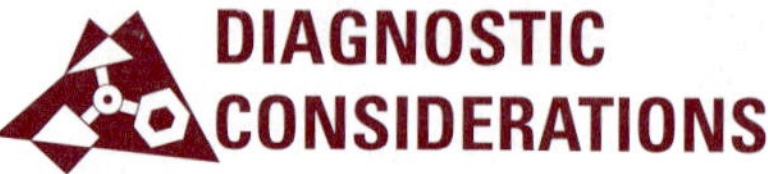

DIAGNOSTIC CONSIDERATIONS

- Pelvic inflammatory disease
- Uterine myomas
- Ovarian neoplasms
- Polycystic ovarian disease
- Appendicitis
- Acute enteritis
- Ruptured corpus luteum cyst

RULE OUT

- Ectopic pregnancy
- Threatened abortion
- Acute appendicitis

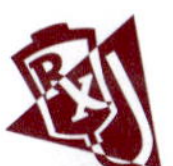

WORK-UP

- Thorough history and physical exam
- Complete pelvic exam
- β-hCG
- Transvaginal US

WHEN TO ADMIT

- Significant abdominal pain and the diagnosis is uncertain

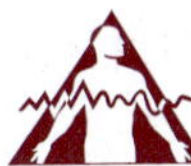

TREATMENT AND MANAGEMENT

- Goal is to ameliorate symptoms and preserve fertility
- Mainstay of therapy is medical inhibition of ovulation
- Laparoscopy/laparotomy to resect the lesions, free adhesions (with or without suspension of the uterus for patients younger than 35 to preserve reproductive function is controversial)
- Foci of endometriosis can be treated laparoscopically by bipolar coagulation or laser vaporization
- Hysterectomy with bilateral salpingo-oopherectomy for patients older than 35 with debilitating pain

SURGERY

Indications

- Definitive diagnosis via laparoscopy
- Failure of medical management

MEDICATIONS

- Gonadotropin-releasing hormone (GnRH) analogs
- Danazol
- Oral contraceptive pills
- Medroxyprogesterone acetate
- NSAIDs during menses

COMPLICATIONS

- Recurrent symptoms
- Infertility

PROGNOSIS

- Prognosis for reproductive function in mild or moderately advanced endometriosis is good with conservative management
- Bilateral oopherectomy is curative in severely affected patients

RESOURCES

REFERENCES

- Reddy S et al. Treatment of endometriosis. *Clin Obstet Gynecol.* 1998;41:387.
- Hoeger KM et al. An update on the classification of endometriosis. *Clin Obstet Gynecol.* 1999;42:611.

Epiphrenic Diverticulum

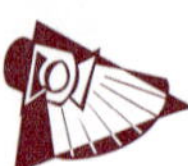

ESSENTIAL FEATURES

- Dysphagia and a sensation of pressure in the lower esophagus after eating
- Intermittent vomiting, substernal pain
- Typical radiologic contour
- Disturbed motility of the lower esophagus
- Associated hiatal hernia on occasion

EPIDEMIOLOGY

- Usually located in the distal 10 cm of the esophagus but may occur as high as the mid thorax
- Usually associated with discordinated smooth muscle activity in the distal esophagus, related to acid reflux, underlying achalasia or diffuse esophageal spasm, which results in segmenting contractions and development of a diverticulum
- Esophagitis may develop at the ostium
  - Peridiverticular localized mediastinitis may be seen, especially if ulceration of the mucosa occurs

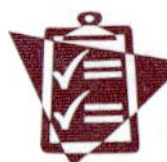

CLINICAL FINDINGS

SYMPTOMS AND SIGNS

- Dysphagia
- Regurgitation
- Aspiration
- Spasm type chest pain
- Heartburn

IMAGING FINDINGS

- **Contrast radiography**
  - Contrast filling of a smooth pouch located in the distal esophagus
  - Distal esophageal narrowing may be observed
- **Manometry**: Simultaneous repetitive contractions (or sometimes high-amplitude, prolonged contractions) in the body of the esophagus and in many cases abnormal lower esophageal sphincter function (ie, high resting pressure, incomplete relaxation with swallowing, or an exaggerated postglutition pressure rise)

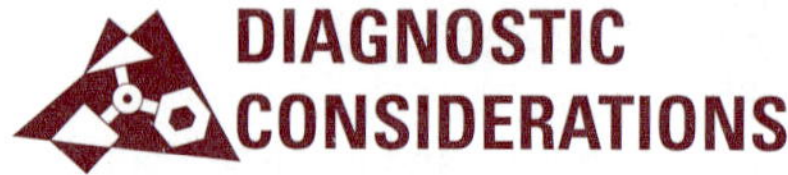

DIAGNOSTIC CONSIDERATIONS

- Esophageal manometry should be performed in every case to evaluate underlying motility disorders and to assess lower esophageal sphincter
- pH monitoring may be added to further evaluate lower esophageal sphincter dysfunction and associated reflux

RULE OUT

- Carcinoma
- Benign strictures
- Esophageal webs
- Achalasia
- Diffuse esophageal spasm

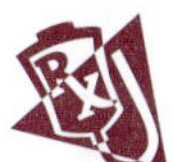

WORK-UP

- Upper GI contrast radiography with fluoroscopy
- Esophagoscopy
- Manometry
- pH monitoring

WHEN TO ADMIT

- Aspiration with pneumonitis
- Perforation with mediastinitis
- Severe dysphagia prohibiting enteral intake

TREATMENT AND MANAGEMENT

- Diverticulectomy and longitudinal myotomy to include the lower esophageal sphincter extending proximally to the level where esophageal function becomes manometrically normal

SURGERY

Indications

- Moderate to severe symptoms
- A loose fundoplication is added to treat or prevent reflux with division of lower esophageal sphincter

COMPLICATIONS

- Esophagitis
- Bleeding from mucosal ulceration
- Aspiration
- Perforation

PROGNOSIS

- Surgery is successful in 80–90% of cases

RESOURCES

REFERENCES

- Thomas ML et al. Oesophageal diverticula. *Br J Surg.* 2001;88:629.
- Tobin RW. Esophageal rings, webs, and diverticula. *J Clin Gastroenterol.* 1998;27:285.

Esophageal Atresia & Tracheoesophageal Fistula (TEF)

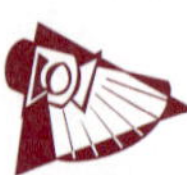

ESSENTIAL FEATURES

- 85% esophageal atresia with distal TEF, 5–7% pure esophageal atresia, 2–6% TEF alone, other configurations more rare
- Risk factors:
  - First pregnancy
  - Advanced maternal age
  - Affected parent
  - Affected siblings

EPIDEMIOLOGY

- 1/2500 to 1/20,000 births affected

CLINICAL FINDINGS

SYMPTOMS AND SIGNS

- Asymptomatic first few hours of life
- Excessive drooling
- Choking, coughing
- Regurgitation
- Respiratory distress
- Cyanosis
- Scaffoid abdomen if pure esophageal atresia

IMAGING FINDINGS

- **Prenatal US:** Polyhydramnios
- **Chest and abdominal x-ray**
  - Blind esophageal pouch when NG inserted
  - Gasless abdomen means no associated TEF
  - Gas filled means associated TEF

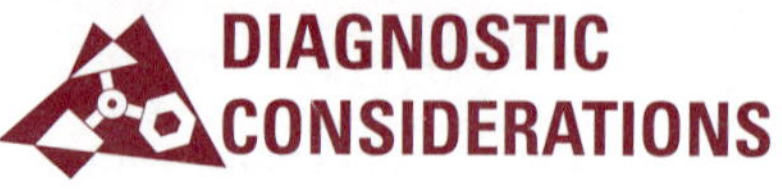

DIAGNOSTIC CONSIDERATIONS

RULE OUT

- Other associated abnormalities (present in 50% of patients)
  - Vertebral
  - Anorectal
  - Cardiac
  - Renal
  - Radial limb

Esophageal Atresia & Tracheoesophageal Fistula (TEF)

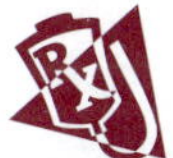

WORK-UP

- History and physical exam
- Chest and abdominal films with presence of NG tube
- Occasionally esophageal contrast study to verify presence of fistula
- Occasionally bronchoscopy or esophagoscopy to verify presence of fistula

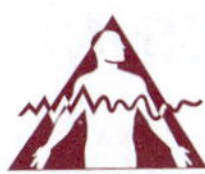

TREATMENT AND MANAGEMENT

SURGERY

- Decompressive gastrostomy if TEF causing gastric distention and subsequent difficulty breathing secondary to compression of diaphragm
- Resection of fistula with primary repair of esophageal atresia

Indications

- Resolution or stabilization of pulmonary or cardiac abnormalities

MEDICATIONS

- Sump suction to esophageal pouch

COMPLICATIONS

- Anastomotic leak, 10–20%
- Stricture, 40%
- Recurrent TEF, 10%
- Gastroesophageal reflux disease, all
- Esophageal dysmotility, all
- Tracheomalacia

PROGNOSIS

- 85–90% survival

RESOURCES

REFERENCES

- Albanese CT et al. Pediatric Surgery. In: Way LW, Doherty GM (editors). *Current Surgical Diagnosis & Treatment,* 11e. New York: McGraw-Hill; 2003:1313–1315.

Esophageal Carcinoma

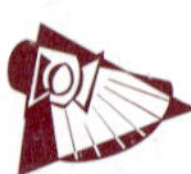

ESSENTIAL FEATURES

- Progressive dysphagia, initially during ingestion of solid foods and later of liquids
- Progressive weight loss and inanition
- Classic radiographic outlines: Irregular mucosal pattern with narrowing, with shelf-like upper border or concentrically narrowed esophageal lumen
- Definitive diagnosis established by endoscopic biopsy or cytologic studies

EPIDEMIOLOGY

- 1% of all malignant lesions and 6% of GI tract cancers
- More common among men
- Associated with alcohol and tobacco use
- Some adenocarcinomas are an upward extension of a gastric tumor but most are related to Barrett epithelium, which has been increasing in frequency
- Squamous cell lesions predominate in the mid esophagus; adenocarcinomas are more common in the lower third
- Direct intramural extension from the gross margin as great as 9 cm in 10% of cases
  - In 15% of patients, there are additional islands of tumor within 5 cm of the gross margin of the lesion
- Metastases to lymph nodes are present at the time of diagnosis in 80% of cases
- Extramural extension is common
- Lung, bone, liver, and adrenal glands are frequent sites of distant metastases

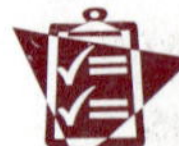

CLINICAL FINDINGS

SYMPTOMS AND SIGNS

- Dysphagia
- Weight loss and weakness
- Difficulty swallowing solid foods initially followed by both solids and liquids
- Pain that may be related to swallowing
  - If pain is constant, the tumor has probably invaded somatic structures
- Regurgitation and aspiration
- Coughing related to swallowing
- Hoarseness most often reflects spread to the recurrent laryngeal nerves

LABORATORY FINDINGS

- Anemia

IMAGING FINDINGS

- **Chest film:** A column of air or air-fluid level in the esophageal lumen
- **Barium swallow**
  - Narrowing of the lumen at the site of the lesion and dilation proximally
  - Tumor appears as an irregular mass
- **Esophagoscopy with biopsy:** Provides a tissue diagnosis in 95% of cases
- **Endoscopic US:** Wall penetration and mediastinal invasion
- **CT scans:** Distant mediastinal and celiac axis nodal metastases
- **Bronchoscopy:** Distortion of the bronchial lumen, blunting of the carina, or intrabronchial tumor

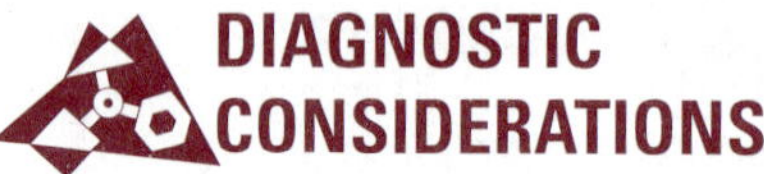

DIAGNOSTIC CONSIDERATIONS

- Angulation of the axis of the esophagus above and below the tumor may be seen on barium swallow, a finding that strongly suggests spread of the lesion to extraesophageal sites
- Because lesions of the upper and mid esophagus may invade the tracheobronchial tree, bronchoscopy is always indicated in the assessment of growths at these levels
- Premalignant states
  - Chronic iron deficiency
  - Esophageal stasis
  - Barrett esophagus
  - Reflux esophagitis
  - Congenital tylosis of the esophagus
- Benign strictures
- Benign papillomas, polyps, or granular cell tumors

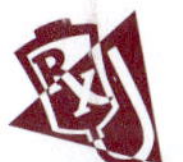

WORK-UP

- Barium swallow
- Esophagoscopy with biopsy
- Endoscopic US
- CT scan
- Bronchoscopy

WHEN TO ADMIT

- Severe pain or dysphagia
- Inability to maintain adequate enteral nutrition
- Severe pain
- Respiratory distress

TREATMENT AND MANAGEMENT

- Preoperative radiation may convert an unresectable growth to a resectable one
- About 50% of tumors are resectable at presentation and about 75% following preoperative radiotherapy and chemotherapy

SURGERY

Indications

- Esophagectomy, for cure or palliation, should be undertaken in suitable candidates without distant metastases with a life expectancy more than a few months

Contraindications

- Distant organ metastases
- Life expectancy less than a few months
- Spread to tracheobronchial tree or aorta
- Vocal cord paralysis

MEDICATIONS

- Preoperative or postoperative chemotherapy and radiation
- Adjuvant radiotherapy has not increased the overall cure rate

TREATMENT MONITORING

- Following preoperative therapy:
  - Esophagoscopy
  - Endoscopic US
  - CT scan

COMPLICATIONS

- Bleeding, rarely massive
- Invasion of mediastinal structures
- Tracheobronchial fistula
- Aspiration pneumonitis

PROGNOSIS

- 5-year survival rate after curative resection is about 30% for patients with squamous cell carcinoma and 10% for patients with adenocarcinoma

RESOURCES

REFERENCES

- Lerut T et al. Treatment of esophageal carcinoma. *Chest.* 1999;116 (6 Suppl):463S.
- Lew JI et al. Long-term survival following induction chemoradiotherapy and esophagectomy for esophageal carcinoma. *Arch Surg.* 2001;136:737.

PRACTICE GUIDELINES

- The National Comprehensive Cancer Network http://www.nccn.org/

CANCER STAGING

- See Esophagus Staging Table on page 747.

STAGE GROUPING

Stage			
0	Tis	N0	M0
I	T1	N0	M0
IIA	T2	N0	M0
	T3	N0	M0
IIB	T1	N1	M0
	T2	N1	M0
III	T3	N1	M0
	T4	Any N	M0
IV	Any T	Any N	M1
IVA	Any T	Any N	M1a
IVB	Any T	Any N	M1b

Esophageal Obstruction

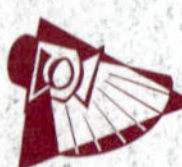

ESSENTIAL FEATURES

- Ingestion of foreign object or bolus of meat
- May be asymptomatic or accompanied by dysphagia, chest pain, or respiratory distress
- Radiopaque objects can be detected on chest x-ray
- Rings, webs, and bands usually detected by endoscopy or contrast radiographic study
- Endoscopic treatment (extraction of foreign objects or dilation of ring, web or band) is usually successful

EPIDEMIOLOGY

- **Foreign objects**
  - 90% pass into the stomach and pass without incident
  - Usually lodge just beyond the cricopharyngeus
  - Most cases occur in children; in adults esophageal meat impaction is most common and many affected patients have underlying esophageal disease
  - 10% require endoscopic removal, and 1% require surgery
  - Button batteries are highly corrosive and should be removed urgently
  - Cocaine smugglers may swallow small packets of cocaine which, if ruptured, can be fatal
- **Congenital bands or webs** may develop at any level but are most frequent in the subcricoid region
- **Schatzki ring:** Narrow mucosal ring at the squamocolumnar junction that occurs with gastroesophageal reflux

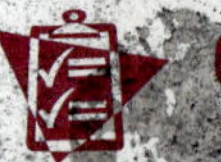

CLINICAL FINDINGS

SYMPTOMS AND SIGNS

- May be asymptomatic
- Dysphagia
- Chest pain
- Respiratory distress

IMAGING FINDINGS

- **Anteroposterior and lateral chest film**
  - If ingested object is radiopaque, determine whether the object is in the esophagus or trachea
  - X-ray small children from the base of the skull to the anus in order to find any additional objects in the gut
- Endoscopy will identify foreign objects suspected of causing esophageal obstruction
- Endoscopy or contrast radiography may identify esophageal rings, bands, or webs that may be associated with esophagitis

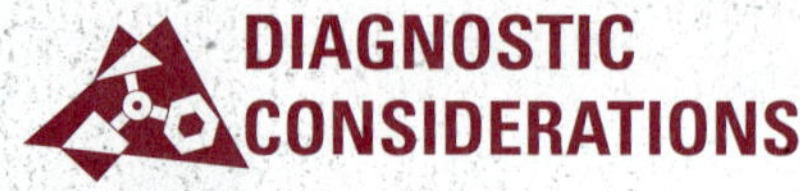

DIAGNOSTIC CONSIDERATIONS

RULE OUT

- Underlying esophageal disease precipitating obstruction, particularly with meat impaction

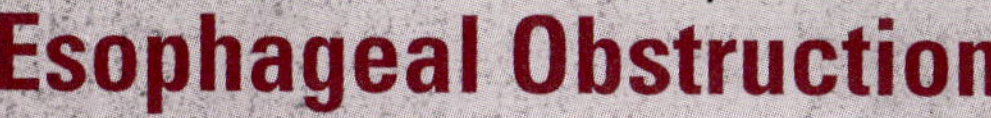

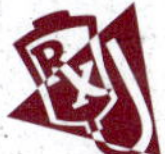

WORK-UP

- If radiopaque foreign object, chest film may be performed
- Most foreign objects as well as webs, rings, or bands can be diagnosed endoscopically

WHEN TO ADMIT

- Suspected esophageal perforation
- Severe respiratory distress
- Need for surgery

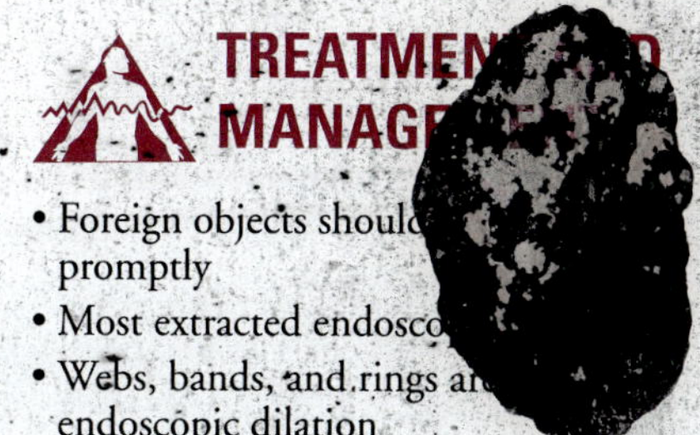

TREATMEN[...] MANAGE[...]

- Foreign objects shoul[...] promptly
- Most extracted endosco[...]
- Webs, bands, and rings a[...] endoscopic dilation

SURGERY

Indications

- Inability to treat endoscopically
- All ingested packets containing cocaine
  - Endoscopic extraction may cause rupture and death

TREATMENT MONITORING

- Subsequent diagnostic endoscopy to exclude underlying esophageal disease

COMPLICATIONS

- Esophagoaortic or esophagotracheal fistula
- Tracheal obstruction and aspiration
- Esophageal ulceration or perforation

PROGNOSIS

- 1500 deaths yearly from complications of ingested foreign bodies
- Most webs, rings, and bands treated effectively by dilation

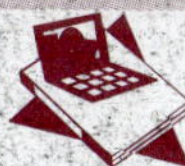

RESOURCES

REFERENCES

- Arana A et al. Management of ingested foreign bodies in childhood and review of the literature. *Eur J Pediatr.* 2001;160:468.
- Buckley K et al. Schatzki ring in children and young adults: clinical and radiologic findings. *Pediatr Radiol.* 1998;28:884.

Esophageal Perforation

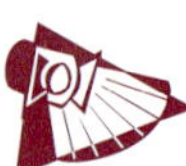

ESSENTIAL FEATURES

- History of recent instrumentation of the esophagus or severe vomiting
- Pain in the neck, chest, or upper abdomen
- Signs of mediastinal or thoracic sepsis within 24 hours
- Contrast radiographic evidence of an esophageal leak
- Crepitus and subcutaneous emphysema of the neck in some cases

EPIDEMIOLOGY

- Esophageal perforations can result from instrumentation, severe vomiting, and external trauma
- Morbidity is principally due infection
- Immediately after injury, infection has not become established
  - Closure of the defect will usually prevent the development of serious infection
- 24 hours after perforation, infection will have occurred and the esophageal defect usually breaks down if it is closed
- Instrumental perforations are most likely to occur in the cervical esophagus
- Spontaneous perforation usually occurs in the left posterolateral aspect 3–5 cm above the gastroesophageal junction and typically involves the pleura
- Thoracic perforations are most common at the level of the left main-stem bronchus and diaphragmatic hiatus
  - Pleural rupture occurs in 75% of cases

CLINICAL FINDINGS

SYMPTOMS AND SIGNS

- Pain
  - In the neck with cervical perforations
  - In the chest or upper abdomen with thoracic perforations
  - May radiate to the back
- **Cervical perforations:** Pain is followed by crepitus in the neck, dysphagia, and signs of infection
- **Thoracic perforations:** Tachypnea, hyperpnea, dyspnea, and hypotension
- With pleural perforation, pneumothorax is produced followed by hydrothorax and, if not promptly treated, empyema
- Escape of air into the mediastinum may result in a "mediastinal crunch"

LABORATORY FINDINGS

- Thoracentesis will reveal cloudy or purulent fluid with elevated amylase content; serum amylase levels may also be high as a result of absorption of amylase from the pleural cavity

IMAGING FINDINGS

- **Radiographs for cervical perforation**
  - Air in the soft tissues, especially along the cervical spine
  - Trachea may be displaced anteriorly by air and fluid
  - Later, widening of the superior mediastinum may be seen
- **Radiographs for thoracic perforations**
  - Mediastinal widening and pleural effusion with or without pneumothorax
  - Mediastinal emphysema takes at least 1 hour to develop
- An esophagogram using water-soluble contrast medium should be performed promptly in order to confirm level and extent of injury

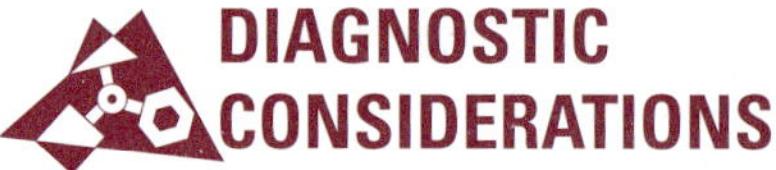

DIAGNOSTIC CONSIDERATIONS

- Diagnosis should occur promptly as timing has a great influence on surgical treatment and patient survival

RULE OUT

- Coexistent esophageal carcinoma, in which case the most appropriate treatment is esophagectomy

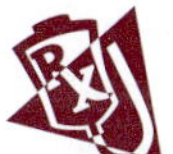

WORK-UP

- Recent history of instrumentation or forceful vomiting along with signs and symptoms of perforation
- Plain chest films
- Esophagogram with water soluble contrast material

WHEN TO ADMIT

- All cases

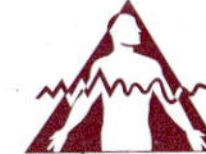

TREATMENT AND MANAGEMENT

- Antibiotics should be given immediately
- Definitive therapy (eg, resection) should be performed in patients with other surgical conditions (carcinoma)

SURGERY

Indications

- All cases
- If < 24 hours, closure and drainage
- If > 24 hours, resect perforation, cervical esophagostomy, close distal esophagus, drain mediastinum, and jejunostomy

Contraindications

- Incomplete rupture
  - Tear is confined to the mucosal layer
  - It dissects distally in the submucosal plane
  - Treatment is with antibiotics and total parenteral nutrition

MEDICATIONS

- Antibiotics

TREATMENT MONITORING

- Upper GI continuity can occur after clearance of infection and resolution of inflammation

COMPLICATIONS

- Mediastinitis
- Empyema

PROGNOSIS

- The survival rate is 90% when surgical treatment is accomplished in < 24 hours
- The survival rate drops to about 50% when treatment is delayed

RESOURCES

REFERENCES

- Younes Z, Johnson DA. The spectrum of spontaneous and iatrogenic esophageal injury: perforations, Mallory-Weiss tears, and hematomas. *J Clin Gastroenterol.* 1999;29:306.

Esophageal Spasm, Diffuse

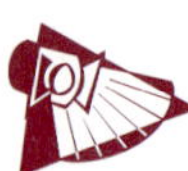

ESSENTIAL FEATURES

- Dysphagia, substernal pain
- Nervousness, intermittent symptoms
- Fluoroscopic, cineradiographic, and manometric evidence of high-amplitude contractions

EPIDEMIOLOGY

- Characterized by nonperistaltic esophageal contractions, often associated with intermittent chest pain
- The cause is not known, although stress can induce similar manometric findings in normal subjects, so stress and psychological disorders might play a role
- The esophagogram is abnormal in 60% of patients
- Sliding hiatal hernia and epiphrenic diverticula may be secondary complications of the uncoordinated and severe contractions of the esophagus

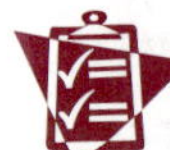

CLINICAL FINDINGS

SYMPTOMS AND SIGNS

- Intermittent chest pain, which varies from slight discomfort to severe spasmodic pain that simulates the pain of coronary artery disease
- Dysphagia for liquids and solids

IMAGING FINDINGS

- **Fluoroscopic studies**
  - Segmental spasms
  - Areas of narrowing
  - Irregular uncoordinated peristalsis
  - A small hiatal hernia or epiphrenic diverticulum may be present
- **Manometry**
  - Repetitive, nonperistaltic (simultaneous) contractions after swallowing
  - The lower esophageal sphincter may fail to relax in response to swallows
  - **Provocative testing** during manometry is positive if the anticholinesterase edrophonium, which causes strong esophageal contractions, elicits pain similar to the spontaneous symptom

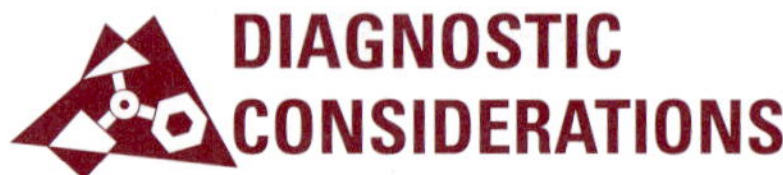

DIAGNOSTIC CONSIDERATIONS

- The diagnosis is made by the characteristic findings on manometry and by eliciting the symptoms with provocative tests

RULE OUT

- Heart disease, particularly coronary ischemia
- Mediastinal masses
- Benign and malignant esophageal tumors
- Scleroderma

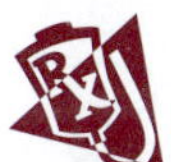

WORK-UP

- Symptoms of dysphagia and intermittent substernal pain
- Manometry and provocative testing
- Esophagoscopy to confirm the absence of intraluminal lesions
- 24-hour pH monitoring may demonstrate reflux, a common associated problem

WHEN TO ADMIT

- Severe symptoms prohibiting adequate enteral nutrition

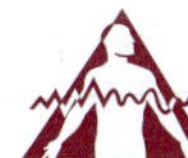

TREATMENT AND MANAGEMENT

- Reassurance and symptomatic therapy are often sufficient
- A soft diet taken in 5 or 6 small feedings per day may be required
- Esophageal dilation is ineffective

SURGERY

Indications

- Esophageal myotomy for symptoms refractory to medical therapy
- Esophagectomy for persistent symptoms after myotomy

MEDICATIONS

- Hydralazine
- Calcium channel blockers
- Long-acting nitrates
- Anticholinergic agents

COMPLICATIONS

- Sliding hiatal hernia
- Epiphrenic diverticula
- Regurgitation
- Aspiration

PROGNOSIS

- Esophageal myotomy is successful in 90% of cases
- Postoperative relief is associated with reduced intraluminal pressure

RESOURCES

REFERENCES

- Ellis FH Jr. Long esophagomyotomy for diffuse esophageal spasm and related disorders: an historical overview. *Dis Esophagus.* 1998;11:210.
- Storr M, Allescher HD. Esophageal pharmacology and treatment of primary motility disorders. *Dis Esophagus.* 1999;12:241.

Esophageal Sphincter Dysfunction, Upper

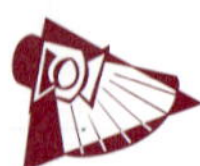

ESSENTIAL FEATURES

- Cervical dysphagia
- Cricopharyngeal bar on barium swallow
- Pharyngoesophageal diverticulum (Zenker diverticulum) in some patients

EPIDEMIOLOGY

- Most often occurs in patients over age 60
- May occur as an isolated abnormality or in association with Zenker diverticulum

CLINICAL FINDINGS

SYMPTOMS AND SIGNS

- Cervical dysphagia, more pronounced for solids than for liquids
- Chronic cough from minor aspirations of saliva and ingested food

IMAGING FINDINGS

- **Upper GI contrast radiography** nearly always shows a prominent cricopharyngeal bar
- **Endoscopy** shows an extrinsic constriction that allows passage of the endoscope as it is advanced
- **Manometry** often reveals imperfect coordination of relaxation of the cricopharyngeal sphincter, occurring at or just after initiation of the pharyngeal contraction, instead of just before

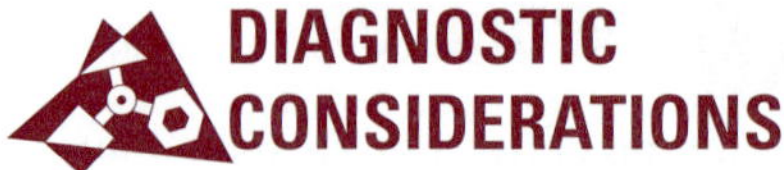

DIAGNOSTIC CONSIDERATIONS

- Patients with symptoms of cervical dysphagia, more pronounced for solids than for liquids, should be evaluated by upper GI contrast radiography, which will usually be diagnostic

RULE OUT

- Esophageal neoplasms
- Reflux resulting from lower esophageal sphincter incompetence

WORK-UP

- Symptoms of cervical dysphagia, more pronounced for solids than for liquids
- Upper GI contrast radiography will usually be diagnostic
- Upper GI endoscopy to rule out esophageal neoplasm
- Cricopharyngeal and esophageal manometry to rule out reflux disease, as indicated

WHEN TO ADMIT

- Severe dysphagia prohibiting adequate enteral nutrition

TREATMENT AND MANAGEMENT

- Myotomy of the cricopharyngeus and upper 3–4 cm of the esophageal musculature, made in the midline posteriorly

SURGERY

Indications

- All confirmed cases of upper esophageal sphincter dysfunction

Contraindications

- Patients with gastroesophageal reflux because of the increased risk of aspiration after myotomy

COMPLICATIONS

- Aspiration

PROGNOSIS

- Relief of symptoms is usually complete and permanent after myotomy

RESOURCES

REFERENCES

- Owen W. ABC of the upper gastrointestinal tract. Dysphagia. *BMJ.* 2001;323:850.
- Hila A et al. Pharyngeal and upper esophageal sphincter manometry in the evaluation of dysphagia. *J Clin Gastroenterol.* 2001;33:355.

Esophageal Tumors, Benign

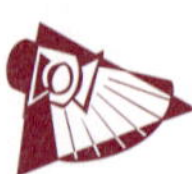

ESSENTIAL FEATURES

- Dysphagia often present but frequently mild
- Sense of pressure in thorax or neck
- Radiographic demonstration of intraluminal or extraluminal mass, smooth in outline

EPIDEMIOLOGY

- May arise in any layer
  - Mucosa
  - Submucosa
  - Muscularis propria
- **Mucosa**
  - Squamous papilloma is small, solitary and sessile; usually in distal esophagus; must be differentiated from squamous cell carcinoma by biopsy
  - Fibrovascular polyps are pedunculated; may extend distally to stomach; associated with regurgitation; granular cell tumor is third most common
- **Submucosa**
  - Lipoma
  - Fibroma
  - Hemangioma
  - May bleed
- **Muscularis propria**
  - Leiomyoma most common
  - Tumor may bleed
  - Biopsy does not penetrate deep enough to sample tumor
  - Rarely malignant
- **Cysts**
  - Second most common
  - Most are congenital foregut cysts
  - May cause airway compromise in children
  - Most become symptomatic by adulthood

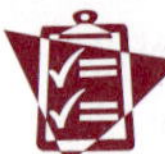

CLINICAL FINDINGS

SYMPTOMS AND SIGNS

- Often asymptomatic
- Mild dysphagia
- Sense of pressure in neck or thorax
- Gastroesophageal reflux
- Chest pain
- Cough
- Dyspnea
- Regurgitation
- Upper GI bleeding

IMAGING FINDINGS

- **Barium swallow:** Reveals a smoothly rounded, often spherical mass that causes extrinsic narrowing of the esophageal lumen
- **Esophagoscopy**
  - Intraluminal growths can usually be recognized and a specific tissue diagnosis should always be obtained
  - Because leiomyomas arise from the deeper muscularis propria, endoscopic biopsy will not penetrate deeply enough to reach the tumor
- **Endoscopic US:** Allows identification of the layer from which the tumor arises and may allow more precise sampling by fine-needle biopsy

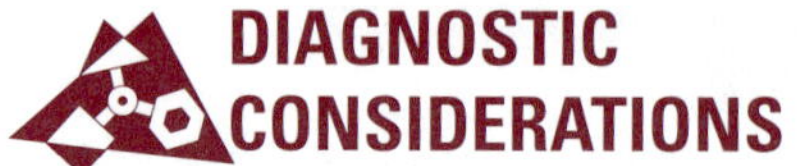

DIAGNOSTIC CONSIDERATIONS

- Most benign lesions are asymptomatic, slow growing, have low malignant potential and are discovered incidentally during upper GI contrast radiography or esophagoscopy
- Leiomyomas and cysts can be distinguished from cancerous growths by their classic radiographic appearance
- Intraluminal papillomas, granular cell tumors and other benign tumors may be indistinguishable radiographically from early carcinoma, so their exact nature must be confirmed histologically

RULE OUT

- Carcinoma

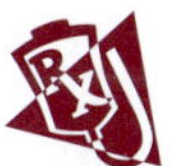

WORK-UP

- Upper GI contrast study
- Esophagoscopy with biopsy
- Endoscopic US with fine-needle aspiration (if not performed previously)

WHEN TO ADMIT

- Severe upper GI bleeding
- Severe dysphagia prohibiting adequate enteral nutrition

TREATMENT AND MANAGEMENT

- Most small benign esophageal tumors can be removed endoscopically
- Larger lesions may require excision or enucleation to confirm diagnosis if symptomatic

SURGERY

Indications

- Inability to exclude carcinoma
- All symptomatic lesions
- All cysts

TREATMENT MONITORING

- Interval endoscopy not indicated for excised lesions unless atypical
- Interval endoscopy indicated for nonexcised, observed lesions

COMPLICATIONS

- Hemorrhage
- Obstruction
- Regurgitation with aspiration
- Respiratory distress

PROGNOSIS

- Low rate of recurrence and excellent prognosis after excision of benign esophageal tumors

RESOURCES

REFERENCES

- Bonavina L et al. Surgical therapy of esophageal leiomyoma. *J Am Coll Surg.* 1995;181:257.
- Takada N et al. Utility of endoscopic ultrasonography in assessing the indications for endoscopic surgery of submucosal esophageal tumors. *Surg Endosc.* 1999;13:228.

Esophagitis, Corrosive

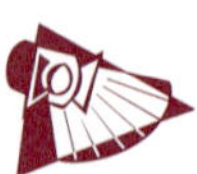

ESSENTIAL FEATURES

- History of ingestion of caustic liquids or solids
- Burns of the lips, mouth, tongue, and oropharynx
- Chest pain and dysphagia

EPIDEMIOLOGY

- Extent of injury depends on degree of exposure to the agent (concentration, duration, and quantity)
- Ingestion of strong alkali produces "liquefaction necrosis," which involves dissolution of protein and collagen, saponification of fats, dehydration of tissues, thrombosis of blood vessels, and severe deep penetrating injuries
- Acids produce a "coagulation necrosis" involving eschar formation, which tends to shield the deeper tissues from injury
  - Greatest injury is to the stomach, with the esophagus remaining intact in over 80% of cases
- Liquid caustics usually produce more extensive esophageal injury than solids
- Oropharyngeal burns are common but do not predict distal esophageal injury
- Esophageal perforation may occur as late as 14 days after injury

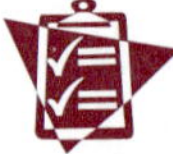

CLINICAL FINDINGS

SYMPTOMS AND SIGNS

- Inflammatory edema of the lips, mouth, tongue, and oropharynx
- Pain on attempted swallowing
- Chest pain
- Dysphagia
- Drooling of large amounts of saliva
- Fever, shock, peritoneal signs with esophageal perforation
- Tracheobronchitis, coughing, and increased bronchial secretions
- Stridor and respiratory distress
- Complete esophageal obstruction due to edema, inflammation, and mucosal sloughing may develop

LABORATORY FINDINGS

- Systemic acidosis and coagulopathy with severe injury

IMAGING FINDINGS

- **Esophagoscopy**
  - Usually within 12 hours of admission after initial resuscitation
  - The scope is inserted far enough to gauge the degree of burn but not beyond the proximal extent of injury
- **Chest film:** May identify pneumomediastinum, pneumoperitoneum or pleural effusion, indicating perforation
- **Laryngoscopy and fiberoptic nasopharyngoscopy:** May show edema, hyperemia, and mucosal sloughing
- Water soluble contrast radiography may be used to detect perforation

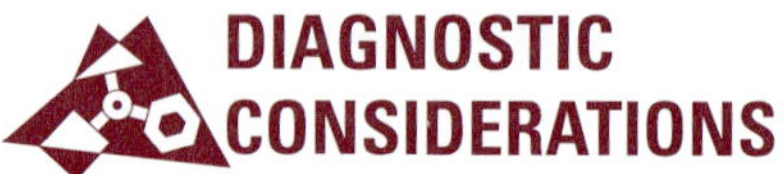

DIAGNOSTIC CONSIDERATIONS

- Esophageal burns can be classified by endoscopic appearance
- Grade I: Superficial mucosal injury
  - Mucosal hyperemia and edema
- Grade II: Partial thickness injury
  - Mucosal sloughing
  - Ulceration
  - Pseudomembranes
  - Grade IIA, patchy injury; grade IIB, circumferential injury
- Grade III: Transmural injury with periesophageal and/or perigastric extension
  - Full thickness necrosis
  - Eschar formation
  - Black or gray ulcers

RULE OUT

- Respiratory distress or severe pharyngeal injury with airway compromise necessitating intubation or tracheostomy
- Simultaneous gastric injury

WORK-UP

- Laryngoscopy
- Fiberoptic nasopharyngoscopy
- Chest film
- Early endoscopy
- Contrast radiography

WHEN TO ADMIT

- All cases
- Mild exposures without symptoms may be discharged after brief observation

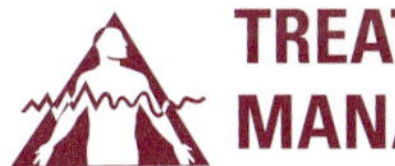

TREATMENT AND MANAGEMENT

- Fluid resuscitation and airway protection

SURGERY

- Laparotomy
- Resection of areas of necrosis
- Cervical esophagostomy
- Oversew distal segment
- Feeding jejunostomy

Indications

- Perforation
- Grade III injury
- Severe grade II injury
- Shock, peritonitis, worsening symptoms

Contraindications

- Grade I injury—observation only

MEDICATIONS

- Do not attempt dilution or induce emesis
- Antibiotics
- Steroids controversial
- H_2 receptor blockers

TREATMENT MONITORING

- Periodic esophagoscopy in late follow up to look for stricture formation, which is treated early by dilation

COMPLICATIONS

- Stricture development (severe grade II and grade III only)
- Perforation
- Increased risk of carcinoma

PROGNOSIS

- Grade III, 20% mortality
- With early endoscopy and aggressive treatment, mortality for less severe injury is low

RESOURCES

REFERENCES

- de Jong AL et al. Corrosive esophagitis in children: a 30-year review. *Int J Pediatr Otorhinolaryngol.* 2001;57:203.
- Huang YC et al. Balloon dilation of double strictures after corrosive esophagitis. *J Pediatr Gastroenterol Nutr.* 2001;32:496.

Felty Syndrome

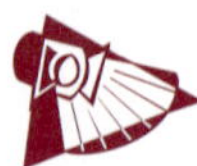

ESSENTIAL FEATURES

- Neutropenia
- Recurrent infections
- Splenomegaly
- Affects patients with seropositive nodular rheumatoid arthritis

EPIDEMIOLOGY

- Affects approximately 1% of patients with rheumatoid arthritis
- High levels of IgG on the surface of neutrophils with evidence of increased granulopoiesis in the bone marrow
- Recurrent infections are due to decreased and dysfunctional neutrophils coated with IgG

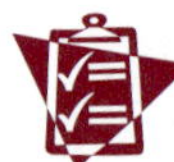

CLINICAL FINDINGS

SYMPTOMS AND SIGNS

- Recurring infections
- Splenomegaly
- Chronic leg ulcers

LABORATORY FINDINGS

- Decreased neutrophil count
- Increased granulopoiesis in the bone marrow
- High levels of IgG on the surface of neutrophils

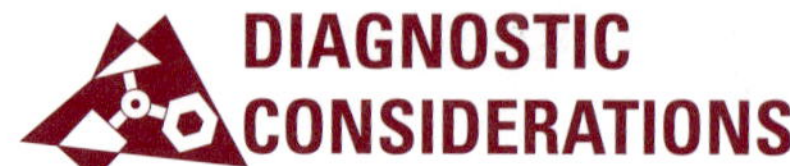

DIAGNOSTIC CONSIDERATIONS

- Pathologic analysis of the spleen in patients with Felty syndrome shows a larger proportionate increase in the white pulp as opposed to most conditions of splenomegaly
- There is evidence of excess accumulation of neutrophils in both the T cell zone of the white pulp as well as the cord and sinuses of the red pulp

RULE OUT

- Other causes of neutropenia
  - Aplastic anemia
  - Pure white cell aplasia
  - Drugs (sulfonamides, procainamide, penicillin, cyclosporines, cimetidine, phenytoin, chlorpropamide)
  - Sepsis
  - Immune mediated

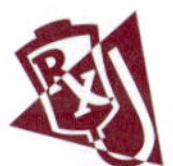

WORK-UP

- CBC count
- Neutrophil count
- Antineutrophil surface IgG
- Bone marrow biopsy

WHEN TO ADMIT

- Severe neutropenia
- Infectious complications

WHEN TO REFER

- All patients should be managed in conjunction with an hematologist

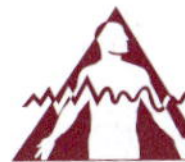

TREATMENT AND MANAGEMENT

- Splenectomy removes source of antibody-mediated neutrophil destruction

SURGERY

Indications

- Patients with recurrent bacterial infections and evidence of IgG on the surface of neutrophils

TREATMENT MONITORING

- Neutrophil counts

COMPLICATIONS

- Infection

PROGNOSIS

- Neutropenia will improve in 60–70% after splenectomy; recurrence possible.
- Splenectomy beneficial even if no postoperative increase in neutrophil count

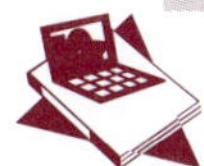

RESOURCES

PREFERENCES

- Logue GL et al. Failure of splenectomy in Felty's syndrome. *N Engl J Med.* 1981;304:580.

Femoral Hernia

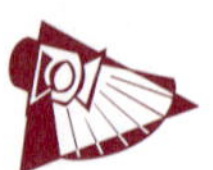

ESSENTIAL FEATURES

- Groin bulge inferior to the inguinal ligament elicited with the Valsalva maneuver
- Differentiation between inguinal and femoral hernias difficult clinically and often not appreciated until the hernia sac is dissected free in the operating room
- Femoral hernia protrudes through the femoral canal, bordered by the inguinal ligament superiorly, pubic ramus inferior-medially, and the femoral vein laterally
- Classification of hernias
  - Reducible: Visceral contents of the hernia sac able to retract into the abdominal cavity
  - Incarcerated: Visceral contents cannot be returned to the abdominal cavity
  - Strangulated: Incarcerated hernia where the blood flow to the entrapped viscera is compromised

EPIDEMIOLOGY

- 1.8:1 female predominance is seen with femoral hernia formation
- Compared with inguinal hernias, femoral hernias more likely to present as incarcerated with or without strangulation
- Femoral hernias are much less common than inguinal hernias

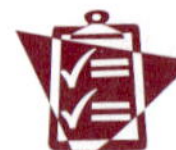

CLINICAL FINDINGS

SYMPTOMS AND SIGNS

- Asymptomatic inguinal bulge most common symptom
- Exam of the groin reveals a bulge inferior to the inguinal ligament that may extend onto the thigh
- The hernia bulge may or may not be reducible
- Patients may complain of a fullness or dragging sensation
- As the hernia enlarges, it is likely to produce a sense of discomfort that may radiate onto the ipsilateral thigh or groin
- Incarcerated (and especially strangulated) inguinal hernia bulge is exquisitely painful
- Coughing or straining will help demonstrate small hernias
- Small bowel obstruction symptoms (nausea, vomiting, abdominal distention) may be present with incarcerated femoral hernias

IMAGING FINDINGS

- **US:** Although rarely needed, can verify the presence of a femoral hernia sac and reliably differentiate between a hernia and inguinal lymphadenopathy

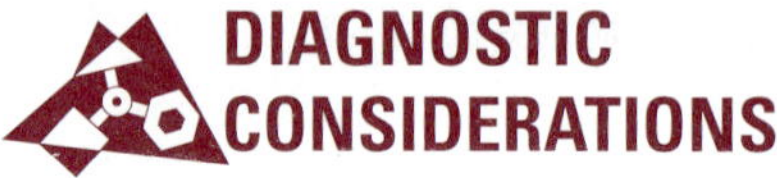

DIAGNOSTIC CONSIDERATIONS

- Inguinal hernia
- Hydrocele
- Cord mass
- Strained groin muscle
- Epididymitis
- Inguinal lymphadenopathy
- Varicocele
- Undescended testes

RULE OUT

- Strained groin muscle (chronic groin pain commonly develops in these following operative intervention)

WORK-UP

- Physical exam usually all that is required to accurately diagnose inguinal hernia
- In equivocal cases, US may be helpful

WHEN TO ADMIT

- Acute hernia incarceration
- Clinical evidence of strangulation
- Associated small bowel obstruction
- Uncomplicated femoral hernia management can be performed as an outpatient

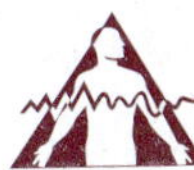

TREATMENT AND MANAGEMENT

- Femoral hernias should be surgically repaired unless there are specific contraindications
- Several successful repairs available including native tissue or prosthetic mesh repair
- Femoral hernia repair may be performed via upper thigh incision or with a standard transverse inguinal incision
- Both open and laparoscopic repairs are commonly used

SURGERY

Indications

- Immediate repair in the case of incarcerated or strangulated femoral hernia repair
- Uncomplicated femoral hernias can be repaired electively as an outpatient

TREATMENT MONITORING

- Physical exam to detect wound/prosthetic infection or hernia recurrence

COMPLICATIONS

- Strangulated femoral hernia with visceral necrosis
- Femoral vein injury
- Recurrence

PROGNOSIS

- Recurrence rates < 5% in most series

RESOURCES

REFERENCES

- Bendavid R. A femoral "umbrella" for femoral hernia repair. *Surg Gynecol Obstet.* 1987;165:153.
- Glassow F. Femoral hernia. Review of 2,105 repairs in a 17 year period. *Am J Surg.* 1985;150:353.

Frostbite

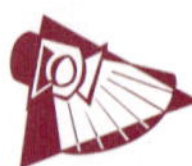

ESSENTIAL FEATURES

- Frostbite involves freezing of tissues
- Ice crystals form between cells and grow at expense of extracellular fluid
- Cellular dehydration and ischemia due to vasoconstriction and increased viscosity are mechanisms of tissue injury
- Caused by cold exposure; effects can be amplified by moisture or wind

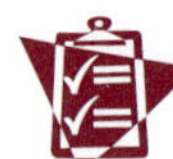

CLINICAL FINDINGS

SYMPTOMS AND SIGNS

- Frostbitten parts are numb, painless, and white or waxy in appearance
- Superficial frostbite is compressible with pressure (unfrozen deep tissues)
- Deep frostbite is woody (frozen deep tissues)

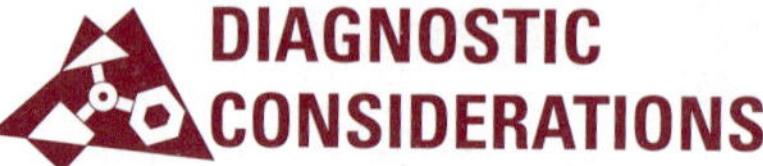

DIAGNOSTIC CONSIDERATIONS

- Evaluate for endocarditis
- Evaluate for secondary LV dysfunction
- After rewarming, frostbitten area becomes mottled blue or purple and painful and tender
- Blisters appear that may take weeks to heal
- Affected part becomes edematous and painful
- Must evaluate for other associated injuries as suggested by history

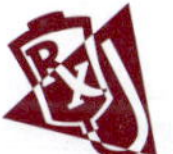

WORK-UP

- Nuclear medicine scans may be useful to delineate tissue viability

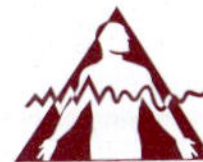

TREATMENT AND MANAGEMENT

- Frostbitten part should be rewarmed in a water bath at 40–42.2 °C for 20–30 min
- Thawing should not be attempted until the victim can be kept permanently warm and at rest
- After thawing, patient should be kept recumbent and with thawed part exposed to air
- Blisters should be left intact
- Skin gently debrided by immersion in whirlpool for 20 min twice daily
- Vasodilating agents and sympathectomy are NOT helpful

SURGERY

Indications

- Constricting eschar

Contraindications

- Expectant management is the rule
- Tissue usually sloughs spontaneously
- Amputation rarely indicated before 2 months

PROGNOSIS

- Excellent if appropriate treatment is provided
- Recovered patients will have increased susceptibility to future frostbite

RESOURCES

REFERENCES

- Farstad M et al. Recovering from accidental hypothermia by extracorporeal circulation: a retrospective study. *Eur J Cardiothorac Surg.* 2001;20:58.
- Peng RY, Bongard FS. Hypothermia in trauma patients. *J Am Coll Surg.* 1999;188:685.

Furuncle, Carbuncle, & Hidradenitis Suppurativa

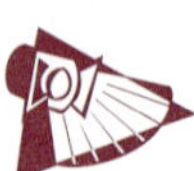

ESSENTIAL FEATURES

- Furuncles and carbuncles: Cutaneous abscess that begin in skin glands and hair follicles
- Furuncles (boils) usually start in infected hair follicles, some caused by retained foreign bodies and other injuries
- Infection can spread as cellulitis or form a subcutaneous abscess
- Furuncles may take a phlegmonous form, ie, extend into the subcutaneous tissue, forming a long, flat abscess
- Furuncles can be multiple and recurrent (furunculosis)
- Carbuncle is a deep-seated mass of fistulous tracts between infected hair follicles
- Staphylococci and anaerobic diphtheroids are most common organisms
- Hidradenitis suppurativa is a serious skin infection of the axillae or groin consisting of multiple abscesses of the apocrine sweat glands

EPIDEMIOLOGY

- Furunculosis usually occurs in young adults and is associated with hormonal changes resulting in impaired skin function
- Carbuncles on the back of the neck are seen almost exclusively in diabetic patients or other relatively immunocompromised patients

CLINICAL FINDINGS

SYMPTOMS AND SIGNS

- Furuncles itch and cause pain
- Skin first becomes red and then turns white and necrotic over the top of the abscess
- Surrounding erythema and induration
- Regional lymphadenopathy
- Carbuncles start as furuncles, with infection dissecting through dermis and subcutaneous tissue in connecting tunnels; extensions open to the surface, giving the appearance of large furuncles with many pustular openings
- Patients may be febrile and mildly toxic
- **Hidradenitis:** Abscesses are concentrated in the apocrine gland areas, ie, the axillae, groin, and perineum

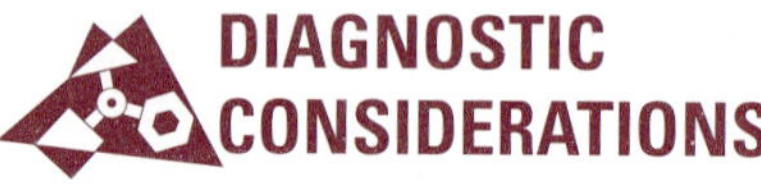

DIAGNOSTIC CONSIDERATIONS

- Rheumatoid nodules
- Gout
- Bursitis
- Sinusitis
- Erythema nodosum
- Fungal infections
- Benign or malignant skin tumors
- Sebaceous or epithelial inclusion cysts

Furuncle, Carbuncle, & Hidradenitis Suppurativa

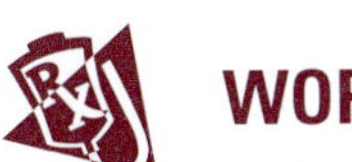

WORK-UP

- History and physical exam

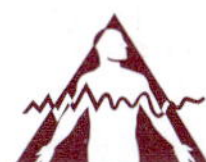

TREATMENT AND MANAGEMENT

- Drainage of abscesses
- Invasive carbuncles treated by excision and antibiotics
- Extensive laundering of all personal clothing
- Excision is continued until sinus tracts are removed, usually far beyond the cutaneous evidence of suppuration
- Hidradenitis is usually treated by drainage of the individual abscess followed by careful hygiene
- Apocrine sweat-bearing skin must be excised; if the deficit is large, closure with a skin graft may be indicated
- Avoidance of antiperspirant and deodorant

SURGERY

Indications

- Diabetic or immunocompromised patients require urgent attention
- Abscesses on the face usually must be treated with antibiotics as well as by prompt incision and drainage

MEDICATIONS

- Use of antibiotics depends on location of the abscess and extent of infection
- Washing with soaps containing hexachlorophene
- Topical and systemic antibiotics may be beneficial

COMPLICATIONS

- Suppurative phlebitis when located near major veins

PROGNOSIS

- Left untreated or inadequately treated may lead to infiltration of adjacent organs and body cavities
- Without adequate excision, hidradenitis may become chronic and disabling

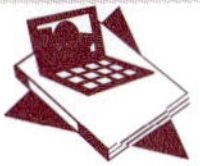

RESOURCES

REFERENCES

- Brown TJ et al. Hidradenitis suppurativa. *South Med J.* 1998;91:1107.

Gallbladder Adenocarcinoma

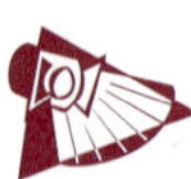

ESSENTIAL FEATURES

- 5% overall survival
- Risk factors
  - Gallstones (70–90% of patients have gallstones)
  - Native American heritage
  - Stones > 3 cm (10-fold increased risk)
  - Porcelain gallbladder (at least 25% develop cancer)
  - Choledochal cyst
  - Gallbladder adenoma > 1 cm
- 0.5% of patients with cholelithiasis have adenocarcinoma
- 1% of patients undergoing elective cholecystectomy have unsuspected adenocarcinoma identified
- Only 25% of patients have chance for curative resection

EPIDEMIOLOGY

- 6000–7000 cases annually
- 3:1 female:male ratio
- Peak incidence in seventh decade
- Risk is at least 5% among Native Americans who have gallstones

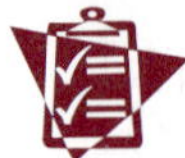

CLINICAL FINDINGS

SYMPTOMS AND SIGNS

- Biliary colic or cholecystitis
- Jaundice
- Weight loss
- Anorexia
- Palpable right upper quadrant mass
- Hepatomegaly
- Ascites

LABORATORY FINDINGS

- Leukocytosis
- Hyperbilirubinemia
- Elevated alkaline phosphatase
- Elevated transaminases
- Elevated carcinoembryonic antigen (CEA)

IMAGING FINDINGS

- **Right upper quadrant US**
  - Gallbladder inflammation and/or gallstones
  - Occasional gallbladder mass
  - Portal or cystic lymphadenopathy
  - Dilated common bile duct (CBD)
  - Direct tumor extension into liver
- **CT or MRI**
  - Gallbladder mass (90% sensitive) with occasional portal lymphadenopathy
  - Hepatic extension of tumor
- **ERCP or percutaneous transhepatic cholangiogram (PTC)**
  - Intraluminal gallbladder mass
  - Occasional CBD dilatation
  - Intraluminal extension of tumor

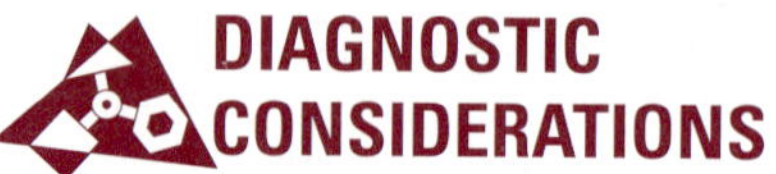

DIAGNOSTIC CONSIDERATIONS

- Lymph node involvement
- Extension into extrahepatic biliary tree
- Extension into hepatic parenchyma

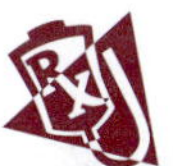

WORK-UP

- History and physical exam
- CBC count
- Liver function tests
- Right upper quadrant US
- Abdominal CT or MRI
- CEA level

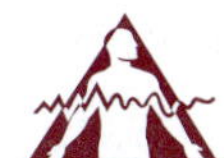

TREATMENT AND MANAGEMENT

SURGERY

- Cholecystectomy (T1 tumors—limited to muscular wall)
- Cholecystectomy with segment 4b, 5 liver resection and portal lymphadenectomy (T2 tumors—invasion to perimuscular tissue but not to serosa)
- Right extended hepatectomy (for some T3 and T4s and recurrence after cholecystectomy or 4b, 5 segmental resection)
- Right extended hepatectomy and resection of CBD followed by hepaticojejunostomy for invasion into CBD

TREATMENT MONITORING

- CEA levels
- US or CT scanning

COMPLICATIONS

- Biliary leak or injury
- Anastomotic leak or stricture
- Liver failure
- Perihepatic infection
- Disease recurrence

PROGNOSIS

- 5-year survival with resection for curative intent, 17%
- > 95% survival for T1 tumors treated with cholecystectomy
- Range from 70% to > 90% for T2 and T3 if 4b and 5 segment resections performed and no nodal involvement

RESOURCES

REFERENCES

- Kondo S et al. Regional and para-aortic lymphadenectomy in radical surgery for advanced gallbladder carcinoma. *Br J Surg.* 2000;87:418.
- Baillie J. Tumors of the gallbladder and bile ducts. *J Clin Gastroenterol.* 1999;29:14.

PRACTICE GUIDELINES

- The National Comprehensive Cancer Network http://www.nccn.org/

CANCER STAGING

- See Gallbladder Staging Table on page 748.

STAGE GROUPING

Stage 0	Tis	N0	M0
Stage IA	T1	N0	M0
Stage IB	T2	N0	M0
Stage IIA	T3	N0	M0
Stage IIB	T1	N1	M0
	T2	N1	M0
	T3	N1	M0
Stage III	T4	Any N	M0
Stage IV	Any T	Any N	M1

Gastric Adenocarcinoma

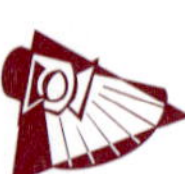

ESSENTIAL FEATURES

- Vague postprandial abdominal heaviness or fullness
- Anorexia and weight loss
- Upper GI endoscopic biopsy and histologic confirmation

EPIDEMIOLOGY

- **Ulcerating (25%):** Ulcer-tumor that extends through all gastric layers
- **Polypoid (25%):** Large, bulky intraluminal growths
- **Superficial spreading (15%):** Confined to the mucosa and submucosa; also known as early gastric cancer
- **Linitis plastica (10%):** Spreading tumor involving all gastric layers
- **Advanced (35%):** Large tumors partly within and partly outside stomach
- 40% in antrum, 30% in the body and fundus, 25% at the cardia, and 5% involve the entire organ
- *Helicobacter pylori* infection carries a 3.6- to 18-fold increased risk of gastric cancer
- Mean age at diagnosis is 63 years
- Majority are adenocarcinoma; squamous cell arises from esophagus
- Intestinal type histology has better prognosis than diffuse type

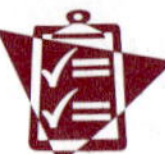

CLINICAL FINDINGS

SYMPTOMS AND SIGNS

- Postprandial abdominal heaviness
- Anorexia develops early; weight loss averages about 6 kg
- Vomiting, often containing blood, is a feature if pyloric obstruction occurs
- Epigastric mass in 25% of cases
- Hepatomegaly in 10% of cases
- In 50% of cases, stool positive for occult blood; melena is seen in a few
- Signs of distant spread
  - Metastases to the neck (Virchow node)
  - Metastases anterior to rectum detectable on rectal examination (Blumer shelf)
  - Metastases to ovaries (Krukenberg tumors)

LABORATORY FINDINGS

- Anemia is present in 40% of patients
- Carcinoembryonic antigen (CEA) levels are elevated in 65% of patients, usually indicating extensive spread of the tumor

IMAGING FINDINGS

- Large gastric carcinomas can usually be identified at endoscopy
- All gastric lesions, whether polypoid or ulcerating, should be examined by taking multiple biopsy and brush cytologic specimens during endoscopy

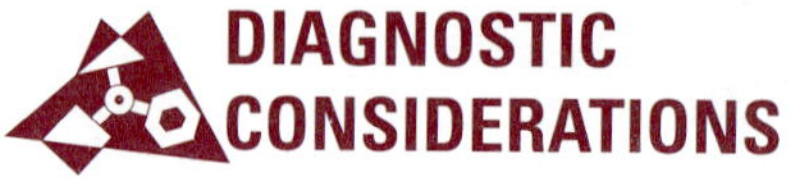

DIAGNOSTIC CONSIDERATIONS

- Vague postprandial abdominal heaviness or fullness, along with anorexia and weight loss should prompt upper GI endocopy and biopsy
- Any endoscopically evident gastric ulcer should be adequately biopsied to rule out carcinoma

RULE OUT

- Benign gastric ulcer

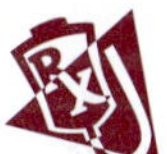

WORK-UP

- Upper GI endoscopy and biopsy will provide histologic diagnosis
- CT scan for staging

WHEN TO ADMIT

- High-grade gastric outlet obstruction preventing adequate enteral nutrition and hydration
- Severe bleeding from ulcer

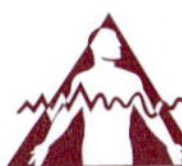

TREATMENT AND MANAGEMENT

- Resect tumor, adjacent margin of stomach (6 cm proximally) and duodenum, regional lymph nodes (no radical lymphadenectomy), and portions of adjacent organs if involved

SURGERY

Indications

- Curative resection if no metastases and reasonable operative risk
- Palliative resection if the stomach is still movable and life expectancy is estimated to be more than 1–2 months

Contraindications

- Limited life expectancy (< 1–2 months) and prohibitive operative risk

MEDICATIONS

- Adjuvant chemotherapy after curative surgery has not been of value
- For advanced disease, chemotherapy has an approximate 20% response rate

COMPLICATIONS

- Post-gastrectomy syndromes (dumping syndrome, fistulae, alkaline gastritis, gastroparesis)

PROGNOSIS

- Overall 5-year survival rate, 12%
- Early gastric cancer: 5-year survival, 90%
- 5-year survival
  - Stage I, 70%
  - Stage II, 30%
  - Stage III, 10%
  - Stage IV, 0%

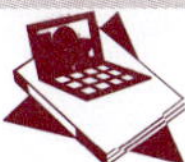

RESOURCES

REFERENCES

- De Vivo R et al. Gastric cancer and *Helicobacter pylori:* a combined analysis of 12 case control studies nested within prospective cohorts. *Gut.* 2001;49:347.

PRACTICE GUIDELINES

- The National Comprehensive Cancer Network http://www.nccn.org/

CANCER STAGING

- See Stomach Staging Table on page 755.

STAGE GROUPING			
Stage 0	Tis	N0	M0
Stage IA	T1	N0	M0
Stage IB	T1	N1	M0
	T2a/b	N0	M0
Stage II	T1	N2	M0
	T2a/b	N1	M0
	T3	N0	M0
Stage IIIA	T2a/b	N2	M0
	T3	N1	M0
	T4	N0	M0
Stage IIIB	T3	N2	M0
Stage IV	T4	N1-3	M0
	T1-3	N3	M0
	Any T	Any N	M1

Gastric Bezoar

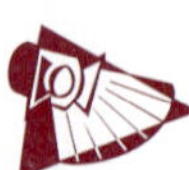

ESSENTIAL FEATURES

- Concretions formed in the stomach, composed of hair or vegetable or fruit fibers, which may cause ulceration of the gastric mucosa with bleeding and perforation

EPIDEMIOLOGY

- **Trichobezoars** are composed of hair and are usually found in young girls who pick at their hair and swallow it
- **Phytobezoars** consist of agglomerated vegetable fibers, orange segments or other fruits that contain a large amount of cellulose
- The postgastrectomy state predisposes to bezoar formation because pepsin and acid secretion are reduced and the triturating function of the antrum is gone
- Large semisolid bezoars of *Candida albicans* have also been found in postgastrectomy patients
- Improper mastication of food is a contributing factor that can sometimes be obviated by providing the patient with properly fitted dentures

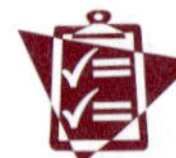

CLINICAL FINDINGS

SYMPTOMS AND SIGNS

- Upper GI bleeding from gastric ulcer caused by pressure from mass
- Gastric perforation
- Abdominal pain

LABORATORY FINDINGS

- Anemia

IMAGING FINDINGS

- Upper GI contrast radiographic study will show mass in lumen of stomach
- Upper GI endoscopy will detect the bezoar and usually allow identification of its contents

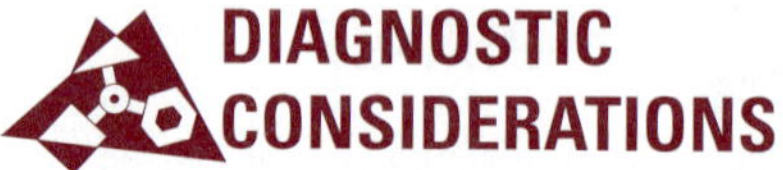

DIAGNOSTIC CONSIDERATIONS

- Diagnosis is usually apparent on upper GI contrast radiographic study or endoscopy

RULE OUT

- Other causes of GI bleeding or perforation

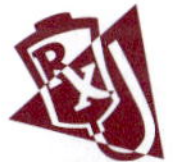

WORK-UP

- Diagnosis is usually apparent on upper GI contrast radiographic
- Upper GI endoscopy is both diagnostic and therapeutic

WHEN TO ADMIT

- Severe GI bleeding
- Gastric perforation
- High-grade obstruction

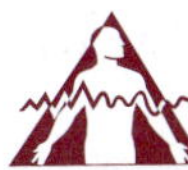

TREATMENT AND MANAGEMENT

- Nearly all gastric bezoars can be broken up and dispersed by endoscopy

SURGERY

Indications

- Inability to extract endoscopically
- Complications of gastric bleeding or perforation

COMPLICATIONS

- Gastric ulceration with bleeding and perforation

PROGNOSIS

- Ulceration and bleeding are associated with a death rate of 20%

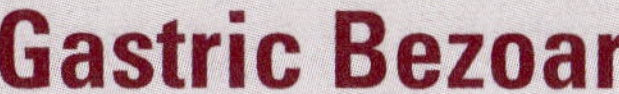

RESOURCES

REFERENCES

- Lee J. Bezoars and foreign bodies of the stomach. *Gastrointest Endosc Clin North Am.* 1996;6:605.

Gastric Lymphoma

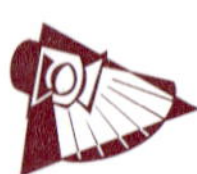

ESSENTIAL FEATURES

- Epigastric pain and weight loss
- Contrast radiographic or upper GI endoscopic evidence of gastric mass
- Endoscopic biopsy provides diagnosis

EPIDEMIOLOGY

- **Gastric lymphoma**
  - Second most common primary cancer of the stomach, representing 2% of the total number
  - Most common site of extranodal lymphoma
  - Almost all are non-Hodgkin lymphomas, generally classified as B cell mucosa-associated lymphoid tissue (MALT) lymphomas
  - Subclassified as low- or high-grade based on nuclear pattern
  - 20% of patients manifest a second primary cancer in another organ
  - Associated with chronic *Helicobacter pylori* infection
- **Gastric pseudolymphoma**
  - Consists of a mass of lymphoid tissue in the gastric wall often associated with an overlying mucosal ulcer
  - Represents response to chronic inflammation and is not malignant

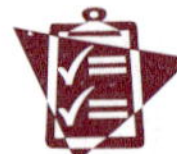

CLINICAL FINDINGS

SYMPTOMS AND SIGNS

- The principal symptoms are epigastric pain and weight loss
- Nausea and vomiting
- Occult GI hemorrhage
- Characteristically, the tumor has attained bulky proportions by the time it is discovered and a palpable epigastric mass is present in 50% of patients
- Pseudolymphoma presents similarly with pain and weight loss

LABORATORY FINDINGS

- Associated with *H pylori* infection
- Anemia

IMAGING FINDINGS

- **Barium x-ray studies** will demonstrate the lesion
- **Gastroscopy with biopsy and brush cytology** provides the correct diagnosis preoperatively in about 75% of cases
- **CT scan and bone marrow biopsy** for preoperative staging

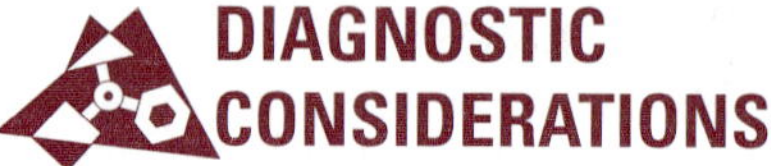

DIAGNOSTIC CONSIDERATIONS

- Epigastric pain and weight loss should prompt upper GI endoscopy, which will reveal the lesion
- Endoscopic biopsy is diagnostic

RULE OUT

- Gastric adenocarcinoma
- Benign gastric ulcer
- Gastric lymphoma in the case of pseudolymphoma

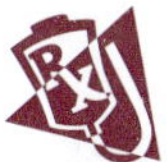

WORK-UP

- Upper GI contrast study will reveal the lesion
- Gastroscopy with biopsy and brush cytology will be diagnostic in most cases; endoscopic US may increase the diagnostic yield
- Preoperative staging
  - CT scan
  - Bone marrow biopsy
  - Biopsy of any enlarged peripheral lymph nodes

WHEN TO ADMIT

- Inability to tolerate enteral nutrition

TREATMENT AND MANAGEMENT

- **Lymphoma:** Surgical resection and staging followed by total abdominal radiotherapy
- **Pseudolymphoma:** Resection; no additional therapy

SURGERY

Indications

- Splenectomy should be performed only if the spleen is directly invaded

Contraindications

- Extension into the duodenum or esophagus should not lead to resection of these organs but to postoperative adjunctive therapy

MEDICATIONS

- Adjuvant radiation and chemotherapy for stage II and higher
- Eradication of *H pylori* for low-grade MALT

COMPLICATIONS

- Occult GI bleeding

PROGNOSIS

- 5-year disease-free survival, 50%; correlates with stage, grade, and extent of penetration of the gastric wall
- 60% of recurrences are extra-abdominal

PREVENTION

- Eradication of *H pylori*

RESOURCES

REFERENCES

- Kolve ME et al. Primary gastric non-Hodgkin's lymphoma: requirements for diagnosis and staging. *Recent Results Cancer Res.* 2000;156:63.

Gastric Ulcer

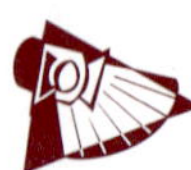

ESSENTIAL FEATURES

- Epigastric pain
- Ulcer demonstrated by endoscopy or radiography
- Acid present on gastric analysis

EPIDEMIOLOGY

- Peak incidence at 40–60 years old
- 85–90% of patients infected with *Helicobacter pylori*
- **Type I ulcers (50%)**
  - Located within 2 cm of the incisura angularis
  - Gastric acid output is normal or low
- **Type II ulcers (20%)**
  - Both ulceration of gastric body and duodenum
  - Increased acid secretion
- **Type III ulcers (20%)**
  - Prepyloric location
  - Increased acid secretion
- **Type IV ulcers (5–10%)**
  - Located high on lesser curvature at or near gastroesophageal junction
  - Gastric acid output is normal or low
- **Type V ulcers (< 5%)**
  - Results from NSAID use

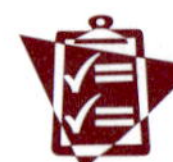

CLINICAL FINDINGS

SYMPTOMS AND SIGNS

- Principal symptom is epigastric pain relieved by food or antacids
- Vomiting, anorexia, and aggravation of pain by eating are also common
- Epigastric tenderness may be present

LABORATORY FINDINGS

- Evaluation for *H pylori* infection

IMAGING FINDINGS

- Radiographic or endoscopic evidence of gastric ulceration

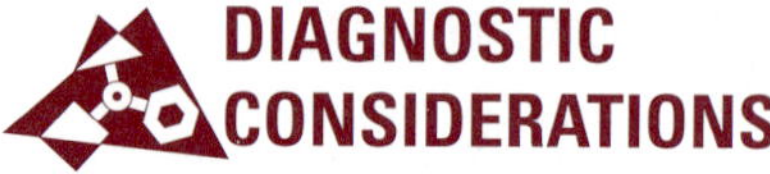

DIAGNOSTIC CONSIDERATIONS

- Signs and symptoms of gastric ulcer should prompt contrast radiography or upper endoscopy for diagnosis

RULE OUT

- Ulcerated malignancy
  - Obtain multiple biopsies from edge of the lesion
  - Rolled-up ulcer margins
  - More common with larger ulcers (> 2 cm)
- Zollinger-Ellison syndrome if disease is severe and refractory or if associated with more distal ulceration

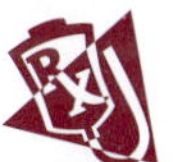

WORK-UP

- Signs and symptoms of gastric ulcer
- Radiographic or endocopic findings consistent with gastric ulcer
- Biopsy to exclude malignancy
- Testing for *H pylori*

WHEN TO ADMIT

- Complications of gastric ulcer (bleeding, perforation, high-grade obstruction, severe pain)

TREATMENT AND MANAGEMENT

- Types I, IV, and V gastric ulcers represent defects in mucosal protection
- Types II and III gastric ulcers are associated with acid hypersecretion and behave similar to duodenal ulcers

SURGERY

- Parietal cell vagotomy
- Truncal vagotomy and antrectomy
- Vagotomy and pyloroplasty

Indications

- Intractibility: Excision of ulcer and acid reduction
- Perforation, bleeding, obstruction

MEDICATIONS

- Treatment of *H pylori*
- Antacids
- H_2 receptor blockers
- Proton pump inhibitors

TREATMENT MONITORING

- Repeat endoscopy after 4–16 weeks to document healing

COMPLICATIONS

- Perforation
- Obstruction
- Bleeding

PROGNOSIS

- < 5% recurrence after vagotomy and antrectomy
- 10–12% recurrence after parietal cell or truncal vagotomy and pyloroplasty

PREVENTION

- Avoidance of NSAIDs

RESOURCES

REFERENCES

- Calam J, Baron JH. ABC of the upper gastrointestinal tract: pathophysiology of duodenal and gastric ulcer and gastric cancer. *BMJ.* 2001;323:980.

Gastric Volvulus

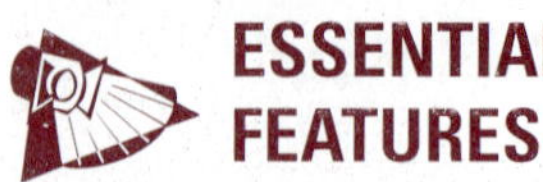

ESSENTIAL FEATURES

Acute

- Severe abdominal pain
- Vomiting followed by retching and then inability to vomit
- Epigastric distention
- Inability to pass an NG tube

Chronic

- May be asymptomatic or associated with intermittent crampy abdominal pain

EPIDEMIOLOGY

- Chronic volvulus is more common than acute
- The stomach may rotate about its longitudinal axis (organo-axial volvulus) or a line drawn from the mid lesser to the mid greater curvature (mesenterioaxial volvulus)
- Organo-axial volvulus is more common than mesenterioaxial volvulus and is often associated with a paraesophageal hiatal hernia
- Volvulus may also be caused by eventration of the left diaphragm, allowing the colon to rise and twist the stomach by pulling on the gastrocolic ligament

CLINICAL FINDINGS

SYMPTOMS AND SIGNS

Acute

- Severe abdominal pain
- Vomiting followed by retching and then inability to vomit
- Epigastric distention
- Inability to pass an NG tube

Chronic

- May be asymptomatic or cause crampy intermittent abdominal pain

IMAGING FINDINGS

- Upper GI contrast radiography will show a block at the point of the volvulus

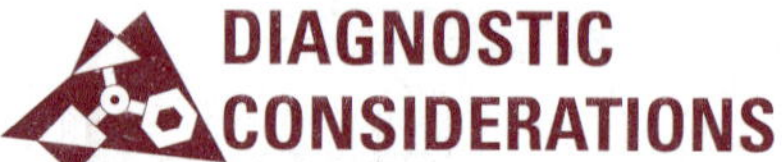

DIAGNOSTIC CONSIDERATIONS

- A high level of suspicion is required for timely diagnosis of acute gastric volvulus to avoid complication of gastric ischemia and necrosis

RULE OUT

- Other causes of upper GI obstruction

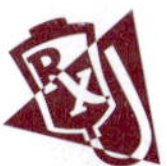

WORK-UP

- Symptoms and signs consistent with gastric volvulus
- Upper GI contrast radiography will provide diagnosis

WHEN TO ADMIT

- All cases of acute volvulus
- Cases of chronic volvulus if severely symptomatic or evidence of possible gastric ischemia and shock

TREATMENT AND MANAGEMENT

- Immediate laparotomy for acute cases
- Cases associated with paraesophageal hiatal hernia should be treated by repair of the hernia and anterior gastropexy

SURGERY

Indications

- All cases of gastric volvulus

COMPLICATIONS

- Gastric ischemia
- Gastric necrosis
- Gastric perforation
- Shock

PROGNOSIS

- Good outcome if diagnosed and treated promptly
- The mortality rate is high with gastric ischemia and necrosis

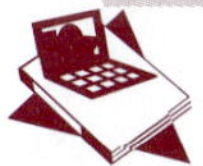

RESOURCES

REFERENCES

- Schaefer DC et al. Gastric volvulus: an old disease process with some new twists. *Gastroenterologist.* 1997;5:41.
- Wasselle JA, Norman J. Acute gastric volvulus: pathogenesis, diagnosis, and treatment. *Am J Gastroenterol.* 1993;88:1780.

Gastrinoma (Zollinger-Ellison Syndrome)

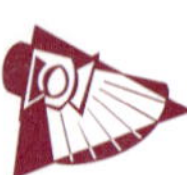

ESSENTIAL FEATURES

- Peptic ulcer disease—often severe
- Gastric hypersecretion
- Elevated serum gastrin
- Gastrin producing non-B islet cell tumor of the pancreas or duodenum (gastrinoma)

EPIDEMIOLOGY

- 95% pancreatic, 60% non-B islet cell carcinomas; 25% solitary adenomas; 10% hyperplasia or microadenomas
- 5% are due to solitary submucosal gastrinomas in the first or second portion of the duodenum
- Rarely found in the antrum or ovary
- About 33% associated with multiple endocrine neoplasia type 1 (MEN 1)—usually multiple benign gastrinomas
- Those without MEN 1 (sporadic cases) usually have solitary gastrinomas that are often malignant
- The tumors may be as small as 2–3 mm; in about 33% of cases, the tumor cannot be located at laparotomy
- Histologic pattern is similar for benign and malignant tumors
  - Diagnosis of cancer can be made only with findings of metastases or blood vessel invasion

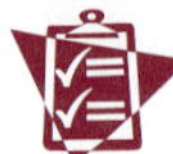

CLINICAL FINDINGS

SYMPTOMS AND SIGNS

- Symptoms are principally a result of peptic ulcer disease from acid hypersecretion
- Ulcer symptoms are often refractory to antacids or H_2 blocking agents.
- Some patients have severe diarrhea from the large amounts of acid entering the duodenum, which can destroy pancreatic lipase and produce steatorrhea, damage the small bowel mucosa, and overload the intestine with gastric and pancreatic secretions

LABORATORY FINDINGS

- Hypergastrinemia (> 500 pg/mL) in the presence of acid hypersecretion(> 15 mEq H^+ per hour).
- Gastrin levels > 5000 pg/mL or α chains of hCG in the serum usually indicates established metastasis
- Secretin provocative test for borderline gastrin values (200–500 pg/mL)
  - A rise in gastrin level of >150 pg/mL within 15 minutes is diagnostic

IMAGING FINDINGS

- **Esophagogastroduodenoscopy:** Usually shows ulceration in the duodenal bulb, distal duodenum, or proximal jejunum
- **CT** or **MRI:** Often detects pancreatic tumors.
- **Somatostatin-receptor scintigraphy:** Very sensitive for detection of gastrinoma primary and metastatic sites
- **Failure of other methods:** Localize with intra-arterial secretin test (infusion of secretin into the artery supplying a functional gastrinoma causes an increase in hepatic vein gastrin levels)

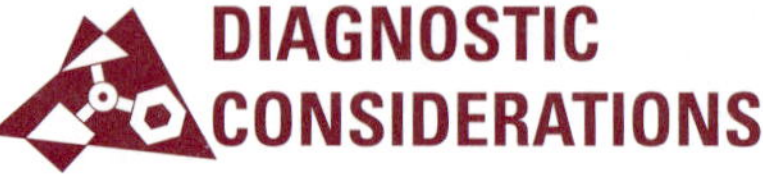

DIAGNOSTIC CONSIDERATIONS

- Serum gastrin levels should be measured in any patient with suspected gastrinoma or ulcer disease severe enough to warrant consideration of surgical treatment
- Discontinue H_2 receptor blocking agents, omeprazole, or antacids several days before measuring gastrin level (may increase serum gastrin concentrations)
- Measure serum calcium (common association with hyperparathyroidism)

RULE OUT

- Hypergastrinemia and gastric acid hypersecretion also seen in gastric outlet obstruction, retained antrum, and antral cell hyperplasia
  - Differentiate with secretin test
- Pernicious anemia, atrophic gastritis, gastric ulcer and postvagotomy state may cause a rise in serum gastrin with decreased gastric acid

Gastrinoma (Zollinger-Ellison Syndrome)

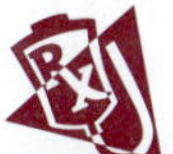

WORK-UP

- Signs and symptoms of peptic ulcer disease
- Endoscopic evidence of peptic ulceration
- Measurement of serum gastrin
- Confirmation of acid hypersecretion
- If diagnosis remains unclear, secretin provocation test

WHEN TO ADMIT

- Complications of peptic ulcer disease (perforation, bleeding, high-grade obstruction, severe pain)

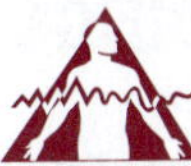

TREATMENT AND MANAGEMENT

- Initial reduction in gastric acid hypersecretion
- Resection is the ideal treatment for gastrinoma
  - Intraoperative US may aid pancreatic localization

SURGERY

Indications

- Resection is indicated in all patients with apparently localized disease and no other significant limitations to their survival

Contraindications

- Unresectible metastatic disease

MEDICATIONS

- H_2 blocking agents
- Proton pump inhibitor
- Maintain gastric H^+ output < 5 mEq in the hour preceding the next dose

COMPLICATIONS

- Perforation
- Bleeding
- Obstruction from peptic ulcer disease

PROGNOSIS

- Cure possible with complete resection
- 70% of patients have biochemical cure
- 30% of patients disease-free after 5 years
- Patients with MEN 1 rarely cured

RESOURCES

REFERENCES

- Norton JA et al. Surgery to cure the Zollinger-Ellison syndrome. *N Engl J Med.* 1999;341:635.
- Pisegna JR. The effect of Zollinger-Ellison syndrome and neuropeptide-secreting tumors on the stomach. *Curr Gastroenterol Rep.* 1999;1:511.

Gastroesophageal Reflux Disease (GERD) & Hiatal Hernia

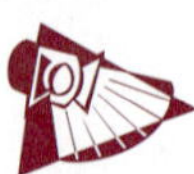

ESSENTIAL FEATURES

- Heartburn, often worse on recumbency
- Regurgitation
- Sliding hiatal hernia on upper GI series
- Endoscopic biopsy evidence of esophagitis
- Decreased resting pressure in lower esophageal sphincter
- Abnormal esophageal acid exposure on prolonged pH monitoring

EPIDEMIOLOGY

- Most patients (80%) with GERD have a sliding hiatal hernia (type I) in which the gastroesophageal junction (GEJ) is displaced upward into the posterior mediastinum, exposing the lower esophageal sphincter to intrathoracic pressure, which is less than intra-abdominal pressure
- The principal barrier to reflux is the lower esophageal sphincter, the competence of which is a function of sphincter pressure, sphincter length, and the length exposed to intra-abdominal pressure
- Bile acids may also play a role in esophagitis, especially in patients with previous gastric surgery
- 15% of patients have severe symptoms refractory to optimal medical treatment and will require surgery

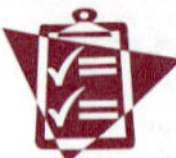

CLINICAL FINDINGS

SYMPTOMS AND SIGNS

- Retrosternal and epigastric burning pain that occurs after eating and while sleeping or lying in a recumbent position and is relieved by drinking liquids, antacids, or by standing or sitting
- Regurgitation of bitter or sour-tasting fluid
- Pulmonary symptoms (wheezing, dyspnea) as the result of aspiration
- Dysphagia, which results from inflammatory edema in the lower esophagus

IMAGING FINDINGS

- **Upper GI contrast radiography**: Protrusion of the stomach upward through the esophageal hiatus
- **Esophagoscopy and biopsy**: Determine the presence and degree of esophagitis and Barrett metaplasia
- **Manometry**: Decreased mean resting pressure in the lower esophageal sphincter
- **Abnormal lower esophageal peristalsis:** Low amplitude and decreased velocity of propagation of the peristaltic wave
- **pH monitoring**: Increased exposure of the lower esophagus to acid, correlating with symptom onset

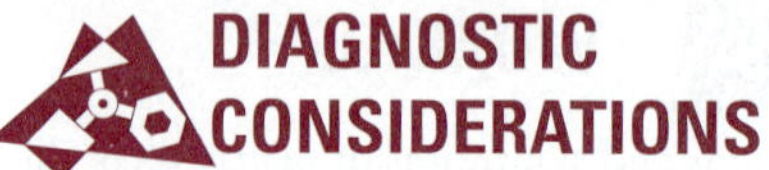

DIAGNOSTIC CONSIDERATIONS

- If sphincter function as measured manometrically seems intact, the possibility of delayed gastric emptying should be assessed by measuring the rate of passage from the stomach of a technetium Tc 99m-labeled solid meal

RULE OUT

- Cholelithiasis
- Diverticulitis
- Peptic ulcer disease
- Achalasia
- Coronary artery disease

Gastroesophageal Reflux Disease (GERD) & Hiatal Hernia

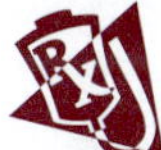

WORK-UP

- Upper GI contrast radiography may indicate a sliding hiatal hernia and evidence of contrast reflux
- Upper GI endoscopy with biopsy to assess presence and degree of esophagitis and evaluate for Barrett metaplasia
- pH monitoring to document acid reflux and association with symptoms
- Manometry to assess status of lower esophageal sphincter and force of peristalsis

WHEN TO ADMIT

- Aspiration pneumonitis

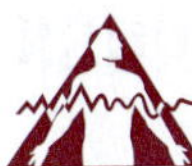

TREATMENT AND MANAGEMENT

- Asymptomatic hiatal hernias require no treatment
- Fundoplication: intra-abdominal placement of GEJ and buttress the gastroesophageal sphincter

SURGERY

Indications

- Persistent or recurrent symptoms despite good medical therapy
- Complete mechanical incompetence of the sphincter (pressure < 6 mm Hg)
- Presence or development of strictures

Contraindications

- Shortened esophagus requires construction of a tubular extension along the lesser curvature for intra-abdominal placement of GEJ (Collis)

MEDICATIONS

- H_2 receptor blockers
- Proton pump inhibitors
- Recurrence is usual when drugs are discontinued

TREATMENT MONITORING

- Interval esophagoscopy to assess healing of esophagitis and monitor Barrett metaplasia

COMPLICATIONS

- Esophageal ulcerations
- Esophageal strictures
- Barrett metaplasia and cancer
- Aspiration
  - Pneumonia
  - Asthma

PROGNOSIS

- 90% of patients experience a good result following surgery
- 80–85% of cases of esophagitis heal after treatment with a proton pump inhibitor

RESOURCES

REFERENCES

- Watson DI et al. The changing face of treatment for hiatus hernia and gastro-oesophageal reflux. *Gut.* 1999;45:791.
- Schowengerdt CG. Standard acid reflux testing revisited. *Dig Dis Sci.* 2001;46:603.

Gastrointestinal Stromal Tumor (GIST), Leiomyomas, & Leiomyosarcomas

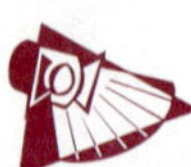

ESSENTIAL FEATURES

- Radiographic or endoscopic evidence of gastric mass
- Often accompanied by upper GI bleeding

EPIDEMIOLOGY

- Represent 1% of all GI malignancies
  - Stomach is most common site
- Difficult to distinguish malignant from benign histologically
- Increased size (> 6–10 cm) correlates with increased risk of malignancy
- In most cases, the tumor arises from the proximal stomach
  - Benign tumors more common on lesser curvature
  - Malignant tumors more common on greater curvature
- Tumors may grow into the gastric lumen, remain entirely on the serosal surface, or even become pedunculated within the abdominal cavity
- Spread is by direct invasion or blood-borne metastases
  - Liver most common site of metastases

CLINICAL FINDINGS

SYMPTOMS AND SIGNS

- Often asymptomatic
- May present with occult or apparent GI bleeding (melena, hematochezia)
- Weight loss
- Nausea and vomiting may be present if tumor obstructs gastric outlet
- Epigastric mass palpable in 20% of patients

LABORATORY FINDINGS

- Anemia

IMAGING FINDINGS

- **Radiology and endoscopy:** Tumor usually contains a central ulceration caused by necrosis from outgrowth of its blood supply
- **CT scans:** Provide useful information on the amount of extragastric extension

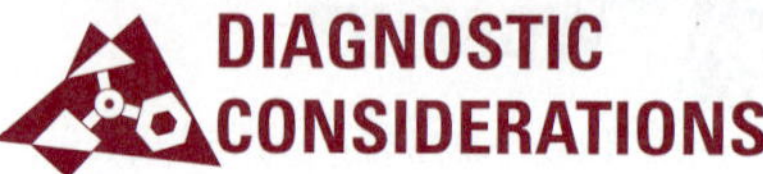

DIAGNOSTIC CONSIDERATIONS

- Contrast radiography or upper GI endoscopy will reveal a gastric mass
- Endoscopic biopsy that penetrates through the gastric mucosa will usually provide diagnosis but not distinguish benign from malignant

RULE OUT

- Adenocarcinoma
- Lymphoma
- Other gastric neoplasm

Gastrointestinal Stromal Tumor (GIST), Leiomyomas, & Leiomyosarcomas

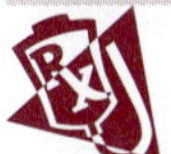

WORK-UP

- Contrast radiography or upper GI endoscopy will reveal a gastric mass
- Endoscopic biopsy, perhaps guided by endoscopic US, will usually be diagnostic
- CT scans provide useful information on the amount of extragastric extension
- Hct to assess anemia and treat accordingly

WHEN TO ADMIT

- Severe anemia or apparent upper GI hemorrhage
- High-grade obstruction

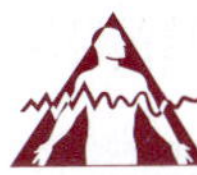

TREATMENT AND MANAGEMENT

- **Leiomyomas:** Enucleation or wedge resection (2–3 cm margin)
- **Leiomyosarcomas:** More radical gastric resection

SURGERY

Indications

- All leiomyomas and leiomyosarcomas
- Complete resection of metastases in addition to the primary may improve the outcome

MEDICATIONS

- Imatinib mesylate

COMPLICATIONS

- GI bleeding
- Gastric outlet obstruction

PROGNOSIS

- **GIST:** 5-year survival rate is 20–55% after resection
- Tumors with 10 or more mitoses in a high-powered field rarely can be cured

RESOURCES

REFERENCES

- DeMatteo RP et al. Two hundred gastrointestinal stromal tumors: recurrence patterns and prognostic factors for survival. *Ann Surg.* 2000;231:51.

PRACTICE GUIDELINES

- The National Comprehensive Cancer Network
  http://www.nccn.org/

Glucagonoma

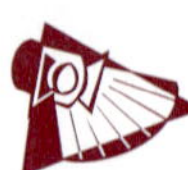

ESSENTIAL FEATURES

- Migratory necrolytic dermatitis, usually involving the legs and perineum
- Weight loss
- Stomatitis
- Thrombophlebitis
- Anemia
- Mild to moderate diabetes mellitus

EPIDEMIOLOGY

- Arise from cells in the pancreatic islets
- Most tumors are solitary and large (> 4 cm) located in the body or tail of the pancreas
- About 25% are benign and confined to the pancreas
  - The remainder has metastasized by the time of diagnosis, most often to the liver, lymph nodes, adrenal gland, or vertebrae
- The age range is 20–70 years, and the condition is more common in women

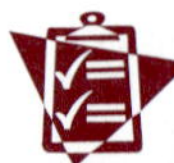

CLINICAL FINDINGS

SYMPTOMS AND SIGNS

- Migratory necrolytic dermatitis, usually involving the legs and perineum
- Weight loss
- Stomatitis
- Thrombophlebitis

LABORATORY FINDINGS

- Elevated serum glucagon level (> 1000 pg/mL)
- Hypoaminoacidemia
- Anemia
- Hyperglycemia

IMAGING FINDINGS

- CT scan or MRI demonstrates the tumor and sites of metastases

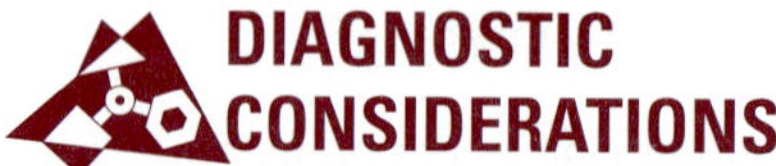

DIAGNOSTIC CONSIDERATIONS

- The diagnosis may be suspected from the distinctive skin lesion
  - In fact, the presence of a prominent rash in a patient with diabetes mellitus should be enough to raise suspicions
- Glucagonoma should also be suspected in any patient with new onset of diabetes after age 60

RULE OUT

- Other causes of dermatitis
- Other pancreatic islet cell tumors

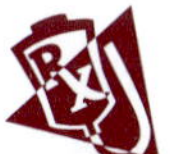

WORK-UP

- Elevated serum glucagon
- Decreased serum amino acids
- CT scan or MRI

WHEN TO ADMIT

- Severe symptoms

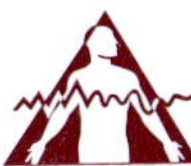

TREATMENT AND MANAGEMENT

- Surgical resection of the primary tumor
  - Location of tumor determines procedure

SURGERY

- Distal subtotal pancreatectomy and splenectomy (for head and body)
- Pancreaticoduodenectomy (for head)
- Debulking of metastases

Indications

- Whenever technically possible
- Preoperative total parenteral nutrition should be administered for malnutrition

MEDICATIONS

- Total parenteral nutrition
- Somatostatin for symptomatic palliation
- Streptozocin and dacarbazine for unresectable lesions

PROGNOSIS

- Good with complete resection of the tumor
- Palliation can be achieved with resection and debulking of metastatic disease

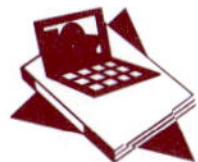

RESOURCES

REFERENCES

- Chastain MA. The glucagonoma syndrome: a review of its features and discussion of new perspectives. *Am J Med Sci.* 2001;321:306.

Goiter, Simple or Nontoxic (Diffuse & Multinodular)

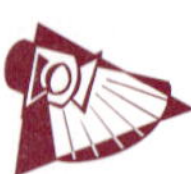

ESSENTIAL FEATURES

- May be a diffuse or a multinodular goiter
- May be physiologic or pathophysiologic
  - Physiologic occurs during puberty, menses, or pregnancy
  - Pathophysiologic is due to iodine-deficiency, congenital defect in thyroid hormone production, or goitrogenic foods or drugs
- Generally assumed to be compensatory response to inadequate thyroid hormone production
- Thyroid growth immunoglobulins may also be important
- Food goitrogens include isothiocyanate and goitrin (in milk products)
- Drugs implicated as goitrogens include:
  - Lithium
  - p-Aminosalicylic acid
  - Aminoglutethimide
  - Sulfonamides
  - Phenylbutazone
- Congenital determined failures in thyroid hormone metabolism include iodine transport defects, abnormal secretion of iodoproteins, and thyroid hormone resistance syndromes

EPIDEMIOLOGY

- Prevalence of about 5%; increases with age and in women

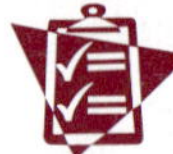

CLINICAL FINDINGS

SYMPTOMS AND SIGNS

- Neck mass
- Inspiratory stridor
- Dyspnea
- Dysphagia
- Symmetrically enlarged thyroid with smooth surface, or enlarged thyroid with multiple nodules
- Enlargement and prominence of the large veins of the neck and upper thorax

LABORATORY FINDINGS

- Thyroid function tests usually normal
- Thyroid-stimulating hormone (TSH) may be suppressed slightly, and radioiodine uptake increased

IMAGING FINDINGS

- US reveals size and extent of goiter; can define focal nodules
- CT or MRI can define retrosternal or intrathoracic extension but are not considered as primary diagnostic tools
- Thyroid scintigraphy can confirm extension and functional status of the gland
- Chest radiograph may demonstrate an anterior mediastinal mass, with or without tracheal deviation, in the setting of a substernal goiter

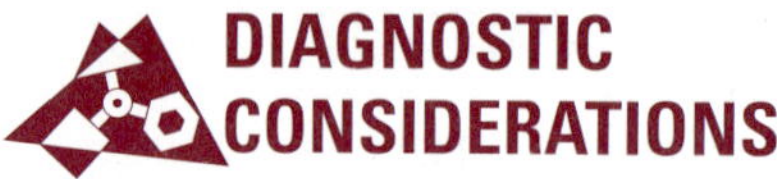

DIAGNOSTIC CONSIDERATIONS

- As the goiter persists, nodules can develop

RULE OUT

- Thyroid malignancy or lymphoma
- Acute suppurative thyroiditis
- Silent thyroiditis
- Subacute thyroiditis
- Reidel thyroiditis

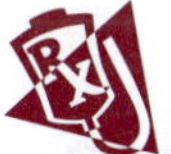

WORK-UP

- Complete history and physical exam
- Thyroid function tests
- Thyroid US
- Fine-needle aspiration biopsy of any concerning nodule

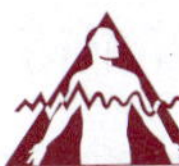

TREATMENT AND MANAGEMENT

- Goiter usually responds favorably to thyroid hormone administration
- Multinodular goiter can be treated with operative removal, thyroid hormone administration, or radioactive iodine therapy
- Operative candidates with tracheal compression or deviation should undergo awake, fiberoptic intubation

SURGERY

Indications

- Relief of local compressive symptoms
- Diagnostic to rule out cancer in areas of hardness or rapid growth
- Proven malignancy

MEDICATIONS

- Suppressive thyroxine (T_4)
- Radioactive iodine 131

TREATMENT MONITORING

- Long-term suppressive/replacement thyroid hormone therapy
- Monitor TSH and T_4

PREVENTION

- Long-term administration in diet (to prevent iodine-deficiency goiter)
- Limit intake of natural or pharmacologic goitrogens

RESOURCES

REFERENCES

- Mack E. Management of patients with substernal goiters. *Surg Clin North Am.* 1995;75:377.
- Petrone LR. A primary care approach to the adult patient with nodular thyroid disease. *Arch Fam Med.* 1996;5:92.
- Shaha A. Surgery for benign thyroid disease causing tracheoesophageal compression. *Otolaryngol Clin North Am.* 1990;23:391.

Graves Disease

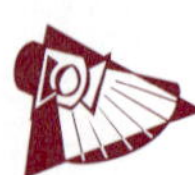

ESSENTIAL FEATURES

- Diffusely hypersecretory goiter with resultant increased levels of thyroid hormone in the blood
- Nervousness, weight loss with increased appetite, heat intolerance, increased sweating, muscular weakness and fatigue, increased bowel frequency, polyuria, menstrual irregularities, infertility
- Goiter, tachycardia, atrial fibrillation, warm moist skin, thyroid thrill and bruit, cardiac flow murmur, gynecomastia
- Eye signs include:
  - Stare
  - Lid lag
  - Exophthalmos
- Thyroid-stimulating hormone (TSH) low or absent
- Increased radioactive iodine uptake
- Increased tri-iodothyronine (T_3) and thyroxine (T_4)
- Abnormal T_3 suppression test
- Elevated thyroid-stimulating immunoglobulin

EPIDEMIOLOGY

- 85% of all hyperthyroid cases
- Peak age of onset is fourth decade
- Incidence: 23 per 100,000
- Female:male ratio of 4:1 to 5:1
- 50% of patients show clinical signs of ophthalmopathy
- 50% of patients have myopathy that presents as proximal muscle weakness

CLINICAL FINDINGS

SYMPTOMS AND SIGNS

- Nervousness, increased diaphoresis, heat intolerance, tachycardia, palpitations, fatigue, and weight loss
- Nodular, multinodular, or diffuse goiter on physical exam
- Flushed and staring appearance
- Warm, thin, and moist skin
- Fine hair
- Possible exophthalmos
- Pretibial myxedema
- Vitiligo
- Shortened Achilles reflex time

LABORATORY FINDINGS

- Suppressed TSH
- Elevated T_3, free T_4, and radioactive iodine uptake
- Failure to suppress radioiodine uptake with exogenous T_3
- Failure of rise in TSH with thyrotropin-releasing hormone (TRH) administration
- High thyroid-stimulating immunoglobulin level
- Low serum cholesterol
- Lymphocytosis
- Occasional hypercalcemia, hypercalciuria, or glycosuria

IMAGING FINDINGS

- Diffuse increased uptake on radioactive iodine scan
- Thyroid US reveals an enlarged gland, with or without nodules, and high vascular flow
- Orbital US, CT, or MRI can evaluate extraocular muscles, retrobulbar soft tissue, and optic nerve

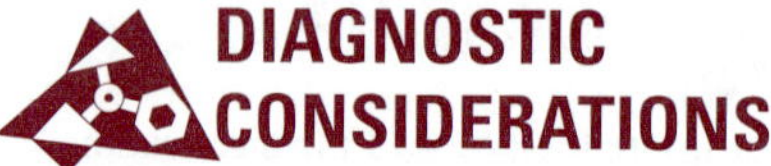

DIAGNOSTIC CONSIDERATIONS

- Clinical manifestations may go through periods of exacerbation and remission
- Graves disease is an autoimmune disease in which antibodies are directed against the TSH receptor
- Pathogenesis of ocular problems in Graves disease is unclear
- Eye complications may begin before and continue after thyroid dysfunction

RULE OUT

- Anxiety neurosis
- Pheochromocytoma
- Primary ophthalmopathy (eg, orbital tumors)
- Thyrotoxicosis factitia
- Thyroiditis

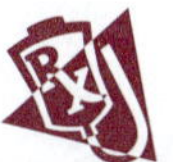

WORK-UP

- Complete history (including family) and physical examof the thyroid gland
- Thyroid function tests

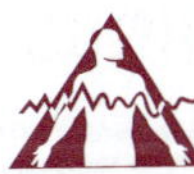

TREATMENT AND MANAGEMENT

- Antithyroid drugs, radioactive iodine, or thyroidectomy
- Treatment of ocular problems of Graves disease include:
  - Maintenance of euthyroid state
  - Protecting the eyes from light and dust
  - Elevating the bed
  - Diuretic use
  - Methylcellulose or guanethidine eye drops
  - Systemic glucocorticoids
  - Ophthalmologic surgery

SURGERY

Indications

- Very large goiter or multinodular goiter with relatively low radioactive iodine uptake
- Thyroid nodule that may be malignant
- Patients with ophthalmopathy
- Pregnant patients or children
- Women who wish to become pregnant within 1 year of treatment
- Patients who for any reason are unable to maintain adequate long-term follow-up evaluation
- Relapse after treatment with antithyroid medication or radioiodine

Contraindications

- Patient is too ill to undergo general anesthesia

MEDICATIONS

- Propylthiouracil
- Methimazole
- Radioiodine (^{131}I)

TREATMENT MONITORING

- TSH and T_4 measurements

PROGNOSIS

- Hypothyroidism develops spontaneously or as a result of treatment in some patients
- If left untreated, Graves disease leads to progressive and profound catabolic disturbances and cardiac damage, which may result in death
- Surgical treatment is associated with < 0.1% mortality

RESOURCES

REFERENCES

- Ljunggren JG et al. Quality of life aspects and costs in treatment of Graves' hyperthyroidism with antithyroid drugs, surgery, or radioiodine: results from a perspective randomized trial. *Thyroid.* 1998;8:653.
- McIver B et al. The pathogenesis of Graves' disease. *Endocrinol Metab Clin North Am.* 1998;27:73.
- Menegaux F et al. The surgical treatment of Graves' disease. *Surg Gynecol Obstet.* 1993;176:277.
- Miccoli P et al. Surgical treatment of Graves' disease: subtotal or total thyroidectomy? *Surgery.* 1996;120:1020.

Gynecomastia

ESSENTIAL FEATURES

- Hypertrophy of normal breast tissue
- Can be divided into 2 categories:
  1. Pubertal hypertrophy (ages 13–17)
  2. Senescent hypertrophy (older than age 50)

EPIDEMIOLOGY

- Associated with some recreational and therapeutic drugs
  - Marijuana
  - Digoxin
  - Thiazides
  - Estrogens
  - Phenothiazines
  - Theophylline

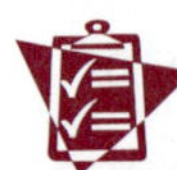

CLINICAL FINDINGS

SYMPTOMS AND SIGNS

- Unilateral or bilateral breast enlargement
- Mass is subareolar, smooth, firm, and discoid
- Rarely painful, but patient may complain of vague breast discomfort

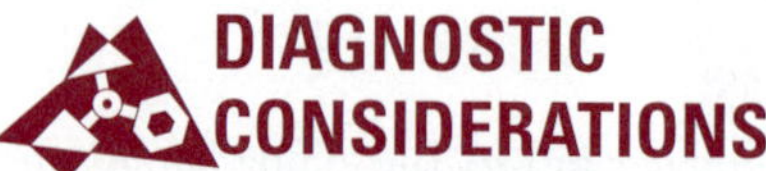

DIAGNOSTIC CONSIDERATIONS

- Frequently no identifiable cause
- Without pain, pubertal gynecomastia frequently regresses as the patient passes into adulthood
- Senescent gynecomastia may also regress spontaneously
- May represent local manifestation of systemic illness such as hepatic or renal insufficiency, or alterations in steroid metabolism

RULE OUT

- Carcinoma of the breast

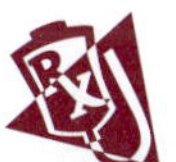

WORK-UP

- History and physical exam
- Observation
- Biopsy of any dominant mass if concern for malignancy

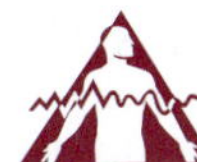

TREATMENT AND MANAGEMENT

- Usually left untreated
- Dominant mass may be biopsied

SURGERY

Indications

- Failure of enlargement to regress and breast is cosmetically unacceptable

TREATMENT MONITORING

- Follow physical exam

RESOURCES

REFERENCES

- Lazala C, Saenger P. Pubertal gynecomastia. *J Ped Endocrinol Metab.* 2002;15:553.
- Daniels IR, Layer GT. Gynaecomastia. *Eur J Surg.* 2001;167:885.

Hashimoto Thyroiditis

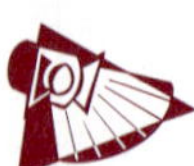

ESSENTIAL FEATURES

- Autoimmune thyroiditis
- Possible initial transient hyperthyroidism
- Possible chronic hypothyroidism

EPIDEMIOLOGY

- Most common form of thyroiditis
- 0.3 to 1.5 cases per 1000 population per year; 10–15 times more common in women
- Approximately 15% of women are affected in the United States; majority are 30–50 years of age

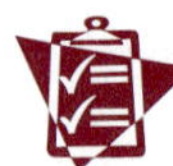

CLINICAL FINDINGS

SYMPTOMS AND SIGNS

- Enlarged, occasionally tender, thyroid
- Atrophic stage, shrunken, firm thyroid
- Dysphagia

LABORATORY FINDINGS

- Elevated thyroid-stimulating hormone (TSH)
- Decreased tri-iodothyronine (T_3) and thyroxine (T_4) levels
- Elevated titers of antimicrosomal and antithyroglobulin antibodies

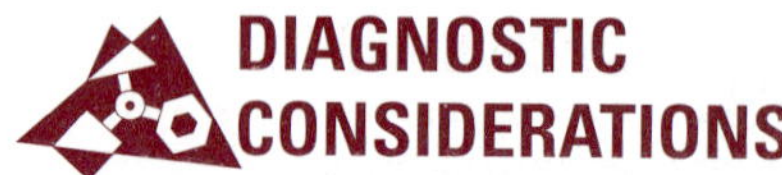

DIAGNOSTIC CONSIDERATIONS

- Patient may have other associated autoimmune conditions
- Associated with HLA-DR3, HLA-DR5, and HLA-B8
- Thyroid neoplasia should be ruled out in the setting of asymmetry or cervical lymphadenopathy

RULE OUT

- Thyroid lymphoma
- Thyroid carcinoma

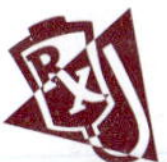

WORK-UP

- History and physical exam
- Serum thyroid function tests and thyroglobulin and microsomal antibody titers
- Needle biopsy if concerned about malignancy

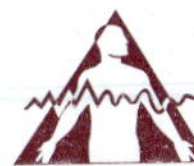

TREATMENT AND MANAGEMENT

- Initial treatment includes administration of exogenous thyroid hormone

SURGERY

Indications

- Local symptoms of pressure
- Suspected malignancy
- Enlarging gland despite a trial of thyroid hormone suppression

MEDICATIONS

- Thyroid hormone
- Occasionally, a β-blocker is required to control symptoms of hyperthyroidism

TREATMENT MONITORING

- TSH, T_3, and T_4 levels

COMPLICATIONS

- Association with thyroid lymphoma

RESOURCES

REFERENCES

- Singer PA. Thyroiditis: acute, subacute and chronic. *Med Clin North Am.* 1991;75:61.

Head & Neck Squamous Cell Cancer

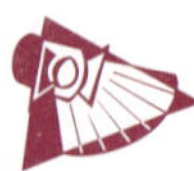

ESSENTIAL FEATURES

- Curable in 80% of cases when detected at an early stage
- Most patients present with locoregional spread
- Most important causative agents are tobacco and alcohol
- A lesion that appears 3 years after a previous cancer is considered a new primary cancer
- Potential sites include:
  - Oral cavity
  - Bucca
  - Mucosa
  - Hard palate
  - Tongue
  - Tonsil
  - Oropharynx
  - Hypopharynx
  - Nasopharynx
  - Paranasal sinus
  - Larynx
  - Glottis
  - False vocal cords
  - External auditory canal

EPIDEMIOLOGY

- Approximately 40,300 new cases per year
- Tobacco and alcohol account for 75% of oral, oropharyngeal, and hypopharyngeal cancers
- Cigarrette smoking causes 80% of laryngeal cancers
- Second primary cancers develop in 10–15% of cases

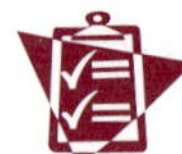

CLINICAL FINDINGS

SYMPTOMS AND SIGNS

- Leukoplakia and erythroplakia are important premalignant lesions
- Pain (location correlates with tumor location)
- Bleeding
- Obstruction
- Mass
- Otalgia
- Odynophagia
- Dysphagia
- Trismus
- Hoarseness
- Loss of hearing
- Horner syndrome

IMAGING FINDINGS

- CT scan of head and neck can demonstrate involvement of the paranasal sinus, the parapharyngeal, and pterygomaxillary spaces; the orbits; and the anterior skull base
- MRI of the head and neck can demonstrate cancer involvement at the skull base, in the parapharyngeal space, and in the orbit

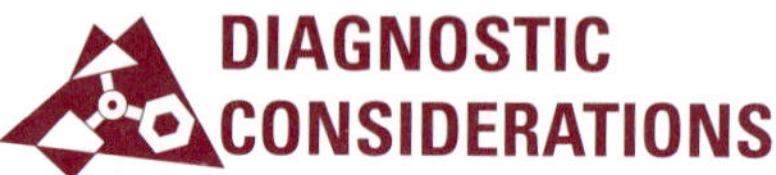

DIAGNOSTIC CONSIDERATIONS

- Complete exam may require topical anesthetic spray
- Most sites are well seen with a headlight and laryngeal mirror
- Flexible fiberoptic exam may be necessary

RULE OUT

- Squamous cell carcinoma of the skin
- Melanoma

WORK-UP

- Biopsy for definitive diagnosis (punch or fine-needle aspiration)
- Exam under anesthesia (including direct laryngoscopy, nasopharyngoscopy, rigid esophagoscopy, and bronchoscopy)
- Chest film
- Barium swallow
- Panorex x-rays
- CT scan of the head and neck
- MRI of the head and neck

TREATMENT AND MANAGEMENT

- Multimodal
  - Surgery
  - Radiation oncology
  - Medical oncology
  - Maxillofacial prosthetics
  - Speech therapy
- Priorities are to eradicate cancer, then to maintain function, then to preserve appearance

SURGERY

Indications

- Almost all should be resected with neck dissections as directed by nodal disease or electively

MEDICATIONS

- Vitamin A and its derivatives have been used to treat oral leukoplakia
- Isotretinoin and fenretinide are potential chemopreventative agents

TREATMENT MONITORING

- Physical exam

COMPLICATIONS

- From radiation:
  - Skin reaction
  - Mucositis
  - Fibrosis
  - Vascular sclerosis
  - Xerostomia
  - Osteoradionecrosis

PROGNOSIS

- Curable in 80% of patients when diagnosed at an early stage
- Depends on stage and tumor location

PREVENTION

- Discontinue tobacco and alcohol use

RESOURCES

REFERENCES

- Beenken SW et al. Work-up of a patient with a mass in the neck. *Adv Surg.* 1996;28:371.

PRACTICE GUIDELINES

- The National Comprehensive Cancer Network http://www.nccn.org/

CANCER STAGING

- See Lip and Oral Cavity Staging Table on page 750.
- See Larynx Staging Table on page 749.
- See Nasal Cavity and Paranasal Sinuses Staging Table on page 753.
- See Pharynx (Including Base of Tongue, Soft Palate, and Uvula) Staging Table on page 753.

Heart Lesions, Congenital

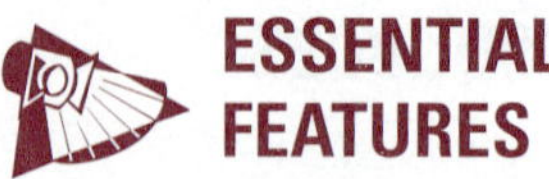

ESSENTIAL FEATURES

Anomalous Left Coronary Artery

- Left coronary artery (LCA) arises from pulmonary artery (PA)
- Causes myocardial ischemia, heart failure, myocardial infarction (MI), heart dilation, and fibrosis
- R coronary normal, supplies entire myocardium, retrograde into L coronary causing large coronary steal

Pulmonary Arteriovenous Fistula (PAF)

- Rare anomaly, associated with Rendu-Osler-Weber syndrome in 50%
- Large AV fistulas not communicating with alveolar capillaries
- Most common in lower lobes
- Pulmonary blood shunts into veins causing cyanosis

Persistent Left Superior Vena Cava (LSVC)

- LSVC connects left jugular and subclavian veins to coronary sinus
- Relatively common anomaly

Endocardial Fibroelastosis

- Nonoperable lesion
- Associated w/ aortic coarctation, aortic stenosis, anomalous LCA, mitral valve disease
- Hyperplasia of subendocardial elastic and collagenous tissue and proliferation of capillaries cause markedly thickened and smooth glistening lining of LV wall
- Trabeculae obliterated, papillary muscles and chordae contracted
- Affects principally LV and LA
- May result from subendocardial ischemia in utero
- Affects 1–2% of patients with congenital heart disease, often without other disease

Cardiac Tumors

- Uncommon; primary tumors more common than metastatic lesions
- > 90% are benign
- **Rhabdomyoma:** Most common benign tumor
  - Most arise from ventricular septum
  - Pale, gray nodules
  - Associated with tuberous sclerosis in 50%
- **Fibroma:** Second most common benign tumor
  - More common in ventricular septum
  - Solid white lesion with distinct borders
- In infants, teratoma more common than fibroma; hamartoma also common
- Myxoma rare in children
- Malignant tumors rare; malignant teratoma and sarcoma most common

EPIDEMIOLOGY

PAF

- 50% associated with multiple telangiectases (Rendu-Osler-Weber syndrome)

Cardiac Tumors

- 0.002–0.008% of patients, uncommon in infancy and childhood

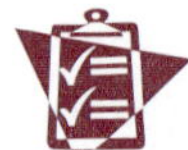

CLINICAL FINDINGS

SYMPTOMS AND SIGNS

LCA

- Pallor, sweating
- Tachycardia, episodic chest pain suggesting angina pectoris

PAF

- Dyspnea, cyanosis, right heart failure occasionally in infants
- Cyanosis, clubbing, polycythemia in late childhood
- Sometimes soft systolic/continuous murmur

LSVC

- Usually asymptomatic

Endocardial Fibroelastosis

- Symptoms and signs of left heart failure

Cardiac Tumors

- Symptoms due to space occupying lesion or involvement of conduction system
- Include failure, outflow tract obstruction, arrhythmias

IMAGING FINDINGS

PAF

- **Chest film:** Irregular opacified lesion in peripheral lung fields at site of fistula
- **Angiography/chest CT:** Confirm diagnosis

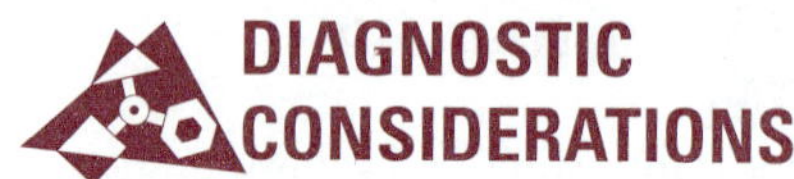

DIAGNOSTIC CONSIDERATIONS

LCA

- Echocardiography and catheterization with angiography make diagnosis

Cardiac Tumors

- Echocardiography, catheterization, MRI all useful

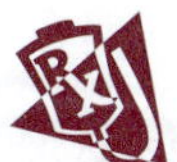

WORK-UP

- Echocardiography
- Angiography if diagnosis unclear

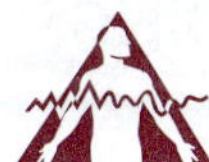

TREATMENT AND MANAGEMENT

LCA

- Anastomose left coronary to aorta

PAF

- Fistula excision
- Local resection or formal lobectomy

LSVC

- If adequate drainage to right side, can ligate LSVC

Endocardial Fibroelastosis

- Cardiac transplantation only available option

Cardiac Tumors

- Transvenous biopsy for asymptomatic or limited symptoms
- Attempt complete removal of tumor, preserving critical structures
- Rhabdomyoma, spontaneous regression considered normal

SURGERY

Indications

LCA

- Diagnosis warrants repair

PAF

- Indicated for symptomatic patients or single lesions, generally not for multiple lesions

LSVC

- Adequate drainage of LSVC to right side of heart via innominate or other connection

Cardiac Tumors

- Significant symptoms warrant removal

PROGNOSIS

Endocardial Fibroelastosis

- Nearly all infants die of left heart failure within 1 year of life

RESOURCES

REFERENCES

- Laks H et al. Aortic implantation of anomalous left coronary artery: an improved surgical approach. *J Thorac Cardiovasc Surg.* 1995;109:519.
- Cooley DA et al. Primary cardiac tumors in infants and children: immediate and long-term operative results. *Ann Thorac Surg.* 1996;62:559.

Heart Lesions, Congenital: Increased Pulmonary Flow

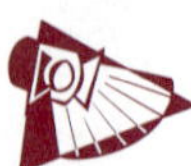

ESSENTIAL FEATURES

- Congenital heart lesion that increases pulmonary artery (PA) blood flow
- Results in the following:
  - Left to right shunt
  - Lung infection
  - Pulmonary vascular congestion
  - PA hypertension
  - Right heart failure
  - Pulmonary vasoconstriction
  - Pulmonary vascular obstructive disease
- **Eisenmenger syndrome:** Increased pulmonary hypertension such that left to right shunt ceases and shunt becomes right to left, requiring heart-lung transplant
- Inhaled nitric oxide, oxygen, or IV tolazoline reverses PA vasoconstriction
- PA band is palliative and can reduce PA flow to alleviate RV failure and progression of pulmonary hypertension

EPIDEMIOLOGY

Ruptured Sinus of Valsalva

- More common in Marfan syndrome or other autoimmune diseases

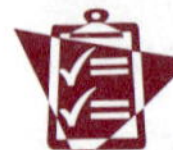

CLINICAL FINDINGS

SYMPTOMS AND SIGNS

Aortopulmonary Window

- Findings similar to patent ductus arteriosus (PDA)
- Early heart failure and pulmonary hypertension

Ruptured Sinus of Valsalva

- Continuous, well localized, parasternal murmur with associated thrill
- Rapid heart failure develops in most patients

Left Ventricular-Right Atrial Shunt

- Heart failure in infancy or late childhood
- Murmur not diagnostic

Coronary Arterial Fistula

- Many asymptomatic
- Myocardial ischemia or heart failure
- Continuous murmur over heart

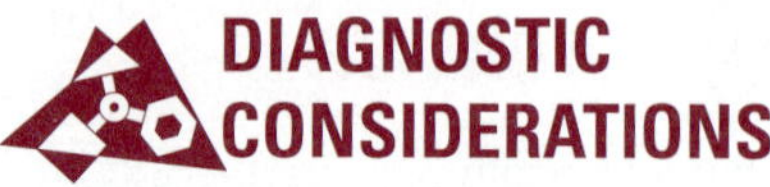

DIAGNOSTIC CONSIDERATIONS

Aortopulmonary Window

- Connection between ascending aorta and main PA, rare anomaly
- 50% associated anomalies (atrial septal defect, ventricular septal defect, interrupted aortic arch)

Ruptured Sinus of Valsalva

- Rupture of thin membranous tissue between aortic sinus of Valsalva and intracardiac chamber (immediate left to right shunt)
- Rupture into RV (70%), into RA (20%)

Left Ventricular-Right Atrial Shunt

- Defect in membranous septum near annulus or septal leaflet of tricuspid valve
- Uncommon, size of shunt variable

Coronary Arterial Fistula

- Fistula between RV and right coronary (60%) or left coronary (40%) artery
- Produces left to right shunt
- Involved coronary artery is dilated
- Fistulous openings may be multiple

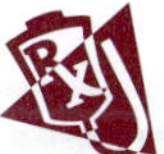

WORK-UP

Ruptured Sinus of Valsalva

- Echocardiography and catheterization needed for precise anatomic diagnosis

Left Ventricular-Right Atrial Shunt

- At catheterization: Oxygen saturation increased in RA
- RA opacifies with injection into LV

Coronary Arterial Fistula

- Angiogram required to determine number and location of fistula

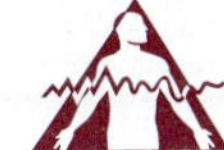

TREATMENT AND MANAGEMENT

Aortopulmonary Window

- Surgical repair with patch closure

Ruptured Sinus of Valsalva

- Early operation warranted

Left Ventricular-Right Atrial Shunt

- Closed primarily on bypass

Coronary Arterial Fistula

- Ligate fistulous connections without interrupting coronary artery

SURGERY

Indications

- Once diagnosed, all of these defects should be repaired

PROGNOSIS

- Low operative mortality for left ventricular-right atrial shunt and coronary artery fistula

RESOURCES

REFERENCES

- Rabinovitch M. Pathobiology of pulmonary hypertension: impact on clinical management. *Semin Thorac Cardiovasc Surg Pediatr Card Surg Annu.* 2000;3:63.

Heat Stroke

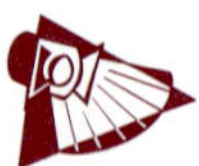

ESSENTIAL FEATURES

- Occurs when body core temperature exceeds 40 °C and produces severe CNS dysfunction
- Result of imbalance between heat production and dissipation
- Humans dissipate heat via skin by radiation, conduction, convection, and evaporation

EPIDEMIOLOGY

- Kills approximately 4000 persons each year in the United States
- Most often affects young people who are exercising in hot environment (military, athletes, laborers, etc.)
- Sedentary heat stroke is disease of the elderly and can be predicted when ambient temperature > 32.2 °C and relative humidity reaches 50–76%
- Predisposing factors include:
  - Dermatitis
  - Use of phenothiazines, β-blockers, diuretics, and anticholinergics
  - Unrelated fever
  - Obesity
  - Alcoholism
  - Heavy clothing

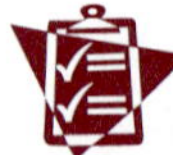

CLINICAL FINDINGS

SYMPTOMS AND SIGNS

- Sudden coma in hot environment
- Patient temperature > 40 °C is diagnostic
- Prodrome of dizziness, headache, nausea, chills, and gooseflesh of arms and chest rarely seen
- Confusion, belligerence, or stupor may precede coma
- Skin is pink or ashen and sometimes, paradoxically, dry and hot
- Profuse sweating also common
- Heart rate ranges from 140 to 170 bpm
- Hyperventilation may reach 60 breaths a minute with respiratory alkalosis
- Pulmonary edema and bloody sputum may develop in severe cases
- Jaundice is common in first few days after onset

LABORATORY FINDINGS

- No characteristic laboratory abnormalities
- Hypocalcemia is common
- Hypophosphatemia may occur
- Aspartate aminotransferase (AST), lactic dehydrogenase (LDH), and creatine kinase (CK) may be elevated in first few days
- Acidosis can result from renal failure or lactic acidosis
- Proteinuria and granular and RBC casts are seen in initial urine specimens
- Disseminated intravascular coagulation (DIC) pattern not uncommon

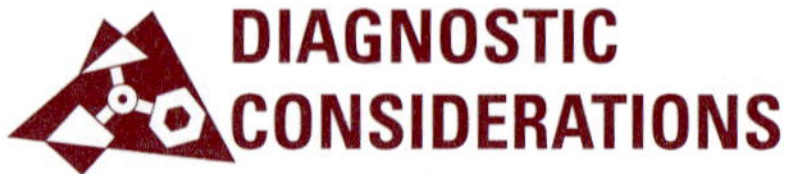

DIAGNOSTIC CONSIDERATIONS

- Temperature must be taken rectally

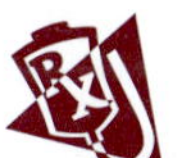

WORK-UP

- Physical exam including rectal temperature
- Serum electrolytes

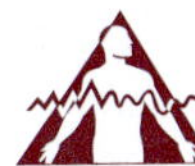

TREATMENT AND MANAGEMENT

- Patient should be cooled rapidly
  - Spraying patient with water that is 15 °C and fanning with warm air is most efficient
  - Immersion in ice water bath also effective
- Monitor the rectal temperature often
- Stop cooling when patient's temperature reaches 38.9 °C
- Shivering controlled with phenothiazines
- Oxygen should be administered, intubate as needed for PaO_2 < 65 mm Hg
- Fluid, electrolyte management guided by frequent laboratory measurements
- IV mannitol early if myoglobinuria present
- DIC may require heparin
- Acute renal failure may require hemodialysis
- Inotropes for cardiac insufficiency

SURGERY

Prognosis

- Bad prognostic indicators:
  - Temperature > 42.2 °C
  - Coma > 2 hours
  - Shock
  - Hyperkalemia
  - AST > 1000 U/L in first 24 hours
- 10% mortality in those treated promptly
- Deaths in first few days due to cerebral damage, late deaths from bleeding or organ failure (kidney, liver, heart)

PREVENTION

- Adherence to graduated schedule of increasing performance that allow acclimatization over 2–3 weeks
- Unrestricted access to drinking water
- Clothing and equipment should be lightened

RESOURCES

REFERENCES

- Bouchama A, DeVol EB. Acid-base alterations in heatstroke. *Intensive Care Med.* 2001;27:680.
- Khosla R, Guntupalli KK. Heat-related illnesses. *Crit Care Clin.* 1999;15:251.

Hemolytic Anemia, Acquired

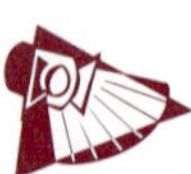

ESSENTIAL FEATURES

- Fatigue, pallor, jaundice
- Splenomegaly
- Persistent anemia and reticulocytosis

EPIDEMIOLOGY

- Autoimmune disorder that is either idiopathic (40–50%) or secondary to drug exposure, connective tissue diseases, or lymphoproliferative disorders
- Classified according to the optimal temperature at which autoantibodies react with the red cell surface (warm or cold antibodies)
  - Warm antibody: IgG autoantibodies directed against the Rh locus on the erythrocyte coat the cell and bind to IgG specific Fc receptors on macrophages in the spleen
  - Cold antibody: IgM autoantibodies are directed against the I red cell antigen; hemolysis occurs intravascularly and not within the spleen
- Most common after age 50; occurs twice as often in women than in men

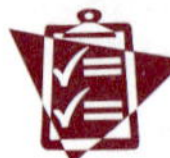

CLINICAL FINDINGS

SYMPTOMS AND SIGNS

- Fatigue
- Mild jaundice
- Fever
- Splenomegaly

LABORATORY FINDINGS

- Acute onset normocytic normochromic anemia
- Reticulocytosis (> 10%)
- Erythroid hyperplasia of the marrow
- Elevation of serum indirect bilirubin
- Serum haptoglobin is usually low or absent
- Positive direct Coombs test

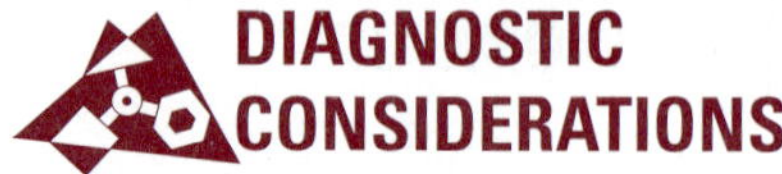

DIAGNOSTIC CONSIDERATIONS

- Rarely, a sudden, severe onset hemolytic anemia produces hemoglobinuria, renal tubular necrosis, and a 40–50% death rate
- May be associated with systemic lupus erythematosus and chronic lymphocytic leukemia
- Drugs commonly implicated include methyldopa, penicillin, quinidine

RULE OUT

- Other causes of hemolytic anemia
  - Hereditary hemolytic anemias
  - Thrombotic thrombocytopenic purpura
  - Disseminated intravascular coagulation
  - Infection

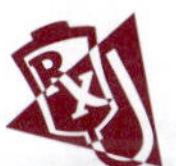

WORK-UP

- CBC count
- Serum bilirubin
- Reticulocyte count
- Peripheral blood smear
- Serum haptoglobin
- Bone marrow biopsy
- Coombs test

WHEN TO ADMIT

- Severe anemia

WHEN TO REFER

- All cases should be managed in conjunction with a hematologist

TREATMENT AND MANAGEMENT

- Drug-induced hemolytic anemia: Terminate exposure to the agent.

SURGERY

- Splenectomy is indicated for patients with warm-antibody hemolysis meeting the following criteria:

Indications

- Failure to respond to 4–6 weeks of high-dose corticosteroid therapy
- Relapse when corticosteroids are withdrawn
- Contraindications to corticosteroid therapy
- Chronic high-dose corticosteroid therapy

Contraindications

- Cold-antibody hemolytic anemia

MEDICATIONS

- Corticosteroids
- IV immune globulin

TREATMENT MONITORING

- CBC count

COMPLICATIONS

- Pigment gallstones

PROGNOSIS

- 75% remission rate with medical treatment; 25% are permanent
- Relapses may occur after splenectomy

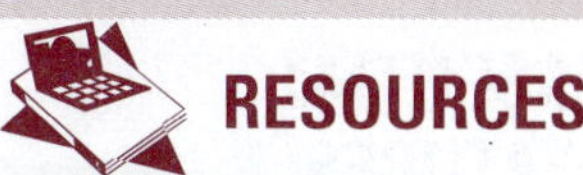

RESOURCES

REFERENCES

- Beutler E et al. Hemolytic anemia. *Semin Hematol.* 1999;36:38.

Hemolytic Anemias, Miscellaneous Hereditary

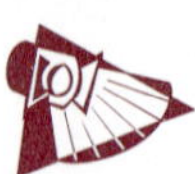

ESSENTIAL FEATURES

- Structural or enzymatic defects in erythrocytes leading to hemolysis
- Anemia, mild to severe
- Splenomegaly

EPIDEMIOLOGY

Hereditary Elliptocytosis

- Elliptical erythrocytes due to defects in cytoskeletal proteins, leading to change in shape, decreased plasticity, and shortened lifespan

Hereditary Nonspherocytic Hemolytic Anemia

- Due to inherited red cell defects that lead to oxidative hemolysis (pyruvate kinase deficiency and glucose 6-phosphate dehydrogenase [G6PD] deficiency)

Thalassemia Major and Minor

- Structural defect in the β-globin chain causes excess α chains to precipitate and cells to pass poorly through the spleen leading to increased splenic destruction and target cells
- Heterozygotes usually have mild anemia (thalassemia minor); however, starting early in infancy, homozygotes have severe chronic anemia

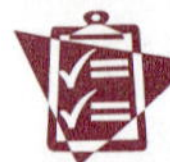

CLINICAL FINDINGS

SYMPTOMS AND SIGNS

- Abdominal pain
- Jaundice
- Splenomegaly

LABORATORY FINDINGS

- Anemia
- Increased serum bilirubin
- Decreased haptoglobin
- Increased reticulocyte count

Hereditary Elliptocytosis

- Elliptical red blood cells on peripheral smear

Thalassemia

- Target cells, nucleated red cells, and a hypochromic microcytic anemia on peripheral smear
- Persistence of fetal hemoglobin (Hb F)

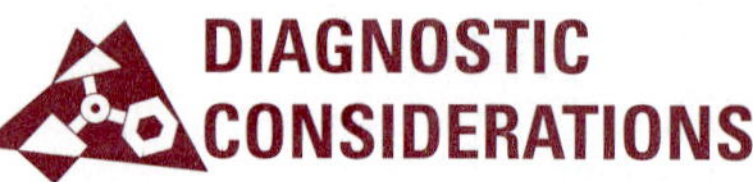

DIAGNOSTIC CONSIDERATIONS

- Laboratory investigation indicated in cases of hemolytic anemia in order to determine whether caused by underlying structural or enzymatic defects
- High incidence pigmented gallstones found in patients with hereditary hemolytic anemia

RULE OUT

- Other causes of hemolytic anemia
  - Autoimmune hemolytic anemias
  - Thrombotic thrombocytopenic purpura,
  - Disseminated intravascular coagulation
  - Infection

WORK-UP

- CBC count
- Peripheral smear
- Serum bilirubin
- Serum haptoglobin

WHEN TO ADMIT

- Severe anemia

WHEN TO REFER

- These disorders should be managed in conjunction with a hematologist

TREATMENT AND MANAGEMENT

- Splenectomy may reduce transfusion requirements and lessen abdominal pain associated with splenomegaly
- If gallstones are present, patient should undergo concurrent cholecystectomy

SURGERY

Indications

- Elliptocytosis
- Nonspherocytic hemolytic anemia
- Thalassemia

Contraindications

- **G6PD deficiency:** Splenectomy is not beneficial, and treatment consists of avoidance of dietary oxidants

MEDICATIONS

- Iron chelation therapy for thalassemia

TREATMENT MONITORING

- CBC count to monitor anemia

COMPLICATIONS

- Pigment gallstones

PROGNOSIS

- Transfusion requirements may be decreased and abdominal pain improved after splenectomy

RESOURCES

REFERENCES

- Silveira P et al. Red blood cell abnormalities in hereditary elliptocytosis and their relevance to variable clinical expression. *Am J Clin Pathol.* 1997;108:391.
- Weatherall DJ. The thalassemias. *BMJ.* 1997;314:1675.

Hemorrhoids

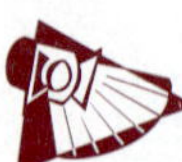

ESSENTIAL FEATURES

- Internal hemorrhoids originate above dentate line, covered by mucosa
- External hemorrhoids are vascular complexes covered by anoderm, below dentate line
- Function as vascular pillows, protect the anal canal during defecation
- No correlation between constipation and hemorrhoids
- Internal hemorrhoids classification:
  - First-degree: Bleed
  - Second-degree: Bleed and prolapse but spontaneously reduce
  - Third-degree: Bleed, prolapse, and require manual reduction
  - Fourth-degree: Incarcerated
- Internal hemorrhoids become symptomatic when chronic engorgement leads to tissue laxity and tissue prolapse into the anal canal
- External hemorrhoids become symptomatic with thrombosis

EPIDEMIOLOGY

- May more commonly develop in younger men and older women
- Hemorrhoids may develop in younger men due to higher resting pressure within the anal canal
- Hemorrhoids may develop in older women due to chronic straining, leading to vascular engorgement and dilatation
- Become engorged with increased intra-abdominal pressure as in obesity, pregnancy, lifting, straining

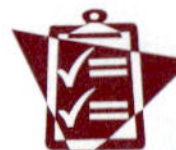

CLINICAL FINDINGS

SYMPTOMS AND SIGNS

- Internal hemorrhoids
  - Cause bright red blood per rectum, mucus discharge
  - Sense of rectal fullness but are painless
  - May prolapse into the anal canal and may become strangulated and necrotic
- External hemorrhoids
  - Sudden, severe perianal pain, itching
  - May be accompanied by a skin tag
- Thrombosed external hemorrhoids
  - Tense, tender subcutaneous mass
  - Purple-black discoloration

LABORATORY FINDINGS

- Chronic bleeding from internal hemorrhoids may cause anemia (rare)

IMAGING FINDINGS

- **Defecography:** May help define cause of obstructed defecation such as rectal prolapse

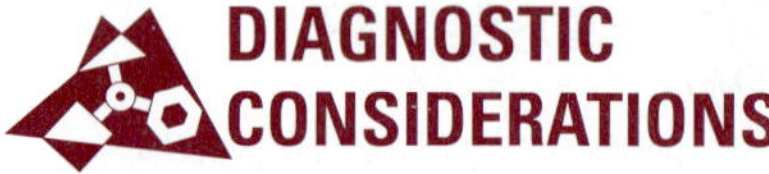

DIAGNOSTIC CONSIDERATIONS

- Anal fissure
- Anal ulcer
- Anorectal malignancy
- Inflammatory bowel disease
- Diverticular disease
- Rectal prolapse
- Condylomata acuminata

RULE OUT

- Other causes of anemia should be ruled out before attributing anemia to hemorrhoids

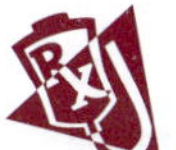

WORK-UP

- Evaluate for GI sources for anemia
- History of straining
- Defecography may be useful to evaluate for obstruction and rectal prolapse

WHEN TO ADMIT

- Infection or impending necrosis of thrombosed hemorrhoid
- Perianal sepsis

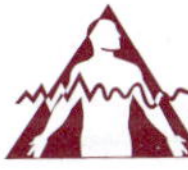

TREATMENT AND MANAGEMENT

- Initial medical management recommended for first- and most second-degree hemorrhoids
- Dietary alteration, addition of bulking agents, stool softeners, increased liquid intake, sitz baths
- Decreasing time spent on commode
- Elastic band ligation:
  - Band placed at base results in sloughing and scar formation
  - Must be placed above dentate line
- Sclerotherapy
  - May be efficacious for bleeding hemorrhoids
  - Sclerosant is injected into submucosal connective tissue to induce inflammation and scarring
- Excisional hemorrhoidectomy
  - For third- and fourth-degree lesions and incarcerated internal hemorrhoids
  - Tissue is excised, vascular pedicle ligated

SURGERY

Indications

- Failure of medical management
- Strangulated, thrombosed hemorrhoids

Contraindications

- Patients receiving anticoagulants should be treated with excisional hemorrhoidectomy instead of band ligation
- Care should be exercised with banding in immunocompromised patients (high risk for perineal sepsis)

MEDICATIONS

- Stool softeners
- Bulking agents

COMPLICATIONS

- Bleeding
- Pain
- Necrosis
- Perianal sepsis
- Anal stenosis
- Internal anal sphincter injury

PROGNOSIS

- Prognosis for recurrence mostly related to changing bowel habits
- Good with increasing fiber and exercise, decreasing constipating foods and time spent on commode; decrease amount of straining

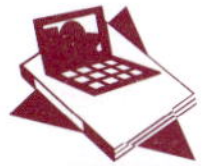

RESOURCES

REFERENCES

- Komborozos VA et al. Rubber band ligation of symptomatic internal hemorrhoids: results of 500 cases. *Dig Surg.* 2000;17:71.
- Loder PB et al. Haemorrhoids: pathology, pathophysiology, and actiology. *Br J Surg.* 1994;81:946.

Hepatic Abscess

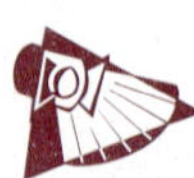

ESSENTIAL FEATURES

- Etiologies include:
  - Benign or malignant obstruction with cholangitis
  - Extrahepatic abdominal sepsis
  - Trauma or surgery to right upper quadrant
  - Hepatic artery thrombosis or hepatic artery chemotherapy
- Multifocal abscesses: Usually due to biliary obstruction and cholangitis
- Unifocal abscess: Usually due to hematogenous spread from abdominal sepsis
- Risk factors:
  - Metastatic cancer
  - Diabetes
  - Alcoholism
- Mortality, 15%

EPIDEMIOLOGY

- Equal incidence among men and women
- Median age onset: In fifth decade

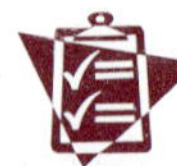

CLINICAL FINDINGS

SYMPTOMS AND SIGNS

- Fever
- Right upper quadrant pain
- Jaundice
- Dyspnea

LABORATORY FINDINGS

- Leukocytosis
- Elevated alkaline phosphatase
- Elevated transaminases
- Hypoalbuminemia

IMAGING FINDINGS

- **US and CT:** Multifocal or unifocal hepatic abscesses unilocular in appearance and contrast enhancement peripherally by CT
- **Chest film:** Right lower lobe infiltrate (atelectasis, effusion, etc)

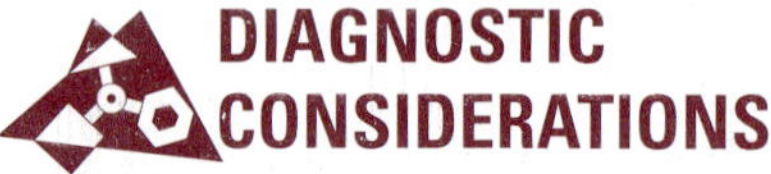

DIAGNOSTIC CONSIDERATIONS

- Other intra-abdominal sepsis
- Other infections, eg, amebic or hydatid disease
- Biliary obstruction

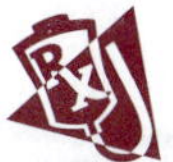

WORK-UP

- History and physical exam
- CBC count
- Liver function tests
- CT scan with contrast
- CT-guided aspiration of abscess for culture
- ERCP or percutaneous transhepatic cholangiogram if biliary obstruction suspected

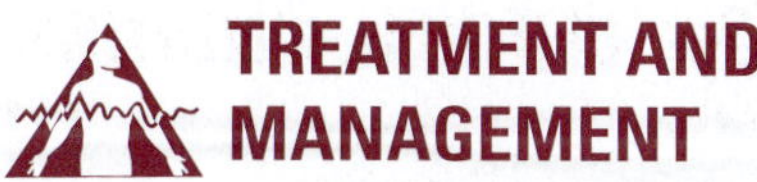

TREATMENT AND MANAGEMENT

SURGERY

- CT-guided aspiration and drainage for abscesses > 2–3 cm and fewer than 3 total abscesses
- Surgical drainage if patient has continued signs of sepsis despite antibiotics and CT-guided drainage or if fevers persist for 2 weeks, or if pus is too viscous for drainage
- Treat biliary obstruction if present

MEDICATIONS

- Empiric antibiotic therapy to cover GI flora with double coverage until culture results are available

COMPLICATIONS

- Recurrent abscess
- Liver failure
- Bile leak

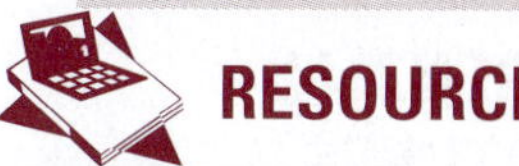

RESOURCES

REFERENCES

- Johannsen EC et al. Pyogenic liver abscesses. *Infect Dis Clin North Am.* 2000;14:547.

Hepatic Failure, Acute

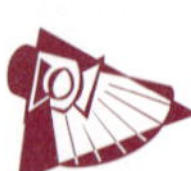

ESSENTIAL FEATURES

- Acute hepatic injury causes sudden loss in hepatocytes due to toxins, ischemia, or inflammatory reaction to liver
- Fulminant hepatic failure defined as onset of encephalopathy within 8 weeks (9–24 weeks for subfulminant) after onset of acute hepatocellular injury
- Etiologies include:
  - Hepatitis viruses
  - Cytomegalovirus (CMV)
  - Epstein-Barr virus (EBV)
  - Varicella
  - Herpesvirus
  - Toxins (acetaminophen, isoniazid most common)
  - Ischemia
  - Fatty liver of pregnancy
  - Reye syndrome
  - Wilson disease
  - Lymphoma
  - Hereditary metabolic disorders

EPIDEMIOLOGY

- 2000 cases of fulminant or subfulminant hepatic failure annually in United States with 80% mortality

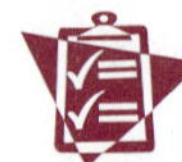

CLINICAL FINDINGS

SYMPTOMS AND SIGNS

- Jaundice
- Right upper quadrant pain
- Bleeding
- Encephalopathy
- Hypotension
- Sepsis
- Renal failure
- Uncal herniation
- Corneal rings

LABORATORY FINDINGS

- Hyperbilirubinemia
- Elevated transaminases
- Prolonged prothrombin time (PT)
- Elevated creatinine

IMAGING FINDINGS

- Head CT can show cerebral edema

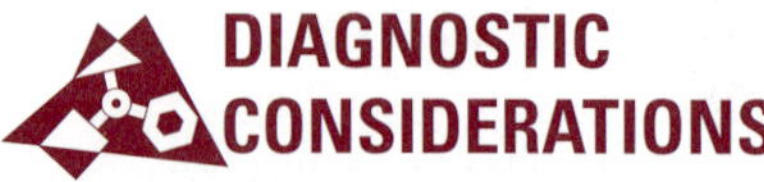

DIAGNOSTIC CONSIDERATIONS

- History of chronic liver disorder
- Family history of liver failure (eg, Wilson disease)
- Exposure to toxins or drugs
- Rapidity of encephalopathy onset

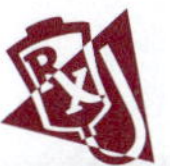

WORK-UP

- History and physical exam
- Serum antibodies for hepatitis viruses, CMV, and EBV
- Ceruloplasmin level (Wilson disease)
- Head CT if grade IV encephalopathy present (coma)
- Temperature

WHEN TO ADMIT

- Any patient with acute hepatic injury, ICU for fulminant cases

WHEN TO REFER

- Transplantation center whenever encephalopathy develops

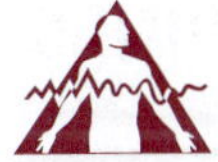

TREATMENT AND MANAGEMENT

SURGERY

- Liver transplantation
- Ventriculostomy for grade IV encephalopathy

Indications

- Fulminant or subfulminant failure unresponsive to medical management

Contraindications

- Medical comorbidities precluding transplantation, active malignancy

MEDICATIONS

- N-acetylcysteine
- Minimizing hypoglycemia
- Broad-spectrum antibiotics for any fever (avoid aminoglycosides)
- Fresh frozen plasma for planned invasive interventions
- Mannitol for elevated intracranial pressure
- Vasopressor support for hypotension
- Mechanical ventilation for grade IV encephalopathy

TREATMENT MONITORING

- Frequent neurologic exams and head CT scans when indicated
- Liver function tests
- PT

COMPLICATIONS

- Primary nonfunction
- Rejection
- Biliary leak or stricture
- hemorrhage
- Hepatic artery thrombosis

PROGNOSIS

- 60–70% 5-year survival following liver transplant
- All patients recover from acute illness in absence of encephalopathy
- Greater than 50% recovery for patients with grade III encephalopathy
- Overall survival correlated with grade of encephalopathy
- Rapid onset associated with more favorable prognosis
- Associated sepsis, acidosis, age < 2 or > 40 years, renal failure, PT > 50 all associated with worse prognosis

RESOURCES

REFERENCES

- Schiodt FV, Lee WM. Fulminant liver disease. *Clin Liver Dis.* 2003;7:331.

Hepatic Neoplasms, Benign

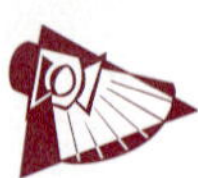

ESSENTIAL FEATURES

- Most hepatic masses are benign
- Major diagnoses:
  - Adenoma
  - Hemangioma
  - Focal nodular hyperplasia
  - Cysts
  - Angiomyolipoma
  - Regenerative nodules
- Estrogens or anabolic steroids can be associated with adenomas, hemangioma growth, and focal nodular hyperplasia

EPIDEMIOLOGY

- Adenomas occur primarily in women 20–40 years of age
- Hemangioma most common benign tumor of liver, affecting 7%

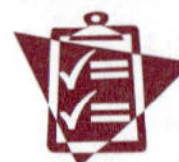

CLINICAL FINDINGS

SYMPTOMS AND SIGNS

- Most asymptomatic and seen on imaging studies performed for other reasons
- Pain (right upper quadrant or epigastric)
- Early satiety
- Hemorrhage
- Jaundice
- Kasabach-Merritt syndrome (consumptive coagulopathy in infantile hemangiomatosis)

LABORATORY FINDINGS

- Mostly normal
- Occasionally, elevated transaminases, bilirubin, thrombocytopenia, or coagulopathy

IMAGING FINDINGS

- **Ademoma:** Homogeneous hyperintense on T1 or T2 MRI or CT, but 10–20% with hemorrhagic areas making appearance heterogenous
  - PET scan with decreased uptake when compared with hepatocellular carcinoma or metastatic disease
- **Hemangioma:** Early peripheral enhancement with IV contrast on CT, MRI, or tagged red cell scan followed by centripetal pooling (MRI and CT- lesion hypodense before contrast)
- **Focal nodular hyperplasia:** CT or MRI showing stellate scar and enhancement with IV contrast, sulfur colloid or superparmagnetic iron oxide uptake (with MRI)
- **Cysts:** Hypointense or water density on US, CT, or MRI with no septations

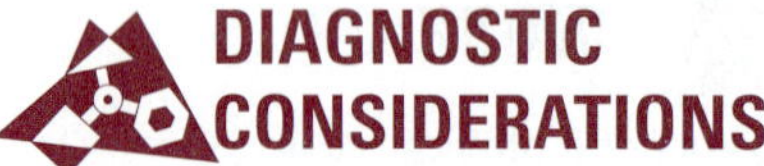

DIAGNOSTIC CONSIDERATIONS

- History of previous malignant disease
- History of previous hepatitis or cirrhosis
- History of other infections (eg, HIV)

RULE OUT

- Malignant hepatic tumor with resection often being necessary to secure diagnosis

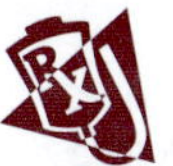

WORK-UP

- CBC count
- Liver function tests
- Alpha-fetoprotein (AFP), CA 19-9, CA 125, carcinoembryonic antigen (CEA)
- History and physical exam
- US, CT, or MRI depending on overall suspicion of diagnosis
- Intraoperative US if resection is planned

WHEN TO ADMIT

- Tumor with symptomatic hemorrhage

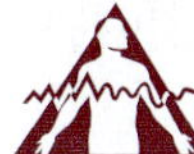

TREATMENT AND MANAGEMENT

SURGERY

- Enucleation if diagnosis is secure
- Formal anatomic resection if diagnosis is in doubt

Indications

- Symptomatic lesions or when diagnosis in doubt
- Adenomas over 5 cm

Contraindications

- Medical comorbidity associated with too high a risk for general anesthesia

MEDICATIONS

- Discontinue estrogens or androgens for suspected adenomas, focal nodular hyperplasia, or hemangiomas

TREATMENT MONITORING

- Individualized based on recurrence of symptoms following resection
- Serial CT scans to verify stability of lesion for presumed benign lesions for 2 years or when symptoms change

COMPLICATIONS

- Liver failure
- Hemorrhage
- Biliary injury
- Perihepatic infection

RESOURCES

REFERENCES

- Bioulac-Sage P et al. Diagnosis of focal nodular hyperplasia: not so easy. *Am J Surg Pathol.* 2001;25:1322.
- Terkivatan T et al. Indications and long-term outcome of treatment for benign hepatic tumors: a critical appraisal. *Arch Surg.* 2001;136:1033.
- Terkivatan T et al. Treatment of ruptured hepatocellular adenoma. *Br J Surg.* 2001;88:207.

Hepatic Trauma

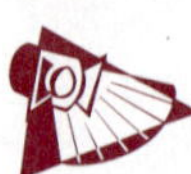

ESSENTIAL FEATURES

- Blunt versus penetrating trauma
- High velocity vs low velocity trauma
- Lacerations vs bursting injuries

EPIDEMIOLOGY

- Liver is most commonly injured organ in blunt abdominal trauma
- Second most common injury in penetrating abdominal trauma

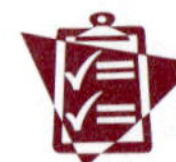

CLINICAL FINDINGS

SYMPTOMS AND SIGNS

- Shock
- Abdominal pain
- Distended abdomen
- Penetrating wounds
- Ecchymosis

LABORATORY FINDINGS

- Leukocytosis
- Anemia (later in course)
- Elevated transaminases

IMAGING FINDINGS

- **Focused abdominal sonography for trauma (FAST) US:** Shows intraperitoneal fluid, hepatic laceration, or hepatic hematoma
- **CT:** Shows extravasation of blood, hematoma, laceration, or parenchyma injury; grade poor predictor of operative findings
- **Angiography:** Helpful in diagnosing and treating active hemorrhage

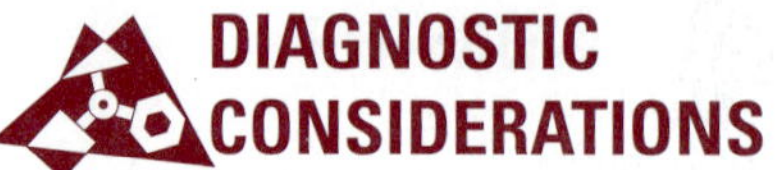

DIAGNOSTIC CONSIDERATIONS

- Retrohepatic cava or hepatic vein injury
- Portal triad injury
- Coagulopathy
- CT grade a poor predictor of outcome unless major vascular injury present

RULE OUT

- Additional abdominal injuries

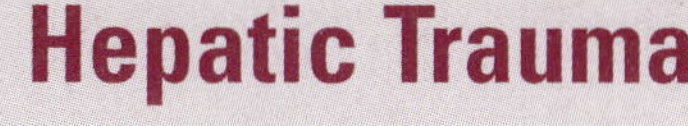

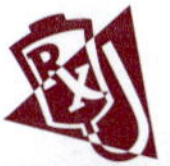

WORK-UP

- FAST US if blunt trauma
- CT if blunt trauma
- Diagnostic peritoneal lavage if blunt trauma not stable for CT
- Laparotomy if penetrating trauma
- Other ATLS protocol
- Angiography occasionally useful for stable patients

WHEN TO ADMIT

- All hepatic traumas
- ICU for unstable patients or those with high injury severity scores

TREATMENT AND MANAGEMENT

- Observation for most blunt trauma without active blood loss (CT grade poor predictor of success)
- Treatment of coagulopathy
- Pringle maneuver to control bleeding

OR

- Other methods to control bleeding include:
  - Drainage
  - Debridement
  - Hemostasis using clips or ligatures
  - Damage control laparotomy with packing of abdomen and plans for later removal of packs
  - Partial hepatic resection
  - Caval-atrial shunt
  - Angiography with embolization

SURGERY

Indications

- Shock and positive FAST or diagnostic peritoneal lavage after blunt trauma
- Penetrating abdominal trauma
- Possible major vascular injury on CT
- Continued active bleeding following blunt trauma and absence of coagulopathy

MEDICATIONS

- Blood products
- Passive and active warming
- Calcium if large transfusion requirement

TREATMENT MONITORING

- ICU monitoring
- Liver function tests
- CT for suspicion of infection or hemorrhage

COMPLICATIONS

- Hemorrhage
- Sepsis
- Liver failure
- Biliary leak
- Multi-organ failure

PROGNOSIS

- 1% mortality for penetrating trauma
- 10–20% mortality for blunt trauma
- 70% mortality if 3 major organs including liver involved

RESOURCES

REFERENCES

- Doherty GM, Way LW. Liver & Portal Venous System. In: Way LW, Doherty GM (editors). *Current Surgical Diagnosis & Treatment,* 11e. New York: McGraw-Hill; 2003:569. (See Table 25–1, Liver Injury Scale.)

PRACTICE GUIDELINES

- ATLS provider manual

Hepatic Tumor, Metastatic

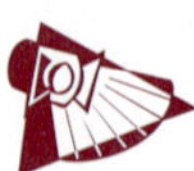

ESSENTIAL FEATURES

- Most common tumors of liver
- 90% with extrahepatic metastases
- 20% of patients with metastatic colon cancer have metastasis isolated to liver
- Common site of metastasis for multiple tumor types; most common candidates for resection include colon, endocrine, melanoma, breast, sarcoma, lung, renal, and other GI tumors

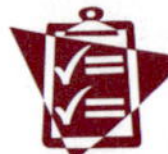

CLINICAL FINDINGS

SYMPTOMS AND SIGNS

- Weight loss
- Fatigue
- Fevers
- Right upper quadrant pain
- Ascites
- Jaundice
- Hepatomegaly
- Portal hypertension

LABORATORY FINDINGS

- Anemia
- Hyperbilirubinemia
- Elevated alkaline phosphatase

IMAGING FINDINGS

- Masses in liver sometimes better visualized with CT by portography or use of MRI

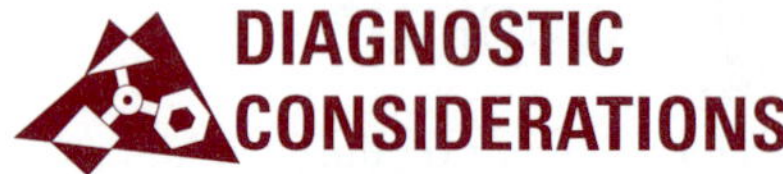

DIAGNOSTIC CONSIDERATIONS

- Site of primary tumor
- Time since resection of primary tumor

RULE OUT

- Extrahepatic disease before consideration of resection

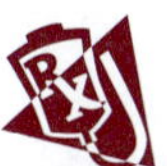

WORK-UP

- History and physical exam
- Liver function tests
- CBC count
- CT with portography
- MRI if CT is nondiagnostic
- Mesenteric angiogram if considering hepatic artery pump for metastatic colon cancer
- Bone scan if markedly elevated alkaline phosphatase
- Carcinoembryonic antigen (CEA), CA 125, CA 19-9, and alpha-fetoprotein (AFP) which aid in distinguishing primary from metastatic tumors
- Intraoperative US if resection is planned

TREATMENT AND MANAGEMENT

SURGERY

- Resection
- Hepatic artery chemotherapy pump (for metastatic colon cancer only)
- Radiofrequency ablation (RFA) or cryotherapy for unresectable lesions

Indications

- No extrahepatic disease
- Disease-free interval of 1 year or more for primary tumors, such as gastric and breast
- Colon cancer metastasis not amenable to resection and no extrahepatic disease (hepatic artery chemotherapy pump)
- Most common resectable tumors:
  - Colon
  - Endocrine
  - Melanoma
  - Breast
  - Sarcoma
  - Lung
  - Prostate
  - Renal
  - Other GI tumors (rarely)

Contraindications

- Extrahepatic disease
- Minimal planned residual liver function
- Multiple bilobar metastasis
- Metastasis involving bilateral portal branches

MEDICATIONS

- 5-fluorouracil for colon cancer
- Other chemotherapy for specific tumor types

TREATMENT MONITORING

- CEA levels for colon cancer
- CT scanning
- Hormonal markers, eg, gastrin for metastatic endocrine tumors

COMPLICATIONS

- Liver failure
- Hemorrhage
- Recurrent disease
- Biliary leak
- Gastroduodenitis (hepatic artery pump)
- Hepatic artery or pump thrombosis (hepatic artery pump)
- Sclerosing cholangitis (hepatic artery pump)
- Perihepatic abscess

PROGNOSIS

- **Colon cancer:** 25% 5-year survival with resection
- **Other metastatic disease:** 10–20% 5-year survival possible
- Marked palliation for metastatic endocrine tumors
- Hepatic artery chemotherapy (colon) increases 2-year survival when compared with systemic therapy

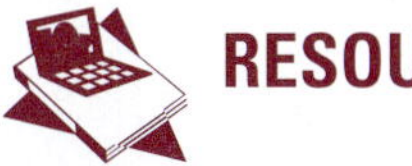

RESOURCES

REFERENCES

- Harmon KE et al. Benefits and safety of hepatic resection for colorectal metastases. *Arch Surg.* 1999;177:402.

Hepatic Tumor, Uncommon Primary

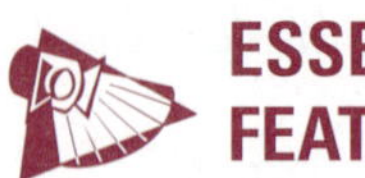

ESSENTIAL FEATURES

- Angiosarcoma
- Hepatoblastoma
- Hepatic adenocarcinoma
- Intrahepatic cholangiocarcinoma

EPIDEMIOLOGY

- Hepatoblastoma mainly in children
- Frequency increased in Beckwith-Wiedemann syndrome hemihypertrophy, fetal alcohol syndrome, and parenteral nutrition
- Angiosarcoma and sarcoma risk factors
  - Vinyl chloride
  - Arsenic
  - Androgenic steroids

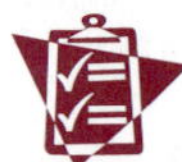

CLINICAL FINDINGS

SYMPTOMS AND SIGNS

- Right upper quadrant pain
- Weight loss
- Hepatomegaly
- Abdominal mass in childhood
- Hepatic bruit
- Ascites
- Distant metastases
- Asymptomatic
- Intraperitoneal hemorrhage
- Decompensated cirrhosis

LABORATORY FINDINGS

- Hyperbilirubinemia
- Elevated transaminases
- Elevated alkaline phosphatase

IMAGING FINDINGS

- **CT scan**
  - Hypervascular tumor (for angiosarcoma)
  - Multi-septate cyst for adenocarcinoma

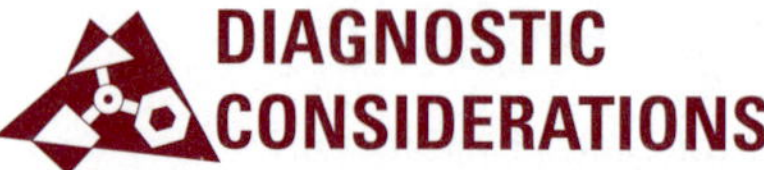

DIAGNOSTIC CONSIDERATIONS

- Biopsy of limited usefulness given high degree of sampling error and risk of tumor seeding
- Overall and planned reserve liver function

RULE OUT

- Metastatic carcinoma
- Benign neoplasms if possible
- Other abdominal malignancy

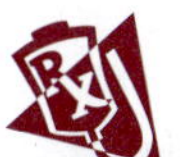

WORK-UP

- CT scan
- US
- Angiography
- Biopsy if unresectable
- Resection for diagnosis and treatment

WHEN TO ADMIT

- Intrahepatic hemorrhage
- Decompensated cirrhosis

TREATMENT AND MANAGEMENT

SURGERY

- Resection

Indications

- Localized tumor

Contraindications

- Poor liver function
- Extrahepatic disease
- Diffuse hepatic disease

MEDICATIONS

- Chemotherapy for unresectable lesions

TREATMENT MONITORING

- CT surveillance

COMPLICATIONS

- Hemorrhage
- Biliary leak
- Abdominal infection
- Liver failure

PROGNOSIS

- **Resectable cholangiocarcinoma:** 5-year survival, 15–20%
- **Angiosarcoma:** Very poor
- **Hepatoblastoma:** Overall survival 50%

RESOURCES

REFERENCES

- Tagge EP et al. Resection, including transplantation, for hepatoblastoma and hepatocellular carcinoma: impact on survival. *J Pediatr Surg.* 1992;27:292.
- Wheatley JM, LaQuaglia MP. Management of hepatic epithelial malignancy in childhood and adolescence. *Semin Surg Oncol.* 1993;9:532.
- Newman KD. Hepatic tumors in children. *Semin Pediatr Surg.* 1997;6:38.

PRACTICE GUIDELINES

- The National Comprehensive Cancer Network http://www.nccn.org/

CANCER STAGING

- See Liver (Including Intrahepatic Bile Ducts) Staging Table on page 750.

STAGE GROUPING

Stage I	T1	N0	M0
Stage II	T2	N0	M0
Stage IIIA	T3	N0	M0
IIIB	T4	N0	M0
IIIC	Any T	N1	M0
Stage IV	Any T	Any N	M1

Hepatitis (Acute & Chronic)

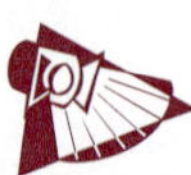

ESSENTIAL FEATURES

- Viral etiology most common cause
- Most common viral etiologies: Hepatitis B, C, and A
- Other viral etiologies include:
  - Hepatitis D and E
  - Cytomegalovirus (CMV)
  - Epstein-Barr
  - HIV
  - Herpes simplex virus
- Other nonviral etiologies include:
  - Alcoholic
  - Drug side effects
  - Environmental toxicity
  - Ischemia
  - Idiopathic
  - Autoimmune

EPIDEMIOLOGY

- Hepatitis B and C most endemic in Asia and Africa
- Hepatitis A most frequent in areas of poor sanitation
- In 40% of hepatitis C cases, no is source identified

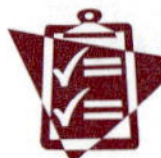

CLINICAL FINDINGS

SYMPTOMS AND SIGNS

- Right upper quadrant pain
- Jaundice
- Liver failure
- Dark urine
- Light colored stools
- Hepatomegaly
- Spider angiomas

LABORATORY FINDINGS

- Elevated transaminases
- Antihepatitis B core Ab (elevated in chronic also), surface antigen, antihepatitis B early antigen Ab
- Antihepatitis C antibodies
- Hyperbilirubinemia
- Antihepatitis A antibodies

IMAGING FINDINGS

- Nonspecific, occasional hepatomegaly

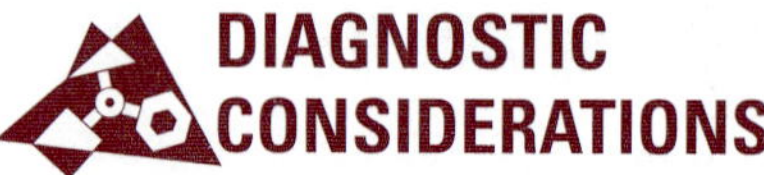

DIAGNOSTIC CONSIDERATIONS

- Onset/duration
- Family history
- Injection drug use
- Transfusion history
- History of alcoholism
- Medications
- Travel history

RULE OUT

- Cholecystitis
- Choledocholithiasis
- Pancreatitis
- Cholangitis

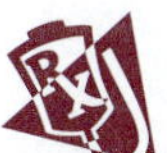

WORK-UP

- Transaminases
- Hepatitis serologies
- Right upper quadrant US
- Serum fractionated bilirubin

WHEN TO ADMIT

- Liver failure

TREATMENT AND MANAGEMENT

SURGERY

- Liver transplantation

Indications

- Fulminant liver failure
- Cirrhosis
- Hepatoma

MEDICATIONS

- Interferon (for hepatitis B and C)
- Ribavirin (for hepatitis C)
- Antihepatitis A Ig
- Lamivudine (for chronic hepatitis B)

TREATMENT MONITORING

- Liver function tests
- Hepatitis C viral load (RNA)

COMPLICATIONS

- Of liver transplantation:
  - Primary nonfunction
  - Rejection
  - Biliary leak or stricture
  - Hemorrhage
  - Hepatic artery thrombosis

PROGNOSIS

- 90% remission or recovery (hepatitis B)
- 10% have chronic hepatitis B (70–90% as carrier only)
- 55–70% chronic hepatitis C

PREVENTION

- Hepatitis B vaccine
- Hepatitis A vaccine (endemic areas)

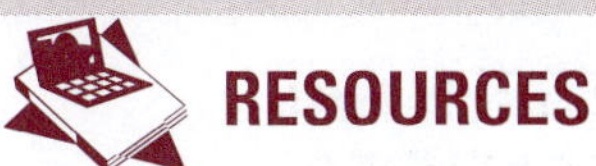

RESOURCES

WEB SITES

- http://www.cdc.gov

Hepatobiliary Infections, Parasitic

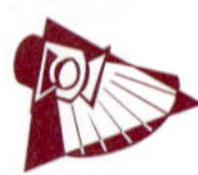

ESSENTIAL FEATURES

- Etiologies include:
  - Amebic
  - Echinococcal
  - Schistosomal
- Risk factors for amebic abscess:
  - HIV
  - Travel to high prevalence area
  - Alcoholism
- Hydatid cysts:
  - Liver (50–70% of cases)
  - Lung (20–30% of cases)

EPIDEMIOLOGY

- 10% of adults in the United States shed amebic cysts in feces without evidence of diarrhea or hepatic abscess
- Schistosomal infection major cause of portal hypertension worldwide

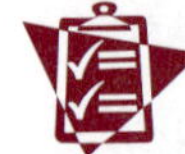

CLINICAL FINDINGS

SYMPTOMS AND SIGNS

- Fever
- Right upper quadrant pain
- Jaundice
- Dyspnea
- Diarrhea in 33% with amebic abscess
- Anaphylaxis (hydatid cyst)
- Palpable hepatic mass (hydatid cyst)
- For schistosomal disease:
  - Maculopapular rash
  - Lassitude
  - Anorexia
  - Diarrhea
  - Headache
  - Fevers
  - Hepatomegaly
  - Splenomegaly
  - Lymphadenopathy
  - Variceal hemorrhage

LABORATORY FINDINGS

- Leukocytosis
- Elevated alkaline phosphatase
- Elevated transaminases
- Hypoalbuminemia rare for amebic abscess
- *Entamoeba histolytica* serologic studies (positive in 95% of cases) in amebic abscess
- Hydatid serologic studies (positive in > 80% of cases)
- Schistosomal ova in feces
- Eosinophilia in hydatid disease

IMAGING FINDINGS

- **CT scan and US for amebic abscess:** Unifocal or multifocal fluid filled areas in liver with peripheral contrast enhancement (not distinguishable from pyogenic)
- **CT scan for hydatid cyst:** Presence of daughter cysts within parent cyst accompanied by calcification

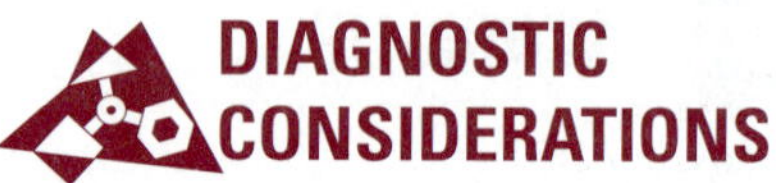

DIAGNOSTIC CONSIDERATIONS

- Pyogenic abscess

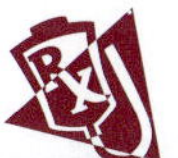

WORK-UP

- History and physical exam
- CBC count
- Liver function tests
- Abdomen CT with contrast
- *E histolytica* serologic studies (positive in 95% of cases) in amebic abscess
- CT-guided aspiration
- Hydatid serologic studies (positive in > 80% of cases)
- Schistosomal ova in feces

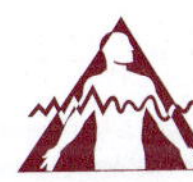

TREATMENT AND MANAGEMENT

SURGERY

- CT-guided drainage of hydatid cysts

MEDICATIONS

- Metronidazole with or without chloroquine for amebic abscess
- Albendazole for 8 weeks for hydatid disease
- Praziquantel for schistosomiasis

COMPLICATIONS

- Rupture of amebic abscess or hydatid cyst
- Secondary bacterial infection of amebic abscess or hydatid cyst
- Hydatid cyst spilling into open peritoneal cavity

PREVENTION

- Improved sanitation in areas of high risk for *E histolytica* infection

RESOURCES

REFERENCES

- Doherty GM, Way LW. Liver & Portal Venous System. In: Way LW, Doherty GM (editors). *Current Surgical Diagnosis & Treatment,* 11e. New York: McGraw-Hill; 2003:593–594.

Hepatocellular Carcinoma

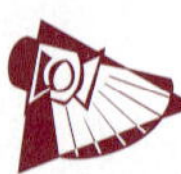

ESSENTIAL FEATURES

- 80% of primary hepatic malignancy
- 50% with fibrous capsule
- 70% with extrahepatic disease
- Metastases most common to hilar and celiac nodes
- Distant metastases most common to lung and peritoneum
- Highly vascular tumors
- Often multicentric with nodular satellite lesions

EPIDEMIOLOGY

- Equal incidence among genders
- 9000 cases/yr in United States
- Incidence increases among persons older than 50 years
- Fibrolamellar variant (not associated with cirrhosis) peak incidence at age 25
- Associated with all etiologies of cirrhosis
- Associated with hepatitis B and C prevalence
- Greatest incidence in Asia and Africa

CLINICAL FINDINGS

SYMPTOMS AND SIGNS

- Right upper quadrant pain
- Weight loss
- Jaundice
- Hepatomegaly
- Hepatic bruit
- Fever
- Ascites
- Gastroesophageal varices
- Distant metastases
- Asymptomatic
- Intraperitoneal hemorrhage
- Decompensated cirrhosis

LABORATORY FINDINGS

- Hyperbilirubinemia (33% of patients)
- Hyperalkaline phosphatase (25% of patients)
- Hepatitis B or C positive (75% of patients)
- Alpha-fetoprotein > 200 ng/mL

IMAGING FINDINGS

- CT with IV portography often shows hypervascular tumor, frequently with multicentric disease
- US hyperechoic tumor
- MRI with or without magnetic resonance cholangiopancreatography (MRCP) shows gadolinium-enhancing lesion
- Combination of CT, US, and MRI is 80% sensitive
- Angiography shows hypervascular tumor

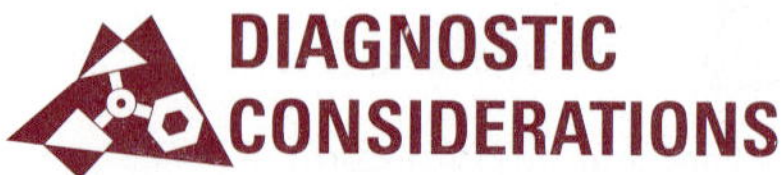

DIAGNOSTIC CONSIDERATIONS

- Biopsy of limited usefulness given high degree of sampling error and risk of tumor seeding
- Overall and planned reserve liver function

RULE OUT

- Metastatic hepatic carcinoma
- Cholangiocarcinoma
- Benign neoplasms if possible
- Other abdominal malignancy

WORK-UP

- Serum alpha-fetoprotein
- CT
- US
- Angiography
- Biopsy in limited circumstances
- Resection for diagnosis and treatment

WHEN TO ADMIT

- Liver failure
- Hemorrhage
- Cholangitis

WHEN TO REFER

- Always to centers of excellence for planned resection or ablative therapy

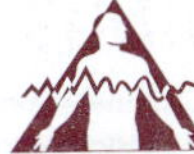

TREATMENT AND MANAGEMENT

SURGERY

- Liver transplantation (treatment of choice in the presence of cirrhosis)
- Partial hepatectomy with at least 0.5 cm margins (25% are candidates)

Contraindications

- Medical comorbidity
- Total tumor volume > 6.5 cm (for liver transplantation)
- Extrahepatic disease or distant metastases
- Bilobar disease and total volume > 6.5 cm
- Poor liver function (class C) and not transplant candidate

PROCEDURES

- Ethyl alcohol ablation (75% complete necrosis)
- Radiofrequency ablation (RFA)
- Chemoembolization (50% response in 25% of patients)

TREATMENT MONITORING

- Alpha-fetoprotein
- CT
- Liver function tests
- Physical exams

COMPLICATIONS

- Hemorrhage
- Biliary leak
- Abdominal infection
- Liver failure

PROGNOSIS

- **Negative prognosis:**
  - Age older than 50
  - Cirrhosis
  - Vascular invasion
  - Portal thrombosis
  - Multilobar or multicentric disease
- Resection: 5-year survival (noncirrhotic), 40%
- Resection: 5-year survival fibrolamellar, 60%
- Transplantation: 5-year survival, 70%

PREVENTION

- Screening with alpha-fetoprotein and US in persons with cirrhosis
- Hepatitis B vaccine
- Education of exposure to ethyl alcohol, hepatitis B and C

RESOURCES

PRACTICE GUIDELINES

- The National Comprehensive Cancer Network http://www.nccn.org/

CANCER STAGING

- See Liver (Including Intrahepatic Bile Ducts) Staging Table on page 750.

STAGE GROUPING

Stage I	T1	N0	M0
Stage II	T2	N0	M0
Stage IIIA	T3	N0	M0
IIIB	T4	N0	M0
IIIC	Any T	N1	M0
Stage IV	Any T	Any N	M1

Herpes Zoster

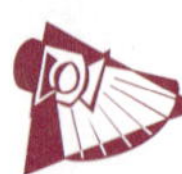

ESSENTIAL FEATURES

- Herpes zoster is an acute vesicular eruption due to reactivation of the varicella-zoster virus
- Focal, often severe, unilateral abdominal wall pain that upon careful questioning follows a dermatomal distribution
- Delayed development (> 48 hours) of classic vesicular lesions along a specific dermatomal distribution
- Positive Tzanck smear
- The diagnosis may become clear in postoperative patients 1–2 days following a negative exploration

EPIDEMIOLOGY

- Usually occurs in adults
- With rare exceptions, patients only suffer 1 attack
- Generalized disease or occurrence in patients < 55-years-old raises the suspicion of an immunosuppressive disorder

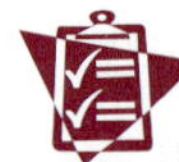

CLINICAL FINDINGS

SYMPTOMS AND SIGNS

- Pain precedes vesicular eruption by 48 hours or more
- Pain may persist and actually increase in intensity after the lesions disappear
- The dermatologic lesions consist of grouped, tense, deep-seated vesicles distributed unilaterally along a dermatome
- Regional lymph nodes may be tender and swollen

LABORATORY FINDINGS

- Multinucleated giant cells on Tzanck smear

IMAGING FINDINGS

- Normal

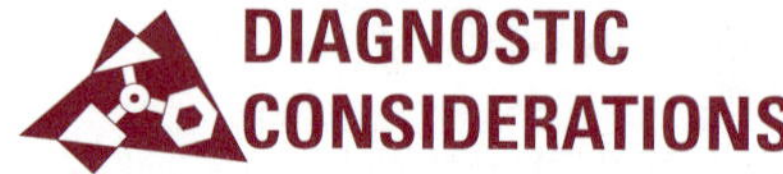

DIAGNOSTIC CONSIDERATIONS

- Because of the severity of abdominal pain and its localized nature as well as the anatomic proximity to affected dermatomes, herpes zoster may be misdiagnosed as the following:
  - Acute cholecystitis
  - Acute appendicitis
  - Incarcerated hernia
  - Ureteral colic
- Generalized vasculitis
- Abdominal wall tumor
- Rectus sheath hematoma
- Thoracolumbar spinal nerve root compression

RULE OUT

- Diseases that may require surgery
  - Prior to vesicle eruption, the diagnosis of zoster is presumptive

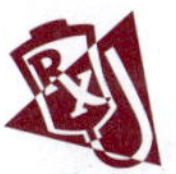

WORK-UP

- CBC count
- Basic chemistries
- Amylase and lipase
- UA
- Abdominal x-rays

WHEN TO ADMIT

- Admit for observation and serial abdominal exams when a surgical diagnosis is contemplated
- Treatment of zoster otherwise performed as an outpatient

WHEN TO REFER

- Dermatology consult to diagnose herpetic rash and perform Tzanck smear
- Chronic pain clinics best manage postherpetic neuralgia

TREATMENT AND MANAGEMENT

- Exclude surgical etiology of abdominal wall pain
- NSAIDs or narcotics for pain
- Early institution of antiviral medications
- Patient is infectious
  - Isolate from immunocompromised patients
- Evaluate for HIV or other immunocompromised states in patients younger than 55

SURGERY

Indications

- None

MEDICATIONS

- Acyclovir, famciclovir, or valacyclovir
- Early medical treatment of zoster may reduce the incidence of postherpetic neuralgia (controversial)
- Nerve blocks for severe pain
- Systemic corticosteroids for severe pain

TREATMENT MONITORING

- Symptomatic improvement

COMPLICATIONS

- Postherpetic neuralgia
- Anesthesia of affected area
- Scarring

PROGNOSIS

- Postherpetic neuralgia develops in 15% of patients

RESOURCES

REFERENCES

- Balfour HH. Antiviral drugs. *N Engl J Med.* 1999;340:1255.

Hirschsprung Disease

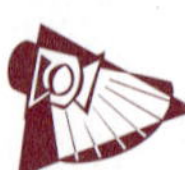

ESSENTIAL FEATURES

- Distal colon aganglionosis resulting in dysfunctional myenteric plexus
- Associated cardiac defects in 2–5%
- Trisomy 21 in 5–15%
- Occasionally preceded by neonatal appendicitis or meconium plug syndrome
- 50% of cases diagnosed in neonates, almost 50% of cases diagnosed in children younger than 2, and rarely in older children or adults

EPIDEMIOLOGY

- 1/5000 births
- 4:1 male:female ratio

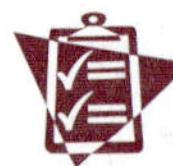

CLINICAL FINDINGS

SYMPTOMS AND SIGNS

- Failure to pass meconium in first 24–48 hours of life
- Feeding intolerance
- Abdominal distention
- Bilious emesis
- Chronic constipation
- Fever (if entercolitis complicating)
- Rectal spasm
- Abdominal pain (if complicated by enterocolitis)
- Diarrhea, occasionally bloody (if enterocolitis present)

IMAGING FINDINGS

- **Abdominal x-ray**
  - Shows intestinal obstruction (occasionally distal transition point visualized)
  - Pneumatosis intestinalis if enterocolitis present
- Contrast enema shows transition zone distally (but may not be present in neonates)
- Anorectal manometry shows failure of relaxation to balloon distention

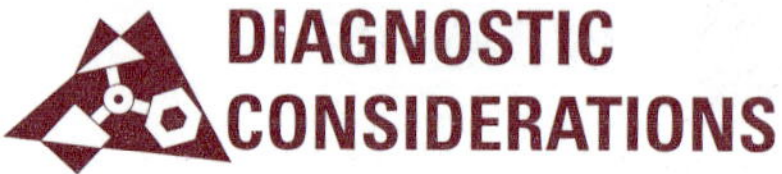

DIAGNOSTIC CONSIDERATIONS

- Causes of low intestinal obstruction in neonates include:
  - Rectal or colonic atresia
  - Meconium plug syndrome
  - Meconium ileus
  - Hypermagnesemia
  - Hypocalcemia
  - Hypokalemia
  - Hypothyroidism

WORK-UP

- History and physical exam
- Abdominal x-ray
- Contrast enema
- Suction rectal biopsy (85–90% sensitive)

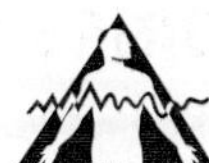

TREATMENT AND MANAGEMENT

SURGERY

- Diverting colostomy for neonates with enterocolitis and Hirschsprung disease (colostomy must contain ganglia)
- Duhamel, Soave, or Swenson procedure at age 9–12 months or once proximal dilation has subsided after diverting colostomy

COMPLICATIONS

- Anastomotic leak or stricture
- Abscess
- Obstruction
- Enterocolitis (10–30%)

PROGNOSIS

- 80–90% maintaining good bowel function

RESOURCES

REFERENCES

- Albanese CT et al. Pediatric Surgery. In: Way LW, Doherty GM (editors). *Current Surgical Diagnosis & Treatment,* 11e. New York: McGraw-Hill; 2003:1321–1322.

Hodgkin Lymphoma

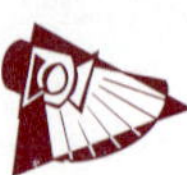

ESSENTIAL FEATURES

- A malignant neoplasm that originates in lymphoid tissue
- Characterized histologically by the presence of Reed-Sternberg cells
- Develops in lymph nodes and spreads in an orderly fashion to contiguous lymph node beds
- Several histologic subtypes exist based on lymphocyte infiltration:
  - Nodular sclerosis: 70%
  - Mixed cellularity: 20%
  - Lymphocyte predominance: 6%
  - Lymphocyte depletion: 2%
- Most important prognostic factor is the disease stage
  - Ann Arbor staging system most accepted classification

EPIDEMIOLOGY

- Bimodal age distribution with first peak occurring in the 20s and the second peak over age 50
- Incidence appears to be higher among patients who meet the following criteria:
  - Fewer siblings
  - Early birth order
  - Siblings with Hodgkin disease
  - Fewer playmates
  - Certain HLA antigens
  - Single-family dwellings
  - Post tonsillectomy
  - Immunodeficiency

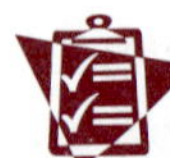

CLINICAL FINDINGS

SYMPTOMS AND SIGNS

- Nontender enlargement of lymph nodes
- Constitutional symptoms that lead to a "B" designation include:
  - Fever
  - Drenching night sweats
  - Weight loss

LABORATORY FINDINGS

- No distinctive basic laboratory findings present, although lymphomas tend to be associated with an elevated lactate dehydrogenase level

IMAGING FINDINGS

- Imaging findings are specific to the location and stage
- **Chest film:** May demonstrate mediastinal adenopathy
- CT scan is the main staging tool used to demonstrate contiguous areas of adenopathy

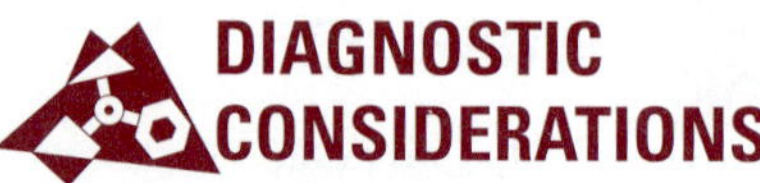

DIAGNOSTIC CONSIDERATIONS

- Hodgkin lymphoma
- Non-Hodgkin lymphoma
- Reactive lymphadenopathy
  - Infectious mononucleosis
  - Cat-scratch disease
  - HIV
  - Drug reactions (eg, phenytoin)
- Tumor metastases

RULE OUT

- Reactive lymphadenopathy
- Metastatic disease to the lymph nodes

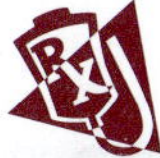

WORK-UP

- Detailed history; ask about risk factors and presence of constitutional B-symptoms
- Thorough physical exam assessing all lymph node beds
- Routine laboratory testing
- Excisional biopsy of enlarged lymph node
- Bone marrow biopsy
- CT scans of the neck, chest, abdomen, and pelvis

WHEN TO ADMIT

- Most patients with lymphadenopathy suspicious for lymphoma are evaluated urgently as an outpatient or admitted to expedite the process

WHEN TO REFER

- Following histologic diagnosis, patients are referred to medical and radiation oncologists for definitive treatment

TREATMENT AND MANAGEMENT

- Treatment of Hodgkin disease involves radiation for localized disease and a combination of radiation and chemotherapy for more advanced disease

SURGERY

- Excisional lymph node biopsy to establish diagnosis
- Rarely, a staging laparotomy is necessary if the anatomic extent of disease in the abdomen is important in guiding therapy

MEDICATIONS

- The 2 common chemotherapy regimens include:
  - MOPP (mechlorethamine, oncovorin, procarbazine, and prednisone)
  - ABVD (adriamycin, bleomycin, vinblastine, and dacarbazine)

TREATMENT MONITORING

- Physical exam to evaluate for lymphadenopathy
- Radiographic evaluation as clinically indicated (eg, with the re-development of constitutional "B" symptoms)

COMPLICATIONS

- Localized radiation-induced complications
- Chemotherapy-induced pancytopenia with the resulting bleeding and infectious complications

PROGNOSIS

- Over 70% of patients may be cured with therapy

RESOURCES

REFERENCES

- Advani RH, Horning SJ. Treatment of early-stage Hodgkin's disease. *Semin Hematol.* 1999;36:270.
- Jox A et al. Hodgkin's disease–new treatment strategies toward the cure of patients. *Cancer Treat Rev.* 1999;25:169.

Hürthle Cell Neoplasms

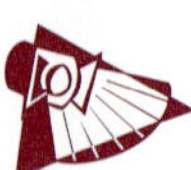

ESSENTIAL FEATURES

- More aggressive variant of follicular thyroid neoplasms
- History of radiation to the neck in some patients
- Painless or enlarging nodule, dysphagia, or hoarseness
- Firm or hard, fixed thyroid nodule; cervical lymphadenopathy
- Normal thyroid function; nodule stippled with calcium (x-ray), solid (US), cold (radioiodine scan), positive or suspicious cytologic studies
- Family history of thyroid cancer

EPIDEMIOLOGY

- Accounts for approximately 2% of all malignant thyroid tumors
- Appears later in life than papillary thyroid cancers, with peak incidence in fifth decade
- More common in women

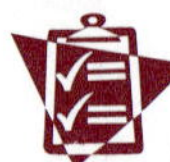

CLINICAL FINDINGS

SYMPTOMS AND SIGNS

- Thyroid nodule: Hard, rubbery, or soft
- Enlarged or hard cervical lymph nodes
- Pain in the thyroid or paralaryngeal neck
- Hoarseness
- Dyspnea
- Stridor
- Dysphagia

LABORATORY FINDINGS

- Normal thyroid-stimulating hormone (TSH)

IMAGING FINDINGS

- Solid or cystic nodule on US
- Nonfunctioning (cold) on radioiodine scan

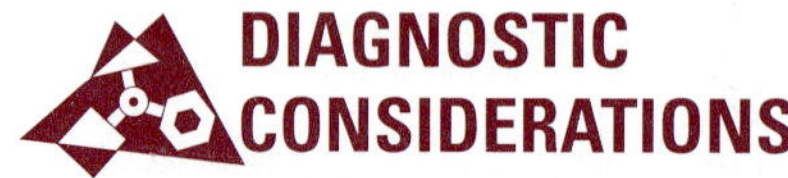

DIAGNOSTIC CONSIDERATIONS

- Fine-needle aspiration (FNA) is unable to reliably differentiate the atypical cells of invasive Hürthle adenocarcinoma from its counterpart benign adenoma
- Sometimes bilateral and multicentric
- Commonly metastasize to cervical lymph nodes
- 95% resistant to radioiodine

RULE OUT

- Concurrent hyperparathyroidism (so that it can be treated during the same operation if necessary)

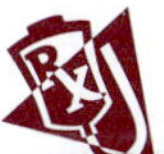

WORK-UP

- Complete history and physical exam
  - With attention to risk factors, family history, palpable characteristics of the nodule, or lymphadenopathy
- Measurement of serum TSH and calcium
- FNA biopsy

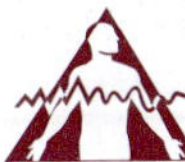

TREATMENT AND MANAGEMENT

- Treatment starts with operative removal
- External beam radiation may palliate nonresectable metastases that are resistant to radioiodine

SURGERY

Indications

- All Hürthle cell neoplasms should be excised unless the Hürthle cell adenoma can be diagnosed with 100% certainty on FNA
- Bulky or palpable nodal recurrences

MEDICATIONS

- Suppressive doses of thyroid hormone after thyroid ablation or thyroidectomy

TREATMENT MONITORING

- Semiannual or yearly neck exams, serum thyroglobulin, thyroglobulin antibodies, and whole body radioiodine scan

COMPLICATIONS

- Neck hematoma
- Superior laryngeal nerve injury
- Recurrent laryngeal nerve injury
- Transient of permanent hypoparathyroidism
- Wound infection

PROGNOSIS

- Worse prognosis predicted by extensive angioinvasion, older age, and presence of distant metastases
- 10-year survival rate, approximately 70%

RESOURCES

REFERENCES

- Cooper D, Schneyer C. Follicular and Hürthle cell carcinoma of the thyroid. *Endocrinol Metab Clin North Am.* 1990;19:577.

PRACTICE GUIDELINES

- The National Comprehensive Cancer Network http://www.nccn.org/

CANCER STAGING

- See Thyroid Staging Table on page 756.

STAGE GROUPING

Separate stage groupings are recommended for papillary or follicular, medullary, and anaplastic (undifferentiated) carcinoma.

Papillary or Follicular
UNDER 45 YEARS

Stage I	Any T	Any N	M0
Stage II	Any T	Any N	M1

Papillary or Follicular
45 YEARS AND OLDER

Stage I	T1	N0	M0
Stage II	T2	N0	M0
Stage III	T3	N0	M0
	T1	N1a	M0
	T2	N1a	M0
	T3	N1a	M0
Stage IVA	T4a	N0	M0
	T4a	N1a	M0
	T1	N1b	M0
	T2	N1b	M0
	T3	N1b	M0
	T4a	N1b	M0
Stage IVB	T4b	Any N	M0
Stage IVC	Any T	Any N	M1

Medullary Carcinoma

Stage I	T1	N0	M0
Stage II	T2	N0	M0
Stage III	T3	N0	M0
	T1	N1a	M0
	T2	N1a	M0
	T3	N1a	M0
Stage IVA	T4a	N0	M0
	T4a	N1a	M0
	T1	N1b	M0
	T2	N1b	M0
	T3	N1b	M0
	T4a	N1b	M0
Stage IVB	T4b	Any N	M0
Stage IVC	Any T	Any N	M1

Hyperadrenocorticism (Cushing Disease/Syndrome)

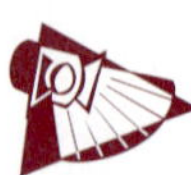

ESSENTIAL FEATURES

- Due to chronic glucocorticoid excess
- Facial plethora, dorsocervical fat pad, supraclavicular fat pad, truncal obesity, easy bruisabilility, purple striae, hirsutism, impotence or amenorrhea, muscle weakness, and psychosis
- Hypertension
- Hyperglycemia
- Includes Cushing disease (excess adrenocorticotropic hormone [ACTH] produced by pituitary adenomas) and Cushing syndrome (ectopic ACTH syndrome or primary adrenal disease resulting in glucocorticoid secretion independent of ACTH stimulation)

EPIDEMIOLOGY

- In children, Cushing syndrome is most commonly caused by adrenal cancers

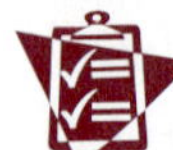

CLINICAL FINDINGS

SYMPTOMS AND SIGNS

- Truncal obesity, hirsutism, moon facies, acne, buffalo hump, purple striae
- Hypertension
- Hyperglycemia
- Weakness
- Depression
- Growth retardation or arrest in children

LABORATORY FINDINGS

- Overnight, low-dose dexamethasone suppression test and measurement of urinary free cortisol establishes diagnosis
  - No suppression and elevated urinary cortisol suggest Cushing syndrome
- Detection of elevated midnight cortisol level suggests Cushing syndrome (midnight plasma level or late-night salivary cortisol sampling)
- Once Cushing syndrome established, measure plasma ACTH level
  - A normal or elevated ACTH level suggests pituitary adenoma or ectopic ACTH secretion
  - Suppressed ACTH is diagnostic of hyperadrenocorticism due to primary adrenal disease
- If ACTH-dependent Cushing disease and no clear pituitary lesion on MRI, may proceed to petrosal sinus sampling with corticotropin-releasing hormone (CRH) stimulation: a central to peripheral ACTH gradient suggests Cushing disease, while no gradient suggests ectopic ACTH secretion

IMAGING FINDINGS

- MRI finding of pituitary lesion suggests Cushing disease
- **Cushing syndrome caused by primary adrenal diseases:** Thin-section CT scan or MRI can detect virtually all adrenal tumors and hyperplasia

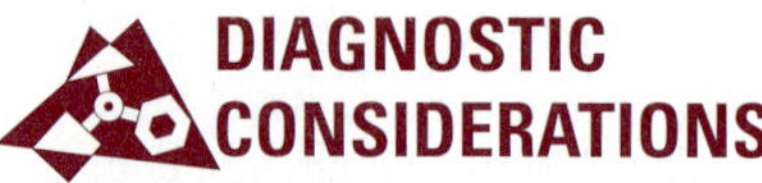

DIAGNOSTIC CONSIDERATIONS

- Rare forms of ACTH-independent Cushing syndrome include macronodular hyperplasia
- Pigmented micronodular hyperplasia is associated with the syndrome of Carney complex (also includes cardiac myxomas and lentigines)
- Rarely, ectopic adrenal tissue can be the source for excess cortisol secretion; most common location is along the abdominal aorta
- Ectopic ACTH syndrome usually caused by small-cell lung cancers or carcinoids but can result from tumors of the pancreas, thyroid, thymus, prostate, esophagus, colon, ovaries, pheochromocytoma, and malignant melanoma
- False-positive dexamethasone suppression tests seen in patients with depression, physiologic stress, marked obesity, renal failure, or taking drugs that accelerate dexamethasone metabolism (phenytoin, rifampin, phenobarbital); estrogens increase cortisol binding globulins and elevate total plasma cortisol concentrations

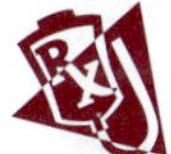

WORK-UP

- Complete history and physical exam
- Overnight, low-dose dexamethasone suppression test
- 24-hour urinary cortisol measurement
- Plasma ACTH level
- Directed imaging including pituitary MRI or abdominal CT or MRI
- Potential role for petrosal sinus sampling to delineate nonvisualized pituitary source for excess ACTH

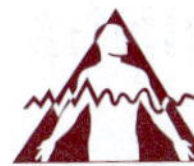

TREATMENT AND MANAGEMENT

- Resection is best treatment for cortisol-producing adrenal tumors or ACTH-producing tumors
- Pituitary irradiation may be necessary if pituitary surgery fails
- Medical treatment may be indicated to control hypercortisolism, or when patients not cured by resection or when complete resection is impossible

SURGERY

Indications

- Transsphenoidal resection if pituitary adenoma
- Bilateral adrenalectomy for Cushing disease if pituitary surgery fails
- Bilateral adrenalectomy when ectopic ACTH-secreting tumor cannot be found or resected
- Bilateral adrenalectomy for patients with bilateral primary adrenal disease, such as pigmented micronodular hyperplasia or macronodular hyperplasia
- Unilateral adrenalectomy for unilateral adrenal adenomas or carcinomas

MEDICATIONS

- Ketoconazole, metyrapone, aminoglutethimide (all control hypercortisolism via inhibiting steroid biosynthesis)
- **Mifepristone (RU 486):** Progesterone and glucocorticoid receptor antagonist
- **Mitotane:** Toxic to adrenal cortex but has serious side effects at effective doses

TREATMENT MONITORING

- Following total adrenalectomy, lifelong corticosteroid maintenance therapy and potentially mineralocorticoid therapy becomes necessary

COMPLICATIONS

- Sustained hypercortisolism can lead to hypertension, cardiovascular disease, stroke, thromboembolism, infections, severe debilitating muscle wasting, weakness
- Psychosis
- Death from underlying tumors
- Truncal obesity and muscle weakness predispose to postoperative pulmonary complications
- Atrophic skin and easy bruisability predict poor wound healing
- Nelson syndrome

PROGNOSIS

- Natural history of Cushing syndrome depends on underlying disease, and varies from mild, indolent disease to rapid progression and death
- Good prognosis after resection of benign adrenal adenoma, pituitary adenoma, or benign ACTH-secreting tumor
- Signs and symptoms of hypercortisolism resolve over period of months
- Cushing disease can recur after excision of a pituitary adenoma
- Residual adrenal tissue or embryonic rests are present in up to 10% of patients and can result in Cushing syndrome if stimulation with ACTH continues
- Extremely poor prognosis in patients with adrenocortical carcinoma and with malignant tumors causing ectopic ACTH syndrome

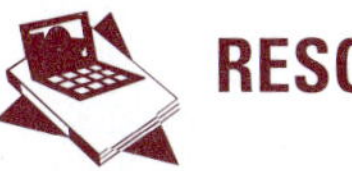

RESOURCES

REFERENCES

- Doherty GM et al. Time to recovery of the hypothalamic-pituitary-adrenal axis after curative resection of adrenal tumors in patients with Cushing's syndrome. *Surgery.* 1990;108:1085.
- Findling JW, Raff H. Newer diagnostic techniques and problems in Cushing's disease. *Endocrinol Metab Clin North Am.* 1999;28;191.

Hypercalcemia

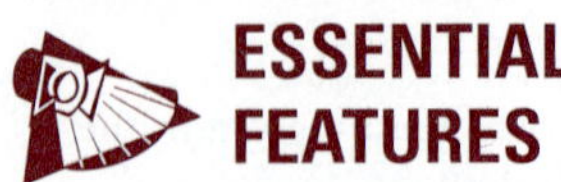

ESSENTIAL FEATURES

- Elevated serum calcium

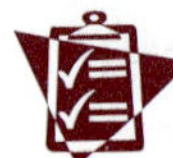

CLINICAL FINDINGS

SYMPTOMS AND SIGNS

- Fatigability
- Muscle weakness
- Depression
- Anorexia
- Nausea
- Constipation
- Polyuria
- Polydipsia
- Metastatic calcification
- Coma

LABORATORY FINDINGS

- Elevated serum calcium

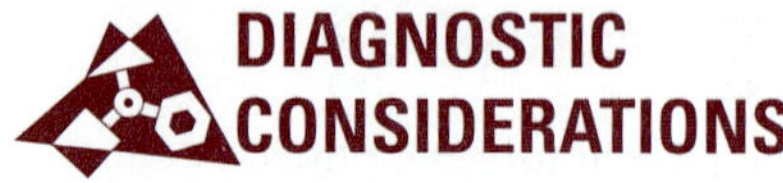

DIAGNOSTIC CONSIDERATIONS

- Hyperparathyroidism
- Cancer with bone metastases
- Ectopic parathyroid hormone (PTH) production
- Vitamin D intoxication
- Hyperthyroidsm
- Milk-alkali syndrome
- Prolonged immobilization
- Thiazide diuretics
- Addison disease

WORK-UP

- Physical exam
- Measure PTH

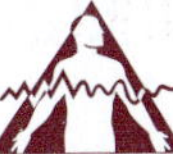

TREATMENT AND MANAGEMENT

- If severe (> 14.5 mg/dL), IV isotonic saline should be given
- Lasix
- IV sodium sulfate
- Plicamycin is useful to treat those with metastatic cancer
- Corticosteroids for sarcoidosis, vitamin D intoxication, and Addison disease
- Calcitonin can be useful for patients with impaired renal or cardiac function who might not tolerate forced diuresis
- Hemodialysis in renal failure

RESOURCES

REFERENCES

- Bilezikian JP. Management of acute hypercalcemia. *N Engl J Med.* 1992;326:1196.
- Body JJ. Current and future directions in medical therapy: Hypercalcemia. *Cancer.* 2000;88(12 Suppl):3054.
- Ziegler R. Hypercalcemic crisis. *J Am Soc Nephrol.* 2001;12(Suppl 17):S3.

Hypercalcemia, Familial Hypocalciuric

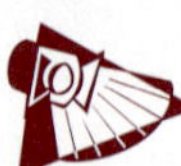

ESSENTIAL FEATURES

- Benign condition of chronic, nonprogressive hypercalcemia with mildly elevated intact parathyroid hormone
- Family history of hypercalcemia, especially in children
- Etiology is a defect in the gene coding for the calcium sensing receptor; transmitted in an autosomal dominant fashion
- Essentially is an elevation in the calcium set point
- Often discovered incidentally with screening laboratory studies

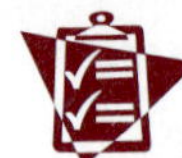

CLINICAL FINDINGS

SYMPTOMS AND SIGNS

- Usually none
- May have polyuria and polydipsia or thirst

LABORATORY FINDINGS

- High serum calcium
- Normal or mildly elevated intact parathyroid hormone level
- Low urinary calcium
- Urinary calcium clearance to creatinine clearance ratio of < 0.01
- Possibly high serum magnesium level

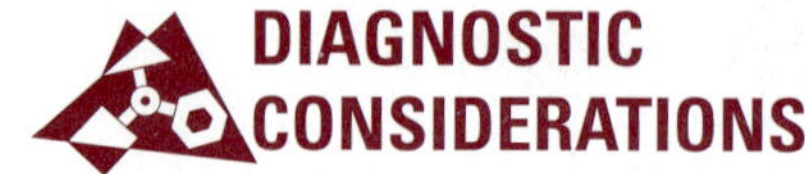

DIAGNOSTIC CONSIDERATIONS

RULE OUT

- Primary hyperparathyroidism

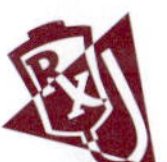

WORK-UP

- Complete history (including family) and physical exam

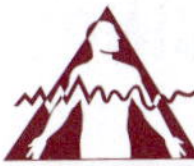

TREATMENT AND MANAGEMENT

- None required
- Operative neck exploration does not alleviate this condition (with the exception of total parathyroidectomy, and surgically induced permanent hypoparathyroidism)
- Genetic counseling important; offspring homozygous for mutation have severe neonatal hyperparathyroidism, which is potentially lethal

RESOURCES

REFERENCES

- Pollak MR et al. Mutations in the human Ca-sensing receptor gene cause familial hypocalciuric hypercalcemia and neonatal severe hyperparathyroidism. *Cell.* 1993;75:1297.
- Marx SJ et al. The hypocalciuric or benign variant of familial hypercalcemia: clinical and biochemical features in fifteen kindreds. *Medicine.* 1998;60:397.

Hypercalcemia of Malignancy, Humoral

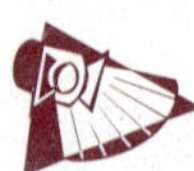

ESSENTIAL FEATURES

- Hypercalcemia due to hormonal product of nonparathyroid cancer
- Most common cause of hypercalcemia in hospitalized patients

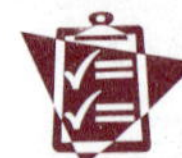

CLINICAL FINDINGS

LABORATORY FINDINGS

- Low intact parathyroid hormone level
- Elevated parathyroid hormone-related protein level
- Anemia
- Elevated serum calcium sometimes (to > 14 mg/dL)
- Increased alkaline phosphatase activity

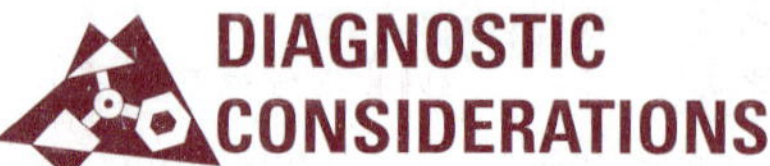

DIAGNOSTIC CONSIDERATIONS

- Most common tumors causing ectopic hyperparathyroidism are the following:
  - Squamous cell carcinoma of the lung
  - Renal cell carcinoma
  - Bladder cancer
- Less common offending tumors are the following:
  - Hepatoma
  - Tumors of the ovary, stomach, pancreas, parotid gland, or colon

RULE OUT

- Primary hyperparathyroidism

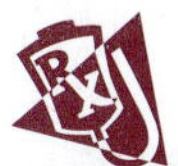

WORK-UP

- History and physical exam
- Laboratory evaluation
- Search for primary malignancy

WHEN TO ADMIT

- Hypercalcemic crisis

TREATMENT AND MANAGEMENT

- Treatment is directed at normalizing serum calcium level
- Treatment of primary tumor treats malignancy-associated hypercalcemia

RESOURCES

REFERENCES

- Strewler GJ, Nissenson RA. Hypercalcemia in malignancy. *West J Med.* 1990;16:791.

Hyperkalemia

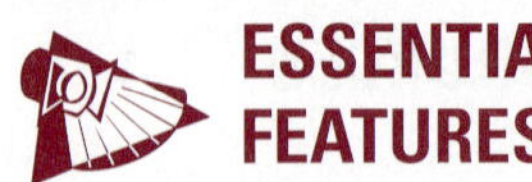

ESSENTIAL FEATURES

- Elevated serum potassium

EPIDEMIOLOGY

- Severe trauma
- Burns
- Crush injuries
- Renal insufficiency
- Marked catabolism
- Addison disease

CLINICAL FINDINGS

SYMPTOMS AND SIGNS

- Nausea
- Vomiting
- Colicky abdominal pain
- Diarrhea

LABORATORY FINDINGS

- Elevated serum potassium
- Peaked T waves
- Wide QRS
- Depressed ST segment

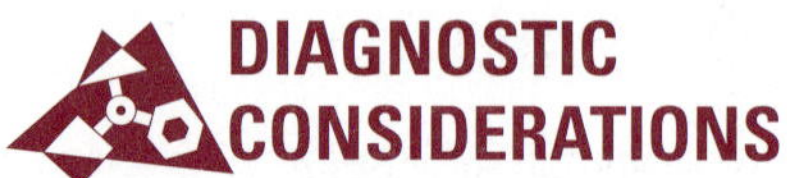

DIAGNOSTIC CONSIDERATIONS

- Addison disease

RULE OUT

- Hemolysis
- Leukocytosis
- Thrombocytosis (> 1,000,000/μL
- Abnormalities of acid-base status (acidosis)
- Addison disease

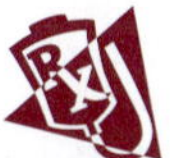

WORK-UP

- Serum electrolytes
- CBC count with platelets

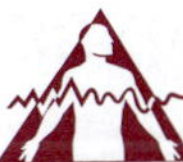

TREATMENT AND MANAGEMENT

- IV 100 mL D_{50} with 20 U regular insulin
- IV $NaHCO_3$
- IV calcium
- Sodium polystyrene sulfonate orally or by enema (40–80 g/d)
- Hemodialysis
- β-Agonists (inhaled)

MEDICATIONS

- D_{50}/insulin
- Calcium
- Sodium polystyrene sulfonate
- $NaHCO_3$
- Albuterol

TREATMENT MONITORING

- Serum electrolytes
- ECG

COMPLICATIONS

- Diastolic cardiac arrest

PROGNOSIS

- Excellent

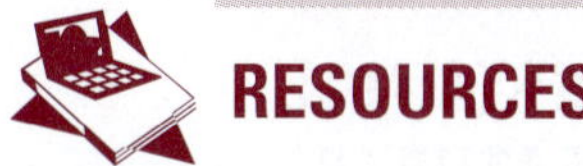

RESOURCES

REFERENCES

- Greenberg A. Hyperkalemia: treatment options. *Semin Nephrol.* 1998;18:46.

Hypermagnesemia

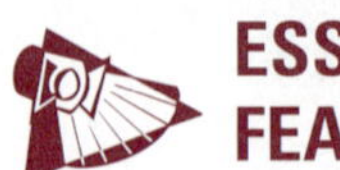

ESSENTIAL FEATURES

- Renal insufficiency
- Elevated serum magnesium

EPIDEMIOLOGY

- Usually occurs in patients with renal disease
- Rare in surgical patients

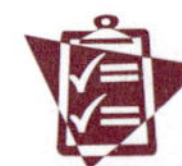

CLINICAL FINDINGS

SYMPTOMS AND SIGNS

- Lethargy
- Weakness
- Widened QRS complex
- Depressed ST segment
- Peaked T waves

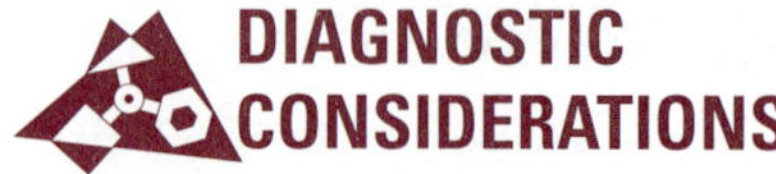

DIAGNOSTIC CONSIDERATIONS

- When serum level reaches 6 mEq/L, deep tendon reflexes are lost
- Levels > 10 mEq/L can lead to somnolence, coma, and death

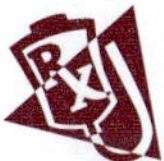

WORK-UP

- Magnesium should be carefully monitored in patients with renal insufficiency
- Serum levels
- ECG

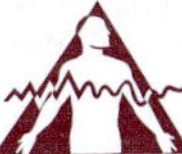

TREATMENT AND MANAGEMENT

- IV isotonic saline to increase renal excretion
- Slow IV infusion of calcium
- Dialysis may be necessary

SURGERY

MEDICATIONS

- Isotonic saline infusion
- Calcium gluconate infusion

TREATMENT MONITORING

- ECG monitoring
- Serum magnesium levels

PROGNOSIS

- Excellent if treated

PREVENTION

- Regulation of magnesium intake in patients with renal insufficiency

RESOURCES

REFERENCES

- Whang R. Clinical disorders of magnesium metabolism. *Compr Ther.* 1997;23:168.

Hypernatremia

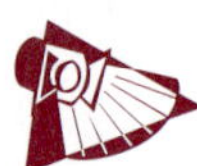

ESSENTIAL FEATURES

- High serum sodium
- Caused by either a loss of water or a gain of hypertonic saline

EPIDEMIOLOGY

- Typically accompanies dehydration/water loss in perioperative or post-trauma patients
- Pure water loss
  - Unreplaced insensible water losses
  - Hypodipsia
  - Neurogenic diabetes insipidus
  - Congenital diabetes insipidus
  - Acquired nephrogenic diabetes insipidus (renal disease, hypercalcemia, hypokalemia, drugs including lithium and amphotericin B)
- Hypotonic fluid loss
  - Renal losses (due to loop diuretics, osmotic diuretics, postobstructive diuresis, polyuric acute tubular necrosis)
  - GI losses (vomiting, NG drainage, enterocutaneous fistula, diarrhea, osmotic cathartic agents)
  - Cutaneous losses (burns, excessive sweating)
- Hypertonic sodium gain
  - Hypertonic sodium bicarbonate infusion
  - Hypertonic feeding solution
  - Sodium chloride ingestion
  - Sea water ingestion/drowning
  - Hypertonic sodium chloride infusion, enemas, intrauterine injection, or dialysate
  - Primary hyperaldosteronism
  - Cushing syndrome

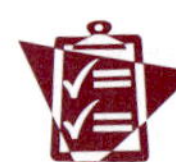

CLINICAL FINDINGS

SYMPTOMS AND SIGNS

- CNS dysfunction; may be very hard to demonstrate in a person with coexisting illness
  - More prominent symptoms with rapid changes in sodium level
- Thirst early, which resolves as hypernatremia becomes more severe

LABORATORY FINDINGS

- High serum sodium

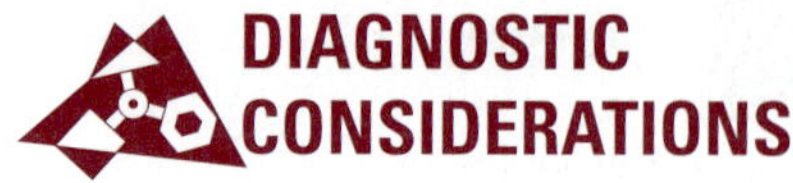

DIAGNOSTIC CONSIDERATIONS

- Must determine intravascular volume status to guide resuscitation

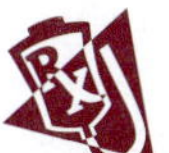

WORK-UP

- Serum electrolytes

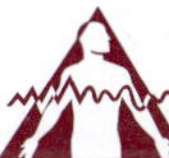

TREATMENT AND MANAGEMENT

- Water replacement and/or sodium restriction
- Change serum sodium no more than 1–2 mEq/L/h
  - More rapid changes risk iatrogenic cerebral edema

TREATMENT MONITORING

- Serum electrolytes

COMPLICATIONS

- Permanent brain damage

PROGNOSIS

- Excellent

PREVENTION

- Judicious IV administration and monitoring of volume status

RESOURCES

REFERENCES

- Adrogue HJ, Madias NE. Hypernatremia. *N Engl J Med.* 2000;342:1493.

Hyperparathyroidism, Primary

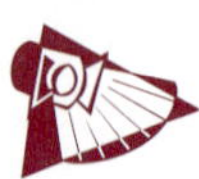

ESSENTIAL FEATURES

- Due to excess secretion of parathyroid hormone (PTH)
- "Stones, bones, abdominal groans, psychic moans, and fatigue overtones"
- Some patients are asymptomatic
- Most common cause of hypercalcemia in the ambulatory patient
- Nonparathyroid cancer is the most common cause of hypercalcemia in the hospitalized patient

EPIDEMIOLOGY

- 0.1–0.3% of the general population
- 83% from single parathyroid adenoma, 6% from multiple adenomas, 10% from 4-gland hyperplasia, 1% from parathyroid carcinoma
- Uncommon before puberty
- Peak incidence is between third and fifth decade
- 2–3 times more common in women than men

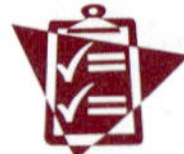

CLINICAL FINDINGS

SYMPTOMS AND SIGNS

- Fatigue, weakness, arthralgias, nausea, vomiting, dyspepsia, constipation, polydipsia, polyuria, nocturia, psychiatric disturbances, renal colic, bone and joint pain
- Nephrolithiasis and nephrocalcinosis, osteopenia, osteitis fibrosa cystica, peptic ulcer disease, gout, chondrocalcinosis, pancreatitis
- Hypertension, band keratopathy
- Neck mass (rare)

LABORATORY FINDINGS

- Elevated serum calcium
- Elevated intact PTH level (although can be inappropriately high normal)
- Elevated chloride; low or normal phosphate
- Serum chloride to phosphate ratio of greater than 33
- Uric acid and alkaline phosphatase sometimes elevated
- Urine calcium increased or normal
- Urine phosphate increased
- Tubular reabsorption of phosphate decreased
- Urine osteocalcin and deoxypyridinoline crosslinks increased
- **Hydrocortisone suppression test:** Reduces serum calcium in most cases of sarcoidosis and vitamin D intoxication but not primary hyperparathyroidism

IMAGING FINDINGS

- Subperiosteal resorption of radial side of phalanges
- Demineralization of skeleton (osteopenia or osteoporosis)
- Bone cysts
- Nephrocalcinosis or nephrolithiasis
- Neck sestamibi scan may localize adenomatous parathyroid gland
- Neck US may localize an abnormally large parathyroid gland
- Bone densitometry can document level of bone demineralization

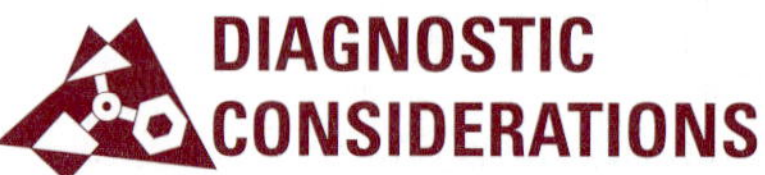

DIAGNOSTIC CONSIDERATIONS

- Primary hyperparathyroidism also is part of the multiple endocrine neoplasia syndromes, type I and IIa
- Other causes of hypercalcemia include:
  - Hyperthyroidism
  - Addison disease
  - Pheochromocytoma
  - Hypothyroidism
  - VIPoma
  - Milk-alkali syndrome
  - Vitamin D or A overdose
  - Thiazides
  - Lithium
  - Aluminum
  - Granulomatous disease
  - Familial hypocalciuric hypercalcemia
  - Paget disease
  - Immobilization
  - Idiopathic hypercalcemia of infancy
  - Dysproteinemias
  - Rhabdomyolysis
- Nonparathyroid tumors that secrete pure PTH are extremely rare
- In patients with previous neck explorations, and negative preoperative localization studies (sestamibi/US), selective venous catheterization with PTH assay is recommended and helps localize tumors in about 80% of patients

RULE OUT

- Parathyroid carcinoma (usually intraoperative discovery)
- Ectopic hyperparathyroidism or nonparathyroid cancer

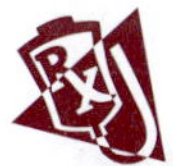

WORK-UP

- Complete history and physical exam
- Serum calcium, PTH, phosphate, chloride, alkaline phosphatase, creatinine, blood urea nitrogen, urinary calcium
- Cervical localization study (sestamibi with or without US)

WHEN TO ADMIT

- Hypercalcemic crisis:
  - Patients need to be hydrated and have hypokalemia and hyponatremia corrected
  - Furosemide can increase calcium excretion in rehydrated patients
  - Glucocorticoids are effective in sarcoid, vitamin D intoxication, and cancer
  - Etidronate, plicamycin, and calcitonin are effective in lowering calcium level for short periods regardless of cause

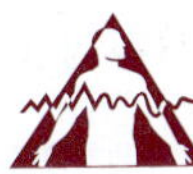

TREATMENT AND MANAGEMENT

- Only successful treatment is parathyroidectomy
- Symptomatic and asymptomatic patients benefit from surgery (both symptomatically and metabolically)

SURGERY

Indications

- All patients

TREATMENT MONITORING

- Serum calcium and intact PTH levels
- Immediately postoperatively, oral calcium and possible calcitriol will be needed for the short term

PROGNOSIS

- Untreated yields increased risk of premature death from cardiovascular or malignant disease
- 80% of treated patients have resolution of symptoms
- Younger patients, and those with less severe disease, return to normal survival curve sooner after treatment than do older patients
- Experienced surgeons have a success rate of 95% at initial surgery

RESOURCES

REFERENCES

- Clark OH. Changing surgical approaches to patients with primary hyperparathyroidism. *Curr Surg.* 2000;57:546.
- Utiger RD. Treatment of primary hyperparathyroidism. *N Engl J Med.* 1999;341:1301.

Hyperparathyroidism, Secondary

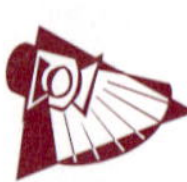

ESSENTIAL FEATURES

- Induced abnormality of endogenous mechanisms that ensure calcium homeostasis
- Increased parathyroid hormone (PTH) secretion in response to low plasma concentration of ionized calcium
- Can see a hyperplasia of parathyroid chief cells

EPIDEMIOLOGY

- Secondary hyperparathyroidism develops in 1–28% of patients who undergo dialysis

CLINICAL FINDINGS

SYMPTOMS AND SIGNS

- Similar symptoms to primary hyperparathyroidism
- Complaints of significant bone pain

LABORATORY FINDINGS

- Elevated intact PTH level
- Low or normal serum calcium level
- Elevated serum phosphorous level (when results from renal disease)
- Normal or low serum phosphorous level (when results from malabsorption or rickets)

IMAGING FINDINGS

- Similar (or more severe) skeletal changes as seen with primary hyperparathyroidism

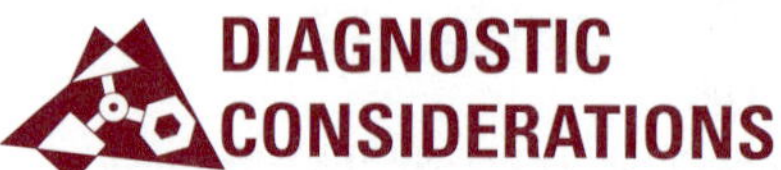

DIAGNOSTIC CONSIDERATIONS

- In patients with secondary hyperparathyroidism, a higher serum calcium concentration is needed to suppress PTH secretion
- Associated with renal disease as well as malabsorption syndromes
- Almost universal complication of hemodialysis and peritoneal dialysis
- When associated with renal disease, often due to phosphate retention, failure of kidneys to generate 1,25 dihydroxyvitamin D, resistance of bones to PTH action, and decreased serum calcium concentration

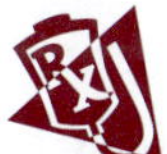

WORK-UP

- Measure serum intact PTH level
- Measure serum calcium and phosphorous level

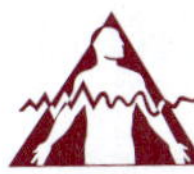

TREATMENT AND MANAGEMENT

- Goal is to decrease stimulation of the parathyroid gland by limiting serum hyperphosphatemia and supplementing both calcium and vitamin D
- Will often resolve after correction of renal function (ie, with renal transplantation)

SURGERY

- Subtotal parathyroidectomy or total parathyroidectomy with parathyroid autograft

Indications

- Hypercalcemia
- Normocalcemia with severe renal osteodystrophy, bone pain, elevated alkaline phosphatase, bone fracture, torn tendon, pruritus, soft-tissue calcification, calciphylaxis, enlarged parathyroid gland

MEDICATIONS

- PO or IV calcitriol
- Adjusting calcium and phosphorous concentration in dialysate solutions
- Limiting phosphorous intake
- Phosphate binders
- Nonhypercalcemic vitamin D derivative and calcimimetics are being developed

TREATMENT MONITORING

- Serum calcium and intact PTH levels

COMPLICATIONS

- Profound hypocalcemia following subtotal parathyroidectomy for renal osteodystrophy, both because of "hungry bones" and because of decreased PTH secretion
- Mortality is < 1% for parathyroidectomy in patients with secondary hyperparathyroidism despite significant comorbidities

PROGNOSIS

- 1–10% of patients who undergo successful kidney grafting have persistent secondary hyperparathyroidism and hypercalcemia

PREVENTION

- Should start early in the course of chronic renal failure when intact PTH is normal or only slightly elevated

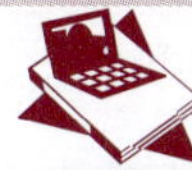

RESOURCES

REFERENCES

- Tominaga Y et al. Indications for parathyroidectomy in renal hyperparathyroidism. *Acta Chir Austriaca.* 1996;124:10.
- Rothmund M et al. Subtotal parathyroidectomy versus total parathyroidectomy and autotransplantation in secondary hyperparathyroidism: a randomized trial. *World J Surg.* 1991;15:745.

Hyperparathyroidism, Tertiary

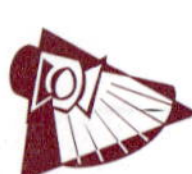

ESSENTIAL FEATURES

- Autonomous, hyperplastic parathyroid glands in a patients with secondary hyperparathyroidism
- Persistent hypercalcemia following normalization of renal function (usually with renal transplantation)

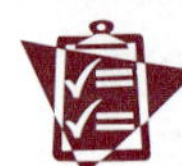

CLINICAL FINDINGS

LABORATORY FINDINGS

- Elevated intact parathyroid hormone levels
- Elevated serum calcium and phosphate levels
- Elevated alkaline phosphatase levels

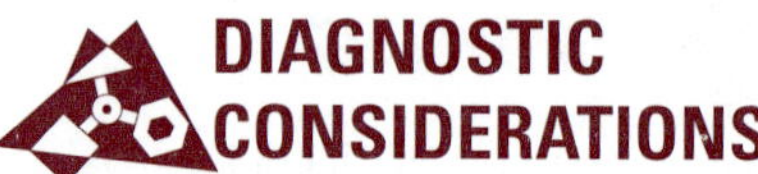

DIAGNOSTIC CONSIDERATIONS

- Consider malignancy in appropriate clinical settings

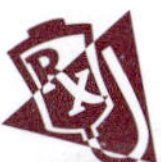

WORK-UP

- Measure serum calcium and intact parathyroid hormone

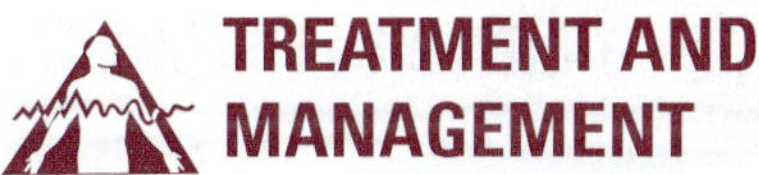

TREATMENT AND MANAGEMENT

SURGERY

- Surgical therapy is withheld until all medical approaches have been exhausted

Indications

- Hyperparathyroidism refractory to all medical therapies
- Calcium-phosphate product greater than 70
- Severe bone pain
- Pruritus
- Extensive soft-tissue calcification with tumoral calcinosis
- Calciphylaxis

MEDICATIONS

- Phosphate binders
- Calcium supplementation
- Vitamin D

TREATMENT MONITORING

- Serum calcium level

PROGNOSIS

- Usually dramatic relief of symptoms once treated (medically or surgically)
- Few patients continue to have bone pain due to osteomalacia
- Few patients can have profound hypoparathyroidism because of remineralization of bones ("hungry bones") and because of decreased parathyroid hormone secretion

RESOURCES

REFERENCES

- Pasieka JL et al. A prospective surgical outcome study assessing the impact of parathyroidectomy on symptoms in patients with secondary and tertiary hyperparathyroidism. *Surgery.* 2000;128:531.

Hyperphosphatemia

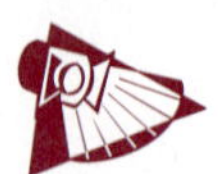

ESSENTIAL FEATURES

- Elevated serum phosphorus

EPIDEMIOLOGY

- Renal insufficiency
- Post-trauma
- Marked tissue catabolism
- Excess intake (rarely)

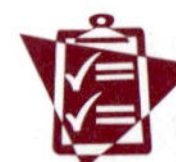

CLINICAL FINDINGS

SYMPTOMS AND SIGNS

- Usually asymptomatic

LABORATORY FINDINGS

- Elevated serum phosphorus
- Decreased serum calcium

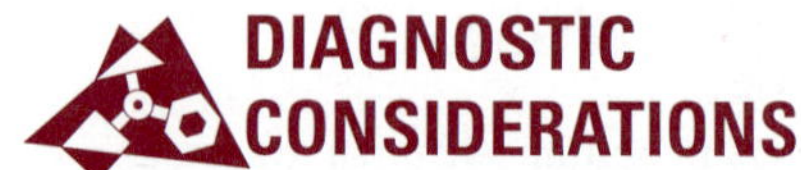

DIAGNOSTIC CONSIDERATIONS

- In perioperative or post-trauma setting, almost always associated with renal insufficiency, even when other factors also present

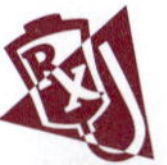

WORK-UP

- Serum electrolytes
- ABG measurements

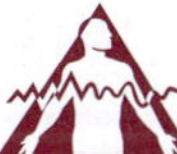

TREATMENT AND MANAGEMENT

- Diuresis
- Phosphate binding antacids
- Dialysis

MEDICATIONS

- Diuretics
- Phosphate binding antacids (aluminum hydroxide)

TREATMENT MONITORING

- Serum electrolytes

PROGNOSIS

- Excellent

RESOURCES

REFERENCES

- Klahr S et al. Acute renal failure. *N Engl J Med.* 1998;338:671.

Hyperthyroidism, Non-Graves

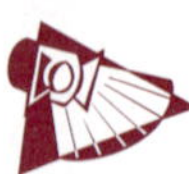

ESSENTIAL FEATURES

- Myriad of causes, that include both increased secretion of thyroid hormone from the thyroid gland and disorders that increase thyroid hormone levels without increasing thyroid gland secretion
  - Solitary toxic adenoma
  - Toxic multinodular goiter (Plummer disease)
  - Jodbasedow disease (thyrotoxicosis that occurs after iodine supplementation)
  - Amiodarone-toxicity
  - Thyroid-stimulating hormone (TSH)-secreting pituitary adenoma
  - hCG-secreting tumor (hydatidiform mole, choriocarcinoma)
  - Postpartum hyperthyroidism
  - Struma ovarii (thyroid tissue in ovarian tumor, usually teratoma)
  - Factitious hyperthyroidism
  - Iatrogenic hyperthyroidism

EPIDEMIOLOGY

- Toxic multinodular goiter found in the elderly, especially women over 60
- Solitary toxic adenomas are 4 times more likely to occur in females than males
- 5–15% of ovarian teratomas with thyroid tissue result in clinical hyperthyroidism

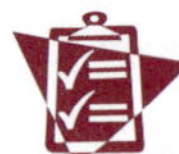

CLINICAL FINDINGS

SYMPTOMS AND SIGNS

- Nervousness, weight loss with increased appetite, heart intolerance, increased sweating, muscular weakness and fatigue, increased bowel frequency, polyuria, menstrual irregularity, infertility
- Goiter, tachycardia, atrial fibrillation, warm moist skin, cardiac flow murmur, gynecomastia

LABORATORY FINDINGS

- Suppressed TSH (except in TSH-secreting pituitary adenoma)
- Elevated tri-iodothyronine (T_3), free thyroxine (T_4), and radioactive iodine uptake
- Failure to suppress radioiodine uptake with exogenous T_3
- Radioactive iodine uptake is generally 35–40% in toxic multinodular goiter

IMAGING FINDINGS

- **Radioiodine scan:** Increased pelvic uptake in cases of struma ovarii

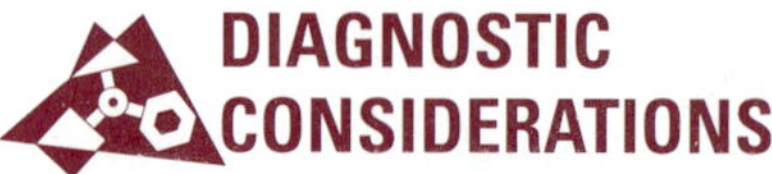

DIAGNOSTIC CONSIDERATIONS

- Toxic multinodular goiter often develops from 1 or more nodule of a nontoxic multinodular goiter becoming autonomous with respect to T_3 and T_4 secretion
- Solitary toxic adenomas may be true adenomas, or colloid nodules with areas of hyperplasia
- Solitary toxic adenomas usually have slow, progressive growth but can have hemorrhage and degeneration
- **Jodbasedow disease:** Iodine deficiency leads to a rise in TSH and thyroid growth; subsequent iodine supplementation can lead to thyrotoxicosis

RULE OUT

- Thyroid cancer

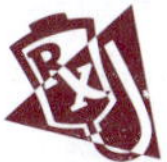

WORK-UP

- Complete history (including family) and physical exam
- Thyroid function tests
- Fine-needle aspiration biopsy of toxic nodules

TREATMENT AND MANAGEMENT

- Treatment often multimodal, including antithyroid medication, radioactive iodine, or thyroid surgery
- Percutaneous ethanol injections in solitary toxic adenoma have been used outside the United States (especially in Italy)

SURGERY

Indications

- Amiodarone-induced hyperthyroidism
- Large goiters with compressive symptoms
- Suspicion of malignancy
- To remove hCG-secreting tumors
- Oopherectomy for struma ovarii

Contraindications

- Patients who will not tolerate general anesthesia

MEDICATIONS

- Propylthiouracil
- Methimazole
- Radioiodine (^{131}I)

TREATMENT MONITORING

- TSH and T_4 measurements

PROGNOSIS

- After treatment of toxic multinodular goiter, 80% are no longer hyperthyroid; 11–16% are hypothyroid

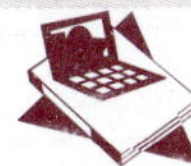

RESOURCES

REFERENCES

- Fradkin JE, Wolff J. Iodide-induced thyrotoxicosis. *Medicine.* 1983;62:1.
- Hamburger JI. Evolution of toxicity in solitary nontoxic autonomously functioning thyroid nodules. *J Clin Endocrinol Metab.* 1980;50:1089.
- Ayhan A et al. Struma ovarii. *Int J Gynaecol Obstet.* 1993;42:143.
- Jensen MD et al. Treatment of toxic multinodular goiter (Plummer's disease): surgery or radioiodine? *World J Surg.* 1986;10:673.

Hypocalcemia

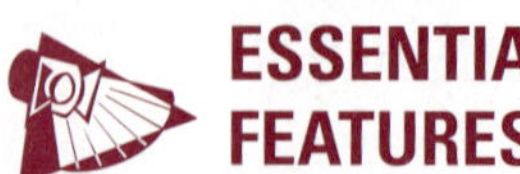

ESSENTIAL FEATURES

- Depressed serum calcium

EPIDEMIOLOGY

- Post thyroidectomy or parathyroidectomy

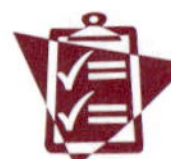

CLINICAL FINDINGS

SYMPTOMS AND SIGNS

- Hyperactive deep tendon reflexes
- Chvostek sign
- Muscle/abdominal cramps
- Carpopedal spasm
- Convulsions

LABORATORY FINDINGS

- Depressed serum calcium
- Hypomagnesemia
- Prolonged QT interval

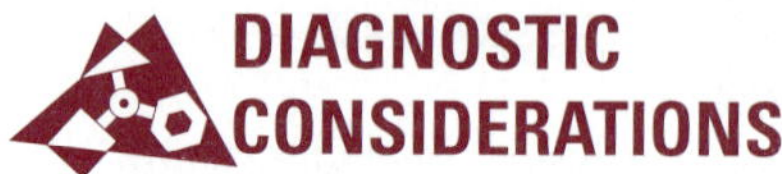

DIAGNOSTIC CONSIDERATIONS

- Hypoparathyroidism
- Hypomagnesemia
- Severe pancreatitis
- Renal failure
- Severe trauma
- Crush injuries
- Necrotizing fasciitis

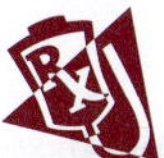

WORK-UP

- Serum calcium, phosphorus, creatinine, and parathyroid hormone (PTH)
- 24-hour urine calcium
- Chest film

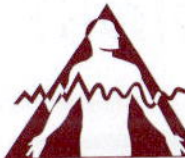

TREATMENT AND MANAGEMENT

- Treat alkalosis if present
- Acutely: Calcium gluconate
- Long-term: Vitamin D, oral calcium, phosphate binders

MEDICATIONS

- Calcium gluconate
  - 6 g in 500 mL D5W
  - Infuse at 1mL/kg/h
  - Monitor serum calcium and adjust infusion as necessary
- Vitamin D
- Oral calcium

TREATMENT MONITORING

- Serum calcium
- Ionized calcium

PROGNOSIS

- Excellent

PREVENTION

- Postoperative calcium surveillance

RESOURCES

REFERENCES

- Lebowitz MR et al. Hypocalcemia. *Semin Nephrol.* 1992;12:146.

Hypokalemia

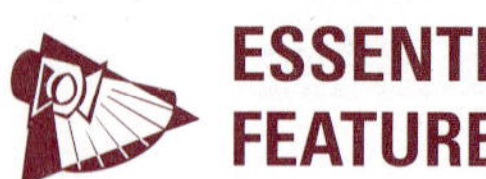

ESSENTIAL FEATURES

- Depressed serum potassium

EPIDEMIOLOGY

- Alcoholics
- Elderly
- Prolonged NPO

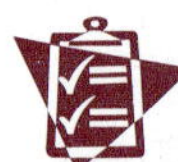

CLINICAL FINDINGS

SYMPTOMS AND SIGNS

- Decreased muscle contractility
- Paralysis

LABORATORY FINDINGS

- Depressed serum potassium
- Alkalosis can contribute
- Hypomagnesemia can contribute to refractoriness

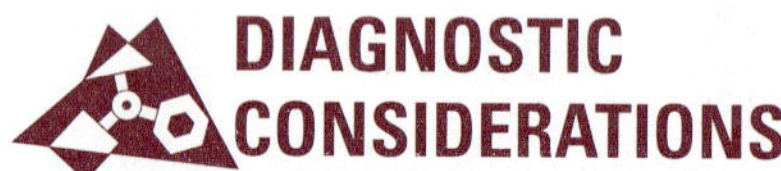

DIAGNOSTIC CONSIDERATIONS

- Laboratory error or difficulty with phlebotomy; blood drawn from above an IV infusion can have spurious results with very low potassium

RULE OUT

- Hypomagnesemia

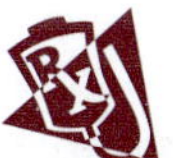

WORK-UP

- Serum electrolytes including magnesium
- ABG (pH) measurement
- Urine potassium losses: (< 30 mEq/d total body deficit, > 30 mEq/d renal wasting)

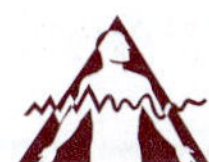

TREATMENT AND MANAGEMENT

- Correct underlying problem
- Potassium repletion
- Magnesium repletion if necessary
- Correct alkalosis if present

MEDICATIONS

- KCl PO if possible, if IV then 20–30 mEq/h by central vein or 10 mEg/h by peripheral vein
- $MgSO_4$

TREATMENT MONITORING

- Serum potassium

COMPLICATIONS

- Hyperkalemia

PROGNOSIS

- Excellent

PREVENTION

- Adequate dietary intake or IV supplements

RESOURCES

REFERENCES

- Kruse JA et al. Rapid correction of hypokalemia using concentrated intravenous potassium chloride infusions. *Arch Intern Med.* 1990;150:613.
- Whang R et al. Refractory potassium repletion: a consequence of magnesium deficiency. *Arch Intern Med.* 1992;152:40.

Hypomagnesemia

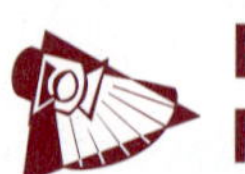

ESSENTIAL FEATURES

• Low serum magnesium

EPIDEMIOLOGY

• Occurs with poor dietary intake, intestinal malabsorption, or excessive losses from the gut
• Can also be caused by excessive urine losses, chronic alcohol abuse, hyperaldosteronism, and hypercalcemia
• Occasionally, develops in acute pancreatitis, diabetic acidosis, burn victims, or with prolonged total parenteral nutrition (TPN) administration

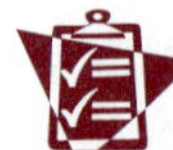

CLINICAL FINDINGS

SYMPTOMS AND SIGNS

• Hyperactive deep tendon reflexes
• Positive Chvostek sign
• Tremors
• Delirium
• Convulsions

LABORATORY FINDINGS

• Low serum magnesium

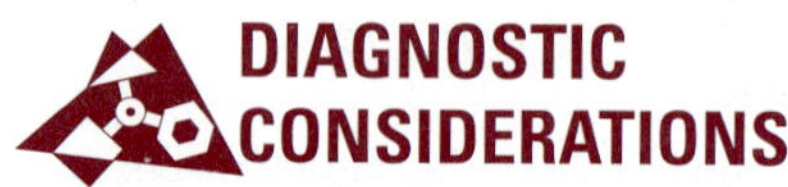

DIAGNOSTIC CONSIDERATIONS

• Depends on clinical suspicion and serum levels

WORK-UP

- Serum levels of calcium, magnesium, and other electrolytes

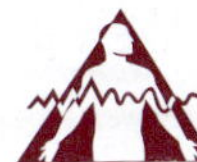

TREATMENT AND MANAGEMENT

- Administering supplemental magnesium
- PO replacement for minor to moderate hypomagenesemia
- For severe deficits: IV magnesium sulfate

COMPLICATIONS

- IV supplementation can quickly lead to hypomagnesaemia in patients with renal insufficiency
- Refractory hypokalemia may accompany hypomagnesemia

PROGNOSIS

- Excellent

PREVENTION

- Adequate daily intake
- Including magnesium in TPN solutions

RESOURCES

REFERENCES

- Kelepouris E et al. Hypomagnesemia: renal magnesium handling. *Semin Nephrol.* 1998;18:58.
- Whang R. Clinical disorders of magnesium metabolism. *Compr Ther.* 1997;23:168.

Hyponatremia

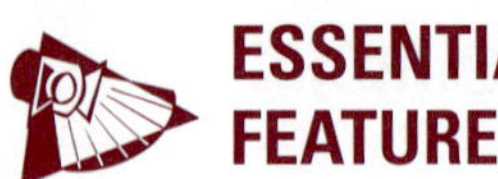

ESSENTIAL FEATURES

- Low serum sodium

EPIDEMIOLOGY

- Postoperative patients
- Premenopuasal women post surgery

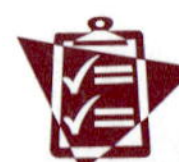

CLINICAL FINDINGS

SYMPTOMS AND SIGNS

- Mental obtundation (sodium < 120 mEq/L)

LABORATORY FINDINGS

- Low serum sodium

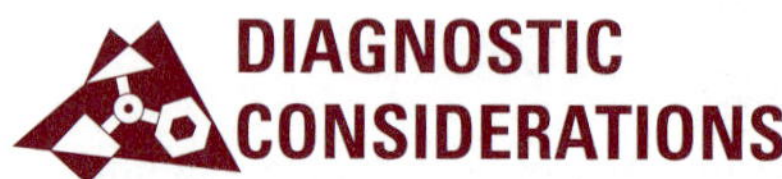

DIAGNOSTIC CONSIDERATIONS

- Must determine intravascular volume status to guide resuscitation

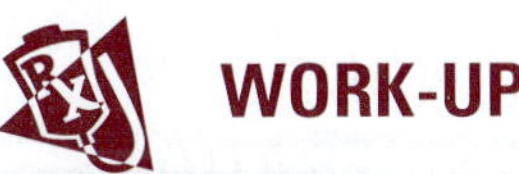

WORK-UP

- Serum electrolytes

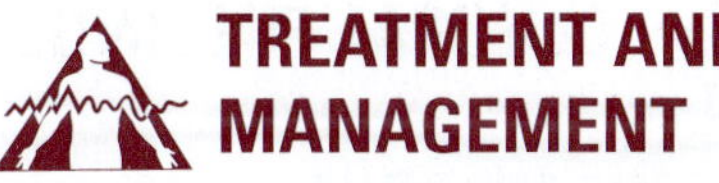

TREATMENT AND MANAGEMENT

- Sodium replacement
- Hypertonic sodium when severe
- Raise serum sodium no more than 1–2 mEq/L/h

TREATMENT MONITORING

- Serum electrolytes

COMPLICATIONS

- Permanent brain damage

PROGNOSIS

- Excellent

PREVENTION

- Judicious IV administration

RESOURCES

REFERENCES

- Adrogue HJ et al. Hyponatremia. *N Engl J Med.* 2000;342:1581.

Hypoparathyroidism

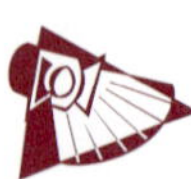

ESSENTIAL FEATURES

- Paresthesias, muscle cramps, carpopedal spasm, laryngeal stridor, convulsions, malaise, muscle and abdominal cramps, tetany, urinary frequency, lethargy, anxiety, psychoneurosis, depression, and psychosis
- History of central neck (thyroid, parathyroid, or laryngeal) resection
- Positive Chvostek and Trousseau signs
- Brittle and atrophied nails, defective teeth, cataracts
- Hypocalcemia and hyperphosphatemia, low or absent urinary calcium, low or absent circulating parathyroid hormone (PTH)
- Calcification of basal ganglia, cartilage, and arteries as seen on x-ray

EPIDEMIOLOGY

- Although uncommon, occurs most often as a complication of thyroid surgery (especially for malignancy or recurrent goiter)
- Idiopathic hypoparathyroidism is an autoimmune process and can be associated with autoimmune adrenocortical insufficiency
- Rare, but possible, after radioiodine therapy for hyperthyroidism
- Neonatal tetany associated with maternal hyperparathyroidism

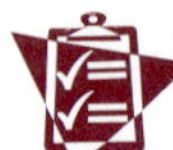

CLINICAL FINDINGS

SYMPTOMS AND SIGNS

- Tetany
- Positive Chvostek or Trousseau signs (or both)
- Paresthesias, circumoral numbness, muscle cramps, irritability, carpopedal spasm, convulsions, opisthotonos, and marked anxiety
- Dry skin, brittle nails, spotty alopecia

LABORATORY FINDINGS

- Low serum calcium
- Elevated serum phosphate
- Low urinary calcium
- Low or absent urinary phosphate
- Low serum PTH
- Low urine hydroxyproline

IMAGING FINDINGS

- Calcification of the basal ganglia, arteries, and external ear

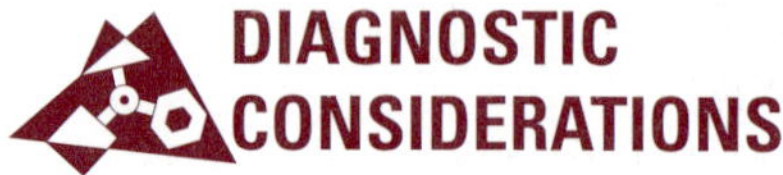

DIAGNOSTIC CONSIDERATIONS

- Most postoperative hypocalcemia is transient

RULE OUT

- Tetany from hyperventilation and alkalosis
- Hypocalcemia from remineralization of bones after therapy for hyperparathyroidism ("hungry bones")
- Hypocalcemia from intestinal malabsorption or renal insufficiency
- Pseudohypoparathyroidsim (X-linked syndrome with defective renal adenylyl cyclase system; associated with round face, thick body, stubby fingers, mental deficiency, and x-ray evidence of calcifications; may have associated thyroid or ovarian dysfunction; patients do not respond with phosphaturia to PTH challenge; serum concentrations of PTH are increased; can be controlled with low dose vitamin D)
- Pseudopseudohypoparathyroidism (thought to be common genetic defect as pseudohypoparathyroidism, but more mild; hypocalcemia only brought out during periods of stress such as pregnancy and rapid growth)

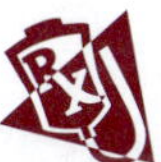

WORK-UP

- History and physical exam
- Special note of prior neck surgery
- Serum and urine tests for calcium, phosphate, and PTH

WHEN TO ADMIT

- In the presence of acute hypoparathyroid tetany

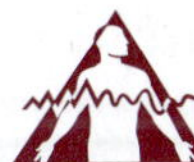

TREATMENT AND MANAGEMENT

- Aim of treatment is to raise serum calcium levels, to bring the patient out of tetany (if present), and to lower serum phosphate levels (to prevent metastatic calcification)
- Treatment is medical (unless parathyroid tissue was cryopreserved at the time of neck operation)

MEDICATIONS

- Oral calcium (calcium, lactate, or carbonate)
- Calcitriol
- IV calcium gluconate for acute tetany (6 g mixed in 500 mL DSW infused at 1 mL/kg/h)
- Magnesium sulfate if also hypomagnesemic
- Phosphorous limited diet, and possibly phosphate binders such as aluminum hydroxide gel

TREATMENT MONITORING

- Symptomatic monitoring
- Serum calcium level

PROGNOSIS

- If postoperative hypocalcemia lasts longer than 2–3 weeks, or if calcitriol therapy is required, the hypoparathyroidism may be permanent

PREVENTION

- Careful identification and protection of parathyroid glands at neck operation

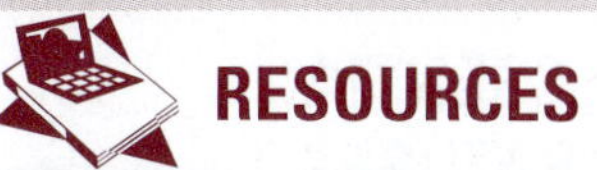

RESOURCES

REFERENCES

- Bergenfelz A et al. Functional recovery of the parathyroid glands after surgery for primary hyperparathyroidism. *Surgery.* 1994;116:827.
- Lebowitz MR et al. Hypocalcemia. *Semin Nephrol.* 1992;12:146.

Hypophosphatemia

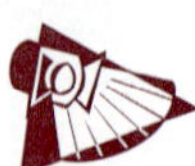

ESSENTIAL FEATURES

- Decreased serum phosphorus

EPIDEMIOLOGY

- Poor dietary intake (especially in alcoholics)
- Hyperparathyroidism
- Phosphate-binding antacid administration
- Refeeding with total parenteral nutrition with insufficient phosphate supplement

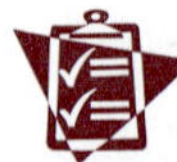

CLINICAL FINDINGS

SYMPTOMS AND SIGNS

- Lassitude, weakness and fatigue may develop with levels below 1 mg/dL
- Severe neuromuscular manifestations can include convulsions and death
- Impaired cardiac contractility and rhabdomyolysis with ongoing severe hypophosphatemia

LABORATORY FINDINGS

- Decreased serum phosphorus
- Anemia from RBC hemolysis

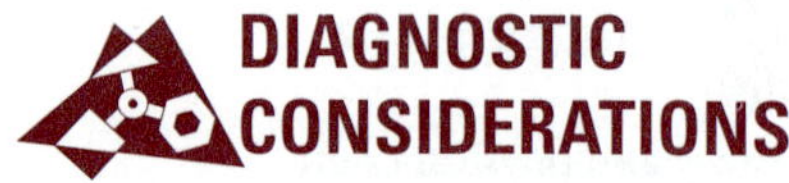

DIAGNOSTIC CONSIDERATIONS

- In perioperative or post-trauma setting, almost always associated with poor nutrition

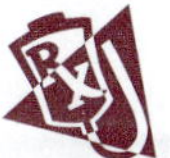

WORK-UP

- Serum electrolytes
- Nutritional assessment

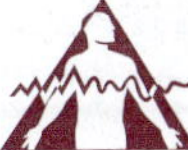

TREATMENT AND MANAGEMENT

- Phosphate replenishment
- Nutritional support

TREATMENT MONITORING

- Serum electrolytes

PROGNOSIS

- Excellent

RESOURCES

REFERENCES

- Subramainan R, Khardori R. Severe hypophosphatemia. Pathophysiologic implications, clinical presentations and treatment. *Medicine.* 2000;79:1.
- Kapoor M, Chan GZ. Fluid and electrolyte abnormalities. *Critical Care Clin.* 2001;17:503.

Hypoplastic Left Heart Syndrome

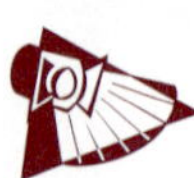

ESSENTIAL FEATURES

- An obstructive congenital heart lesion
- Spectrum of underdevelopment of left-sided structures (mitral and aortic valves, left ventricle, ascending aorta, and arch)
- Commonly associated with the following:
  - Mitral and aortic valve atresia
  - LV hypoplasia
  - Ascending aorta measures 2–3.5 mm
- Coronary arteries may be stenotic
- Other common anomalies:
  - Ventricular septal defect
  - Double-outlet right ventricle
- 25% may have CNS anomalites
- Uniformly fatal without operative treatment
- Entire cardiac output delivered from right heart, maintaining oxygenation through pulmonary flow and systemic oxygen delivery
- Ductus closure/inadequate interarterial communication worsens disease

EPIDEMIOLOGY

- 5–7% of congenital cardiac anomalies
- Accounts for 25% of cardiac mortality in first few days of life

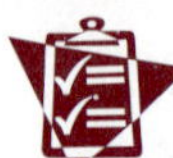

CLINICAL FINDINGS

SYMPTOMS AND SIGNS

- With closure of ductus: Respiratory failure, hemodynamic failure, acidosis, multisystem organ failure

IMAGING FINDINGS

- Echocardiography: Sufficient to make diagnosis

WHEN TO REFER

- These patients should be referred to tertiary center with expertise

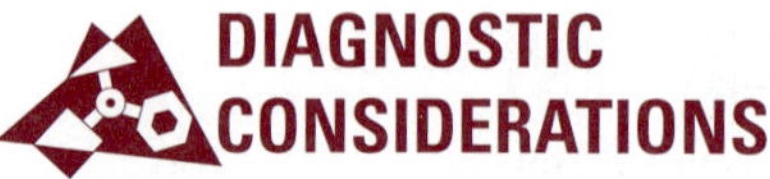

DIAGNOSTIC CONSIDERATIONS

- Evaluate for other cardiac and extracardiac anomalies

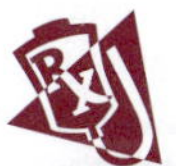

WORK-UP

- Physical exam
- Echocardiography

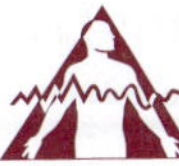

TREATMENT AND MANAGEMENT

- Initial management: Mechanical ventilation, fluid, pressor and HCO_3 resuscitation
- Maintain ductal patency with PGE_1
- If inadequate mixing: Balloon atrial septostomy

SURGERY

- 2 operative choices:
  1. Staged procedure: Norwood, followed by Glenn or hemi-Fontan at 6–8 mos, followed by Fontan at 1–1.5 yrs
  2. Cardiac transplantation

Indications

- Surgical intervention necessary for survival

TREATMENT MONITORING

- Frequent echocardiography and angiography

PROGNOSIS

- Improved recently: 5-year survival, 40–70%
- Most deaths occur soon after first stage

RESOURCES

REFERENCES

- Weldner PW et al. The Norwood operation and subsequent Fontan operation in infants with complex congenital heart disease. *J Thorac Cardiovasc Surg.* 1995;109:654.

Hypothermia, Accidental

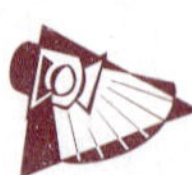

ESSENTIAL FEATURES

- Uncontrolled lowering of core body temperature below 35 °C by exposure to cold
- EtOH facilitates induction of hypothermia by producing sedation (inhibiting shivering) and cutaneous dilation
- Heart is most sensitive organ to cooling and is subject to ventricular fibrillation or asystole when temperature drops to 21–24 °C

EPIDEMIOLOGY

- Elderly patients living alone in inadequately heated homes
- Alcoholics exposed to the cold during a binge
- People engaged in winter sports
- People lost in cold weather
- Predisposing diseases include:
  - Myxedema
  - Hypopituitarism
  - Adrenal insufficiency
  - Cerebral vascular insufficiency
  - Mental impairment
  - Cardiovascular disorders

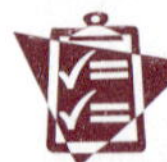

CLINICAL FINDINGS

SYMPTOMS AND SIGNS

- Mentally depressed (somnolent, stuporous, or comatose)
- Cold
- Pale or cyanotic
- Shivering absent below 32 °C
- Slow and shallow respirations
- Usually normotensive and bradycardic
- At temperatures < 32 °C, patients may appear to be dead
- Frostbitten or frozen extremities

LABORATORY FINDINGS

- Severe hypoglycemia is common
- Elevated serum amylase in 50%
- Elevations of aspartate aminotransferase (AST), lactic dehydrogenase (LDH), and creatine kinase (CK) enzymes
- ECG shows PR lengthening, pathognomonic J wave at junction of the QRS and ST segment

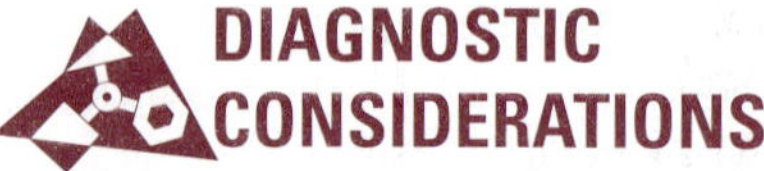

DIAGNOSTIC CONSIDERATIONS

- Patients should never be considered dead until all measures for resuscitation have failed
- Mild hypothermia (32–35 °C) can be treated by passive rewarming with continuous monitoring of rectal or esophageal temperatures
- Active rewarming is indicated for temperatures below 32 °C, cardiovascular instability, or failure of passive rewarming
- Methods for rewarming include:
  - Immersion in warm water
  - Inhalation of heated air
  - Pleural and peritoneal lavage
  - Extracorporeal blood warming

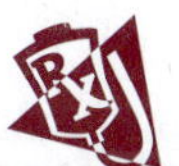

WORK-UP

- Physical exam
- Temperature
- ECG
- Central venous pressure and pulmonary capillary wedge pressure should be kept below 12–14 cm H_20 to minimize edema

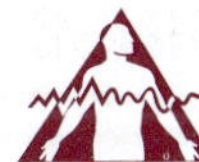

TREATMENT AND MANAGEMENT

- Immersion in warm water (40–42 °C) will raise body temperature 1–2 °C per hour
- Pleural irrigation via 2 right thoracostomy tubes (anterior, posterior) with warm saline (40–42 °C)
- Peritoneal lavage involves giving warm (40–45 °C) crystalloid solutions at 6 L/h which will raise temperature 2–4 °C per hour
- Partial cardiopulmonary bypass (CPB) is the most efficient technique and is indicated for ventricular fibrillation, severe hypothermia, or frozen extremities
- Partial CPB with flows of 6–7 L/min can raise core temperature 1–2 °C every 3–5 minutes
- Endotracheal intubation and mechanical ventilation are often necessary
- Bretylium tosylate 10 mg/kg is best drug for ventricular fibrillation
- Antibiotics are often indicated for pneumonitis
- Hypoglycemia should be treated with IV D50

TREATMENT MONITORING

- Continuous temperature monitoring
- Careful observation for unsuspected disease masked by hypothermia

COMPLICATIONS

- Increased capillary permeability may lead to generalized and pulmonary edema upon rewarming
- Coagulopathies (including disseminated intravascular coagulation) are seen occasionally
- Pancreatitis and acute renal failure (ARF) common in < 32 °C
- Failure to respond to treatment should suggest adrenal insufficiency

PROGNOSIS

- Survival in 50% of patients when core temperature below 32.2 °C
- Coexisting disease (stroke, myocardial infarction, cancer) increase mortality to 75% or more
- Death may be result of pneumonitis, heart failure, or ARF

RESOURCES

REFERENCES

- Farstad M et al. Recovering from accidental hypothermia by extracorporeal circulation: a retrospective study. *Eur J Cardiothorac Surg.* 2001;20:58.
- Peng RY, Bongard FS. Hypothermia in trauma patients. *J Am Coll Surg.* 1999;188:685.

Hypovolemic Shock

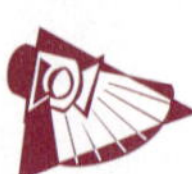

ESSENTIAL FEATURES

- Inadequate circulating blood volume
- Inadequate end organ perfusion

EPIDEMIOLOGY

- Hemorrhage
- Protracted vomiting
- Protracted diarrhea
- Fluid sequestration in gut lumen
- Loss of plasma into tissues (burns, trauma)

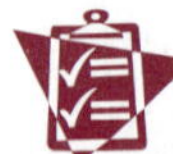

CLINICAL FINDINGS

SYMPTOMS AND SIGNS

- Postural hypotension
- Cutaneous vasoconstriction
- Sweating
- Neck vein collapse
- Concentrated urine
- Oliguria (< 0.5 mL/kg/h in adult)
- Decreasing Hct with fluid administration
- Delayed capillary refill (> 2 seconds)
- Thirst
- Hypotension (degree varies with severity of volume loss)
- Confusion, restlessness, lethargy
- Irregular heart rate
- Little correlation between heart rate and severity of hypovolemia

LABORATORY FINDINGS

- Concentrated urine
- Initial Hct is of no value in acute blood loss
- ST depression, Q waves

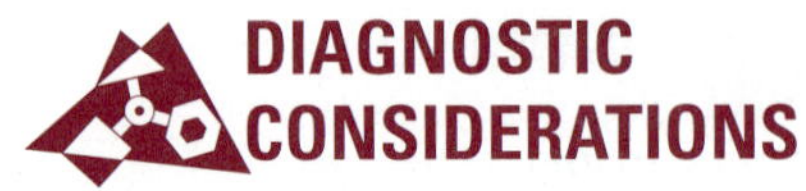

DIAGNOSTIC CONSIDERATIONS

RULE OUT

- Intoxication
- Hypoglycemia

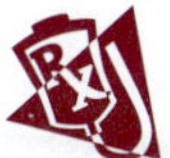

WORK-UP

- Physical exam/trauma work-up
- Serial Hct
- ABG measurements
- UA
- Blood glucose

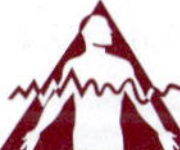

TREATMENT AND MANAGEMENT

- Establish airway
- Nasal oxygen at minimum
- Control external hemorrhage
- Preparations for surgery for patients with internal bleeding
- Large bore venous catheters
- 2 L crystalloid (normal saline or lactated Ringer's solution) wide open for initial resuscitation of severe shock
- Third liter of crystalloid over 10 min should be adequate in patients in whom bleeding has been controlled
- In general, blood should be withheld until bleeding has been controlled
- Blood should be started in those who remain unstable after 3 L of crystalloid

SURGERY

Indications

- Evidence of internal bleeding
- Unstable vitals despite resuscitation
- Ongoing fluid requirements

TREATMENT MONITORING

- Blood pressure monitoring
- Urinary output
- ECG

PROGNOSIS

- Varies with etiology and severity

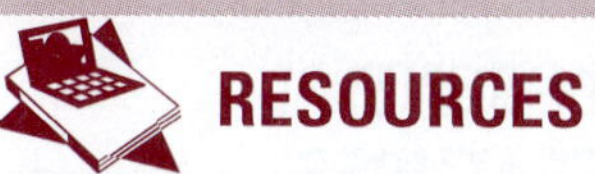

RESOURCES

REFERENCES

- Chang MC et al. Redefining cardiovascular performance during resuscitation: ventricular stroke work, power, and the pressure-volume diagram. *J Trauma.* 1998;45:470.
- Ventilation with lower tidal volumes as compared with traditional tidal volumes for acute lung injury and the acute respiratory distress syndrome. Acute Respiratory Distress Syndrome Network. *N Engl J Med.* 2000;342:1301.
- Velmahos GC et al. Endpoints of resuscitation of critically injured patients: normal or supranormal? A prospective randomized trial. *Ann Surg.* 2000;232:409.

Ileus

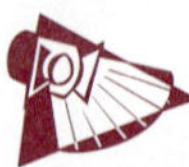

ESSENTIAL FEATURES

- Adynamic ileus is a functional obstruction due to dysmotility of the bowel
- Distinguished from postoperative ileus following abdominal surgery (distinction is based on time since operation and clinical circumstances)
- May present with signs and symptoms of bowel obstruction
- Must differentiate ileus from mechanical bowel obstruction
- Thought to occur as a result of dysfunction due to a combination of neural, hormonal, and metabolic factors
- Occurs with intra-abdominal processes such as pancreatitis, abscess, hemorrhage, peritonitis
- Sympathetic hyperactivity is thought to be a potential contributing factor
- Diagnosis of exclusion

EPIDEMIOLOGY

- Common following abdominal surgery, trauma
- May be induced by medication:
  - Narcotics
  - Psychotropic
  - Anticholinergics
- May result from metabolic/electrolyte abnormalities such as hypokalemia and hypercalcemia or hypocalcemia and hypomagnesemia, uremia, diabetic ketoacidosis

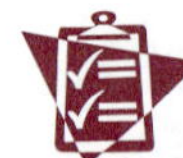

CLINICAL FINDINGS

SYMPTOMS AND SIGNS

- Abdominal tenderness
- Abdominal distention
- Hypoactive to absent bowel sounds
- Absence of flatus or passage of stool

LABORATORY FINDINGS

- Nonspecific
- May have electrolyte derangements (hypokalemia, hyponatremia)

IMAGING FINDINGS

- **Abdominal x-ray**
  - Dilated loops of bowel with air throughout the GI tract
  - No evidence of cut off or transition point suggesting mechanical obstruction
  - Air-fluid levels may or may not be present

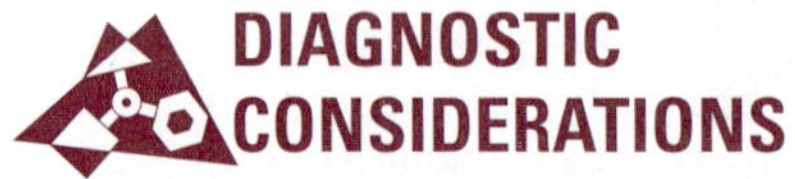

DIAGNOSTIC CONSIDERATIONS

- Mechanical bowel obstruction (eg, neoplasm, hernia, adhesions)

RULE OUT

- Mechanical causes of bowel obstruction

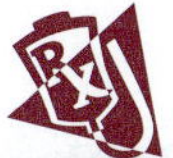

WORK-UP

- History and physical exam
- Digital rectal exam
- History of trauma, recent surgery
- Review medications
- Draw serum chemistry, CBC count, thyroid function tests
- Must rule out mechanical obstruction
- Diagnosis of exclusion
- Obtain upright abdominal and chest films
- Obtain contrast enema or CT scan to rule out mechanical etiology as well as evaluate for intra-abdominal pathology contributing to ileus

WHEN TO ADMIT

- Ileus is a diagnosis of exclusion requiring mechanical sources to be ruled out as a cause of obstruction, which likely requires admission
- Dehydration

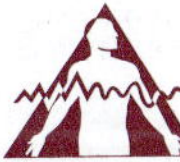

TREATMENT AND MANAGEMENT

- Treatment is conservative
- NPO
- NG decompression
- IV hydration
- Correct electrolyte abnormalities
- Discontinue or substitute for narcotic pain medications or psychotropic medications if possible

SURGERY

Indications

- Treatment of ileus is nonoperative
- Conditions contributing to ileus such as abscesses or hemorrhage may require operative intervention

MEDICATIONS

- Prokinetic agents such as metoclopramide and erythromycin

TREATMENT MONITORING

- Repeat physical exam
- Failure of ileus to resolve after a prolonged period of time may warrant repeat GI contrast study and/or CT scan

COMPLICATIONS

- Dehydration
- Malnutrition

PROGNOSIS

- Time and correction of underlying contributing factors should result in resolution of ileus

PREVENTION

- Measures to prevent prolongation of ileus include meticulous technique in the operating room, minimal use of narcotics for analgesia, correction of electrolyte or metabolic imbalances, and early recognition of septic complications

RESOURCES

REFERENCES

- Shelton AA et al. Small Intestine. In: Way LW, Doherty GM (editors). *Current Surgical Diagnosis & Treatment,* 11e. New York: McGraw-Hill; 2003:683–687.

Iliac Aneurysms

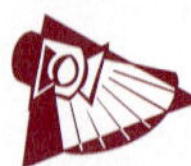

ESSENTIAL FEATURES

- Occur with abdominal aortic aneurysms (AAA) in 20%
- Natural history of these aneurysms unknown
- Rupture occurs frequently but believed to be rare in aneurysms < 3 cm
  - Size most important determinant of rupture risk

EPIDEMIOLOGY

- Isolated iliac aneurysms rare
- Occurs in < 1% of population over age 50
- Solitary iliac aneurysms of common iliac artery, 70% of cases; of internal iliac, 20% of cases; of external iliac, 10% of cases

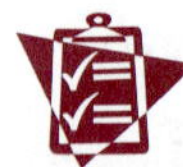

CLINICAL FINDINGS

SYMPTOMS AND SIGNS

- 50% of patients are symptomatic
  - Compression or erosion into surrounding structures
  - Rupture
- Sepsis from ureteral obstruction causing pyelonephritis
- Erosion or rupture into ureter or bladder can cause hematuria, possibly massive
- Neurologic symptoms
  - Compression of femoral, obturator, sciatic nerves
- Massive leg swelling
  - Rupture of iliac artery into iliac vein causing AV fistula
- Most symptomatic iliac aneurysms palpable on abdominal or rectal exam
- Perianal ecchymosis and decreased sphincter tone seen in cases of rupture

IMAGING FINDINGS

- US, CT scan, MRI, arteriography can diagnose
- US depth of arteries in pelvis, overlying intestinal gas may limit study
- CT scan and MRI excellent
- Arteriography may look normal because of mural thrombus; done to evaluate pelvic circulation prior to repair

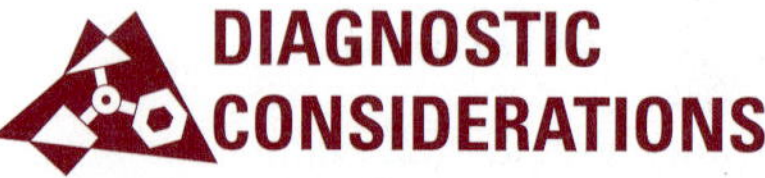

DIAGNOSTIC CONSIDERATIONS

- Evaluate for other sites of peripheral aneurysms

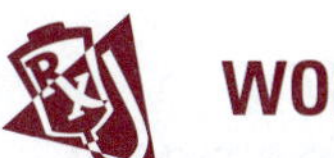

WORK-UP

- CT scan and MRI
- Arteriography

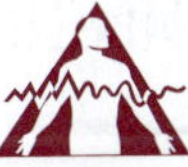

TREATMENT AND MANAGEMENT

- **Solitary aneurysms:**
  - Retroperitoneal approach
  - Hypogastric artery can be safely ligated if contralateral artery is normal
  - If ipsilateral hypogastric aneurysmal, open saci and ligate branches
- **Bilateral common iliac artery aneurysm:**
  - Bifurcated interposition graft
- Currently, many are being treated with endovascular repair

SURGERY

Indications

- Iliac aneurysms > 3 cm with good operative risk, consider repair

RESOURCES

REFERENCES

- Parsons RE et al. Midterm results of endovascular stented grafts for the treatment of isolated iliac artery aneurysms. *J Vasc Surg.* 1999;30:915.
- Sahgal A et al. Diameter changes in isolated iliac artery aneurysms 1 to 6 years after endovascular graft repair. *J Vasc Surg.* 2001;33:289.

Immune Thrombocytopenia Purpura (ITP)

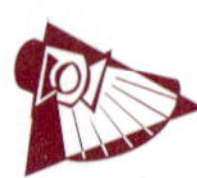

ESSENTIAL FEATURES

- Autoimmune destruction of platelets
- Petechiae, ecchymoses, epistaxis, easy bruising
- No splenomegaly
- Decreased platelet count, prolonged bleeding time, poor clot retraction, normal coagulation time

EPIDEMIOLOGY

- The pathogenesis involves a circulating antiplatelet IgG autoantibody; the spleen is both the site of platelet destruction and a significant source of autoantibody production
- Idiopathic or secondary to the following:
  - Lymphoproliferative disorder
  - Drugs or toxins
  - Bacterial or viral infection (especially in children)
  - Systemic lupus erythematosus
  - Other conditions
- The acute form is most common in children, usually occurring before age 8, and often begins 1–3 weeks after a viral upper respiratory tract illness
- The chronic form, which may start at any age, is more common in women

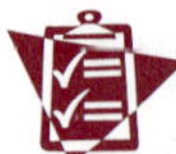

CLINICAL FINDINGS

SYMPTOMS AND SIGNS

- Ecchymoses or showers of petechiae
- Bleeding gums
- Vaginal bleeding
- GI bleeding
- Hematuria

LABORATORY FINDINGS

- Platelet count < 100,000/μL
- Bone marrow shows increased numbers of large megakaryocytes
- Bleeding time is prolonged
- Partial thromboplastin time, prothrombin time, and coagulation time are normal
- Iron deficiency anemia as a result of bleeding

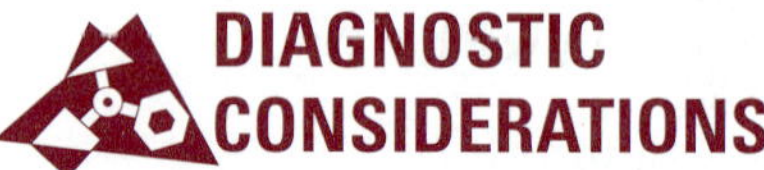

DIAGNOSTIC CONSIDERATIONS

- Symptoms develop when platelet count is < 50,000/μL
- Recurrent thrombocytopenia after splenectomy should be evaluated by imaging with indium-labeled platelets to identify accessory spleens
- Chronic ITP characterized by:
  - An insidious onset
  - A history of easy bruisability and menorrhagia
  - Showers of petechiae, especially over pressure areas
  - Cyclic remissions and exacerbations, which may continue for several years
- Specific determinations of antiplatelet antibody titers may aid in diagnosis

RULE OUT

- Other causes of nonimmunologic thrombocytopenia:
  - Leukemia
  - Aplastic anemia
  - Macroglobulinemia
- Thrombocytopenia and purpura may be caused by:
  - Ineffective thrombocytopoiesis (pernicious anemia)
  - Nonimmune platelet destruction (septicemia, disseminated intravascular coagulation, hypersplenism)

Immune Thrombocytopenia Purpura (ITP)

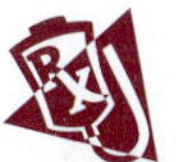

WORK-UP

- Platelet count
- Bone marrow biopsy
- Peripheral blood smear
- Antiplatelet autoantibody titers if diagnosis remains unclear

WHEN TO ADMIT

- Severe thrombocytopenia with active bleeding

WHEN TO REFER

- All patients should be managed in conjunction with a hematologist

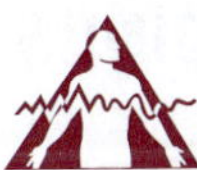

TREATMENT AND MANAGEMENT

- Patients with mild or no symptoms need no specific therapy
- Splenectomy is most effective therapy
- No platelet transfusions unless actively bleeding

SURGERY

Indications

- Failure to respond to corticosteroids
- Relapse after initial remission on corticosteroids
- Corticosteroid dependence

MEDICATIONS

- Corticosteroids
- Intravenous immunoglobulin (IVIG) for temporary treatment
- Azathioprine, vincristine

TREATMENT MONITORING

- Platelet count

COMPLICATIONS

- Bleeding

PROGNOSIS

- **Splenectomy:** Sustained remission in 60–90% of patients
- **Corticosteroids:** Response in 70–80%; sustained remissions in 20% of adults

RESOURCES

REFERENCES

- George JN et al. Idiopathic thrombocytopenic purpura: diagnosis and management. *Am J Med Sci.* 1998;316:87.
- Lilleyman JS. Management of childhood idiopathic thrombocytopenic purpura. *Br J Haematol.* 1999;105:871.

Imperforate Anus

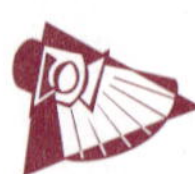

ESSENTIAL FEATURES

- **High imperforate anus:** Above the striated muscle complex or levator ani
- **Low imperforate anus:** Rectal pouch descending into striated muscle complex and therefore have more favorable prognosis following reconstruction
- Male patients most commonly have low imperforate anus with a perineal fistula or high anorectal agenesis with a rectoprostatic urethral fistula
- Female patients most commonly have low imperforate anus and fistula from the blind-ending rectal pouch to perineal body or vaginal vestibule
- 70% associated with other abnormalities such as the VACTERL abnormalities
  - **V**ertebral abnormalities
  - **A**nal atresia
  - **C**ardiac abnormalities
  - **T**racheoesophageal fistula and/or esophageal atresia
  - **R**enal agenesis and dysplasia
  - **L**imb (defects)

EPIDEMIOLOGY

- 1/2500–1/5000 births
- High imperforate anus 2-fold more common in males

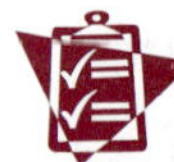

CLINICAL FINDINGS

SYMPTOMS AND SIGNS

- Distended abdomen
- Bilious emesis
- Irritability
- Failure to pass meconium
- Fecaluria (if rectovesicular or rectourethral fistula)
- **High imperforate anus:** Absence of dimple or absence of gluteal fold
- **Low imperforate anus:**
  - Presence of anal membrane, dimple, or fold (usually)
  - External fistula to perineum or vestibule

IMAGING FINDINGS

- **Plain lateral pelvic film:** Shows gas filled rectal stump and relative location
- **Pelvic US:** Shows relation of rectal stump to striated muscle complex
- **CT or MRI:** Delineates the relation between the rectal stump and the striated muscle complex

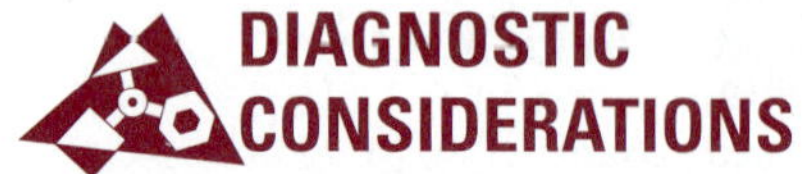

DIAGNOSTIC CONSIDERATIONS

- Differentiating between low and high imperforate anus

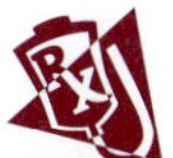

WORK-UP

- History and physical exam
- Abdominal pelvic x-ray
- Pelvic US
- Voiding cystourethrogram
- Echocardiogram
- Spinal MRI or US
- Renal US
- Upper GI

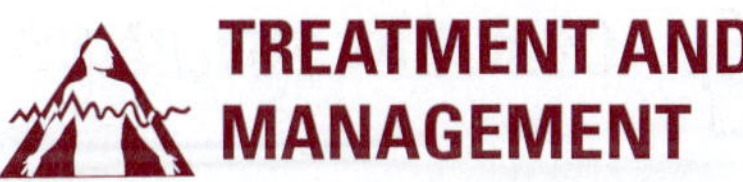

TREATMENT AND MANAGEMENT

SURGERY

- **Low imperforate anus:** Cutback anoplasty (circumferential mobilization of anterior fistula and transposition to center of external anal sphincter)
- **High imperforate anus:** Diverting colostomy until at least 12 months of age followed by (most commonly) posterior sagittal anorectoplasty and closure of rectourinary fistula

COMPLICATIONS

- Leak or stricture, 5–10%
- 30–80% have minimal problems with continence, remainder with significant problems with continence

PROGNOSIS

- 18.7% mortality secondary to other abnormalities

RESOURCES

REFERENCES

- Albanese CT et al. Pediatric Surgery. In: Way LW, Doherty GM (editors). *Current Surgical Diagnosis & Treatment,* 11e. New York: McGraw-Hill; 2003:1324–1327.

Incisional (Ventral) Hernia

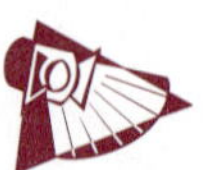

ESSENTIAL FEATURES

- Bulge elicited by the Valsalva maneuver immediately over or adjacent to a laparotomy incision
- Main complaint associated with ventral hernias is the cosmetic appearance
- Patients may note discomfort or a heaviness sensation associated with the hernia bulge
- Small incisional hernia defects appear to be most dangerous and are more commonly associated with an incarcerated presentation
- The fascial defects progressively increase in size and may result in loss of abdominal domain
- Classification of incisional hernias:
  - **Reducible:** Visceral contents of the hernia sac able to retract into the abdominal cavity
  - **Incarcerated:** Visceral contents cannot be returned to the abdominal cavity
  - **Strangulated:** Incarcerated hernia where the blood flow to the entrapped viscera is compromised

EPIDEMIOLOGY

- 11% of all laparotomies result in incisional hernia formation
- Incidence of this iatrogenic hernia is not diminishing despite awareness of the many causative factors
- Highest incidence associated with midline and transverse incisions

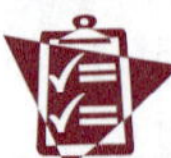

CLINICAL FINDINGS

SYMPTOMS AND SIGNS

- Asymptomatic bulge associated with prior laparotomy incision most common presentation
- Patients may complain of a discomfort, fullness or heaviness associated with the hernia bulge
- The fascial defects progressively increase in size
- Hernia bulge may or may not be reducible
- Incarcerated hernias are exquisitely painful to palpation
- Patients with a strangulated hernia may present with an acute abdomen
- Small bowel obstructive symptoms may be present with incarcerated incisional hernias

IMAGING FINDINGS

- Plain films are typically normal
- US can be used to detect fascial defects as well as differentiate between an incarcerated incisional hernia and a solid mass
- Abdominal pelvic CT scan is excellent in the detection of incisional hernias and characterization of involved viscera
  - CT is particularly useful in diagnosing acute incarceration in morbidly obese patients in whom physical exam is difficult and unreliable

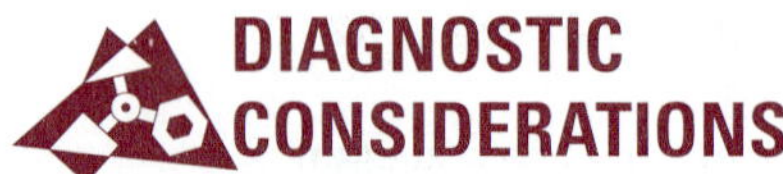

DIAGNOSTIC CONSIDERATIONS

- Diastasis recti
- Stitch granuloma
- Epigastric hernia
- Incisional metastasis
- Desmoid tumor
- Parastomal hernia
- Chronic incisional seroma

RULE OUT

- Incarcerated or strangulated hernia
- Incisional metastasis or other primary abdominal wall neoplasm

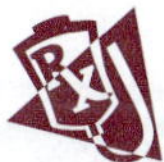

WORK-UP

- Thorough history and physical exam usually will accurately diagnosis incisional hernia
- Abdominal CT scan when diagnosis is in doubt or to anatomically define the adjacent intestinal viscera in complicated cases

WHEN TO ADMIT

- Depends on the magnitude of repair and comorbidities
  - Patients may require postoperative hospitalization

WHEN TO REFER

- Plastic surgery referral may be advantageous in instances where alloplastic reconstruction contraindicated:
  - Infected wound
  - Fistula present
  - No omentum present to bridge between bowel and mesh

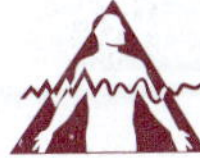

TREATMENT AND MANAGEMENT

- Minimize or eliminate medications deleterious to wound healing, such as corticosteroids
- Weight loss in obese patients
- Preoperative pulmonary conditioning in patients with large hernias who smoke or are chronically debilitated
- Consider native tissue reconstruction in complex abdominal wall defects

SURGERY

- Repair can be performed laparoscopically or open

Indications

- Incisional hernias should be fixed in all patients without medical contraindications
- Laparoscopic repair is preferred for smaller primary defects

Contraindications

- Patients with significant pulmonary disease (the major complication following large incisional hernia formation is respiratory failure)
- Medically unfit for large laparotomy

TREATMENT MONITORING

- Clinical evidence of recurrence

COMPLICATIONS

- Postoperative wound or mesh infection
- Respiratory failure and/or abdominal compartment syndrome (following repair of large hernia defects)
- Recurrence

PROGNOSIS

- Recurrence rate following mesh repair is > 20%
- Recurrence rate following suture repair is > 40% for large hernias
- Recurrence rates increase with each subsequent incisional hernia repair

RESOURCES

REFERENCES

- Holzman MD et al. Laparoscopic ventral and incisional hernioplasty. *Surg Endosc.* 1997;11:32.
- Toy FK et al. Prospective, multicenter study of laparoscopic ventral hernioplasty: preliminary results. *Surg Endosc.* 1998;12:955.

Inguinal Hernia

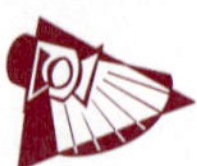

ESSENTIAL FEATURES

- Groin bulge elicited with the Valsalva maneuver
- Types of inguinal hernias
  - **Indirect:** Patent processus vaginalis extension lateral to the inferior epigastrics in the anterior-medial position of the spermatic cord
  - **Direct:** Developed weakness in the abdominal wall located at Hesselbach triangle (inguinal ligament inferiorly, lateral edge of the rectus medially, and the inferior epigastric vessels superior-laterally)
  - **Pantaloon hernia** is a combined direct and indirect inguinal hernia
- Classification of hernias
  - **Reducible:** Visceral contents of the hernia sac able to retract into the abdominal cavity
  - **Incarcerated:** Visceral contents cannot be returned to the abdominal cavity
  - **Strangulated:** Incarcerated inguinal hernia where the blood flow to the entrapped viscera is compromised
  - **Sliding:** Abdominal viscera present in hernia sac; on the left, most commonly the sigmoid colon and bladder, and on the right, most commonly the cecum and bladder

EPIDEMIOLOGY

- 5–10% of the world population will develop an inguinal hernia in their lifetime
- Premature infants most likely to develop inguinal hernia (> 10%)
- Nearly all hernias in infants, children, and young adults are indirect
- Indirect inguinal hernias develop more commonly on the right
- Acute complications from inguinal hernias are more likely to develop in infants and children
- Most common etiology of small bowel obstruction in children is incarcerated inguinal hernia
- Second most common cause of small bowel obstruction in adults is incarcerated inguinal hernia

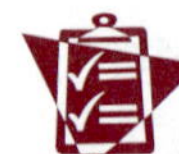

CLINICAL FINDINGS

SYMPTOMS AND SIGNS

- Asymptomatic inguinal bulge most common symptom
- Exam of the groin reveals a bulge adjacent to the ipsilateral pubic tubercle that may extend into the scrotum
- The hernia bulge may or may not be reducible
- Patients may complain of a fullness or dragging sensation
- As a hernia enlarges, it is likely to produce a sense of discomfort that may radiate into the ipsilateral groin
- Sharp ilio-inguinal groin pain without a detectable groin bulge is most commonly a strained groin muscle
- Incarcerated/strangulated inguinal hernia is exquisitely painful
- Coughing or straining will help demonstrate small hernias
- Small bowel obstruction symptoms (nausea, vomiting, abdominal distention) may be present with incarcerated inguinal hernias

IMAGING FINDINGS

- US, although rarely needed, can verify the presence of a hernia sac and reliably differentiate between a hernia, solid cord mass, hydrocele, or lymphadenopathy

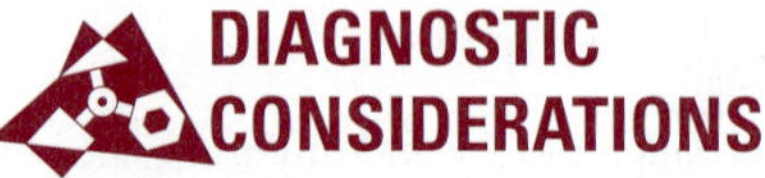

DIAGNOSTIC CONSIDERATIONS

- Femoral hernia
- Hydrocele
- Cord mass
- Strained groin muscle
- Epididymitis
- Inguinal lymphadenopathy
- Varicocele
- Undescended testes

RULE OUT

- Strained groin muscle (chronic groin pain commonly develops in these patients following operative intervention)

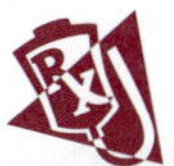

WORK-UP

- Physical exam usually all that is required to accurately diagnose inguinal hernia
- In equivocal cases, US may be helpful

WHEN TO ADMIT

- Uncomplicated inguinal hernia management can be performed as an outpatient
- Indications for admission include:
  - Acute hernia incarceration
  - Clinical evidence of strangulation
  - Associated small bowel obstruction

WHEN TO REFER

- Neonatal and young pediatric hernia repairs performed with less morbidity by experienced pediatric surgeons

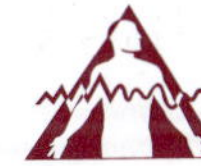

TREATMENT AND MANAGEMENT

- Inguinal hernias should be surgically repaired unless there are specific contraindications

SURGERY

- Several successful approaches available including native tissue or prosthetic repair
- Both open and laparoscopic approaches are commonly used

Indications

- Incarcerated or strangulated hernias warrant immediate repair
- Uncomplicated inguinal hernias can be repaired electively as an outpatient

Contraindications

- Cirrhosis with uncontrolled ascites and indirect hernia is relative contraindication

TREATMENT MONITORING

- Physical exam to detect wound/prosthetic infection or hernia recurrence

COMPLICATIONS

- Strangulated inguinal hernia with visceral necrosis
- Progressive enlargement of the hernia defect with loss of abdominal domain in the case of giant inguinal-scrotal hernias
- Recurrence
- Damage to vas deferens
- Ischemic orchitis

PROGNOSIS

- Recurrence rates < 5% in most series

RESOURCES

REFERENCES

- Amid PK et al. Open "tension-free" repair of inguinal hernias: the Lichtenstein technique. *Eur J Surg.* 1996;162:447.
- Kark AE et al. 3175 primary inguinal hernia repairs: advantages of ambulatory open mesh repair using local anesthesia. *J Am Coll Surg.* 1998;186:447.
- Liem MSL et al. Comparison of conventional anterior surgery and laparoscopic surgery for inguinal hernia repair. *N Engl J Med.* 1997;336:1541.

Insulinoma

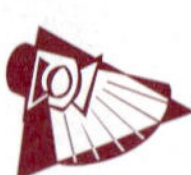

ESSENTIAL FEATURES

- Hypoglycemic symptoms produced by fasting
- Blood glucose below 50 mg/dL during symptomatic episodes
- Relief of symptoms by IV administration of glucose

EPIDEMIOLOGY

- Insulinomas have been reported in all age groups
- 75% are solitary and benign
- 10% are malignant; metastases are usually evident at the time of diagnosis
- Most are sporadic, solitary, benign lesions < 2 cm, occurring in equal distribution throughout the pancreas
- 15% are manifestations of multifocal pancreatic disease—either adenomatosis, nesidioblastosis, or islet cell hyperplasia
- In patients with multiple endocrine neoplasia 1 (MEN 1), insulinomas are typically multifocal

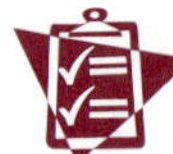

CLINICAL FINDINGS

SYMPTOMS AND SIGNS

- Palpitations
- Sweating
- Tremulousness
- Weight gain
- Bizarre behavior
- Memory lapse
- Unconsciousness

LABORATORY FINDINGS

- Fasting hypoglycemia in the presence of inappropriately high levels of insulin
  - Ratio of plasma insulin:glucose > 0.3 is diagnostic
- Proinsulin levels > 40% suggest a malignant islet cell tumor
- Elevated C-peptide levels exclude self-administration of insulin
- Absent urine sulfonylurea levels exclude oral hypoglycemics

IMAGING FINDINGS

- **High-resolution CT and MRI scans** demonstrate about 40% of tumors
- **Endoscopic US** exam of the pancreas successfully identifies 80–95% of tumors preoperatively
- **Intraoperative US** can identify a pancreatic tumor in nearly all cases and is the gold standard
- More invasive techniques, such as transhepatic portal venous sampling and arteriography with selective calcium infusion are best used for reexploration after unsuccessful intraoperative localization

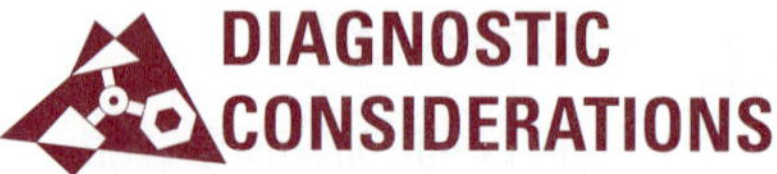

DIAGNOSTIC CONSIDERATIONS

- After diagnosis has been made by demonstration of fasting hypoglycemia and elevated insulin levels, the next step is localization of the insulinoma
- Attempts at preoperative localization should be limited to noninvasive techniques (CT scan or MRI and endoscopic US)

RULE OUT

- Non-islet cell tumors associated with hypoglycemia (hemangiopericytoma, fibrosarcoma, leiomyosarcoma, hepatoma, adrenocortical carcinoma)
- Surreptitious self-administration of insulin
  - Circulating C peptide levels are normal in these patients but elevated in most patients with insulinoma

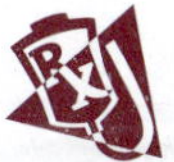

WORK-UP

- Fasting determination of blood glucose and insulin levels; hypoglycemia with elevated insulin level
- Preoperative localization
  - CT scan or MRI
  - Endoscopic US
- Control of hypoglycemia
- Intraoperative US

WHEN TO ADMIT

- Severe, symptomatic hypoglycemia

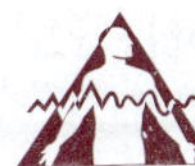

TREATMENT AND MANAGEMENT

- The tumor may be enucleated if it is superficial, or resected as part of a partial pancreatectomy if it is deep-seated
- Resection of metastatic lesions is warranted if technically feasible

SURGERY

Indications

- All patients with technically resectible lesions

MEDICATIONS

- Diazoxide or octreotide to suppress insulin release
- Streptozocin is the best chemotherapeutic agent

COMPLICATIONS

- Permanent cerebral damage
- Obesity

PROGNOSIS

- Patients with benign sporadic insulinomas are cured with resection
- 60% of patients with malignant disease live up to 2 additional years

RESOURCES

REFERENCES

- Grant CS. Surgical aspects of hyperinsulinemic hypoglycemia. *Endocrinol Metab Clin North Am.* 1999;28:533.
- Dolan JP, Norton JA. Occult insulinoma. *Br J Surg.* 2000;87:385.
- Grant CS. Insulinoma. *Surg Oncol Clin North Am.* 1998;7:819.

Intestinal Ischemia, Nonocclusive

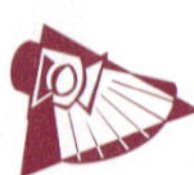

ESSENTIAL FEATURES

- No embolic or thrombotic cause of vascular obstruction
- Associated low flow state (sepsis, cardiac dysrhythmia)
- Severe, diffuse abdominal pain
- Gross or occult intestinal bleeding
- Minimal physical findings

EPIDEMIOLOGY

- In about 25% of patients with intestinal ischemia, vascular occlusion does not involve a major artery or vein (although arterial stenosis is usually present)
- In the presence of some other acute disease such as a cardiac dysrhythmia or sepsis, splanchnic vasoconstriction occurs, and the intestine becomes ischemic because of low perfusion pressure and flow
  - Arterial blood is shunted away from the villi in these circumstances, and the ischemic villi are destroyed if the condition persists

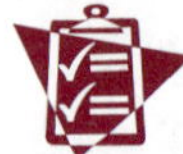

CLINICAL FINDINGS

SYMPTOMS AND SIGNS

- Severe, poorly localized abdominal pain that is often out of proportion to physical findings
- Nausea and vomiting
- Diarrhea
- Shock
- GI bleeding
- Abdominal distention
- Abdominal tenderness
- Peritonitis

LABORATORY FINDINGS

- Leukocytosis
- Serum amylase is elevated
- Significant base deficits
- Increased serum phosphate
- Anemia
- Increased serum lactate

IMAGING FINDINGS

- **Abdominal x-ray**
  - Nonspecific
  - Absence of intestinal gas
  - Diffuse distention with air-fluid levels
- **Specific findings occur late:** Intramural gas and gas in the portal venous system
- **GI contrast radiography:** May reveal "thumbprinting" and disordered motility
- **CT scan**
  - Diffuse distention with air-fluid levels
  - Intestinal wall thickening
  - Intramural gas and gas in the portal venous system
- **Arteriography:** Documents the absence of major vascular occlusion but is not otherwise diagnostic in most cases

DIAGNOSTIC CONSIDERATIONS

- The diagnosis is suspected when acute abdominal pain develops in a potentially susceptible patient
  - Clinical picture is similar to that of arterial thrombosis, but the onset is less often sudden
- Ischemia is most pronounced on the antimesenteric border, and the mucosa may be extensively involved before abnormalities are visible on the serosal surface
  - There are often ischemic areas in other organs such as liver and spleen

RULE OUT

- Intestinal ischemia due to embolic or thrombotic processes
- Acute pancreatitis
- Intestinal obstruction

WORK-UP

- CBC count
- Serum electrolytes
- Serum amylase
- Serum lactate
- ABG measurements
- Abdominal x-ray
- CT scan
- Arteriography

WHEN TO ADMIT

- All cases

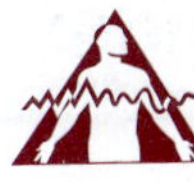

TREATMENT AND MANAGEMENT

- Resection of all involved gut
  - A second-look operation is performed 12–24 hours later if marginally viable bowel was left
- Vascular reconstruction is ineffective

SURGERY

Indications

- Suspected mesenteric ischemia

Contraindications

- Necrotic bowel should be resected unless the extent of damage is so great that satisfactory life could not be expected

MEDICATIONS

- Massive volume support and antibiotics
- Intra-arterial infusion of papaverine

TREATMENT MONITORING

- A second-look operation is performed 12–24 hours after initial operation if marginally viable bowel was left

COMPLICATIONS

- Short gut syndrome
- Sepsis
- Multi-organ failure
- Death

PROGNOSIS

- Mortality rate is near 90%

RESOURCES

REFERENCES

- Gennaro M et al. Acute mesenteric ischemia after cardiopulmonary bypass. *Am J Surg.* 1993;166:231.
- Inderbitzi R et al. Acute mesenteric ischaemia. *Eur J Surg.* 1992;158:123.
- Stoney RJ, Cunningham CG. Acute mesenteric ischemia. *Surgery.* 1993;114:489.

Intra-Abdominal Abscess

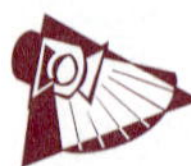

ESSENTIAL FEATURES

- Fever and chills
- Tachycardia
- Leukocytosis
- Focal abdominal tenderness
- Predisposing condition

EPIDEMIOLOGY

- Most common causes are
  - GI perforations
  - Postoperative complications
  - Penetrating trauma
  - Genitourinary infections
- Abscess forms as sequelae of generalized peritonitis in 33% of cases
- Intra-abdominal abscess forms adjacent to diseased viscus (eg, perforated appendicitis) or as a result of external contamination (subphrenic abscess)
- Broadly classified based on anatomic location:
  - Subdiaphramatic
  - Subhepatic
  - Pericolic
  - Pelvic
  - Interloop abscesses

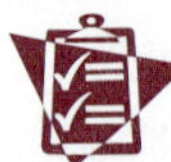

CLINICAL FINDINGS

SYMPTOMS AND SIGNS

- Fever and chills
- Tachycardia
- Focal abdominal tenderness
- Prolonged ileus or sluggish postoperative recovery
- Mass seldom appreciated
- Irritation of contiguous structures manifesting symptoms such as:
  - Lower chest pain
  - Dyspnea
  - Referred shoulder pain or hiccup
  - Basilar atelectasis or effusion
  - Diarrhea
  - Urinary frequency
- Severe peritoneal sepsis with multiple organ failure may develop in patients with advanced cases

LABORATORY FINDINGS

- Leukocytosis
- Bacteremia
- Abnormal liver profile, renal function tests, or ABG measurements
- Elevated ESR and C-reactive protein levels

IMAGING FINDINGS

- **Abdominal x-ray:** Suggest abscess in up to 50% of cases via nonspecific findings, such as
  - Ileus pattern
  - Air-fluid levels
  - Soft-tissue mass
  - Free or mottled gas pockets
  - Effacement of preperitoneal or psoas outlines
  - Displacement of viscera
- **US**
  - Diagnose intra-abdominal abscesses in up to 80% of cases
  - Most useful when an abscess is suspected in the right upper quadrant
  - Bowel gas, stomas, and incisions interfere with the study
- Water-soluble contrast study sensitive in detecting a perforated viscus
- Abdominal pelvic CT scan with IV and PO contrast is the best diagnostic study with > 95% sensitivity, particularly in postoperative patients
  - Percutaneous drainage procedures can often be performed at the same setting

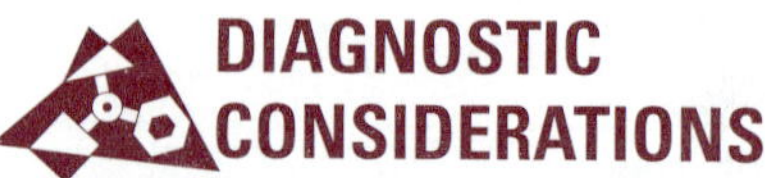

DIAGNOSTIC CONSIDERATIONS

- Sterile fluid collection
- Hematoma
- Biloma
- Urinoma
- Neoplasm
- Other common infectious/inflammatory sources that manifest with fever, leukocytosis, and abdominal pain:
  - Pancreatitis
  - Pyelonephritis
  - Lower lobe pneumonia
  - Deep wound infection
- Bacteremia/line sepsis
- Evaluate for source of abscess:
  - GI anastomotic leak
  - Perforated appendicitis
  - Perforated diverticulitis
  - Crohns enterocolitis
  - Perforated peptic ulcer
  - Pelvic inflammatory disease/tubo-ovarian abscess

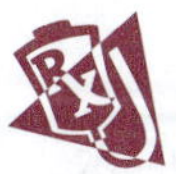

WORK-UP

- CBC count
- Basic chemistries
- Amylase and lipase
- UA
- Blood cultures
- Sputum culture and Gram stain
- Chest film
- Abdominal x-ray
- Abdominal pelvic CT scan with IV and PO contrast

WHEN TO ADMIT

- All patients with an intra-abdominal abscess should be admitted (if not already) for drainage and initiation of IV antibiotics

WHEN TO REFER

- Most patients with intra-abdominal abscesses should be managed by a general surgeon
- Postoperative abscesses ideally should be addressed by the operative surgeon

TREATMENT AND MANAGEMENT

- IV antibiotic therapy may initially be attempted for small abscesses < 1–2 cm if the patient is clinically stable
- Treatment of most abscesses consists of prompt and complete drainage, control of the primary cause, and adjunctive use of antibiotics
- Percutaneous drainage is the preferred drainage method for well-localized, accessible intra-abdominal abscesses that do not have a fistulous communication or contain solid debris
  - Success rate 80% in simple abscesses but < 50% in complex multiloculated abscesses
- Culture and antibiotic sensitivity testing should be performed on the abscess material to narrow antibiotic treatment

SURGERY

Indications

- Percutaneously inaccessible abscesses
- Persistent focus of infection that needs to be controlled, such as an anastomotic leak or perforated diverticulitis
- Failure of percutaneous drain to evacuate abscess
- Complex multiloculated abscesses with solid debris present

MEDICATIONS

- Initial empiric IV antibiotic coverage for enteric aerobic and anaerobic organisms
- Focused antibiotic therapy based on culture results
- PO antibiotic combinations such as a quinolone plus metronidazole or clindamycin may be appropriate in select cases

TREATMENT MONITORING

- Satisfactory drainage is usually evidenced by clinical improvement within 48–72 hours
- Serial US or CT evaluations can be obtained to verify cavity obliteration but are usually unnecessary

COMPLICATIONS

- Inadequate drainage
- Recurrent abscess formation
- Contamination of adjacent peritoneal cavity
- Abdominal sepsis and death

PROGNOSIS

- Mortality rate of serious intra-abdominal abscesses is about 30%
- Death is related to the underlying cause, delay in diagnosis, multiple organ failure, incomplete drainage, and comorbid diseases
- Decompensation of 2 organ systems is associated with a mortality rate of 50%

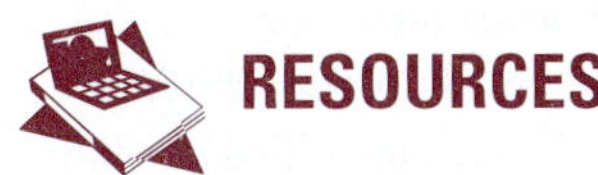

RESOURCES

REFERENCES

- Farthmann EH et al. Epidemiology and pathophysiology of intraabdominal infections (IA). *Infection.* 1998;25:329.

Intussusception, Adult

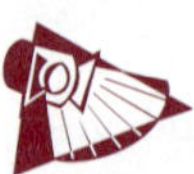

ESSENTIAL FEATURES

- Invagination of proximal intestine into adjacent distal bowel, resulting in luminal obstruction
- Can occur in the small bowel, or anorectum (rectal prolapse)
- Prolonged obstruction can lead to vascular compromise, first venous, then arterial, eventual bowel infarction
- Less common in adults than children
- A lead point is often identified in adults and must be sought out in those in whom this condition develops

EPIDEMIOLOGY

- Rectal prolapse more common in older multiparous women

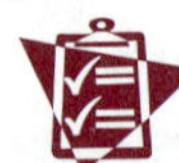

CLINICAL FINDINGS

SYMPTOMS AND SIGNS

- Patients present with clinical evidence of bowel obstruction
  - Colicky abdominal pain
- Vomiting
- Hyperperistaltic bowel sounds

LABORATORY FINDINGS

- No specific findings
- Leukocytosis, acidosis suggestive of bowel compromise

IMAGING FINDINGS

- Barium enema may be both diagnostic and therapeutic: "coiled spring" sign
- After radiographic resolution of obstruction (which is often not possible in adults) the patient must be evaluated thoroughly to identify the anatomic lead point

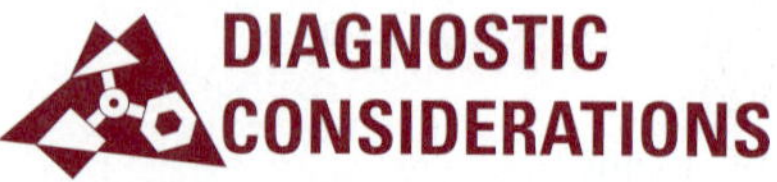

DIAGNOSTIC CONSIDERATIONS

- Other causes for bowel obstruction:
  - Neoplasm
  - Hernia
  - Adhesions
- Diverticulitis
- Appendicitis

RULE OUT

- Neoplasm as lead point for intussusception

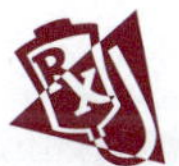

WORK-UP

- Barium enema

WHEN TO ADMIT

- Diagnosis of intussusception requires admission even if successfully reduced nonoperatively
  - This is rarely possible in adults, and the diagnosis usually requires operation for resolution

TREATMENT AND MANAGEMENT

- Operation for reduction
- IV hydration
- NG decompression
- IV broad-spectrum antibiotics
- Barium or air-constrast enema

SURGERY

Indications

- Intussusception should be reduced by pushing the lead point, avoiding pulling
- If reduction cannot be carried out without creating serosal tears, resection and anastomosis should be performed

MEDICATIONS

- IV antibiotics
- Glucagon may assist in reduction efforts

COMPLICATIONS

- Hypovolemia/shock
- Sepsis
- Strangulation of bowel, infarction/necrosis

PROGNOSIS

- Recurrence rates vary from 1–3% whether barium or operative reduction performed
- Deaths are rare but do occur if treatment of gangrenous bowel is delayed

RESOURCES

REFERENCES

- Shelton AA et al. Small Intestine. In: Way LW, Doherty GM (editors). *Current Surgical Diagnosis & Treatment,* 11e. New York: McGraw-Hill; 2003:683–688.

Intussusception, Pediatric

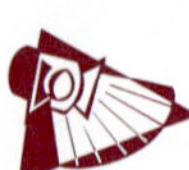

ESSENTIAL FEATURES

- 95% idiopathic, but most commonly involves ileocecal valve

EPIDEMIOLOGY

- Peak age 6–9 mos old but ranges from 3 months to 3 years of age
- 1–4/1000 births
- 3:2 male:female predominance

CLINICAL FINDINGS

SYMPTOMS AND SIGNS

- Abdominal pain (colicky)
- Vomiting
- Bloody stool
- Palpable mass in right abdomen (80–90% cases)
- Heme positive stool in 80–90%

IMAGING FINDINGS

- **Abdominal x-ray:** Shows paucity of gas in right lower quadrant, later air-fluid levels in small intestine with absence of gas distally
- **Contrast enema:** 100% sensitive showing lead point of intussusception and is often therapeutic when performed under pressure
- **CT and US:** Show "bullseye"

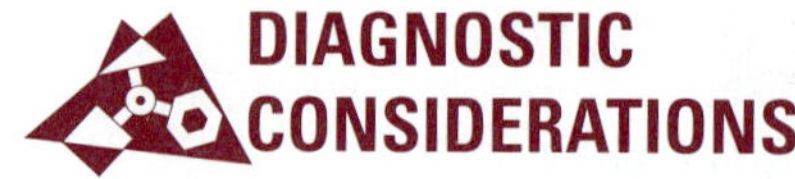

RULE OUT

- Peritonitis

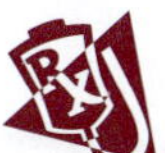

WORK-UP

- History and physical exam
- Abdominal x-ray
- CT or US
- Barium enema in children should be attempted after adequate resuscitation

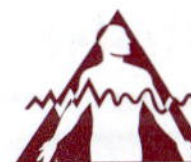

TREATMENT AND MANAGEMENT

SURGERY

- Laparotomy and resection of intussusception if ischemic necrosis present
- Laparoscopic reduction of intussusception if enema unsuccesful

Indications

- Failure to reduce with barium enema

MEDICATIONS

- Contrast enema to reduce (60–80% successful)
  - Pneumatic preferred

COMPLICATIONS

- Recurrence after enema (5%)

PROGNOSIS

- Spontaneously resolve in 20–30%

RESOURCES

REFERENCES

- Albanese CT et al. Pediatric Surgery. In: Way LW, Doherty GM. *Surgical Diagnosis & Treatment,* 11e. New York: McGraw-Hill; 2003:1323–1324.

Islet Cell Tumors, Nonfunctioning

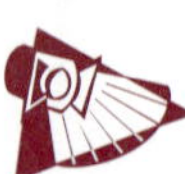

ESSENTIAL FEATURES

- No overt clinical syndrome
- Pancreatic mass on CT scan
- Elevated serum levels of chromogranin A, pancreatic polypeptide, and hCG
- Overall worse prognosis than other pancreatic islet cell tumors

EPIDEMIOLOGY

- Account for 30–50% of pancreatic endocrine tumors
- Elevated serum levels of chromogranin A, pancreatic polypeptide, and hCG are common, without any accompanying clinical syndrome
- Most nonfunctioning tumors are large, malignant, and located in the head of the pancreas
- Metastases are present at the time of diagnosis in 80% of patients

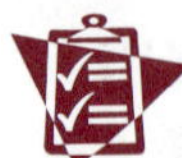

CLINICAL FINDINGS

SYMPTOMS AND SIGNS

- Abdominal and back pain
- Weight loss
- Jaundice
- Nausea and vomiting
- Palpable abdominal mass

LABORATORY FINDINGS

- Elevated serum bilirubin
- Elevated serum chromogranin A
- Elevated serum pancreatic polypeptide
- Elevated serum hCG

IMAGING FINDINGS

- **CT scan**
  - Shows a pancreatic mass, which is typically hypervascular
  - Also useful for detection of metastases
- **Octreotide scintigraphy** may also be useful

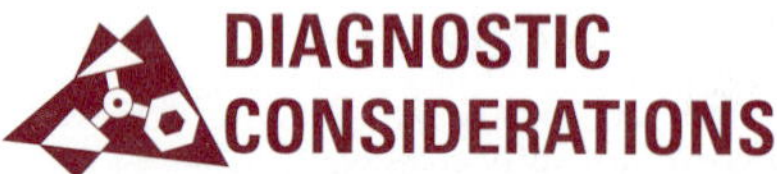

DIAGNOSTIC CONSIDERATIONS

- The histologic pattern on biopsy specimens is diagnostic of islet cell tumor, but whether or not the lesion is malignant rests on evidence of invasiveness or metastases, not the appearance of the cells
- Immunohistochemical staining of the tissue is positive for chromogranin and neuron-specific enolase (markers of APUD tumors)

RULE OUT

- Functional islet cell tumors
- Adenocarcinoma of the head of the pancreas
- Chronic pancreatitis

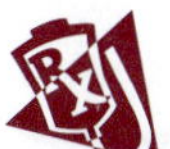

WORK-UP

- CT scan or somatostatin receptor scintigraphy
- Serum levels of chromogranin A, pancreatic polypeptide, and hCG

WHEN TO ADMIT

- Severe symptoms

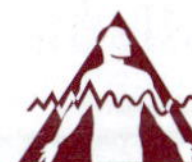

TREATMENT AND MANAGEMENT

SURGERY

- Resection of primary tumor (head, pancreaticoduodenectomy; body and tail, distal pancreatectomy) and debulking of metastases

Indications

- All cases of completely respectable disease

MEDICATIONS

- Streptozocin and doxorubicin for unresectable tumor

COMPLICATIONS

- Biliary obstruction
- Duodenal obstruction

PROGNOSIS

- 5-year disease-free survival rate is 15%

RESOURCES

REFERENCES

- Bartsch DK et al. Management of nonfunctioning islet cell carcinomas. *World J Surg.* 2000;24:1418.
- Somogyi L, Mishra G. Diagnosis and staging of islet cell tumors of the pancreas. *Curr Gastroenterol Rep.* 2000;2:159.

Jaundice

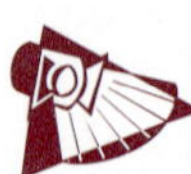

ESSENTIAL FEATURES

- Classified as obstructive (conjugated bilirubinemia) or nonobstructive (unconjugated bilirubinemia)
- Adult etiologies include:
  - Obstruction due to benign or malignant causes (stones, tumors, strictures)
  - Sludge or stasis due to infection or total parenteral nutrition (TPN)
  - Hemolysis or hepatocellular dysfunction
- Neonatal etiologies include:
  - Physiologic
  - Biliary atresia
  - Choledochal cyst
  - TPN
  - Hemolysis
  - Alagille syndrome
  - Intrahepatic bile duct paucity
  - Byler syndrome

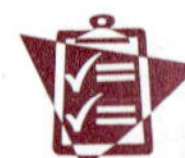

CLINICAL FINDINGS

SYMPTOMS AND SIGNS

- Jaundice
- Malaise
- Anorexia
- Fatigue
- Pruritus
- Encephalopathy
- Kernicterus

LABORATORY FINDINGS

- Hyperbilirubinemia (conjugated or unconjugated)
- Associated elevation of liver function tests if hepatocellular dysfunction
- Anemia if associated sepsis, bleeding, or hemolysis

IMAGING FINDINGS

- **US:** Shows biliary dilatation if obstruction present
- **CT:** Shows biliary obstruction present and accompanying mass
- ERCP, magnetic resonance cholangiopancreatography (MRCP), or percutaneous transhepatic cholangiogram (PTC): Shows biliary obstruction if mass present and proximal and distal extent

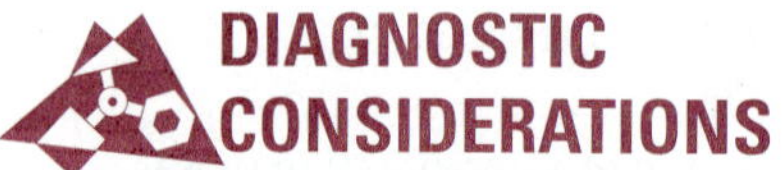

DIAGNOSTIC CONSIDERATIONS

- Conjugated hyperbilirubinemia in neonate

RULE OUT

- Anatomical obstruction to bile flow

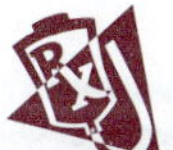

WORK-UP

- History and physical exam
- Bilirubin (conjugated and unconjugated)
- US
- CT
- ERCP, MRCP, or PTC

WHEN TO ADMIT

- Cholangitis
- Obstructive jaundice in neonate
- Encephalopathy

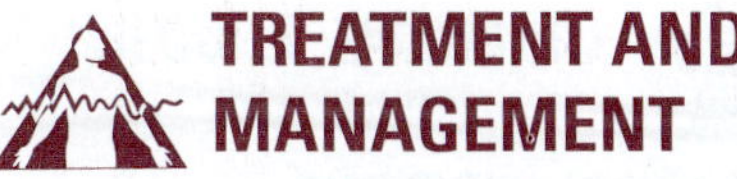

TREATMENT AND MANAGEMENT

SURGERY

- Resolution of bilary tract stone disease by cholecystectomy and decompression of common bile duct by operative, radiologic or endoscopic intervention
- Resection with biliary reconstruction of mass causing obstruction
- Biliary-enteric bypass if benign stricture or unresectable malignant disease

INDICATIONS

- Biliary obstruction

Contraindications

- Medical comorbidity precluding resection or general anesthesia
- Extrahepatic disease if malignant cause

MEDICATIONS

- Ursodiol
- Phototherapy (neonate)
- Exchange transfusion (neonate)

TREATMENT MONITORING

- Serum bilirubin

COMPLICATIONS

- Biliary-enteric anastomotic leak or stricture

RESOURCES

REFERENCES

- Doherty GM, Way LW. Biliary Tract. In: Way LW, Doherty GM (editors). *Current Surgical Diagnosis & Treatment,* 11e. New York: McGraw-Hill; 2003:601–603.

Lipoma

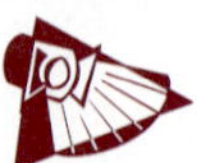

ESSENTIAL FEATURES

- Lipomas are slow growing, benign adipose tumors, most often found in the subcutaneous tissues
- Lipomas may also be found in the deeper tissues such as the intramuscular septa, thoracic cavity, abdominal organs, and the GI tract
- Histologically, lipomas are composed of mature adipocytes arranged in lobules, surrounded by a fibrous capsule
- Infiltrating lipomas are non-encapsulated benign lesions with extensions into muscle
- Variants of lipomas include angiolipoma, pleomorphic lipoma, spindle cell lipoma, and adenolipoma

EPIDEMIOLOGY

- Lipomas are identified in all age groups but most commonly appear first between the ages of 40 and 60
- Multiple lipomas (lipomatosis) associated with hereditary syndromes:
  - Gardner syndrome
  - Madelung disease
- Hereditary multiple lipomatosis
  - Adiposis dolorosa (Dercum disease)
  - Multiple endocrine neoplasia type 1

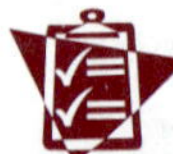

CLINICAL FINDINGS

SYMPTOMS AND SIGNS

- Nontender, oval, mobile subcutaneous masses
- Characteristic soft, doughy texture
- Overlying skin normal
- Deeply positioned lipomas typically present as nontender, nonmobile, soft-tissue masses

IMAGING FINDINGS

- **MRI**
  - Demonstrates the extent of the lesion
  - May be able to differentiate between lipoma and liposarcoma
  - Useful for deep lesions and/or when malignancy is suspected

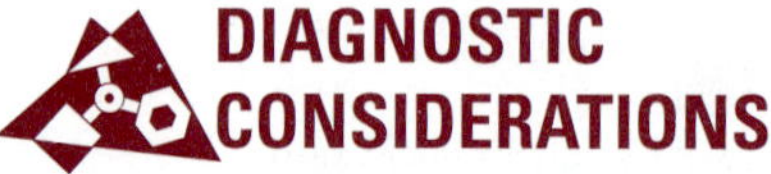

DIAGNOSTIC CONSIDERATIONS

- Lipoma
- Fibroma
- Epidermoid cyst
- Hemangioma
- Desmoid tumor
- Soft-tissue sarcoma (especially liposarcoma)
- Cutaneous metastases
- Nodular subcutaneous fat necrosis

RULE OUT

- Soft-tissue sarcoma

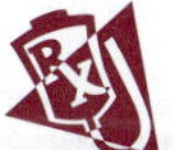

WORK-UP

- Thorough history and physical exam
- When malignancy is suspected, a MRI may be indicated, especially for large or deep-seated lesions

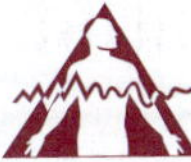

TREATMENT AND MANAGEMENT

- Surgical excision of symptomatic or enlarging lesions
- Lesions > 4 cm should be approached with an incisional biopsy to confirm benign histology prior to complete excision

SURGERY

Indications

- Symptomatic lipoma
- Enlarging soft-tissue mass
- Cosmetic considerations

MEDICATIONS

- Kenalog steroid injection is an alternative to excision (results in fat atrophy)

TREATMENT MONITORING

- Physical exam to detect "recurrence"

COMPLICATIONS

- Surgical infection
- Ecchymosis
- Hematoma

PROGNOSIS

- Uniformly excellent

RESOURCES

REFERENCES

- Jablons D et al. Thoracic Wall, Pleura, Mediastinum, & Lung. In: Way LW, Doherty GM (editors). *Current Surgical Diagnosis & Treatment,* 11e. New York: McGraw-Hill; 2003;354.

Lung Abscess

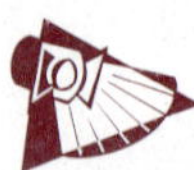

ESSENTIAL FEATURES

- Localized collection of pus
- Acute: < 6 wks
- Chronic: > 6 wks

Primary

- Aspiration of oropharyngeal contents
- Acute necrotizing pneumonia *(Staph, Klebsiella)*
- Chronic pneumonia due to fungi, TB
- Opportunistic infection in immunocompromised person

Secondary

- Bronchial obstruction (cancer, foreign body)
- Cavitating pulmonary lesions (cancer)
- Direct extension (amebiasis, subphrenic abscess)
- Hematogenous dissemination

EPIDEMIOLOGY

- Increased incidence with AIDS, transplantation, and chemotherapy
- Pathogens typically found in cultures include:
  - *Staphylococcus*
  - *Streptococcus*
  - *Klebsiella*
  - *E coli*
  - *Pseudomonas*
  - *Clostridium*
  - *Bacteroides*
- Pathogens found in immunocompromised patients:
  - *Candida*
  - *Legionella*
  - Pneumocystis carinii

CLINICAL FINDINGS

SYMPTOMS AND SIGNS

- Cough, fever, dyspnea, pleuritic chest pain
- Malaise, weight loss if chronic
- On exam: Clubbing; signs of pleural effusion; cachexia; and rarely, draining chest wound (empyema necessitatis)

LABORATORY FINDINGS

- Elevated WBC, with left shift
- Positive sputum culture

IMAGING FINDINGS

- **Chest film:** Area of intense consolidation or rounded density; with or without air-fluid level
- **CT scan:** Helpful in cases of suspected bronchial obstruction

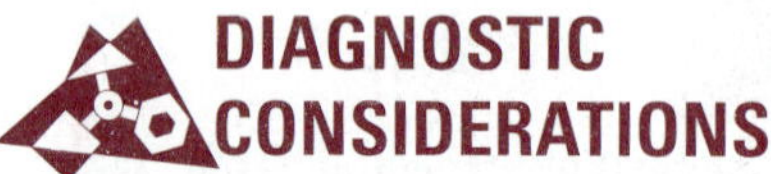

DIAGNOSTIC CONSIDERATIONS

- Evaluate for primary structural diseases of lungs, including cancer

WORK-UP

- WBC, sputum culture
- Chest film, possibly chest CT scan
- Bronchoscopy in patients with unexplained reason for lung abscess
- Fine-needle aspiration (FNA) of abscess cavity identifies pathogens in 94% of cases
  - Bronchoalveolar lavage (BAL) identifies organism in only 3%
- FNA important to identify unusual organisms in immunocompromised patients

TREATMENT AND MANAGEMENT

- Antibiotics mainstay of treatment
- Penicillin and clindamycin commonly used
- Trimethoprim-sulfamethoxazole, pentamidine, erythromycin, or amphotericin B often indicated in immunocompromised patients
- Continue antibiotics until complete resolution (3–6 mos)
- Chest physiotherapy, bronchoscopy with drainage may be necessary

SURGERY

Indications

- Poor response to above medical regimen, percutaneous drainage
- Tense abscess (mediastinal shift, shift of diaphragm, etc)
- Evidence of contralateral lung contamination
- Signs of sepsis after 72 hrs of antibiotic therapy
- Abscess size > 4 cm or enlarging
- Rising fluid level
- Persistent ventilatory dependency

COMPLICATIONS

- Rupture into bronchus
- Rupture into pleural space resulting in pyopneumothorax
- Massive hemoptysis

PROGNOSIS

- **Percutaneous drainage:** 1.5% mortality, 10% morbidity
- **Overall mortality rate:** 5–20%
- **Medical therapy success:** 75–88%
- **Operative patients:** Cured 90% of time, 1% mortality
- **Mortality in immunocompromised patients:** 28%

RESOURCES

REFERENCES

- Bartlett JG. Antibiotics in lung abscess. *Semin Respir Infect.* 1991;6:103.
- Lambiase RE et al. Percutaneous drainage of 335 consecutive abscesses: results of primary drainage with 1-year follow-up. *Radiology.* 1992;184:167.

Lung Cancer, Primary

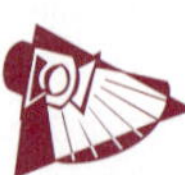

ESSENTIAL FEATURES

- Typically spread by local extension, metastasis to lymph nodes, lung, liver, bone, brain, adrenals

Non–Small-Cell Lung Carcinoma (NSCLC)

- 80% of cases
- Classified as:
  - Early without mediastinal involvement (stage I/II)
  - Locally advanced (stage IIIA/B)
  - Metastatic (stage IV)

Squamous Cell Carcinoma

- 20% of cases
- Keratinization, cellular stratification, and intercellular bridges seen pathologically
- 67% located centrally, 33% located peripherally
- Growth and metastasis rate slower than other lung tumors
- Classified into 2 groups:
  1. Disease in ipsilateral thorax (including lymph nodes)
  2. Disease beyond thorax (extensive)

Adenocarcinoma

- 30% of cases
- 3 subtypes
  - Acinar (columnar lined glands secreting mucin)
  - Papillary
  - Bronchoalveolar (intraluminal papillary fragments in alveoli)
- Increasing frequency, may be spread by aerosol transmission

Large Cell Carcinoma

- Uncommon
- Large polygonal spindle/oval cells in sheets or nests
- Tumors seen peripherally

Small Cell (Oat Cell) Carcinoma

- 15% of cases
- Small round nuclei with nuclear chromatin and cytoplasm
- Biologically and clinically distinct from others
- Occur centrally, early metastasis, highly resistant to treatment

Adenosquamous Tumors

- Show both cellular features
- More aggressive than NSCLC

EPIDEMIOLOGY

- Number 1 cause of cancer-death in men and women
- 170,000 new cases each year: 157,000 deaths each year
- Incidence stable among males, increasing among females
- 85% of cases due to smoking tobacco
- Asbestos exposure implicated in 23% of lung cancer cases, radon increases risk
- Occurs more frequently in right lobe than in left
- Upper lobes affected more than lower or middle lobes
- Increased risk to develop other cancers:
  - Upper respiratory tract
  - Esophagus
  - Bladder
  - Kidney
- No survival benefit from mass screening

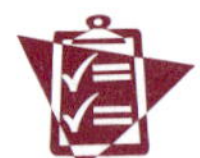

CLINICAL FINDINGS

SYMPTOMS AND SIGNS

- **Central tumors:** Cough, hemoptysis, respiratory distress, pain, pneumonia
- **Peripheral tumors:** Cough, chest wall pain, pleural effusions, pulmonary abscess, Horner syndrome, Pancoast syndrome
- **Symptoms from regional spread:** Hoarseness (recurrent nerve paralysis), dyspnea (phrenic nerve paralysis), dysphagia (esophageal compression), tamponade (pericardial invasion)
- **Systemic symptoms:** Anorexia, weight loss, weakness, malaise
- **Classic paraneoplastic syndromes:**
  - Small cell: Eaton-Lambert (myasthenia), SIADH, ACTH, carcinoid
  - SCC: Hypercalcemia
  - Adenocarcinoma: acanthosis nigricans

LABORATORY FINDINGS

- Elevated alkaline phosphatase suggests bony metastases

IMAGING FINDINGS

- **Chest film:** Vary from nodule to unresolving infiltrate to total atelectasis
- **Chest CT scan:** Evaluation of infiltrate, nodule

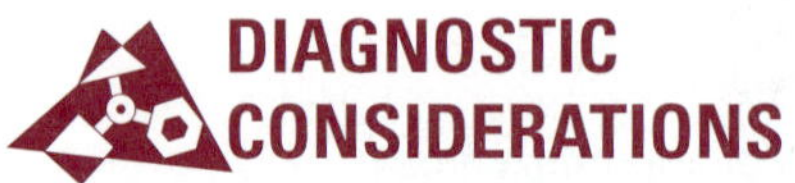

DIAGNOSTIC CONSIDERATIONS

- Definitive diagnosis obtained in 90% with bronchoscopy or fine-needle aspiration (FNA)

RULE OUT

- Metastatic disease with imaging (see below) and thoracentesis

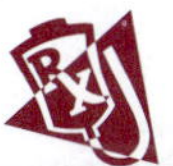

WORK-UP

- Chest film often done for routing physical or for symptoms
- CT chest/abdomen: to rule out common sites of metastasis, such as liver and adrenals
- If serum alkaline phosphatase is elevated, do bone scan
- Brain CT scan if neurologic symptoms
- PET may be important staging test
- Thoracentesis if pleural effusion to rule out malignant pleural effusion
- Determine classifications (see Essential Features)
- Adequate cardiac evaluation prior to operative intervention necessary

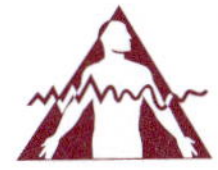

TREATMENT AND MANAGEMENT

Small Cell Carcinoma

- Treatment typically chemoradiotherapy
- For early disease T1-T2 lesions: Resection with chemotherapy may improve local control and survival
- Resect small peripheral tumors with aggressive postoperative chemotherapy to increase local control

NSCLC

- Treatment varies with stage
  - Stages I-IIIA: Resectable
  - Stage IIIB/ IV: Often nonresectable
- For early disease, goal is complete resection
  - Lobectomy with 1 cm normal bronchus margin, sleeve resection if upper lobe involved
  - Pneumonectomy with or without sleeve for proximal bronchial lesions
- For advanced disease:
  - Preoperative chemoradiotherapy
  - Solitary brain/adrenal metastasis candidates for resection
  - Laser resection of proximal obstructing tumors may palliate

SURGERY

Indications

- Chamberlain procedure if no evidence of metastatic disease, and cancer in left lung, for staging
- Cervical mediastinoscopy if limited to thorax for staging
- Stage I/II (now combined with chemotherapy)
- Stage IIIA: Surgery with chemoradiation
- Solitary brain or adrenal metastasis

Contraindications

- Myocardial infarction in previous 3 mos (20% perioperative mortality with lung resection)
- Superior vena cava (SVC) syndrome
- Bilateral endobronchial tumor
- Contralateral lymph node metastases
- Malignant pleural effusion
- Distant metastases (except solitary brain or adrenal)
- FEV_1 (0.8 L), $PaCO_2 > 45$ mm Hg, $PaO_2 < 50$ mm Hg are relative contraindications

MEDICATIONS

NSCLC

- Chemotherapy
  - Used in combination with radiation therapy in locally advanced and metastatic disease
  - Preoperative chemotherapy appears beneficial, postoperative chemotherapy has limited benefit
- Radiation therapy
  - Stage I/II can be curative in patients not surgical candidates
  - Important adjuvant in later stages

Small Cell Carcinoma

- Chemotherapy
  - 80-90% response
  - Cyclophosphamide, doxorubicin, vincrinstine are optimal drugs
- Radiation therapy
  - Improved local control
  - Minimal improved survival with chemotherapy and radiotherapy in early stage
  - No benefit in extensive disease other than palliation for symptoms

PROGNOSIS

- Perioperative mortality 2% for lobectomy, 6% for pneumonectomy

NSCLC

- 5-year survival rates
  - Stage I: 43–64%
  - Stage II: 20–40%
  - Stage IIIA: 15–25%
  - Stage IIIB: 5–7%
  - Stage IV: < 2%

Small Cell Carcinoma

- Limited disease: 2-year survival rate, 5–25%
- Extensive: 2-year survival rate, 1–3%

RESOURCES

REFERENCES

- Schiller JH et al. Comparison of four chemotherapy regimens for advanced non-small cell lung cancer. *N Engl J Med.* 2002;346:92.
- Sugarbaker DJ et al. Results of Cancer and Leukemia Group B protocol 8935: a multiinstitutional phase II trimodality trial for IIIA N2 non-small cell lung cancer. *J Thorac Cardiovasc Surg.* 1995;109:473.
- Friedel G et al. Neoadjuvant chemoradiotherapy of stage III non-small cell lung cancer. *Lung Cancer.* 2000;30:175.

PRACTICE GUIDELINES

- The National Comprehensive Cancer Network http://www.nccn.org/

CANCER STAGING

- Accurate staging essential as treatment plan varies with staging
- See Lung Staging Table on page 751.

STAGE GROUPING			
Occult Carcinoma	TX	N0	M0
Stage 0	Tis	N0	M0
Stage IA	T1	N0	M0
Stage IB	T2	N0	M0
Stage IIA	T1	N1	M0
Stage IIB	T2	N1	M0
	T3	N0	M0
Stage IIIA	T1	N2	M0
	T2	N2	M0
	T3	N1	M0
	T3	N2	M0
Stage IIIB	Any T	N3	M0
	T4	Any N	M0
Stage IV	Any T	Any N	M1

Lung Infection, Aspergillosis

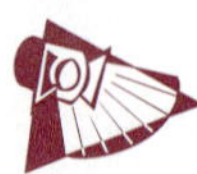

ESSENTIAL FEATURES

- Infection via inhalation of conidia into areas of lung with impaired mucociliary function (ie, tuberculous cavities)
- 3 types of aspergillosis infections:
  1. Allergic bronchopulmonary aspergillosis
  2. Invasive aspergillosis
  3. Aspergilloma (fungus balls)

Allergic Bronchopulmonary Aspergillosis

- Occurs in patients with asthma or cystic fibrosis
- Fungal growth leads to dilated airways filled with mucus and fungus
- 5 stages of infection:
  1. Acute infection
  2. Corticosteroid-induced remission
  3. Asymptomatic worsening of laboratory and x-rays
  4. Onset of corticosteroid-dependent asthma
  5. End-stage fibrosis

Invasive Aspergillosis

- Found only in immunocompromised patients
- Patients with leukemia: 50–70% of cases
- Dissemination frequent
- 3 types of pulmonary disease described
  1. Tracheobronchitis: Larger airways with mucosal ulceration, fungal plugs
  2. Necrotizing bronchopneumonia
  3. Hemorrhagic infarction: Occlusion of arteries with necrosis

Aspergilloma (Fungus Balls)

- Divided into 2 types:
  1. Simple, thin-walled cysts with ciliated epithelium surround by normal lung
  2. Complex cavities with abnormal surrounding lung tissue
- Most often in upper lobes, multiple (22%), calcification and air-fluid levels rare
- Associated with cavitary lung disease (TB, histoplasmosis, sarcoidosis, bronchiectasis, etc)

EPIDEMIOLOGY

- Pulmonary fungal infections are rising due to widespread use of broad-spectrum antibiotics, immunosuppressive drugs, and HIV infection
- Occur anywhere in world, some with characteristic endemic areas

Aspergillosis

- *Aspergillus fumigatus* (most common), *Aspergillus niger, Aspergillus flavus, Aspergillus glaucus*
- Second most common opportunistic fungal infection after candidiasis
- Third most common fungal infection requiring hospital care

CLINICAL FINDINGS

SYMPTOMS AND SIGNS

Allergic Bronchopulmonary Aspergillosis

- Cough, fever, wheezing, dyspnea, pleuritic pain, hemoptysis

Invasive Aspergillosis

- Cough, dyspnea, wheezing, aspergilloma
- Hemoptysis (50–80%), can be multiple recurrent episodes

IMAGING FINDINGS

Allergic Bronchopulmonary Aspergillosis

- **Chest film:** Homogenous densities in "gloved finger," inverted "Y," or "cluster of grapes" pattern

Invasive Aspergillosis

- **Chest film:** Patchy areas of atelectasis secondary to bronchial obstruction, cavitation common, "air crescents" of mycotic lung

Aspergilloma

- **Chest film:** 3–6 cm round, mobile density with crescent of air

DIAGNOSTIC CONSIDERATIONS

- Definitive diagnosis: Demonstration of hyphal tissue invasion or documentation of hyphae on silver stain in suspected aspergilloma
- Diagnosis suggested: Culturing uniform septate hyphae with dichotomous branching at 45 degrees, detection of specific IgG or IgE antibodies

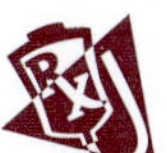

WORK-UP

- Chest film
- Chest CT scan
- Sputum culture

TREATMENT AND MANAGEMENT

Allergic Bronchopulmonary Aspergillosis

- Medical therapy (corticosteroids)

Invasive Aspergillosis

- Amphotericin B (mortality still 90%)

Aspergillomas

- Surgery indicated for complications of aspergillous infections
- Wide resection (lobectomy) required
- In some high risk patients, cavernostomy + muscle flap closure
- Intracavitary amphotericin B if not candidates for resection

SURGERY

Indications

- Hemoptysis secondary to aspergilloma
- Cavitation secondary to invasive aspergillosis

PROGNOSIS

Invasive Aspergillosis

- Mortality 90%

RESOURCES

REFERENCES

- Johnson P, Sarosi G. Current therapy of major fungal diseases of the lung. *Infect Dis Clin North Am.* 1991;5:635.

Lung Infection, Blastomycosis

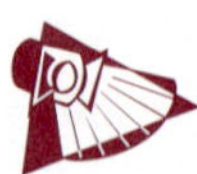

ESSENTIAL FEATURES

- Inhalation of spores causes germination, caseation; occasionally infection occurs through skin inoculation
- Manifestations can occur in many organs
  - Lungs
  - Skin
  - Bone
  - Genitourinary tract
  - CNS
- Pulmonary infection
  - Predilection for upper lobes
  - Hilar mediastinal adenopathy unusual (unlike histoplasmosis and coccidioidomycosis)

EPIDEMIOLOGY

- Pulmonary fungal infections are rising due to widespread use of broad-spectrum antibiotics, immunosuppressive drugs, and HIV
- Occur anywhere in world, some with characteristic endemic areas
- *Blastomycosis dermatitidis* found in warm, wet, nitrogen-rich soil in east, Midwest, and south (except Florida and New England)
  - Characteristically in males (10:1 male:female ratio), from 30- to 60-years-old generally
  - Risk factors include poor hygiene, poor housing

CLINICAL FINDINGS

SYMPTOMS AND SIGNS

- **Pulmonary infection:** Asymptomatic or flu-like symptoms (cough, weight loss, pleuritic pain, fever, hemoptysis, erythema nodosum)
- Evidence of pneumonia or pleurisy may occur

IMAGING FINDINGS

- **Chest film:** Homogeneous, patchy consolidation in nonsegmental distribution with pleural effusions, cavitation (15–35%)
  - Pulmonary masses may mimic malignancy

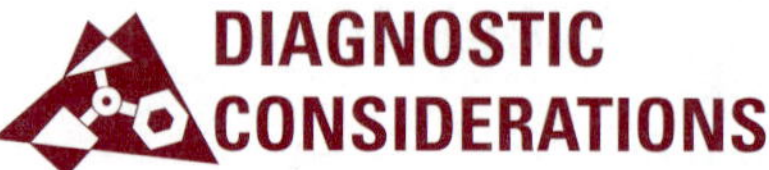

DIAGNOSTIC CONSIDERATIONS

- No accurate skin test
- Culture and identification of yeast form
- Culture of myceal form hazardous
- Yeast form found in sputum (33%), bronchoalveolar lavage (38%), biopsies (21%), fine-needle aspiration (7%)
- Yeast does not have large capsule (unlike *Cryptococcus*), does not grow intracellulary (unlike histoplasmosis)

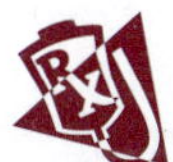

WORK-UP

- Chest film
- Chest CT scan
- Sputum microscopy and culture

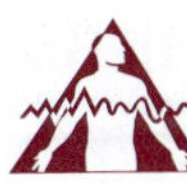

TREATMENT AND MANAGEMENT

- No treatment needed for limited disease and asymptomatic
- Antifungals first-line therapy

SURGERY

- Resect involved tissue, likely lobectomy

Indications

- Rarely necessary except when malignancy cannot be ruled out

MEDICATIONS

- Nonmeningeal disease: Itraconazole for 3 mos (> 80% response)
- Meningeal disease or failed therapy: Amphotericin B

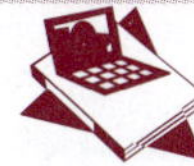

RESOURCES

REFERENCES

- Johnson P, Sarosi G. Current therapy of major fungal diseases of the lung. *Infect Dis Clin North Am.* 1991;5:635.

Lung Infection, Coccidioidomycosis

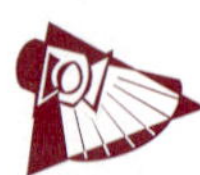

ESSENTIAL FEATURES

- Infection occurs by inhalation of 1–10 spores, germination, and rupture causing spread of infection
- Persistent infection 6–8 wks after primary classified into 5 types:
  1. Persistent pneumonia
  2. Chronic progressive pneumonia
  3. Miliary coccidioidomycosis
  4. Coccidioidal nodules
  5. Pulmonary cavities

EPIDEMIOLOGY

- Pulmonary fungal infections are rising due to widespread use of broad-spectrum antibiotics, immunosuppressive drugs, and HIV infection
- Occur anywhere in world, some with characteristic endemic areas
- *Coccidioides immitis* is endemic to Sonoran life zone (UT, CA, AZ, NV, NM), associated with creosote brush
  - Dry heat with brief intense rain essential for fungus
  - Spread by strong winds
  - In endemic areas, 30–50% of all pulmonary nodules are coccidiomas

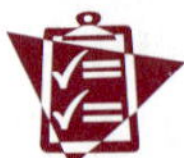

CLINICAL FINDINGS

SYMPTOMS AND SIGNS

- Primary infection is asymptomatic in 60%
- "Desert fever": Fever, productive cough, pleuritic chest pain, pneumonitis, rash
- "Desert rheumatism": Desert fever with arthralgias
- Eosinophilia common (66%)
- Persistent pneumonia
  - Fever
  - Productive cough
  - Pleuritic chest pain
  - Consolidation on chest film
  - Resolves < 8 mos
- Chronic progressive pneumonia
  - Fever
  - Cough
  - Dyspnea
  - Hemoptysis
  - Weight loss
  - Bilateral apical nodules and multiple cavities
  - Lasting > 10 yrs
- Miliary coccidioidomycosis: Occurs early and rapidly with bilateral diffuse infiltrates (mortality: 50%)
- Coccidioidal nodules: 50% asymptomatic; coccidiomas (noncalcified nodular densities) in middle and upper lung fields range from 1 to 4 cm
- Pulmonary cavities
  - Affects 15% of patients
  - Typically solitary, thin-walled, located in upper lobes, and < 6 cm
  - 50% close spontaneously within 2 yrs
- Uncommonly, can disseminate in immunocompromised, third trimester pregnancy, darker-skinned people

LABORATORY FINDINGS

- Acutely elevated IgM titers
- Rising serum IgG titers (seroconversion of 4× rise)

IMAGING FINDINGS

- **Chest film:** Hilar adenopathy (20%), small pleural effusions (2–20%)

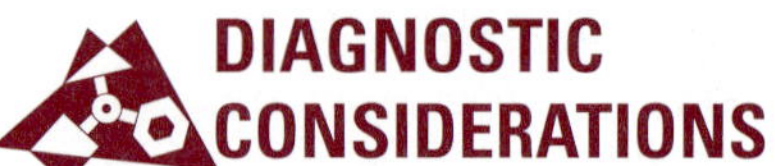

DIAGNOSTIC CONSIDERATIONS

- Acutely elevated IgM titers
- Rising serum IgG titers (seroconversion of 4× rise)
- Skin tests (coccidioidin and spherulin) good for epidemiologic studies, not for diagnosis of acute disease
- *C immitis* early to grow in culture but hazardous to handle
- Spherule identification in tissue, lavage samples helpful in diagnosis
- Pap staining most sensitive (Gram stains fail to demonstrate spherules)

RULE OUT

- Histoplasmosis
- TB

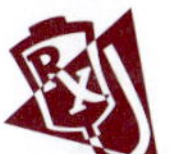

WORK-UP

- Chest film
- Chest CT scan
- Sputum microscopy and culture

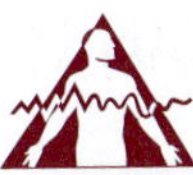

TREATMENT AND MANAGEMENT

- Medical therapy not indicated in asymptomatic patients
- Persistent illness or those at risk for dissemination treat with antifungals

SURGERY

- Resection all diseased tissue, usually with lobectomy

Indications

- Coccidiomas or cavities where cancer is concern on radiographic imaging
- Complications of cavities: Hemoptysis, pyopneumothorax

MEDICATIONS

- Amphotericin B is standard treatment
- Fluconazole, ketoconazole, itraconazole for long-term maintenance

COMPLICATIONS

- 25–50% of those requiring antifungals relapse

PROGNOSIS

- Disseminated and miliary coccidioidomycosis: Mortality, 50%

RESOURCES

REFERENCES

- Johnson P, Sarosi G. Current therapy of major fungal diseases of the lung. *Infect Dis Clin North Am.* 1991;5:635.

Lung Infection, Cryptococcosis

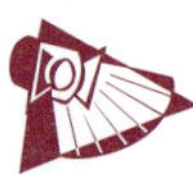

ESSENTIAL FEATURES

- Most common sites of infection are lungs and CNS
- Predilection for lower lobes of lungs

EPIDEMIOLOGY

- Pulmonary fungal infections are rising due to widespread use of broad-spectrum antibiotics, immunosuppressive drugs, and HIV infection
- Occur anywhere in world, some with characteristic endemic areas
- *Cryptococcus neoformans:* Found in pigeon excreta, grasses, trees, plants, fruits, insects, birds, dairy products
  – Exists also on skin and in nasopharynx, GI tract, and vagina

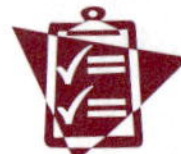

CLINICAL FINDINGS

SYMPTOMS AND SIGNS

Pulmonary Infection

- Many asymptomatic
- If symptoms, cough, pleuritic chest pain, fever

CNS Infection

- Usually follows asymptomatic pulmonary infection
- Symptoms vary since many patients are immunocompromised
- Many do not manifest usual signs of meningitis or cerebritis

LABORATORY FINDINGS

- Elevated serum antigen (via complement fixation tests)

IMAGING FINDINGS

- Chest film: Can appear as 3–10 cm pleural-based mass without smooth borders, areas of consolidation, or as disseminated miliary nodular infiltrate

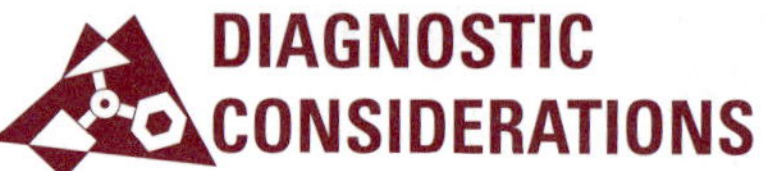

DIAGNOSTIC CONSIDERATIONS

- Elevated serum antigen (via complement fixation tests)
- Histology: India ink stain
- Culture is extremely time consuming
- No skin test exists

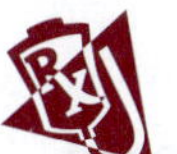

WORK-UP

- Chest film
- Chest CT scan
- Sputum microscopy and culture

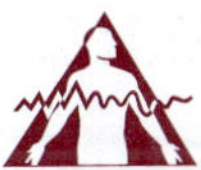

TREATMENT AND MANAGEMENT

- Medical therapy warranted in most cases of pulmonary infection even if asymptomatic
- Surgical resection rarely necessary
- Open lung biopsy if diagnosis is equivocal

SURGERY

Indications

- To exclude malignancy
- Determine etiology of undiagnosed diffuse pulmonary infiltrate

MEDICATIONS

- Amphotericin B is treatment of choice combined with flucytosine
- Fluconazole and itraconazole are useful for long-term maintenance therapy

RESOURCES

REFERENCES

- Johnson P, Sarosi G. Current therapy of major fungal diseases of the lung. *Infect Dis Clin North Am.* 1991;5:635.

Lung Infection, Histoplasmosis

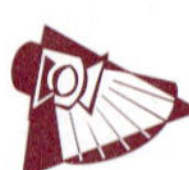

ESSENTIAL FEATURES

- Infection occurs after inhalation of spores with male:female ratio of 3:1
- In lungs, fungus germinates into yeast; cause caseating necrosis and calcification

Acute Infection

- Several different presentations:
  - Flu-like syndrome
  - Flu-like syndrome but limited to lungs
  - Diffuse nodular disease

Chronic Infection

- Several presentations:
  - Asymptomatic solitary nodule < 3 cm with central calcifications in lower lobes (histoplasmoma)
  - In patients with chronic obstructive pulmonary disease, cavitary histoplasmosis 3
  - Mediastinal granulomas resulting in broncholithiasis, esophageal traction diverticula, superior vena cava (SVC) compression, transesophageal (TE) fistulas
  - Fibrosing mediastinitis with SVC, tracheal, or esophageal compression

EPIDEMIOLOGY

- Pulmonary fungal infections are rising due to widespread use of broad-spectrum antibiotics, immunosuppressive drugs, and HIV infection
- Occur anywhere in world, some with characteristic endemic areas
- *Histoplasma capsulatum* is found in fowl and bat excreta, pigeon roosts, chicken houses, caves, hollow trees, attics and lofts
  - Endemic to fertile river valleys, such as Mississippi, Missouri, and Ohio Rivers

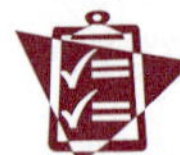

CLINICAL FINDINGS

SYMPTOMS AND SIGNS

- Immunocompetent patients, asymptomatic
- Cough, malaise, hemoptysis, fever, weight loss (30% have coexistent TB)

Acute Infection

- Ranging from flu-like illness to diffuse nodular disease

Chronic Infection

- Variety of presentations:
  - Histoplasmoma most common
  - Local mediastinal compression can occur
- Disseminated disease (acute, subacute, and chronic form): Fever, abdominal pain, hepatosplenomegaly, pancytopenia
- Solitary pulmonary nodules: 15–20% are from histoplasmosis
- Constrictive pericarditis if pericardium involved

LABORATORY FINDINGS

- High or rising serum titers
- Tissue cultures, sputum cultures

IMAGING FINDINGS

- **Chest film:** Hilar adenopathy common, diffuse interstitial pneumonitis (25%)
- In acute presentation, chest film ranges from upper lobe opacities to diffuse 3–4 mm nodules
- Cavitation indicates advanced disease

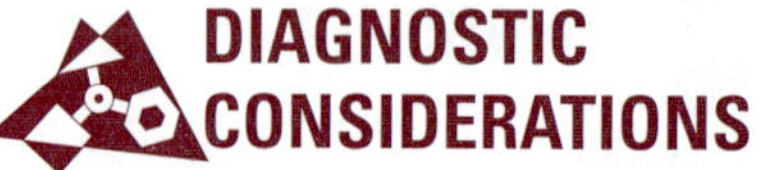

DIAGNOSTIC CONSIDERATIONS

- High/rising serum titers (> 1:32 or elevated 4×)
- Histoplasmin skin test (positive in 2–6 wks)
- Sputum cultures positive in 10%, tissue cultures more reliable

RULE OUT

- TB

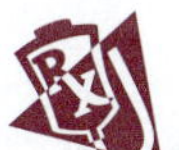

WORK-UP

- Chest film
- Chest CT scan
- Sputum microscopy and cultures

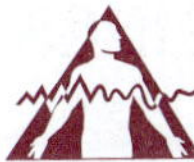

TREATMENT AND MANAGEMENT

- Medical therapy is indicated in immunocompromised hosts or in cavitary or severe disease

SURGERY

- Operative therapy only for complications:
  - Broncholithectomy + pulmonary resection
  - Repair of TE fistula
  - Decompression of mediastinal granulomas
  - Saphenous vein bypass for severe SVC compression

Indications

- Complications of histoplasmosis

MEDICATIONS

- Ketoconazole/itraconazole (6 mos) for cavitary disease
- Amphotericin B for more serious infections or in immunocompromised patients

RESOURCES

REFERENCES

- Johnson P, Sarosi G. Current therapy of major fungal diseases of the lung. *Infect Dis Clin North Am.* 1991;5:635.

Lung Infection, Mucormycosis

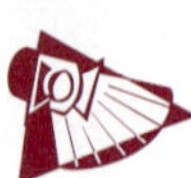

ESSENTIAL FEATURES

- Infection occurs after inhalation of sporangiospores, germination in a hyphal form
- Pulmonary infection occurs in immunocompromised persons, follows a fulminant pattern
- Distinct clinical syndromes:
  - Rhinocerebral infection: Direct extension in CNS from paranasal sinus infection
  - Cutaneous infection: Burn patients
  - GI infection: Children with protein-calorie malnutrition
  - Disseminated infection: Uremic patients receiving deferoxamine therapy

EPIDEMIOLOGY

- Pulmonary fungal infections are rising due to widespread use of broad-spectrum antibiotics, immunosuppressive drugs, and HIV infection
- Occur anywhere in world, some with characteristic endemic areas
- *Rhizopus arrhizus* (most common), absidia species, rhizomucor species
  - Infection occurs in patients with diabetes, leukemia, immunosuppression
  - Common in decaying fruit, vegetables, soil, and manure

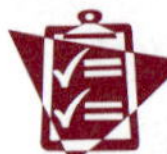

CLINICAL FINDINGS

SYMPTOMS AND SIGNS

- Pulmonary infection: Fever, cough, pleuritic chest pain, hemoptysis

IMAGING FINDINGS

- **Chest film:** 3 distinct patterns
  1. Limited disease with involvement of single lobe
  2. Diffuse or disseminated disease
  3. Endobronchial disease with obstruction and secondary bacterial infection
- **Chest CT scan:** Characteristic halo sign, ring enhancement, and air-crescent sign

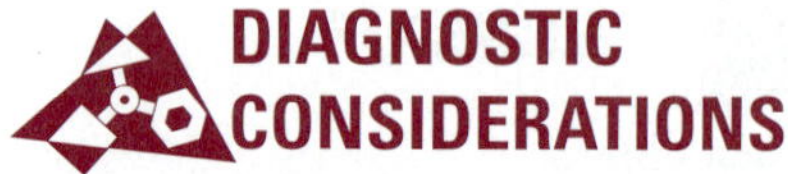

DIAGNOSTIC CONSIDERATIONS

- Demonstrating organism in symptomatic patients
- No skin or serologic test
- Fungi grow in culture as broad irregular nonseptate hyphae branch at 90-degree angles
- Diagnosis most commonly made by histology
- Sine qua non: Hyphal vascular invasion between internal elastic membrane and media of blood vessels causing thrombosis and infarction

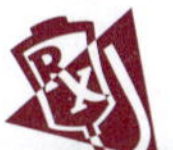

WORK-UP

- Chest film
- Chest CT scan
- Sputum microscopy and culture

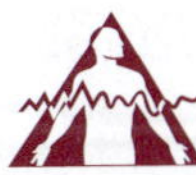

TREATMENT AND MANAGEMENT

- Amphotericin B is standard treatment
- Small group of patients have limited disease: Aggressive surgical resection + amphotericin B
- Endobronchial form: Successful treatment with transbronchoscopic resection using laser therapy

PROGNOSIS

- Mortality is 90% despite best treatment; death from fungal sepsis, pulmonary dysfunction, and hemoptysis
- Those surgically treatable: Mortality 50%
- Endobronchial treatment is generally successful

RESOURCES

REFERENCES

- Johnson P, Sarosi G. Current therapy of major fungal diseases of the lung. *Infect Dis Clin North Am.* 1991;5:635.

Lung Lesions, Metastatic

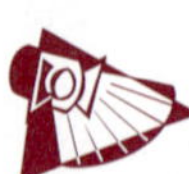

ESSENTIAL FEATURES

- Pulmonary metastases occur via hematogenous spread from primary site; lymphatic and transbronchial spread are rare
- Secondary metastatic spread to pulmonary and mediastinal lymph nodes may occur
- Known extrathoracic primary cancers:
  - Multiple pulmonary lesions: Metastatic disease
  - Solitary lesions: Benign disease, 18%; new primary lung cancer, 18%; metastatic disease, 64%
- Solitary squamous cell nodules should be addressed as a new primary lung cancer

EPIDEMIOLOGY

- 30% of patients with malignancies develop pulmonary metastases
- 12% of isolated lung disease is totally resectable
- 10% of patients (1.2% of all patients) have solitary lung metastases

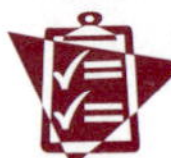

CLINICAL FINDINGS

SYMPTOMS AND SIGNS

- Most asymptomatic
- Cough, hemoptysis, fever, dyspnea, and pain

IMAGING FINDINGS

- Chest film or CT scan identifies nodule(s)

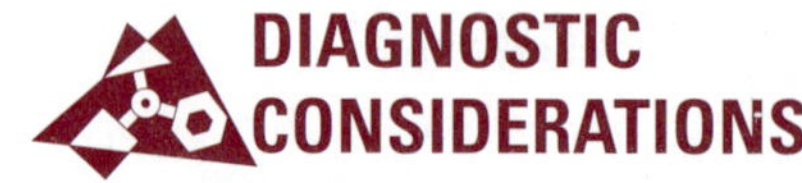

DIAGNOSTIC CONSIDERATIONS

- Pathologic diagnosis is essential

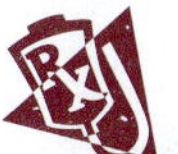

WORK-UP

- Chest film
- Chest CT to assess lungs for other nodules
- CT scans detects 3 mm nodules, with false-positive rate of 55%
- Pathologic diagnosis is essential: obtained at the time of resection, via fine-needle aspiration, or bronchoscopy
- Thorough search for other sites of metastasis including bone scan, head CT, or MRI

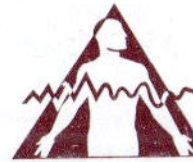

TREATMENT AND MANAGEMENT

- If complete resection not possible, resection should not be offered

SURGERY

- Wedge resection treatment of choice unless lesion is solitary squamous cell carcinoma or adenocarcinoma—treated as primary lung cancers with lobectomy and mediastinal lymph node dissection
- Lobectomy or even pneumonectomy occasionally required if proximal pulmonary artery or bronchus involved

Indications

- Primary tumor controlled or imminently controllable
- No other sites of disease exist
- No other therapy can offer comparable results
- Low operative risk

PROGNOSIS

- Best prognosis
  - Testicular: 51% 5-year survival
  - Head-neck cancers: 47% 5-year
- Osteogenic, sarcomas, renal cell, colon: 20–35%
- Melanoma: 10–15% survival
- Rectal cancer with isolated pulmonary metastasis: 55% 5-year
- Poor prognosis:
  - Multiple or bilateral lesions
  - > 4 lesions on CT
  - Tumor doubling time < 40 days
  - Short disease-free interval
  - Advanced age

RESOURCES

REFERENCES

- Pogrebniak HW, Pass HI. Initial and reoperative pulmonary metastasectomy: indications, technique, and results. *Semin Surg Oncol.* 1993;9:142.
- Todd TR. Pulmonary metastectomy: current indications for removing lung metastases. *Chest.* 1993;103(4 Suppl):401S.

Lung Neoplasms, Benign

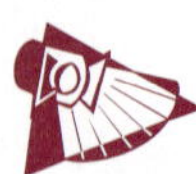

ESSENTIAL FEATURES

- Uncommon
- < 1% of pulmonary tumors
- Include:
  - Fibromas
  - Leiomyomas
  - Neurofibromas
  - Myoblastomas
  - Benign metastasizing leiomyomas
- Most lesions peripheral

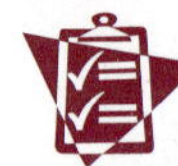

CLINICAL FINDINGS

SYMPTOMS AND SIGNS

- Peripheral: Asymptomatic
- Central lesions: Cough, wheezing, hemoptysis, recurrent pneumonia

IMAGING FINDINGS

- **Chest film:** 1–2 cm well-circumscribed, bosselated lower lung nodule with calcifications in 10–30%

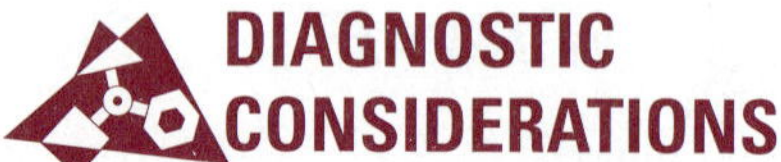

DIAGNOSTIC CONSIDERATIONS

- May be difficult to distinguish from malignant lesions; distinction may occur only after excision

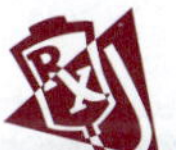

WORK-UP

- Chest film
- Bronchoscopy may be needed for central lesions
- Pathologic diagnosis obtained by surgery or fine-needle aspiration

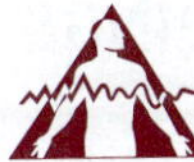

TREATMENT AND MANAGEMENT

- Wedge resection
- Lobectomy if involves proximal airway and associated with infections or bronchiectasis

SURGERY

Indications

- Tissue diagnosis, if unobtainable by bronchoscopy

PROGNOSIS

- Excellent

RESOURCES

REFERENCES

- Gould MK et al. Accuracy of positron emission tomography for diagnosis of pulmonary nodules and mass lesions: a meta-analysis. *JAMA.* 2001;285:914.
- Swanson SJ et al. Management of the solitary pulmonary nodule: role of thoracoscopy in diagnosis and therapy. *Chest.* 1999;116(6Suppl):523S.

Lymphedema & Lymphangitis

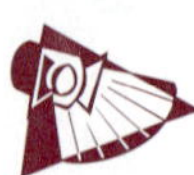

ESSENTIAL FEATURES

- 2 primary diseases: Lymphedema and lymphangitis

Lymphedema

- Little known about fluid dynamics of lymphatic system
- Lymph propulsion occurs from lymphatic smooth muscle contractions
- 2–4 L/d drain into subclavian vein daily
- Mechanism for lymphedema: Impaired flow out of extremity
- Primary disease
  - Abnormal lymphatic development
  - Classified by age: Congenital (< 1 year old), familial (Milroy disease), lymphedema praecox (adolescence, unilateral), lymphedema tarda (> 35 years old)
- Secondary disease
  - Disease that causes obstruction to lymphatic system
  - Most common cause: Surgical excision, also radiation or axillary, inguinal areas
  - Less common causes: Bacterial, fungal infections, trauma
  - Developing countries: Filariasis (*Wuchereria bancrofti*)
  - Chronic lymphedema can result in lymphangiosarcoma (Stewart-Treeves syndrome)

Lymphangitis

- Caused by hemolytic strep or staph infection in area of cellulites near open wound
- Multiple long red streaks seen coursing toward lymph nodes
- Can lead to sepsis and death if untreated

EPIDEMIOLOGY

Lymphedema

- Lymphedema praecox: 3.5:1 female predominance

CLINICAL FINDINGS

SYMPTOMS AND SIGNS

Lymphedema

- Slowly progressive and painless
- In early stages, edema is pitting; with time, fibrosis occurs and edema becomes nonpitting
- Centered around ankle, pronounced around dorsum of foot and toes
- Thickened skin, hyperkeratosis
- Chronic eczematous dermatitis
- History often defines cause
- Painless edema in adolescent girl with family history = primary lymphedema
- History of surgery, radiation, parasite infection suggests secondary cause

Lymphangitis

- Pain at wound site, often red streaks along lymphatics toward lymph nodes
- Regional lymph node enlargement
- High fevers, sepsis

LABORATORY FINDINGS

Lymphangitis

- Elevated WBC count
- Blood and wound cultures

IMAGING FINDINGS

Lymphedema

- **Venous duplex:** Exclude venous insufficiency
- **Lymphangiography:** Rarely used because can damage lymphatics
- **Lymphoscintigraphy:** May confirm diagnosis if ambiguous
- **CT/MRI:** Can diagnose unknown malignancy as a secondary cause

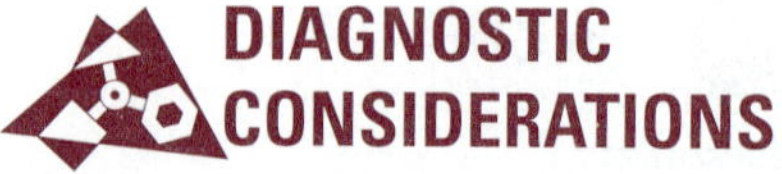

DIAGNOSTIC CONSIDERATIONS

RULE OUT

- Congestive heart failure, chronic renal insufficiency, chronic liver insufficiency
- Congenital vascular malformations
- Chronic venous insufficiency
- Reflex sympathetic dystrophy

Lymphangitis

- Superficial thrombophlebitis
- Cat scratch fever
- Cellulitis

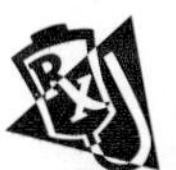

WORK-UP

- Physical exam
- Duplex US
- Lymphoscintigraphy (rarely)

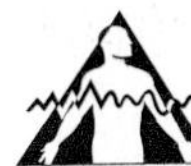

TREATMENT AND MANAGEMENT

Lymphedema

- No cure, goal of therapy to reduce complications
- Pneumatic compression is first-line therapy
- Leg elevation, manual lymphatic drainage massage, low-stretch wrapping
- Skin care to prevent infection
- Moisturizing lotions to prevent cracks
- Rarely, surgical reduction of lumb bulk
  - Sistrunk procedure: Staged excision of subcutaneous tissue
  - Thompson procedure: Lymphatic reconstruction, using omental free flaps to stimulate new lymphatic channels

Lymphangitis

- Elevate extremity, warm compresses
- Aggressive IV antibiotics
- Analgesics, possible debridement

MEDICATIONS

- Diuretics may decrease acute exacerbation of edema

PROGNOSIS

Lymphangitis

- Delayed therapy can lead to sepsis and death

RESOURCES

REFERENCES

- Ko DS et al. Effective treatment of lymphedema of the extremities. *Arch Surg.* 1998;133:452.
- Pain SJ et al. Lymphoedema following surgery for breast cancer. *Br J Surg.* 2000;87:1128.

Mallory-Weiss Tear

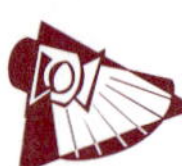

ESSENTIAL FEATURES

- Hematemesis or coffee ground emesis following forceful vomiting or retching
- Epigastric pain

EPIDEMIOLOGY

- Responsible for about 10% of cases of acute upper GI hemorrhage
- Lesion consists of a 1- to 4-cm longitudinal tear in the gastric mucosa near the esophagogastric junction, extending through the mucosa and submucosa but not usually into the muscularis mucosae
- About 75% of these lesions are confined to the stomach; 20% straddle the esophagogastric junction; and 5% are entirely within the distal esophagus
- 67% of patients have a hiatal hernia
- In about 90% of patients, the bleeding stops spontaneously
- The majority of patients are alcoholics

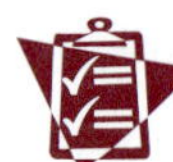

CLINICAL FINDINGS

SYMPTOMS AND SIGNS

- The patient first vomits food and gastric contents, followed by forceful retching and then bloody vomitus
- Epigastric pain
- Epigastric tenderness

LABORATORY FINDINGS

- Hct may be unchanged because of acute blood loss
- Obtain CBC count, type and cross, prothrombin time (PT), partial thromboplastin time (PTT), international normalized ratio (INR)

IMAGING FINDINGS

- **Upper GI endoscopy:** Evidence of gastric and/or distal esophageal mucosal tear with bleeding

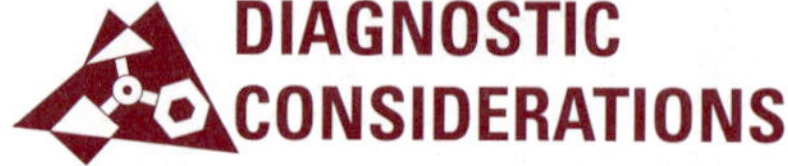

DIAGNOSTIC CONSIDERATIONS

- As in any case of acute upper GI bleeding, endoscopy should be performed emergently for diagnosis and possible treatment

RULE OUT

- Boerhaave syndrome: Actual rupture of the distal esophagus produced by vomiting
- Other causes of upper GI hemorrhage

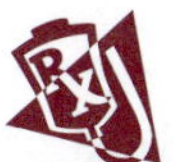

WORK-UP

- Admission to ICU
- Laboratory tests (type and cross, CBC, PT, PTT, INR)
- NG lavage
- Upper GI endoscopy

WHEN TO ADMIT

- All cases of acute GI hemorrhage should be admitted

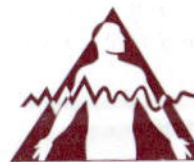

TREATMENT AND MANAGEMENT

- The bleeding can sometimes be controlled by endoscopic therapy
- Surgical repair by gastrotomy and oversewing the tears

SURGERY

Indications

- Persistent or recurrent bleeding after endoscopic treatment

MEDICATIONS

- H_2 blockers, proton pump inhibitors to possibly decrease risk of rebleeding

TREATMENT MONITORING

- Serial Hct to evaluate for ongoing blood loss

COMPLICATIONS

- Recurrent or ongoing bleeding after endoscopic treatment

PROGNOSIS

- Postoperative recurrence is rare

RESOURCES

REFERENCES

- Kortas DY. Mallory-Weiss tear: predisposing factors and predictors of a complicated course. *Am J Gastroenterol.* 2001;96:2863.

Malrotation

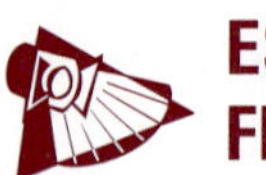

ESSENTIAL FEATURES

- Varying degrees of failure or absence of rotation with the small intestine being on the right and colon on the left with narrow superior mesenteric artery pedicle and Ladd bands lying across duodenum
- 50–75% present in first month of life

EPIDEMIOLOGY

- 5% incidence of some variant in population

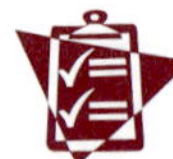

CLINICAL FINDINGS

SYMPTOMS AND SIGNS

- Bilious emesis
- Abdominal distention
- Feeding intolerance
- Irritability
- Hematemesis
- Hypotension
- Shock

LABORATORY FINDINGS

- Heme positive stool (if ischemia present)

IMAGING FINDINGS

- **Abdominal x-ray:** Shows proximal duodenal and gastric distention with paucity of gas distally
- **Upper GI series:** Shows duodenojejunal junction to right of midline and some duodenal narrowing

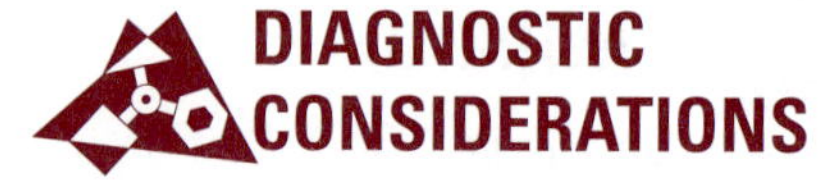

DIAGNOSTIC CONSIDERATIONS

RULE OUT

- Volvulus with ischemia by emergent laparotomy if malrotation is suspected and symptomatic

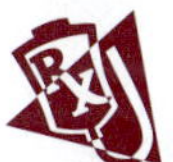

WORK-UP

- History and physical exam
- Abdominal x-ray
- Upper GI series
- Fecal hemoccult test

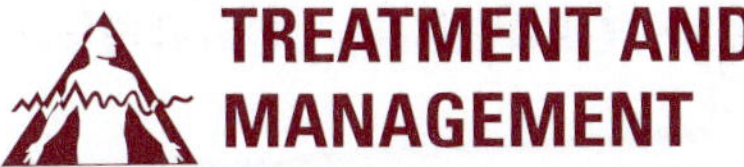

TREATMENT AND MANAGEMENT

SURGERY

- Ladd procedure, resection of any necrotic bowel, and appendectomy

COMPLICATIONS

- Small bowel obstruction in 1–10%

PROGNOSIS

- Excellent

RESOURCES

REFERENCES

- Albanese CT et al. Pediatric Surgery. In: Way LW, Doherty GM (editors). *Current Surgical Diagnosis & Treatment,* 11e. New York: McGraw-Hill; 2003:1318–1320.

Mechanical Pulmonary Failure

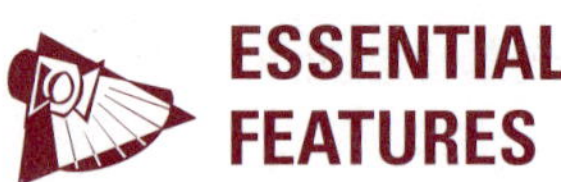

ESSENTIAL FEATURES

- Hypoxemia
- Hypercarbia
- Mechanical insufficiency

EPIDEMIOLOGY

- Trauma
- Pain/weakness postoperatively
- Debility of long-term illness
- Bronchopleural fistula

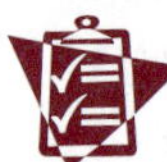

CLINICAL FINDINGS

SYMPTOMS AND SIGNS

- Hypoxemia
- Evidence of chest trauma
- Chest pain
- Free-floating chest wall segment
- Large air leak via wound or chest tube
- Poor ventilatory effort (pain, debility)

LABORATORY FINDINGS

- Hypoxemia
- Hypercarbia

IMAGING FINDINGS

- **Chest film:** Multiple rib fractures

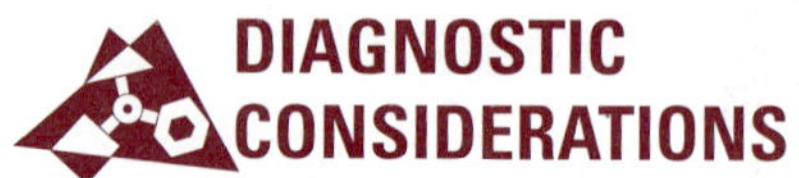

DIAGNOSTIC CONSIDERATIONS

- Often multifunctional basis, for example combination of injury, anesthetic, pain medications and muscle weakeners from catabolism; all factors must be addressed

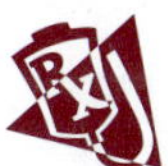

WORK-UP

- ABG measurements
- Chest film

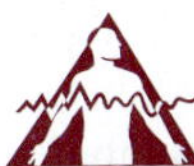

TREATMENT AND MANAGEMENT

- Mechanical ventilation
- Analgesia
- Chest tube decompression
- Chest wall stabilization
- Occlusion of bronchopleural fistulas
- Weaning and nutritional support (debility)
- Tracheostomy (debility)

SURGERY

Indications

- Large bronchopleural fistula

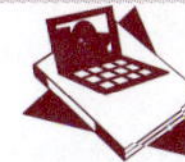

RESOURCES

REFERENCES

- Esteban A et al. A comparison of four methods of weaning patients from mechanical ventilation. *N Engl J Med.* 1995;332:345.
- Tobin MJ. Weaning from mechanical ventilation: what have we learned? *Respir Care.* 2000;45:417.

Mediastinal Masses

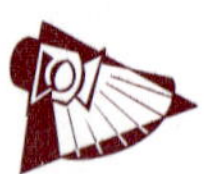

ESSENTIAL FEATURES

Malignant and Benign Lesions

- Divided into 3 regions
  - Anterior
  - Middle (great vessels, heart, trachea, and esophagus)
  - Posterior
- Neurogenic tumors most common masses in children (50–60%);
  - In children younger than 4 years, masses are invariably malignant (neuroblastomas)
- Neurogenic tumors most common mediastinal mass in adults
  - Posterior compartment typical
  - Well circumscribed, calcified, benign
- Anterior masses:
  - More often malignant than neurogenic tumors
  - Thymoma most common then lymphoma

Neurogenic Tumors

- Posterior mediastinum, often superiorly from intercostal or sympathetic nerves
- Nerve sheath tumors (eg, schwannoma and neurofibroma) most common (40–65%)
- Usually benign, 10% malignant
- Malignant tumors arise from nerve cells (neuroblastoma); more common in children
- May be multiple or dumbbell shape

Mediastinal Cystic Lesions

- Arise from pericardium, bronchi, esophagus, or thymus
- 75% located near cardiophrenic angles, 75% on right side
- 10% are diverticula of pericardial sac that communicate with pericardial space
- Bronchogenic cysts arise below carina
- Enterogenous cysts arise along esophagus, may be incorporated, and associated with vertebral anomalies
- 10% nonspecific without identifiable lining

Germ Cell Tumors

- Common in anterior mediastinum
- Both solid and cystic, may contain teeth or hair
- Ectodermal, endodermal, mesodermal elements present
- Most metastatic from retroperitoneal disease; < 5% are primary tumors
- Seminoma (40%), embryonal carcinomas and nongestational choriocarcinomas (20%), yolk sac (20%), and teratomas (20%) can have both benign and malignant components

Lymphomas

- Usually disseminated disease
- Anterior compartment most common but can be anywhere in mediastinum
- Second most common mass in anterior mediastinum

EPIDEMIOLOGY

- Mediastinal masses account for < 20% of all thoracic tumors
- Most masses in adults are benign, with recent shift toward more malignant tumors
- Prevalence: Substernal goiter is most common, then neurogenic tumors (26%), cysts (21%), teratodermoids (16%), thymomas (12%), lymphomas (12%)
- 25% of masses are malignant

CLINICAL FINDINGS

SYMPTOMS AND SIGNS

- Symptoms more common in malignant lesions
- 50% of patients have cough, wheezing, dyspnea, or recurrent pneumonias
- Hemoptysis, chest pain, weight loss, and dysphagia less common, each occurring in 10% of patients
- Myasthenia, fever, superior vena cava (SVC) obstruction, each occurring in 5%
- Cancer suggested if following symptoms are present:
  - Hoarseness
  - Horner syndrome
  - Severe pain
  - SVC obstruction
  - Chylothorax (lymphoma)
- Fever in Hodgkin disease
- **Thymoma:** Myasthenia (15–20%), hypogammaglobulinemia, Whipple disease, red blood cell aplasia, Cushing disease
- **Hypoglycemia:** Rarely in mesothelioma, teratoma, fibroma
- Hypertension and diarrhea in pheochromocytoma and ganglioneuroma
- Neurologic deficits from neurogenic tumors

LABORATORY FINDINGS

- > 90% of germ cell tumors produce bhCG, alpha-fetoprotein (AFP), lactic dehydrogenase (LDH)

IMAGING FINDINGS

- **Chest film: Demonstrates mass**
- **Chest CT:** Diagnostic test of choice
- **MRI**
  - Useful to assess vascular or spinal cord extension
  - In neurogenic tumors, determines intraspinal extension
- **Barium swallow:** Evaluates esophageal lesions or displacement
- **Myelography:** In neurogenic tumors may help plan operative management
- **Bronchography:** Differentiate lung tumors from mediastinal mass
- **Thyroid scintiscan:** Evaluates substernal goiter (can be removed via cervical incision)
- **MIBG scan:** For pheochromocytomas

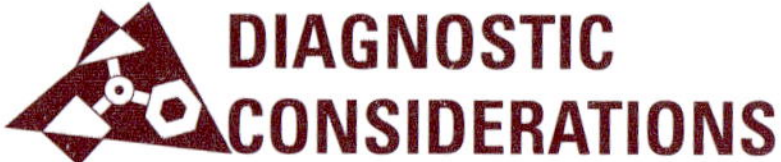

DIAGNOSTIC CONSIDERATIONS

- Extensive work-up often unnecessary as excision required for diagnosis and treatment

RULE OUT

- Lung tumors
- Lymph node lesions

Middle Mediastinum

- Aneurysms, vascular lesions
- Lipoma
- Myxoma
- Bronchogenic cysts
- Pericardial cysts
- Esophageal lesions
- Pheochromocytomas

Anterior Mediastinum

- Thymoma
- Lymphoma
- Teratoma
- Stem cell tumor
- Thyroid goiter
- Parathyroid tumor
- Lipoma

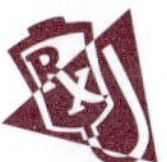

WORK-UP

- Tissue diagnosis via fine-needle aspiration or core biopsy appropriate for metastatic lesions

TREATMENT AND MANAGEMENT

- Complete resection is treatment of choice, often needed for diagnosis
- Excisional biopsy preferred to prevent cancer dispersion
- **Mediastinoscopy/biopsy:** Use cautiously in potentially curable lesions
- Median sternotomy for anterior masses, thoracotomy for middle and posterior mediastinal masses
- Postoperative radiation may decrease local recurrence
- Chemoradiation and surgery combination therapy for germ cell tumors, neurogenic tumors, thymomas

SURGERY

Indications

- For germ cell tumors after chemoradiation has normalized elevated tumor markers

PROGNOSIS

- **Nonseminomatous germ cell tumor:** 50% 5-year survival
- **Seminomas:** 90% 5-year survival
- **Benign lesions:** > 95% cure rate
- **Malignant lesions:** < 50% cure rate

RESOURCES

REFERENCES

- Hagberg H et al. Value of transsternal core biopsy in patients with a newly diagnosed mediastinal mass. *Acta Oncol.* 2000;39:195.
- Gossot D et al. Thoracoscopy or CT-guided biopsy for residual intrathoracic masses after treatment of lymphoma. *Chest.* 2001;120:289.
- Park HS et al. Thymoma. A retrospective study of 87 cases. *Cancer.* 1994;73:2491.
- Cooper JD. Current therapy for thymoma. *Chest.* 1993;103(4 Suppl):3345.

Mediastinitis

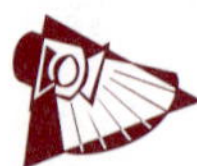

ESSENTIAL FEATURES

- 4 sources
  1. Direct contamination
  2. Hematogenous/lymphatic spread (granulomatous)
  3. Extension of infection from neck/retroperitoneum
  4. Extension from lung/pleura
- Empyema loculates to form paramediastinal abscess; true mediastinal involvement uncommon
- Mediastinitis often involves pleura
- Esophageal perforation is most common form of direct contamination (90% of cases)
- Secondary causes include:
  - Oral surgery
  - Trauma to pharynx
  - Tracheostomy
  - Mediastinoscopy
  - Thyroidectomy
- Pneumothorax after upper endoscopy indicates esophageal perforation

EPIDEMIOLOGY

- Acute: Esophageal, cardiac or other mediastinal operations
- Rarely, direct infection by suppurative conditions involving ribs or vertebrae
- Most cases caused by pyogenic organisms
- Continuous involvement from cervical infection common (along fascial planes)
- Retroperitoneum less commonly involved
- Esophageal perforation caused by:
  - Boerhaave syndrome
  - Iatrogenic trauma (dilation, esophagogastroduodenoscopy, etc)
  - External trauma
  - Cuffed endotracheal tubes
  - Ingestion of corrosives
  - Carcinoma

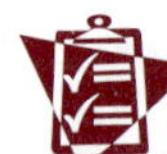

CLINICAL FINDINGS

SYMPTOMS AND SIGNS

- History of vomiting
- Severe boring pain in substernal, left or right chest, or epigastric regions, radiation to back
- Chills, fever, shock, tachycardia
- Dyspnea, pain in shoulder if involves pleura
- Swallowing worsens pain; dysphagia
- 60% have pneumomediastinum/subcutaneous emphysema
- Pericardial crunching with systole (Hamman sign) is late finding
- 50% have pleural effusion or hydropneumothorax
- Neck tenderness, crepitance found in cervical perforation

IMAGING FINDINGS

- Hypaque esophagogram (use water soluble media)
- **CT chest:** With PO and IV contrast, may help determine level of perforation, degree of soilage, underlying pathology

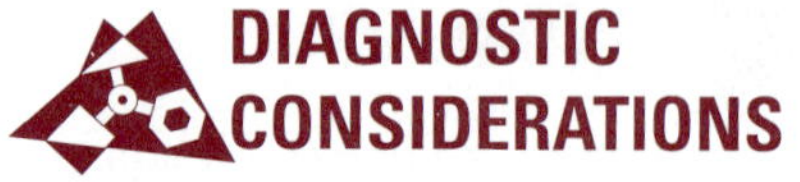

DIAGNOSTIC CONSIDERATIONS

RULE OUT

- Myocardial infarction
  - Often confused with esophageal perforation

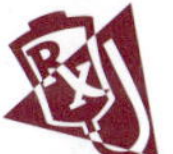

WORK-UP

- History and physical exam
- Hypaque esophagogram (use water soluble media)
- Chest CT with PO or IV contrast

TREATMENT AND MANAGEMENT

- Underlying cause determines treatment
- **Initial management:** Immediate drainage of pleural contamination with chest tube
- Broad-spectrum antibiotics initiated with fluid hydration

SURGERY

- **Right thoracotomy:** Best access to most of intrathoracic esophagus (including distal portion)
- **Left thoracotomy:** Useful for perforation secondary to distal esophageal stricture
- **Iatrogenic perforation (< 24 hrs):** 2-layer closure (mucosal layer with interrupted absorbable sutures and muscle closure), buttress with pleura or muscle flap, wide irrigation and drainage
- **Perforations > 48 hrs:** Wide drainage, resect esophagus
- **Perforation secondary to cancer, severe reflux stricture, achalasia:** Resect esophagus with gastric pull-up if stable and < 24 hrs; if unstable, divert *or* resect without reconstruction

Indications

- All intrathoracic leaks should be explored

MEDICATIONS

- Broad-spectrum antibiotics (including aminoglycosides)

PROGNOSIS

- 30–60% mortality with esophageal perforation

RESOURCES

REFERENCES

- Marty-Ane CH et al. Descending necrotizing mediastinitis. Advantage of mediastinal drainage with thoracotomy. *J Thorac Cardiovasc Surg.* 1994;57:55.

Melanoma

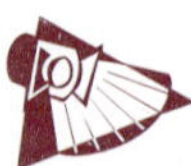

ESSENTIAL FEATURES

- Predominately a disease of fair-skinned whites
- Only 15% of melanomas develop in preexisting nevi, the remainder arise de novo
- Most important prognostic factors include:
  - Vertical height of melanoma
  - Sentinel lymph node status
  - Number of positive lymph nodes
  - Presence of metastatic disease
- Melanoma typically metastasizes by the lymphatic route in a predictable and orderly fashion
- 4 histologic categories of melanoma:
  - Superficial spreading, 70% of cases
  - Nodular melanoma, 15% of cases
  - Lentigo maligna melanoma, 4–10% of cases
  - Acral lentiginous melanoma, 2–8% of cases
- Melanoma most commonly metastasizes to the lungs, liver, and brain but can also involve the bone, adrenals, heart, and bowel

EPIDEMIOLOGY

- 3-fold increase in the incidence of melanoma in the United States in the past decade
- Risk factors include:
  - UV exposure
  - Multiple or dysplastic nevi
  - First sunburn at an early age
  - Freckles
  - Fair complexion
  - Reddish or blond hair
  - Blue eyes
  - First-degree relative with melanoma
- 90% of melanomas are cutaneous lesions, while the remainder occurs in the pigmented cells of the retina, or the mucous membranes of the nasopharynx, vulva, and anal canal
- 2% of melanomas present as metastatic disease to regional lymph nodes or distant sites without a known primary
- 10% of melanomas occur in patients with familial dysplastic nevi syndrome

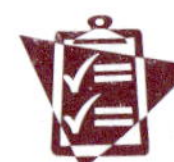

CLINICAL FINDINGS

SYMPTOMS AND SIGNS

- Lesions that are suspicious for melanoma can be identified by their clinical characteristics:
  - Asymmetry
  - Border irregularity
  - Color (variable or dark pigmentation)
  - Diameter (> 6 mm)
- Other clinical signs of melanoma include:
  - Itching
  - Bleeding
  - Ulceration
  - Changes in a preexisting benign mole
- Lymphadenopathy may be present in regional lymph node basins

IMAGING FINDINGS

- **CT or MRI:** Most useful to detect metastatic disease, or in the evaluation of noncutaneous melanomas
- **PET scan:** May demonstrate areas of metastatic disease not detected with conventional CT or MRI

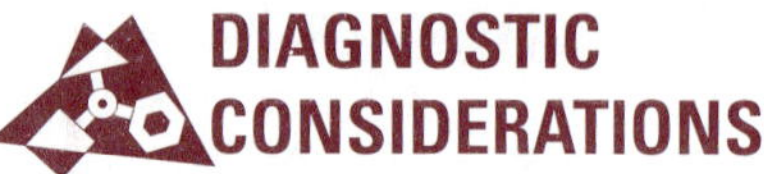

DIAGNOSTIC CONSIDERATIONS

- Melanoma
- Dysplastic nevi
- Benign mole
- Nonmelanotic skin cancer:
  - Basal cell carcinoma
  - Squamous cell carcinoma
  - Merkel cell carcinoma
  - Dermatofibrosarcoma protuberans
  - Sarcomas

RULE OUT

- Synchronous melanoma lesions
- In-transit melanoma metastases
- Evidence of regional lymphadenopathy
- Nonmelanotic skin cancer

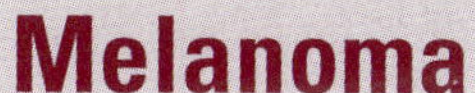

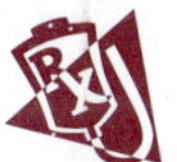

WORK-UP

- Complete history with emphasis on risk factors
- Thorough physical exam including regional lymph node basin assessment
- Excisional biopsy (1–2 mm margins) or punch biopsy of the suspicious lesion
- Fine-needle aspiration of palpable lymph nodes suspected of representing melanoma metastases
- Chest film to evaluate for evidence of pulmonary metastases
- Obtain more thorough radiographic evaluation (head, chest and/or abdominal CT) in high-risk patients that present with bulky lymph node metastatic disease (clinical stage III)

WHEN TO REFER

- All patients diagnosed with melanoma should be evaluated by a dermatologist to assess for synchronous melanomas or other atypical nevi
- Patients with lymph node or regional metastases should be evaluated by a medical oncologist for consideration of adjuvant interferon therapy

TREATMENT AND MANAGEMENT

- Wide local excision of the melanoma
  - < 1-cm lesion: 1-cm margin
  - 2- to 4-cm lesions: 2-cm margin
  - > 4-cm lesion: At least 2 cm
- Sentinel lymph node biopsy for lesions > 0.75 mm thick or thinner lesions with high-risk pathology (ulcerated, many mitoses, etc)
- Full regional lymph node dissection in patients with evidence of lymph node involvement
- Adjuvant immunotherapy in patients with lymph node involvement or metastatic disease
- Resection of solitary metastatic disease
- Radiation therapy to lymph node basins for patients with > 10 positive lymph nodes or evidence of extracapsular invasion
- Radiation therapy for systemic metastases, most commonly to the brain

SURGERY

Indications

- Excisional or punch biopsy for diagnosis
- Therapeutic wide local excision
- Sentinel lymph node biopsy in all lesions > 0.75 mm thick
- Full regional lymph node dissection in patients with evidence of lymph node involvement
- Resection of solitary metastases

MEDICATIONS

- Adjuvant interferon-α_2 has been shown to improve tumor-relapse rate and overall survival for patients with deep primary (IIB) or node positive disease (III)
- Adjuvant vaccine therapy is a promising therapy currently under investigation

TREATMENT MONITORING

- Physical exam for evidence of local or regional recurrence
- Radiographic evaluation for specific symptoms only

COMPLICATIONS

- Local recurrence
- Extremity lymphedema following lymph node dissection
- Metastatic disease

PROGNOSIS

- Depends on stage at presentation
- Most important prognostic factor is lymph node positivity

PREVENTION

- Frequent dermatologic evaluation in patients with dysplastic nevi syndrome
- UV-protective sunscreen

RESOURCES

REFERENCES

- Balch CM et al. Efficacy of 2-cm surgical margins for intermediate-thickness melanomas (1 to 4 mm). Results of a multi-institutional randomized surgical trial. *Ann Surg.* 1993;218:262.
- Reintgen D et al. Lymphatic mapping and sentinel node biopsy in patients with malignant melanoma. 1997;84:188.
- Reintgen D, Kirkwood J. The adjuvant treatment of malignant melanoma. *J Fla Med Assoc.* 1997;84:147.

PRACTICE GUIDELINES

- The National Comprehensive Cancer Network http://www.nccn.org/

CANCER STAGING

- See Melanoma of the Skin Staging Table on page 752.

Ménétrier Disease

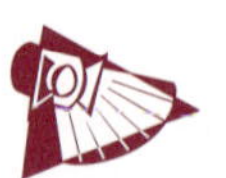

ESSENTIAL FEATURES

- Giant hypertrophy of the gastric rugae with excessive loss of protein from the thickened mucosa into the gut, with resulting hypoproteinemia

EPIDEMIOLOGY

- High, normal, or low acid secretion
- Excessive loss of protein from the thickened mucosa into the gut, with resulting hypoproteinemia
- In children, the disease characteristically is self-limited and benign
- There is an increased risk of adenocarcinoma of the stomach in adults with Ménétrier disease
- Associated with *Helicobacter pylori* infection

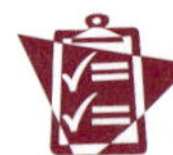

CLINICAL FINDINGS

SYMPTOMS AND SIGNS

- Diarrhea
- Indigestion
- Anorexia
- Weight loss
- Skin rash
- Edema from hypoproteinemia
- Symptomatic anemia

LABORATORY FINDINGS

- Hypoproteinemia
- Anemia

IMAGING FINDINGS

- The hypertrophic rugae present as enormous filling defects on upper GI contrast studies and are frequently misinterpreted as carcinoma
- Hypertrophic rugae apparent on upper GI endoscopy

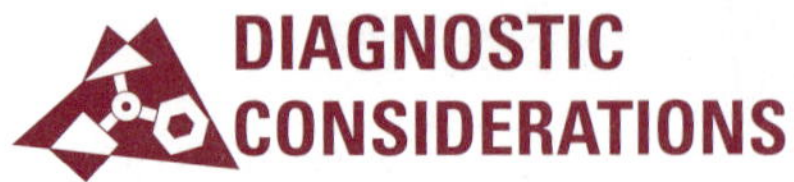

DIAGNOSTIC CONSIDERATIONS

- Radiographic or endoscopic evidence of hypertrophic gastric rugae with hypoproteinemia is strongly suggestive of diagnosis

RULE OUT

- Adenocarcinoma

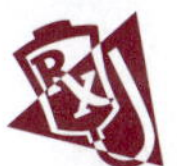

WORK-UP

- Upper GI contrast radiographic study
- Upper GI endoscopy
- Serum protein, Hct

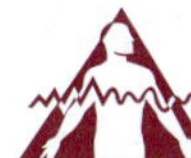

TREATMENT AND MANAGEMENT

- Goal is to reduce protein loss

SURGERY

- Total gastrectomy

Indications

- Rarely indicated for severe intractable hypoproteinemia, anemia, or inability to exclude cancer

MEDICATIONS

- Protein leak may respond to atropine, hexamethonium bromide, eradication of *H pylori,* H_2 blocking agents, or omeprazole

TREATMENT MONITORING

- Endoscopic surveillance for development of adenocarcinoma

COMPLICATIONS

- Hypoproteinemia

PROGNOSIS

- Despite medical management, gastric abnormalities and hypoproteinemia may persist

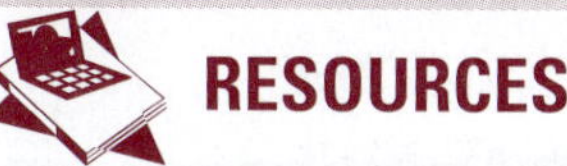

RESOURCES

REFERENCES

- Madsen LG et al. Ménétrier's disease and *Helicobacter pylori:* normalization of gastrointestinal protein loss after eradication therapy. *Dig Dis Sci.* 1999;44:2307.

Mesenteric & Omental Cysts

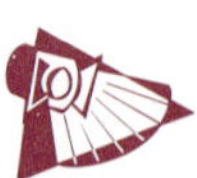

ESSENTIAL FEATURES

- Rare developmental lesions thought to result from the sequestration of lymphatic tissue during development
- Characterized by thin walls lined with endothelial cells without surrounding smooth muscle
- Lesions located in the mesentery, omentum, or retroperitoneum
- Cysts may be filled with serous lymphatic fluid (common in the mesocolon and omentum), or chyle (common in the small bowel mesentery)
- Most lesions are benign
- Cysts often become extraordinarily large before producing symptoms
- Bleeding, rupture, torsion, and infection of the cyst may occur

EPIDEMIOLOGY

- Mesenteric cysts twice as common as omental cysts
- 33% of lesions are detected in children, the remainder in adults
- Symptomatic cysts are usually diagnosed in children before age 10
- Commonly discovered incidentally on imaging study obtained for other reasons

CLINICAL FINDINGS

SYMPTOMS AND SIGNS

- Soft, mobile abdominal mass
- Chronic abdominal pain
- Acute abdomen
- Obstructive symptoms
  - Nausea
  - Vomiting
  - Abdominal distention

IMAGING FINDINGS

- **Abdominal x-ray:** May demonstrate displacement of the viscera by the cyst
- Contrast study may help differentiate between an intestinal duplication and a mesenteric or omental cyst
- **US:** Demonstrates a thin-walled hypoechoic homogenous mass that may be uniloculated or multiloculated
- **CT scan:** Demonstrates a thin-walled fluid density mass that may be uniloculated or multiloculated

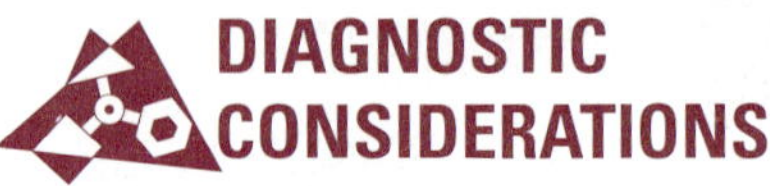

DIAGNOSTIC CONSIDERATIONS

- Pancreatic pseudocysts
- Enteric duplication
- Echinococcal cysts
- Inflammatory cysts
- Retroperitoneal tumors
- Tumor metastasis
- Abscess (especially from perforated appendicitis)
- Large ovarian cysts
- Localized fluid collection
- Hematoma
- Biloma
- Urinoma
- Ascites
- Mesenteric lipodystrophy
- Primary peritoneal mesothelioma
- Pseudomyxoma peritonei

RULE OUT

- Abscess
- Primary or metastatic neoplasm

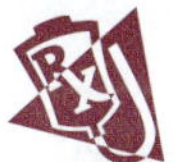

WORK-UP

- Thorough history assessing for abdominal trauma, symptoms and risk factors for pancreatitis (alcoholism, cholelithiasis) or constitutional symptoms (such as weight loss and fatigue)
- CBC count
- Basic chemistries
- Amylase and lipase
- UA
- Abdominal pelvic CT scan with IV and PO contrast

WHEN TO ADMIT

- Acute complications only
- Asymptomatic cyst can be managed as outpatient

WHEN TO REFER

- Children best managed operatively by a pediatric surgeon

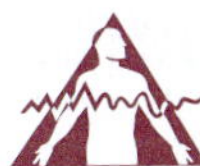

TREATMENT AND MANAGEMENT

- Simple excision of the cyst without resection of adjacent organs or major neurovascular structures
- Partial excision with marsupialization alternative when complete excision not possible
- Internal intestinal drainage also an option, particularly if cyst is adjacent to the intestinal wall and there is concern that the cyst may actually be an enteric duplication

SURGERY

Indications

- Definitive diagnosis and treatment

Contraindications

- Patients medically unfit for operation

TREATMENT MONITORING

- Abdominal exam for mass redevelopment
- Consider US screening for patients in which entire cyst not removed and thus higher chance of recurrence

COMPLICATIONS

- Volvulus of cyst with vascular compromise and infarction of the adjacent intestine
- Bleeding into the cyst
- Cyst rupture into the abdominal cavity
- Cyst infection

PROGNOSIS

- Excellent

RESOURCES

REFERENCES

- Doherty GM, Boey JH. Peritoneal Cavity. In: Way LW, Doherty GM (editors). *Current Surgical Diagnosis & Treatment,* 11e. New York: McGraw-Hill; 2003:531.

Mesenteric Ischemia

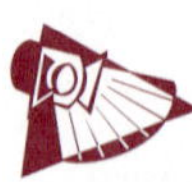

ESSENTIAL FEATURES

- Blood supply to gut:
  - Celiac artery
  - Superior mesenteric artery (SMA)
  - Inferior mesenteric artery (IMA)
  - Internal iliac artery
- Multiple occlusions often well tolerated due to extensive collateral vessels

Chronic Mesenteric Ischemia

- Also known as "intestinal angina"
- Results in ischemia upon "stressing" the gut with food bolus, etc

Acute Mesenteric Ischemia

- Either embolic or thrombotic
- Eventually results in irreversible bowel ischemia
- Due to embolus most often in SMA

EPIDEMIOLOGY

- Stenosis of celiac or SMA caused by
  - Atherosclerosis
  - Vasculitis (lupus, Takayasu)
- Women aged 25–50 years may develop median arcuate ligament syndrome, causing external compression of celiac artery

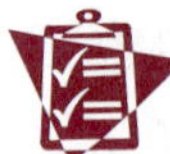

CLINICAL FINDINGS

SYMPTOMS AND SIGNS

Chronic Mesenteric Ischemia

- Postprandial pain 15–30 min after eating
- Epigastric pain, radiating to left upper quadrant/right upper quadrant
- Weight loss from fear of eating
- 80% have epigastric bruit
- Pain out of proportion to physical exam

IMAGING FINDINGS

- Arteriography in anteroposterior and lateral views necessary
  - Patients should be well hydrated to prevent risk of hypercoagulability and bowel infarction
- Duplex and magnetic resonance angiography used to screen but may have low sensitivity and specificity

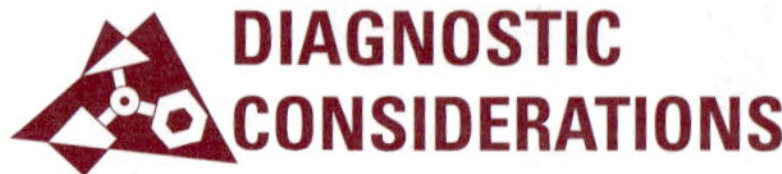

DIAGNOSTIC CONSIDERATIONS

- Angiogram necessary prior to operative repair

RULE OUT

- Should have high clinical suspicion of acute mesenteric ischemia
- For chronic mesenteric ischemia, rule out other causes of postprandial pain
- Peptic ulcer disease
- Gastroesophageal reflux disease
- Cholecystitis

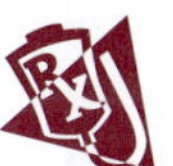

WORK-UP

- Physical exam
- MRI of mesenteric vasculature
- Angiography

TREATMENT AND MANAGEMENT

Acute Mesenteric Ischemia

- Identify occluded vessel, arteriotomy, pass Fogarty, may need bypass
- If bowel not viable, bowel resection

Chronic Mesenteric Ischemia

- **Atherosclerotic lesion:** Surgical revascularization via endarterectomy or bypass
- **Median arcuate ligament syndrome:** Divide ligament with or without arterial bypass
- **Avoid operation if due to vasculitis:** Treat with corticosteroids and immunosuppressive drugs
- Percutaneous transluminal angioplasty + stent for focal, nonorificial stenosis

SURGERY

Indications

- Acute mesenteric ischemia
- Chronic symptomatic ischemia with flow limiting lesion(s)

PROGNOSIS

- **Chronic ischemia:** If surgical revascularization is not performed, high risk of bowel infarction or initiation
- **Acute ischemia:** Early diagnosis essential or outcome is poor
- **Median arcuate ligament compression:** Do well with surgical repair

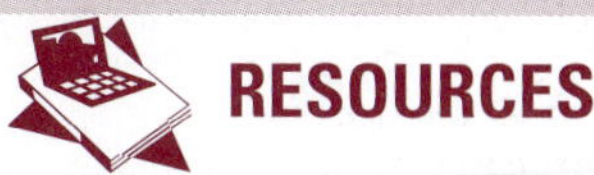

RESOURCES

REFERENCES

- Foley MI et al. Revascularization of the superior mesenteric artery alone for treatment of intestinal ischemia. *J Vasc Surg.* 2000;32:37.
- Kazmers A. Operative management of chronic mesenteric ischemia. *Ann Vasc Surg.* 1998;12:299.

Mesenteric Vascular Occlusion, Acute

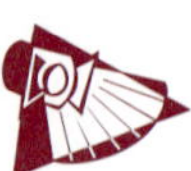

ESSENTIAL FEATURES

- Severe, diffuse abdominal pain
- Gross or occult intestinal bleeding
- Minimal physical findings
- Radiographic findings of vascular occlusion
- Operative findings of ischemic bowel

EPIDEMIOLOGY

- Predominantly a disease of the elderly
- Tissue injury is caused by both ischemia itself as well as reperfusion
- **Mesenteric arterial emboli** (50%): Commonly originate from mural thrombus in an infarcted LV or clot in a fibrillating LA
- **Thrombosis of a mesenteric artery** (25%): The end result of atherosclerotic stenosis; often a history of intestinal angina
- Rare causes of acute arterial occlusion include:
  - Dissecting aortic aneurysm
  - Connective tissue disorders
  - Cocaine ingestion
- **Thrombosis of mesenteric veins** (5%): Associated with portal hypertension, abdominal sepsis, hypercoagulable states, or trauma
- Nonocclusive mesenteric ischemia accounts for the remaining 20% of cases of mesenteric ischemia

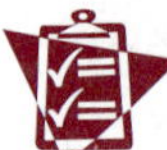

CLINICAL FINDINGS

SYMPTOMS AND SIGNS

- Severe, poorly localized abdominal pain that is often out of proportion to physical findings
- Nausea and vomiting
- Diarrhea
- Shock
- GI bleeding
- Abdominal distention
- Abdominal tenderness
- Peritonitis

LABORATORY FINDINGS

- Leukocytosis
- Serum amylase is elevated
- Significant base deficits
- Increased serum phosphate
- Anemia
- Increased serum lactate
- Antithrombin III deficiency and other abnormalities of coagulation should be sought in cases of venous thrombosis

IMAGING FINDINGS

- **Abdominal x-ray:**
  - Nonspecific
  - Absence of intestinal gas
  - Diffuse distention with air-fluid levels
- **Specific findings occur late**
  - Intramural gas
  - Gas in the portal venous system
- **GI contrast radiography:** Thumbprinting and disordered motility
- **CT scan**
  - Diffuse distention with air-fluid levels
  - Intestinal wall thickening
  - Intramural gas
  - Gas in the portal venous system
- **Mesenteric arteriography:** The gold standard showing disrupted intestinal arterial blood flow or absence of a venous phase

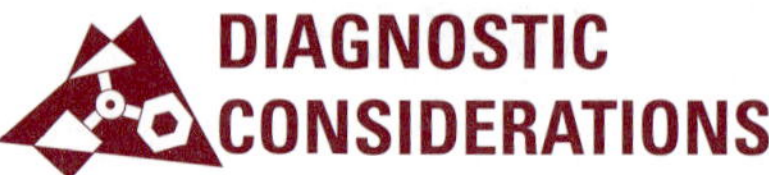

DIAGNOSTIC CONSIDERATIONS

- Survival depends on diagnosis and operative treatment within 12 hours after onset of symptoms
- In the early stages, there is a striking paucity of abdominal findings
- Pain out of proportion to the objective findings is a hallmark of mesenteric vascular occlusion
- Later in the disease course, abdominal distention and tenderness occur
- Shock and generalized peritonitis eventually develop
- Causes of hypercoagulability should be sought postoperatively in cases of venous thrombosis

RULE OUT

- Acute pancreatitis
- Strangulation obstruction
- Nonocclusive intestinal ischemia

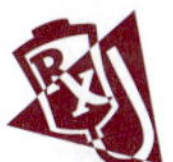

WORK-UP

- CBC count
- Serum electrolytes
- Serum amylase
- Serum lactate
- ABG measurements
- Abdominal x-ray
- CT scan
- Arteriography
- Hypercoagulable studies (venous thrombosis)

WHEN TO ADMIT

- All cases

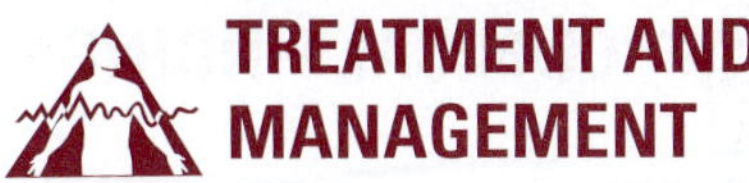

TREATMENT AND MANAGEMENT

SURGERY

- Resection of all involved gut; revascularization of proximal stenosis indicated to salvage viable bowel; thrombectomy usually unsuccessful
- Role of angioplasty is yet to be defined

Indications

- Acute arterial embolism or thrombosis
- Acute venous thrombosis

Contraindications

- Necrotic bowel should be resected unless the extent of damage is so great that satisfactory life could not be expected

MEDICATIONS

- Massive volume support and antibiotics
- Intra-arterial infusion of papaverine
- Heparin and warfarin in cases of venous thrombosis

TREATMENT MONITORING

- A second-look operation is performed 12–24 hours after initial operation if marginally viable bowel was left

COMPLICATIONS

- Sepsis
- Short gut syndrome
- Multi-organ failure
- Death

PROGNOSIS

- Mortality rate
  - Arterial occlusion, 45%
  - Venous thrombosis, 30% with 25% rethrombosis without coumadin

RESOURCES

REFERENCES

- Boley SJ, Brandt LJ. Intestinal ischemia. *Surg Clin North Am.* 1992;72:1.
- Wade TP et al. Mesenteric venous thrombosis: modern management and endoscopic diagnosis. *Surg Endosc.* 1992;6:283.

Middle Lobe Syndrome

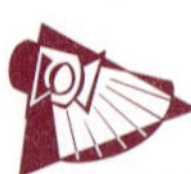

ESSENTIAL FEATURES

- Relapsing lateral pneumonia of right middle pulmonary lobe (RML) caused by intermittent obstruction
- Obstruction most often extrinsic
- Consider diagnosis with repeated right-sided pneumonia
- May be caused by compression/erosion of bronchus by adjacent diseased lymph nodes
- Poor natural drainage and lack of collateral ventilation explain frequency of involvement of RML

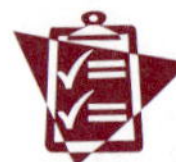

CLINICAL FINDINGS

SYMPTOMS AND SIGNS

- Repeated right-sided pneumonias

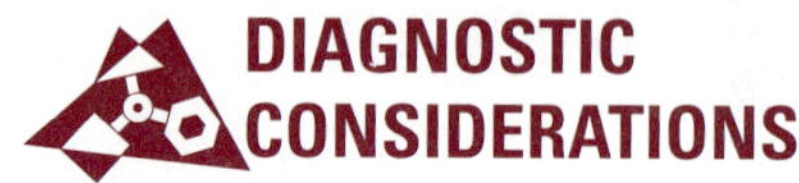

DIAGNOSTIC CONSIDERATIONS

RULE OUT

- Other causes of obstruction (neoplasm, foreign body)

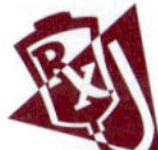

WORK-UP

- Bronchoscopy to rule out endobronchial tumors and foreign bodies

TREATMENT AND MANAGEMENT

- Intensive medical therapy usually adequate treatment

SURGERY

- RML lobectomy

Indications

- Bronchiectasis
- Fibrosis of RML
- RML abscess
- Intractable recurrent pneumonia
- Suspicion of neoplasm

RESOURCES

REFERENCES

- Ring-Mrozik E et al. Clinical findings in middle lobe syndrome and other processes of pulmonary shrinkage in children (atelectasis syndrome). *Eur J Pediatr Surg.* 1991;1:266.

Mitral Regurgitation (MR)

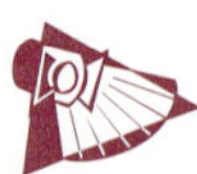

ESSENTIAL FEATURES

- Fibrous annulus of mitral valve (MV) is thin, incomplete ring of fibrous tissue
- Most MVs have anterior and posterior leaflets, attached by thin fibrous chordae tendineae to papillary muscle
- Closed during systole via action of papillary muscle contraction, open during diastole when LA pressure higher than LV pressure
- Etiology includes:
  - Rheumatic heart disease
  - Idiopathic MV calcification
  - Mitral valve prolapse (MVP)
  - Infective endocarditis
  - Ischemic MR
- **Postinfarction papillary muscle rupture:** 0.1% of coronary artery disease; congestive heart failure with new murmur days after myocardial infarction
- MR results in LA hypertension, resulting in pulmonary congestion, dyspnea, pulmonary hypertension, RV failure
- LV is subjected to chronic volume overload causing LV failure (unlike mitral stenosis)

EPIDEMIOLOGY

- Causes of valve disease include:
  - Rheumatic carditis (most common)
  - Valve collagen degeneration
  - Infection
- Less common causes include:
  - Collagen-vascular disease
  - Tumors
  - Carcinoid
  - Marfan syndrome
- Valvular heart disease: 89,000 hospital discharges in 1998
- 40% of MR caused by rheumatic disease
- Risk factors of idiopathic MV calcification include:
  - Hypertension
  - Aortic stenosis
  - Diabetes
  - Chronic renal failure
- MVP is present in 3–4% of general population; 5% of patients with MVP have significant MR
- Infective endocarditis accounts for 5% of MR cases
- 3% of patients with severe coronary disease have ischemic MR; affects posterior leaflet primarily

CLINICAL FINDINGS

SYMPTOMS AND SIGNS

- Exertional dyspnea, orthopnea, fatigue
- Symptoms do not correlate with degree of MR
- Hemoptysis
- Atrial fibrillation (75% of severe cases)
- Malaise, fever, chills in this setting: consider infective endocarditis
- Angina is rare
- Apical impulse displaced to left, palpable thrill at apex
- High pitched holosystolic murmur radiating to axilla and back

LABORATORY FINDINGS

- ECG: LV hypertrophy; if sinus rhythm P mitrale may be present

IMAGING FINDINGS

- **Chest film**
  - LA and LV enlargement
  - RV enlargement
  - Pulmonary edema
  - Kerley B lines
- Transesophageal echocardiography identifies site of regurgitation jet
- Cardiac catheterization demonstrates LA v waves, elevated LV pressure
- Cardiac index < 2.0 L/min/m^2, wide AV oxygen difference indicate severe impairment

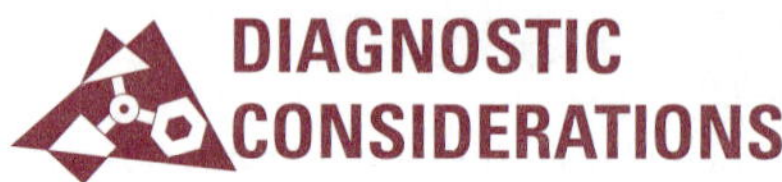

DIAGNOSTIC CONSIDERATIONS

- Evaluate for endocarditis
- Evaluate for secondary LV dysfunction

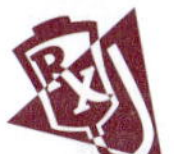

WORK-UP

- 3 determinants of clinical severity:
  1. Degree of regurgitation
  2. LV function
  3. Etiology of valve disease

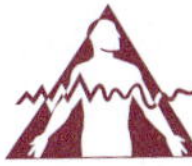

TREATMENT AND MANAGEMENT

- Preload reduction (diuretics), afterload reduction (ACE inhibitors): Helps increase forward output, decrease regurgitation
- Operation: Repair vs replacement
- Virtually all MVP can be repaired (posterior leaflet reconstruction and annuloplasty)
- Ischemic regurgitation: Ring annuloplasty + coronary artery bypass grafting
- Rheumatic disease, valve calcification, or endocarditis: Prosthetic valve replacement

SURGERY

Indications

- Symptomatic heart failure (NYHA class II or greater)
- Asymptomatic, ejection fraction (EF) < 60%, end-systolic dimension > 45 mm, pulmonary hypertension exists, or new atrial fibrillation

Contraindications

- Significant LV dysfunction (EF < 45%) has higher operative mortality, worse long-term outcome

MEDICATIONS

- Diuresis
- ACE inhibitors: Reduce afterload and decrease regurgitation

PROGNOSIS

- Operative mortality, 2–5%
- 5- to 10-year survival, 80% and 65%, respectively
- Survival better for MV repair than for replacement

RESOURCES

REFERENCES

- Enriquez-Sarano M et al. Echocardiographic prediction of survival after surgical correction of organic mitral regurgitation. *Circulation.* 1994;90:830.
- Enriquez-Sarano M et al. Valve repair improves the outcome of surgery for mitral regurgitation. A multivariate analysis. *Circulation.* 1995;91:1022.
- Grigioni F et al. Ischemic mitral regurgitation: long-term outcome and prognostic implications with quantitative Doppler assessment. *Circulation.* 2001;103:1759.
- Ling KH, Enriquez-Sarano M. Long-term outcomes of patients with flail mitral valve leaflets. *Coron Artery Dis.* 2000;11:3.

Mitral Stenosis

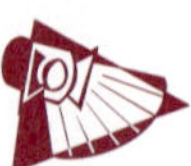

ESSENTIAL FEATURES

- Fibrous annulus of mitral valve (MV) is thin, incomplete ring of fibrous tissue
- Most MVs have anterior and posterior leaflets, attached by thin fibrous chordae tendineae to papillary muscle
- Closed during systole via action of papillary muscle contraction, open during diastole when LA pressure higher than LV pressure
- Mitral stenosis (MS) is fibrosis, narrowing of valvular area causing ventricular inflow obstruction during diastole
- **Early valvular disease of rheumatic fever:** Acute inflammatory infiltrate that heals by fibrous organization
- Leaflets become fibrotic and thickened causing reduced pliability and surface area
- Fusion of leaflets at commissures
- Calcification may occur in leaflets
- Chordae thickened, shortened, and fibrotic
- Mitral complex becomes “fish mouth”
- Results in pulmonary congestion, thickening of pulmonary capillaries, intimal fibrosis of arterioles
- Pulmonary hypertension progresses with time

EPIDEMIOLOGY

- Causes of valve disease include:
  - Rheumatic carditis (most common)
  - Valve collagen degeneration
  - Infection
- Less common causes include:
  - Collagen-vascular disease
  - Tumors
  - Carcinoid
  - Marfan syndrome
- **Valvular heart disease:** 89,000 hospital discharges in 1998
- Number 1 cause of MS is rheumatic fever associated with group A streptococcal pharyngitis
- Death due to heart failure in up to 70%

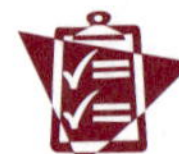

CLINICAL FINDINGS

SYMPTOMS AND SIGNS

- Dyspnea (initially with exertion), orthopnea
- Atrial fibrillation with atrial dilation; often with clinical deterioration due to dependence on atrial kick (20% of cardiac output) and tachycardia
- Thin cachectic “mitral facies”
- Jugular pulsations from fluid overload
- v waves observed if in atrial fibrillation
- Peripheral edema and hepatic enlargement with “hepatojugular reflux”
- Pulmonary component of S_2 pronounced and may be palpable
- Opening snap of MV common due to tensing of leaflets by chordae (heard best at apex)
- Diastolic low pitched rumbling murmur (heard best at apex), accentuated if in sinus rhythm with atrial contraction

LABORATORY FINDINGS

- ECG
  - 90% in sinus rhythm exhibit broad, notched P wave (P mitrale)
  - Later stages: Atrial fibrillation and RV hypertrophy

IMAGING FINDINGS

- **Chest film**
  - Left atrial enlargement
  - Engorged pulmonary veins and arteries
  - Kerley B lines
  - Pulmonary edema if severe congestive heart failure (CHF)
- **Echocardiography:** Provides information on valve anatomy and area
- **Catheterization:** Measure transvalvular gradients/valve area: normal mitral area = 3 cm^2/m^2 BSA; significant MS $\leq$ 1 cm^2/m^2 BSA

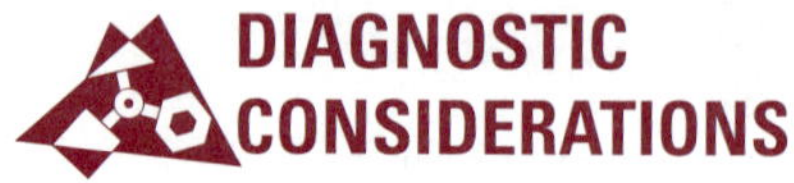

DIAGNOSTIC CONSIDERATIONS

- Echocardiography
- Catheterization

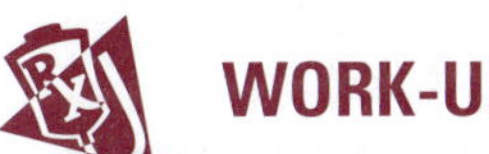

WORK-UP

- Echocardiography
- Catheterization

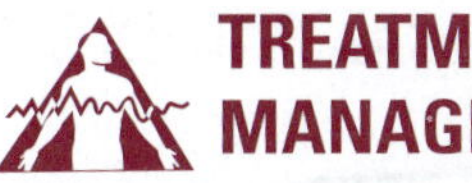

TREATMENT AND MANAGEMENT

- Treat asymptomatic patients medically (control heart rate, anticoagulation therapy for atrial fibrillation)

SURGERY

- Percutaneous balloon valvotomy-moderate to severe symptomatic MS; ideal for minimally calcified, no MR
- Surgical commissurotomy (50%):
  - Absence of leaflet calcification, better candidate
  - Complete incision of commissures
  - Thickened chordae resected
  - Papillary muscles divided to lengthen
- MV replacement: If calcified or fibrous retraction, maintain subvalvular attachments to maintain geometry

Indications

- All symptomatic patients considered
- Significant pulmonary hypertension, pulmonary edema, new onset atrial fibrillation, episodes of thromboembolism

COMPLICATIONS

- **Percutaneous balloon valvotomy:** MR or persistent MS = 2–10%

PROGNOSIS

- 10-year survival in asymptomatic patients > 80%
- Survival for symptomatic MS = 15%
- **Percutaneous balloon valvotomy:** Restenosis-free survival at 10 years = 56%
- **Open commissurotomy:** Results in larger mitral valve area, better functional recovery, and lower incidence of late MR than with balloon valvotomy
- Operative mortality for isolated MV procedures, 1–5%
- Repeat operations necessary in 2–4% per year
- Atrial fibrillation < 1 year significant change of reverting to sinus rhythm

RESOURCES

REFERENCES

- Bonow RO et al. Guidelines for the management of patients with valvular heart disease: executive summary. A report of the American College of Cardiology/American Heart Association Task Force on Practice Guidelines (Committee on Management of Patients with Valvular Heart Disease). *Circulation.* 1998;98:1949.

Mitral Valve Disease, Congenital

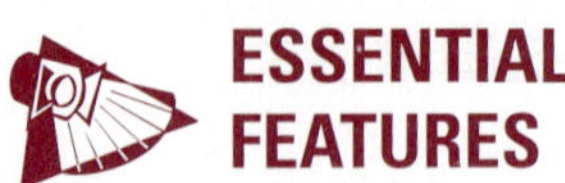

ESSENTIAL FEATURES

Congenital Mitral Valve Disease

- Mitral valve disease uncommon in children
- Can result in stenosis or insufficiency
- Wide spectrum of disease, most have associated pathology
- Associated with ventricular septal defect, atrial septal defect, coarctation
- **Insufficiency:** Dilated annulus, shortened chordae, leaflets restricted
- **Stenosis:** Supravalvular ring, parachute valve, commissural fusion, decreased interpapillary distance
- **Shone syndrome:** Supravalvular ring, parachute mitral valve, subaortic stenosis, aortic coarctation

Cor Triatriatum

- Rare anomaly
  - Pulmonary veins enter accessory venous chamber demarcated from true LA by a diaphragm
- Obstructive orifice connecting chamber to LA
  - Less commonly, chamber connects to RA
- Left-sided superior vena cava (SVC) common
- Results in pulmonary venous hypertension, pulmonary congestion, elevated pulmonary artery pressures
- Respiratory compromise soon ensues

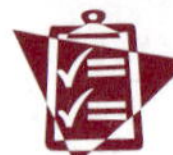

CLINICAL FINDINGS

SYMPTOMS AND SIGNS

- Obstructive symptoms including heart failure, ventricular hypertrophy

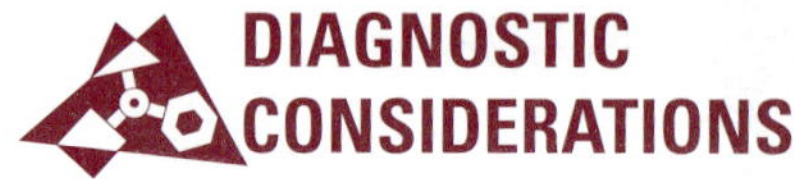

DIAGNOSTIC CONSIDERATIONS

- Evaluate for other cardiac or extracardiac anomalies

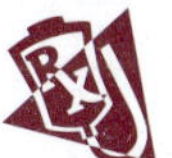

WORK-UP

- Physical exam
- Echocardiography

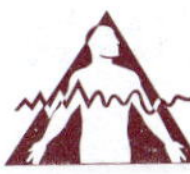

TREATMENT AND MANAGEMENT

Congenital Mitral Valve Disease

- Surgical treatment: Repair preferred over replacement if possible
- Ensure adequate heart function prior to leaving operating room

Cor Triatriatum

- Surgical excision of membrane corrects abnormality

SURGERY

Indications

- Severe symptoms

TREATMENT MONITORING

- Replacement commits patient to anticoagulation therapy and repeat replacement
- Repair may need reintervention in 25–50%

PROGNOSIS

- Good for cor triatriatum

RESOURCES

REFERENCES

- Yoshimura N et al. Surgery for mitral valve disease in the pediatric age group. *J Thorac Cardiovasc Surg.* 1999;118:99.

Mondor Disease (Thrombophlebitis of the Thoracoepigastric Vein)

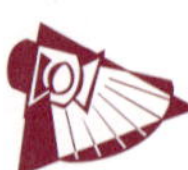

ESSENTIAL FEATURES

- Thrombophlebitis of the thoracoepigastric vein over breast or upper abdomen
- More common in women
- Self-limited, often within 3 wks
- Little to no risk of thromboembolism

EPIDEMIOLOGY

- Occasionally follows radical mastectomy

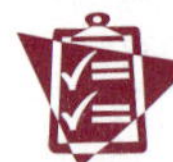

CLINICAL FINDINGS

SYMPTOMS AND SIGNS

- Breast pain
- Superficial abdominal pain
- Localized tender, cord-like structure in subcutaneous tissue of abdomen, thorax, or axilla

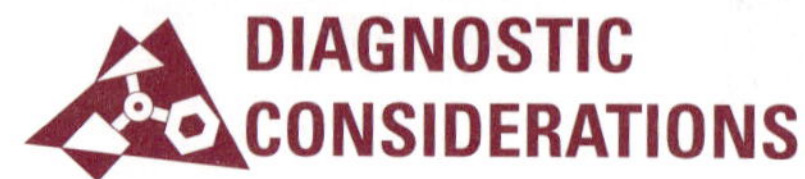

DIAGNOSTIC CONSIDERATIONS

RULE OUT

- Infectious process
- Stasis of venous return due to neoplasm

Mondor Disease (Thrombophlebitis of the Thoracoepigastric Vein)

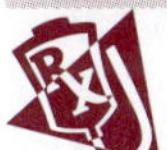

WORK-UP

- Physical exam
- Occasionally, soft-tissue US; usually not necessary

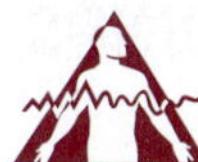

TREATMENT AND MANAGEMENT

- Supportive symptomatic treatment only
- Warm compresses

SURGERY

Indications

- Only if concern for malignancy

MEDICATIONS

- NSAIDs

PROGNOSIS

- Good

RESOURCES

REFERENCES

- Bejanga BI. Mondor's disease: analysis of 30 cases. *J R Coll Surg Edinb.* 1992;37:322.

Multiple Endocrine Neoplasia Type 1 (MEN 1)

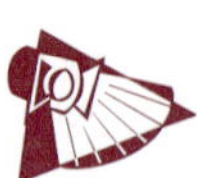

ESSENTIAL FEATURES

- Also known as Wermer syndrome
- Characterized by tumors of the parathyroid, anterior pituitary, and pancreas
- Tumors may develop synchronously or metachronously, may be benign or malignant, and may be hyperplasia, adenomas, or carcinoma
- Pancreatic tumors include functioning and nonfunctioning islet tumors such as gastrinoma, insulinoma, glucagonoma, VIPoma, somatostatinoma, pancreatic polypeptide tumors (PPomas)
- Other tumors in MEN 1 can include adrenocortical tumors, thymic or bronchial carcinoid tumors, multiple lipomas, cutaneous angiofibromas and collagenomas
- Syndrome is transmitted as autosomal dominant trait
- Most common mutation is in the menin gene on 11q13
- Trait has 100% penetrance but variable expressivity

EPIDEMIOLOGY

- Syndrome often develops in the third and fourth decade of life
- Male:female ratio is 1:1
- No known racial predilection
- 90–97% of patients have biochemical evidence of hyperparathyroidism
- 30–80% manifest pancreatic islet cell tumors
- 15–50% develop pituitary tumors
- Gastrinomas with MEN 1 account for 20% of all cases of Zollinger-Ellison syndrome

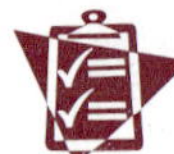

CLINICAL FINDINGS

SYMPTOMS AND SIGNS

- Presentation depends on endocrine tissue involved and the overproduction of a specific hormone; symptoms may arise from tumor mass itself
- Dyspepsia, abdominal pain, hematemesis
- Syncope, tremulousness, diaphoresis, confusion, dizziness (hypoglycemia)
- Symptoms of hypercalcemia, renal stones
- Headaches, visual field defects, amenorrhea, galactorrhea, hypogonadism, acromegaly (pituitary dysfunction)

LABORATORY FINDINGS

- Elevated serum calcium and intact parathyroid hormone
- Elevated gastric acid secretion; elevated fasting serum gastrin level
- Supervised fast with resultant hypoglycemia, elevated serum insulin level, and elevated serum C-peptide level
- Elevated prolactin level
- Direct genetic testing generally offered only for probands with definitive evidence of the MEN 1 syndrome; once the mutation is known, then direct genetic testing of at-risk family members is useful

IMAGING FINDINGS

- Gastrinomas and other pancreatic islet cell tumors can be localized with CT scanning, angiography, or somatostatin receptor scintigraphy

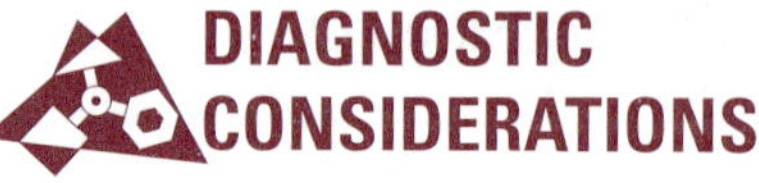

DIAGNOSTIC CONSIDERATIONS

- Hyperparathyroidism is due to multiple parathyroid adenomas with 4 gland involvement
- MEN 1–related hyperparathyroidism occurs earlier in life than nonfamilial primary hyperparathyroidism

Multiple Endocrine Neoplasia Type 1 (MEN 1)

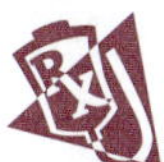

WORK-UP

- CT scanning, angiography, or somatostatin receptor scintigraphy to evaluate for pancreatic islet cell tumors
- Sestamibi scan, cervical US, CT, or selective venous sampling to evaluate location of abnormality for persistent or recurrent hyperparathyroidism
- Annual surveillance for adult gene carriers should include:
  - History and physical exam
  - Calcium and parathyroid hormone measurement for hyperparathyroidism
  - Gastrin, pancreatic polypeptide, abdominal CT scan and somatostatin receptor scintigraphy for pancreatic tumor detection
  - Prolactin level for pituitary adenoma
  - Chest CT scan for thymic carcinoid tumor detection

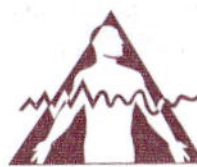

TREATMENT AND MANAGEMENT

- Parathyroid disease treated with surgery
- Treat parathyroid disease first
- Pituitary tumors may require surgical ablation or irradiation but usually are managed medically

SURGERY

Indications

- Biochemical evidence of hyperparathyroidism
- To remove/limit tumor growth of pancreatic tumors (as they are very often malignant)
- To remove insulinomas
- Pituitary tumors

MEDICATIONS

- H_2-receptor antagonist and proton pump inhibitors (for excess gastric acidity from gastrinomas)
- Streptozocin, diazoxide, or octreotide may treat disseminated insulinoma
- Bromocriptine can treat prolactinomas

TREATMENT MONITORING

- Serum calcium and intact parathyroid levels
- Serum levels of pancreatic tumor or pituitary tumor hormones

PROGNOSIS

- After operation, recurrent hyperparathyroidism is seen in up to 40% of cases; permanent hypoparathyroidism is seen in up to 25% of cases

RESOURCES

REFERENCES

- Brandi ML et al. Guidelines for diagnosis and therapy of MEN type 1 and type 2. *J Clin Epidem Metab.* 2001;86:5658.
- Doherty GM et al. Lethality of multiple endocrine neoplasia type 1. *World J Surg.* 1998;22:581.
- Lairmore TC et al. Duodenopancreatic resections in patients with multiple endocrine neoplasia type 1. *Ann Surg.* 2000;231:909.

Multiple Endocrine Neoplasia Type 2 (MEN 2)

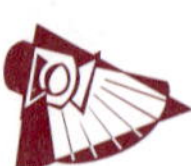

ESSENTIAL FEATURES

- Family of syndromes including:
  - MEN 2A (Sipple syndrome)
  - MEN 2B
  - Familial medullary thyroid carcinoma (FMTC)
- MEN 2A is characterized by:
  - Medullary thyroid carcinoma (MTC)
  - Pheochromocytomas
  - Parathyroid hyperplasia
- MEN 2B consist of MTC, pheochromocytoma, mucosal neuromas, gangliomatosis of the GI tract, and a distinctive marfinoid habitus
  - Also have high incidence of skeletal abnormalities, such as congenital dislocation of the hip, pes planus or cavus, kyphosis, and pectus excavatum
- Transmitted as mendelian autosomal trait, but can occur de novo (especially MEN 2B)
- Common mutation is in the *Ret* proto-oncogone (tyrosine kinase), which maps to the centromeric region of chromosome 10
- Families with hereditary MTC need to be identified with an aggressive screening program because early diagnosis and thyroidectomy renders MTC curable in a large percentage of patients

EPIDEMIOLOGY

- MEN 2A and 2B are transmitted with 100% penetrance but variable expressivity
- Nearly every affected person with MEN 2A and 2B develop bilateral, multicentric MTC
- Pheochromocytomas are present in 50% of MEN 2A patients
- Parathyroid hyperplasia is present in 25% of MEN 2A patients
- MTC occurs earlier and is more aggressive in patients with MEN 2B than those with MEN 2A
- 20% of MTC occurs in a familial setting
- Peak incidence of MTC in setting of FMTC, MEN 2A, or MEN 2B is second or third decade of life
- Pheochromocytomas appear in second or third decade of life; 60% are bilateral

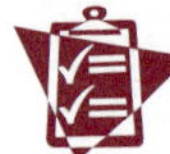

CLINICAL FINDINGS

SYMPTOMS AND SIGNS

- Diarrhea
- Palpable thyroid nodule, or multinodular thyroid gland
- Enlarged, firm cervical nodes (if metastatic disease)
- Hoarseness, dysphagia

LABORATORY FINDINGS

- Calcitonin level is elevated (either basally, or after stimulation with calcium and pentagastrin)
- Elevated plasma metanephrines; elevated urinary catecholamines
- Elevated serum calcium and intact parathyroid hormone

IMAGING FINDINGS

- **Neck x-rays:** May show irregular, dense calcifications
- **Chest film:** May show calcified metastatic hilar and mediastinal nodes
- **Abdominal CT scan:** Can demonstrate adrenal masses
- **MIBG scan:** Can localize pheochromocytomas

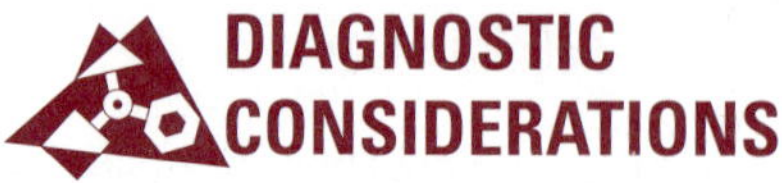

DIAGNOSTIC CONSIDERATIONS

- MTC is usually the first abnormality expressed in MEN 2A and 2B
- Pheochromocytomas are nearly always limited to the adrenal medulla and are nearly always benign
- Most patients are asymptomatic with respect to parathyroid disease
- Pheochromocytoma should be excluded prior to operative neck exploration
- Genetic testing is available for *Ret* mutations

Multiple Endocrine Neoplasia Type 2 (MEN 2)

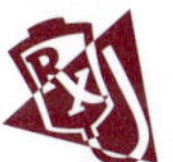

WORK-UP

- Complete history (including family) and physical exam
- Serum calcitonin, calcium, parathyroid hormone, metanephrine levels
- Genetic screening for all patients with MTC

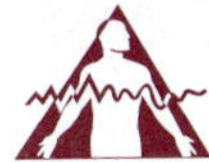

TREATMENT AND MANAGEMENT

SURGERY

Indications

- Elevation of calcitonin level or as soon as diagnosis of FMTC, MEN 2A, or MEN 2B is made
- Presence of pheochromocytoma
- Hypercalcemia

TREATMENT MONITORING

- Calcitonin level
- Routine radiologic and biochemical screening for pheochromocytoma

PROGNOSIS

- Course of MEN 2A and 2B is that of the thyroid lesion

RESOURCES

REFERENCES

- Lairmore TC et al. Management of pheochromocytomas in patients with multiple endocrine neoplasia type 2 syndromes. *Ann Surg.* 1993;217:595.
- Lairmore TC et al. Familial medullary thyroid carcinoma and multiple endocrine neoplasia type 2B map to the same region of chromosome 10 as multiple endocrine neoplasia type 2A. *Genomics.* 1991;9:181.
- Brandi ML et al. Guidelines for diagnosis and therapy of MEN type 1 and type 2. *J Clin Epidem Metab.* 2001;86:5658.

Neck Injuries

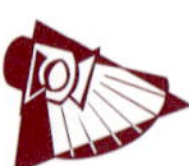

ESSENTIAL FEATURES

- All neck injuries are potentially life-threatening
- Classified as blunt or penetrating with different treatments for each
- Penetrating injuries are divided into zones I, II, and III
- Blunt trauma rarely requires surgery but may cause fracture or dislocation of the cervical vertebrae, occlusion of the carotid arteries, cerebrospinal fluid cysts, or laryngotracheal injuries

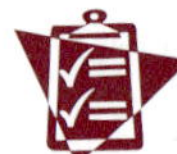

CLINICAL FINDINGS

SYMPTOMS AND SIGNS

- Injuries to the larynx and trachea may be asymptomatic or cause hoarseness, stridor, or dyspnea
- Subcutaneous emphysema may occur with disruption of larynx or trachea
- Severe chest pain and dysphagia with esophageal perforation (may be late appearing)
- Cervical pain or tenderness
- Decreased level of consciousness
- Visible blood loss and hematoma usual with vascular injuries
- Vascular bruit may suggest arterial injury
- Subclavian artery injuries are best approached through a combined cervicothoracic incision
- Venous injuries are best managed by ligation
- Esophageal injuries should be sutured and drained, systemic antibiotics indicated
- Minor tracheal/laryngeal injuries do not require treatment
- Immediate tracheotomy for airway obstruction
- With significant injury to tracheal cartilage silastic stent should be used for support
- Tracheal lacerations should be closed after debridement and distal tracheostomy
- Circumferential tracheal injuries require resection and anastomosis or reconstruction with synthetic material
- Primary neurorrhaphy should be attempted for nerve injury

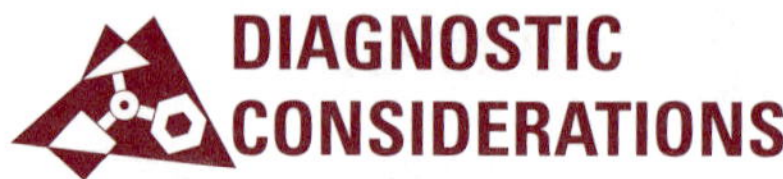

DIAGNOSTIC CONSIDERATIONS

- Zone I injuries occur at the thoracic outlet, extending from clavicles to cricoid cartilage
- Zone II injuries occur in the area between the cricoid and the angle of the mandible
- Zone III injuries occur between the angle of the mandible and the base of the skull
- Zone I includes proximal carotid arteries, subclavian vessels, major vessels in the chest; proximal control will require thoracotomy
- Zone III injuries are difficult to approach and may require disarticulation of the mandible
- Esophageal injuries rarely occur in isolation and may be asymptomatic initially

WORK-UP

- If stable, diagnostic studies should be considered
- Arteriography recommended for patients with zones I and III injuries to help with surgical approach
- Classical approach to any zone II injury penetrating the platysma is operative exploration
- Alternatively, work-up in stable patient should include arteriography or duplex Doppler, rigid endoscopy and rigid bronchoscopy as well as contrast study of esophagus to rule out high esophageal injuries that are easily missed on endoscopy
- Plain films of soft tissues and cervical spine
- Vertebral injuries should be suspected when bleeding from posterior or lateral wound cannot be controlled with pressure, or associated cervical transverse process fracture

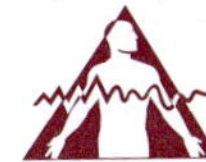

TREATMENT AND MANAGEMENT

- Any injury that penetrates the platysma requires prompt surgical exploration or angiography to rule out major vascular injury
- In zone II injuries, color Doppler may be acceptable alternative
- Neurologic deficit related to arterial injury requires ligation of vessel rather than repair
- Arteries damaged by high velocity missiles require debridement
- If end-to-end anastomosis is not possible, autogenous vein graft can be used
- Vertebral artery injury often requires ligation of vessel (2–3% mortality)

SURGERY

Indications

- Shock
- Expanding hematoma
- Uncontrolled hemorrhage
- Evidence of injury amenable to surgery on work-up of stable patient
- Any zone II injury that penetrates platysma (classic teaching)

COMPLICATIONS

- Untreated injury to larynx and trachea can lead to acute airway obstruction, tracheal stenosis, and sepsis
- Esophageal injuries can result in cervicomediastinal sepsis
- Carotid injuries can cause death from hemorrhage, brain damage, and AV fistula with cardiac decompensation
- Major venous injuries can result in exsanguination, air embolism, and AV fistula formation
- Cervical fracture can result in paraplegia, quadriplegia, or death

PROGNOSIS

- Severance of cervical spinal cord results in paralysis
- Injuries to the soft tissues of the neck, trachea, and esophagus have a good to excellent prognosis if promptly treated
- Major vascular injuries have good prognosis if promptly treated before shock or neurologic deficit
- Overall mortality 10%

RESOURCES

REFERENCES

- Eddy VA. Zone 1 Penetrating Neck Injury Study Group: is routine arteriography mandatory for penetrating injury to zone 1 of the neck? *J Trauma.* 2000;48:208.
- Grossman MD et al. National survey of the incidence of cervical spine injury and approach to cervical spine clearance in U.S. trauma centers. *J Trauma.* 1999;47:684.

Necrotizing Enterocolitis

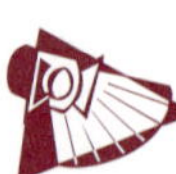

ESSENTIAL FEATURES

- Most frequent surgical condition in a neonate
- Associated with multiple comorbidities in neonate resulting in mucosal injury of the intestine
- Most commonly affecting terminal ileum and right colon

EPIDEMIOLOGY

- 1–3/1000 births and in 30/1000 of low-birth-weight babies

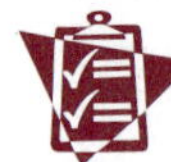

CLINICAL FINDINGS

SYMPTOMS AND SIGNS

- Abdominal distention
- Feeding intolerance
- Bilious emesis
- Occult or gross blood in stool
- Abdominal tenderness
- Abdominal wall edema, crepitus, or discoloration (suggest perforation)
- Temperature instability
- Apnea
- Bradycardia

LABORATORY FINDINGS

- Hypoxemia
- Acidosis
- Thrombocytopenia

IMAGING FINDINGS

- **Abdominal x-ray:** Shows pneumatosis intestinalis from 20% to 98% of time, thickened loops of bowel, ascites, and portal venous gas; possible pneumoperitoneum

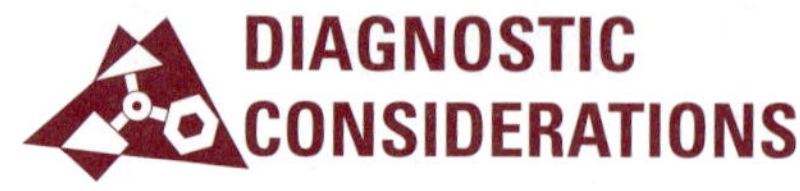

DIAGNOSTIC CONSIDERATIONS

RULE OUT

- Perforation

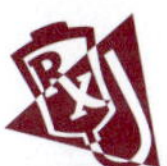

WORK-UP

- History and physical exam
- ABG measurements
- CBC count
- Electrolytes
- Abdominal x-ray

TREATMENT AND MANAGEMENT

SURGERY

- Exploratory laparotomy if patient decompensates or does not improve after 24–72 hours of medical management, pneumoperitoneum, portal venous gas, abdominal wall erythema, or crepitus; resection of necrotic bowel, proximal enterostomy, and distal mucous fistula

MEDICATIONS

- 90% can be managed medically with NG decompression, bowel rest, broad-spectrum antibiotics, and correction of other comorbid conditions

COMPLICATIONS

- 20–40% complication rate including leak, stomal necrosis, fistula formation, and stricture

PROGNOSIS

- Mortality rate, 20–40%

RESOURCES

REFERENCES

- Andorsky DJ et al. Nutritional and other postoperative management of neonates with short bowel syndrome correlates with clinical outcomes. *J Pediatr.* 2001;139:27.
- Ladd AP et al. Long-term follow-up after bowel resection for necrotizing enterocolitis: factors affecting outcome. *J Pediatr Surg.* 1998;33:967.

Necrotizing Fasciitis

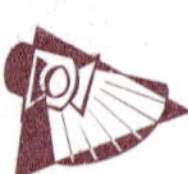

ESSENTIAL FEATURES

- Usually caused by multiple bacterial pathogens
- Infection usually mixed flora, including streptococci, staphylococci, anaerobes, gram-negative aerobes
- Typically begins in localized area (puncture wound, incision)
- Spreads along fascial planes
- Results in thrombosis of penetrating vessels and tissue necrosis
- Area of fascial necrosis usually more extensive than skin appearance indicates

EPIDEMIOLOGY

- More common in patients who are immunosuppressed or debilitated and in those who have diabetes or cancer
- 1000 cases reported in United States per year
- May also develop more frequently in obese patients, following penetrating trauma, postpartum women, injection drug abusers

CLINICAL FINDINGS

SYMPTOMS AND SIGNS

- Hemorrhagic bullae
- Crepitus may be present
- Skin may be anesthetic, edematous
- Fever, pain
- Tachycardia
- Undermining and dissection of the subcutaneous tissue, liquefaction of fat, preservation of overlying skin
- "Dishwater" exudate from wound
- Skin necrosis/gangrene seen in advanced disease

LABORATORY FINDINGS

- Elevated WBC count
- Positive wound culture, Gram stain
- Biopsy of infected tissue reveals:
  - Necrosis
  - Polymorphonuclear leukocyte (PMN) infiltration
  - Thrombi of arteries and veins passing through fascia
  - Angiitis

IMAGING FINDINGS

- Plain x-ray may reveal subcutaneous air

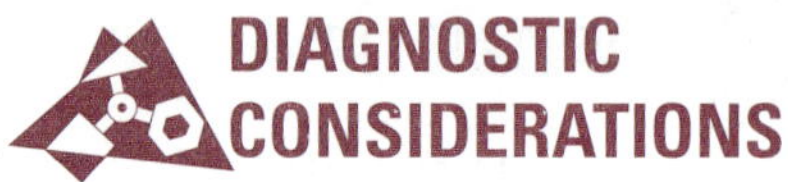

DIAGNOSTIC CONSIDERATIONS

- Superficial cellulitis
- Abscess
- Fistula
- Have high index of suspicion; delay in treatment augments morbidity and mortality significantly

WORK-UP

- High index of suspicion required for diagnosis
- Obtain tissue biopsy/wound aspirate and culture may help direct antimicrobial therapy

WHEN TO ADMIT

- Patients require aggressive resuscitation and surgical treatment

TREATMENT AND MANAGEMENT

- Wide surgical debridement is mainstay of therapy
- Aggressive resuscitation
- Broad-spectrum IV antibiotics
- Multiple debridements may be required

SURGERY

Indications

- Surgical emergency
- High index of suspicion required
- Aggressive debridement of devitalized soft tissue
- Fascial compartments should be decompressed
- Amputation may be required if evidence of diffuse myositis, complete loss of blood supply, and if debridement would clearly leave a useless limb

Contraindications

- Patients should be as aggressively resuscitated as possible prior to operation

MEDICATIONS

- IV broad-spectrum antibiotics: penicillin+aminoglycoside+clindamycin or imipenem-cilastatin
- Intravenous immunoglobulin (IVIG) may be useful for streptococcal toxic shock syndrome
- Aggressive resuscitation required for potential large volume deficits

TREATMENT MONITORING

- Wounds may require further debridement either at bedside or in operating room
- Wound cultures likely to be polymicrobial
- May need to change antibiotic regimen based on wound cultures and sensitivities

COMPLICATIONS

- Sepsis
- Devitalization of entire limb/limb loss

PROGNOSIS

- Potentially lethal
  - 20% with necrotizing fasciitis die
  - > 50% mortality with streptococcal toxic shock syndrome
- Deaths occur when treatment delayed or in the face of other medical comorbidities
- Limbs affected with myonecrosis often become useless, may warrant amputation
- Mortality doubles when > 24 hours elapses between diagnosis and operation

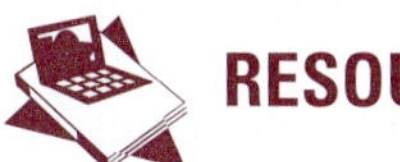

RESOURCES

REFERENCES

- Cobb JP et al. Inflammation, Infection, & Antibiotics. In: Way LW, Doherty GM (editors). *Current Surgical Diagnosis & Treatment,* 11e. New York: McGraw-Hill; 2003:123–125.

Neuroblastoma

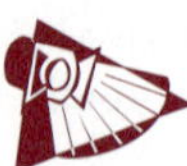

ESSENTIAL FEATURES

- Most common extracranial solid tumor and most common abdominal solid malignancy
- Associated with the following:
  - Neurofibromatosis type I
  - Beckwith-Wiedemann syndrome
  - Hirschsprung disease
  - Musculoskeletal and cardiovascular malformation
  - Turner syndrome
- Factors that place patient at high risk include:
  - Age > 1 year
  - Stage 3 and 4
  - Unfavorable Shimada classification (histology)
  - N-myc amplification
  - No trk expression
  - Diploid
  - 1p deletion
  - > 142 ferritin ng/mL
  - > 1500 LDH IU/L

EPIDEMIOLOGY

- Incidence is approaching 7%
- Median age of diagnosis is age 2, with 80% being younger than 4 years

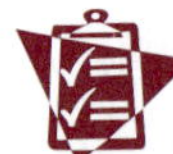

CLINICAL FINDINGS

SYMPTOMS AND SIGNS

- Cervical mass
- Airway compression
- Abdominal mass
- Horner syndrome
- Recurrent urinary tract infections
- Hydronephrosis
- Constipation
- Periorbital ecchymosis
- Opsoclonus-myoclonus
- Secretory diarrhea

LABORATORY FINDINGS

- 24-hour urine collection showing elevated metanephrine, dopamine, and vanillylmandelic acid (VMA)

IMAGING FINDINGS

- **CT or MRI:** Demonstrate extent of disease and location of primary tumor, which can be found anywhere along sympathetic chain
- **Bone scan:** Occasionally shows cortical involvement or marrow involvement
- **MIBG scan:** Shows nodal or metastatic disease

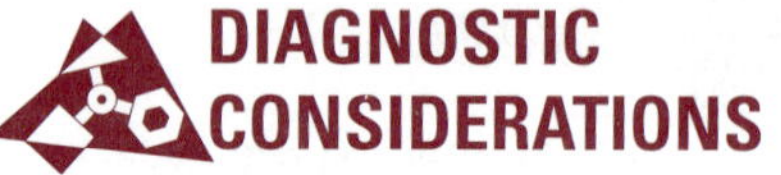

DIAGNOSTIC CONSIDERATIONS

- Stage, high-risk factors, and major vessel involvement

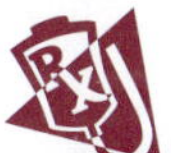

WORK-UP

- History and physical exam
- CT or MRI
- Bone scan
- Bone marrow biopsy
- MIBG scan

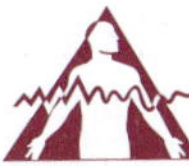

TREATMENT AND MANAGEMENT

SURGERY

- Resection of all gross tumor and regional nodes as well as vascular dissection
- Second debulking resection for high-risk tumors following chemotherapy and radiation therapy is controversial but may be indicated in some cases

MEDICATIONS

- Chemotherapy and radiation for high-risk tumors

TREATMENT MONITORING

- Urinary catecholamines
- CT scanning

COMPLICATIONS

- Damage to neurovascular structures

PROGNOSIS

- 10–30% overall survival for high-risk tumors
- 3-year survival ranging from 40% to 97% (dependent on stage)

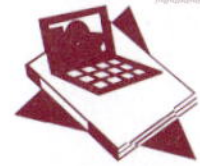

RESOURCES

REFERENCES

- Grosfeld JL. Risk-based management: current concepts of treating malignant solid tumors of childhood. *J Am Coll Surg.* 1999;189:407.
- Shimada H et al. International neuroblastoma pathology classification for prognostic evaluation of patients with peripheral neuroblastic tumors: a report from the Children's Cancer Group. *Cancer.* 2001;92:2451.

Non-Hodgkin Lymphoma

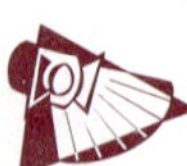

ESSENTIAL FEATURES

- The diagnosis of non-Hodgkin lymphoma encompasses a wide spectrum of lymphoid-derived tumors
- More than 10 distinct tumor subtypes with variable biologic behavior
- Non-Hodgkin lymphoma may originate from B cells, T cells, or histiocytes
- In contrast to Hodgkin lymphoma, lymph node tumor involvement is more likely to spread in a noncontinous fashion in non-Hodgkin lymphoma
- Prognosis and treatment is more dependent on the grade and type of malignancy in contrast to the importance of clinical stage in Hodgkin lymphoma
- Functionally separated into low-grade and high-grade groups
- 33% of cases arise outside of the lymph nodes: oropharynx, paranasal sinuses, thyroid, GI tract, liver, testicles, skin, bone marrow, and CNS
- Most common extranodal site is the stomach, accounting for 50% of all GI lymphomas
- Most accepted classification system is the Revised European-American Lymphoma (REAL) classification

EPIDEMIOLOGY

- Risk factors for the development of lymphoma:
- Ataxia-telangiectasia
- Wiscott-Aldrich syndrome
- Celiac disease
- Prior chemotherapy
- History of radiation therapy
- Immunosuppressive therapy
- HIV
- Human T-cell lymphotropic virus type 1 infection
- Sjögren syndrome
- Extranodal lymphoma risk factors:
  - Gastric lymphoma: *Helicobacter pylori* infection
  - Thyroid lymphoma: Hashimoto thyroiditis

CLINICAL FINDINGS

SYMPTOMS AND SIGNS

- Nontender enlargement of lymph nodes
- Constitutional symptoms:
  - Fever
  - Drenching night sweats
  - Weight loss
- Gastric lymphoma symptoms and signs include epigastric pain, weight loss, and frequently a palpable epigastric mass

LABORATORY FINDINGS

- No distinctive basic laboratory findings present, although lymphomas tend to be associated with an elevated lactic dehydrogenase

IMAGING FINDINGS

- Imaging findings are specific to the location and type of lymphoma
- **Chest film:** May demonstrate mediastinal adenopathy
- **CT scan:** Main staging tool used to demonstrate areas of adenopathy

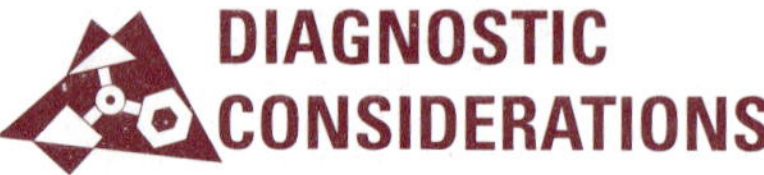

DIAGNOSTIC CONSIDERATIONS

- Hodgkin lymphoma
- Non-Hodgkin lymphoma
- Reactive lymphadenopathy
  - Infectious mononucleosis
  - Cat-scratch disease
  - HIV
  - Drug reactions (eg, phenytoin)
- Tumor metastases

RULE OUT

- Reactive lymphadenopathy
- Metastatic disease to the lymph nodes

WORK-UP

- Detailed history of risk factors and presence of constitutional symptoms
- Thorough physical exam assessing all lymph node beds
- Routine laboratory testing
- Excisional biopsy of enlarged lymph node
- Bone marrow biopsy
- CT scans of the neck, chest, abdomen, and pelvis
- Gastric lymphoma work-up also includes esophagogastroduodenscopy with biopsy and brush cytology

WHEN TO ADMIT

- Most patients with lymphadenopathy that is suspicious for lymphoma are worked-up urgently as an outpatient or admitted to expedite the process

WHEN TO REFER

- Following histologic diagnosis, patients are referred to medical and radiation oncologists for definitive treatment

TREATMENT AND MANAGEMENT

- Treatment depends on grade and stage of the lymphoma:
  - Low-grade localized: Radiation with or without adjuvant chemotherapy
  - Low-grade systemic: "Watch and wait" approach; when more aggressive disease develops, single agent palliative chemotherapy is instituted
  - High-grade localized: Radiation and adjuvant chemotherapy
  - High-grade systemic: Chemotherapy with or without radiation (to areas of bulky disease)
- Gastric lymphoma: Systemic chemotherapy (vs surgical resection and radiation therapy, which are controversial)
- Thyroid lymphoma: Surgical resection followed by combined chemotherapy and neck irradiation

SURGERY

Indications

- Excisional lymph node biopsy to establish diagnosis
- Some centers perform gastric resections for gastric lymphoma to prevent chemotherapy-related perforation or hemorrhage although this practice is controversial and significantly delays beginning therapeutic chemotherapy

MEDICATIONS

- Chemotherapy: Classically, the CHOP regimen (cyclophosphamide, doxorubicin, oncovorin, and prednisone) for high-grade systemic disease and extranodal lymphomas
- Monoclonal antibodies to non-Hodgkin lymphoma tumor-specific antigens are being used in clinical trials

TREATMENT MONITORING

- Physical exam to evaluate for lymphadenopathy
- Radiographic evaluation as clinically indicated (eg, with the redevelopment of constitutional symptoms)

COMPLICATIONS

- Localized radiation-induced complications
- Chemotherapy-induced pancytopenia with the resulting bleeding and infectious complications

PROGNOSIS

- Although the course of low-grade lymphomas is typically indolent, they are difficult to cure and most patients eventually die; median survival times 6–12 years
- High-grade lymphomas are associated with an increased rate of early disease-related mortality but are often curable with aggressive chemotherapy regimens

RESOURCES

REFERENCES

- Mounter PJ, Lennard AL. Management of non-Hodgkin's lymphomas. *Postgrad Med J.* 1999;75:2.
- Patte C. Non-Hodgkin's lymphoma. *Eur J Cancer.* 1998;34:359.

PRACTICE GUIDELINES

- The National Comprehensive Cancer Network
  http://www.nccn.org

Ogilvie Syndrome

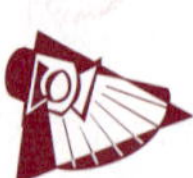

ESSENTIAL FEATURES

- Massive colonic distention in the absence of mechanical obstruction
- Severe form of ileus
- May result from autonomic imbalance
- Aerophagia and impairment of colonic motility by drugs are contributing factors
- Diagnosis of exclusion
  - Must rule out mechanical obstruction

EPIDEMIOLOGY

- Most common in bedridden, elderly patients; following orthopedic injuries; in patients taking psychotropic medications or narcotics
- Associated with metabolic disorders:
  - Hypothyroidism
  - Diabetes
  - Renal failure
- Associated with collagen vascular diseases:
  - Lupus
  - Amyloidosis
  - Scleroderma

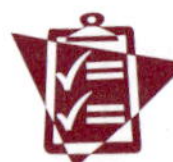

CLINICAL FINDINGS

SYMPTOMS AND SIGNS

- Abdominal distention without pain or tenderness initially
- Later symptoms may mimic obstruction: abdominal pain, tenderness
- Tympanitic abdomen to percussion
- Peritoneal signs indicate bowel compromise and/or perforation
- Bowel sounds often diminished or absent

LABORATORY FINDINGS

- May reveal electrolyte abnormalities (especially magnesium and potassium)
- WBC count usually normal, but an elevation may indicate bowel compromise

IMAGING FINDINGS

- **Abdominal x-ray:** Marked gaseous distention of colon, especially right colon
- **Contrast enema:** Absence of mechanical obstruction

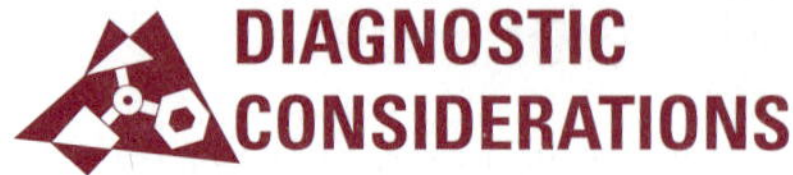

DIAGNOSTIC CONSIDERATIONS

- Mechanical obstruction
  - Carcinoma
  - Hernia
  - Stricture
  - Adhesions
  - Diverticulitis
  - Volvulus
  - Intussusception
- Hirschsprung disease
- Toxic megacolon
- Fecal impaction

RULE OUT

- Mechanical obstruction

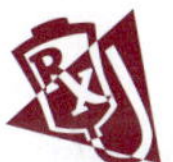

WORK-UP

- Rule out mechanical obstruction
- Review medication history
- Obtain abdominal x-ray
- Contrast enema to determine presence of mechanical obstruction

WHEN TO ADMIT

- Must rule out other etiologies for bowel obstruction and perform serial exams

TREATMENT AND MANAGEMENT

- NG decompression and aggressive enema regimen: Resolution in 86% of patients
- Bowel rest
- Rectal tube placement
- Correct metabolic abnormalities
- Discontinue medications that decrease motility
- Colonoscopic decompression if cecum dilated > 9–10 cm
- If performing colonoscopy, use minimal to no air insufflation
- May place long decompression tube at colonoscopy (Miller or Cantor tube)
- Ensure adequate volume status
- Remove or drain septic collections/abscesses

SURGERY

Indications

- Failure to reduce dilation following conservative measures and endoscopic intervention
- Laparotomy should be performed in patients with peritonitis, nonviable bowel
- Perforated cecum may require ileocecectomy, end ileostomy, and mucus fistula
- Nonperforated cecum may be managed with tube cecostomy

Contraindications

- Ogilvie syndrome occurs most frequently in patients with severe medical comorbidities; early recognition is essential to decrease the need for surgical therapy for complications (perforation/peritonitis)

MEDICATIONS

- Neostigmine (anticholinesterase) may be efficacious in decompressing colon (must be used in monitored setting)

TREATMENT MONITORING

- Serial abdominal exam
- Serial abdominal x-rays following colonoscopic decompression

COMPLICATIONS

- Bowel ischemia/necrosis
- Perforation/peritonitis/sepsis

PROGNOSIS

- Most cases resolve with conservative measures
- If colonoscopic decompression is required, 90% successful
- Recurrence is common following colonoscopic decompression (25%)
- Cecal perforation carries high mortality rate (40%)

RESOURCES

REFERENCES

- Paran H et al. Treatment of acute colonic pseudo-obstruction with neostigmine. *J Am Coll Surg.* 2000;190:315.

Osteitis Fibrosa Cystica

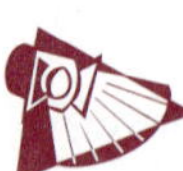

ESSENTIAL FEATURES

- End-stage skeletal manifestation of severe hyperparathyroidism
- Rarely seen now in industrialized societies
- Consists of bone cysts, osteoporosis, and brown tumors (result of excessive osteoclastic bone resorption)

EPIDEMIOLOGY

- Historically, 15% of hyperparathyroid patients presented with bone disease

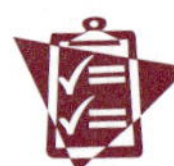

CLINICAL FINDINGS

SYMPTOMS AND SIGNS

- Pain
- Pathologic fractures
- Paraplegia (secondary to vertebral collapse)

LABORATORY FINDINGS

- Elevated serum calcium
- Elevated intact parathyroid hormone level

IMAGING FINDINGS

- Bone radiographs demonstrate osteoporosis, fractures, cysts
- Subperiosteal resorption of the radial aspect of the index and long fingers
- Increased uptake on bone scan

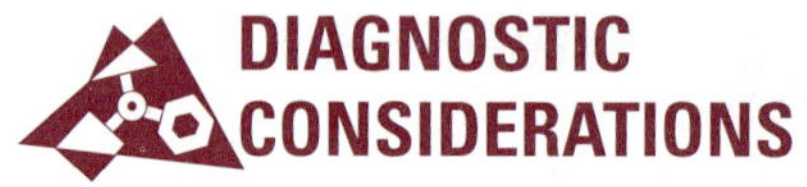

DIAGNOSTIC CONSIDERATIONS

RULE OUT

- Parathyroid carcinoma

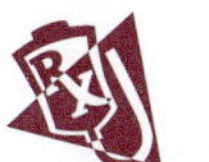

WORK-UP

- Bone scan

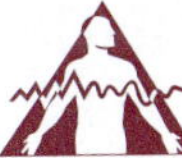

TREATMENT AND MANAGEMENT

- Only effective treatment is the localization and excision of all abnormal parathyroid tissue

SURGERY

Indications

- All patients with osteitis fibrosa cystica should have a parathyroidectomy

MEDICATIONS

- Calcium and vitamin D supplementation postoperatively to aid in bone remineralization

TREATMENT MONITORING

- Monitor serum calcium and intact parathyroid hormone level

PROGNOSIS

- Reversal of bone loss is common after parathyroidectomy, but recovery of bone mass to normal is rare

RESOURCES

REFERENCES

- Agarwal G et al. Recovery pattern of patients with osteitis fibrosa cystica in primary hyperparathyroidism after successful parathyroidectomy. *Surgery.* 2002;132:1075.
- Parisien M et al. Bone disease in primary hyperparathyroidism. *Endocrinol Metab Clin North Am.* 1990;19:19.
- Raeburn CD et al. End-stage skeletal manifestations of severe hyperparathyroidism. *Surgery.* 2002;132:896.

Paget Disease

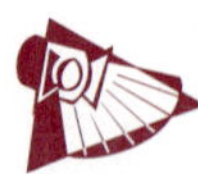

ESSENTIAL FEATURES

- Also known as osteitis deformans
- Nonmalignant disease involving accelerated bone resumption followed by deposition of dense, disorganized, and ineffectively mineralized bone matrix
- Etiology is unknown, although posited to be infectious; hereditary causes possible as well
- 3 phases of disease:
  - Intense bone resorption
  - Production of abundant woven bone with ineffective mineralization
  - Deposition of sclerotic, chaotic cortical and trabecular bone

EPIDEMIOLOGY

- Second most common bone disorder, behind osteoporosis
- Male:female ratio is 1:1
- Affects 3% of persons in the United States
- Affects 10% of persons older than 80 years
- Up to 40% of patients have positive family history for Paget disease
- 1–10% malignant degeneration of pagetic bones

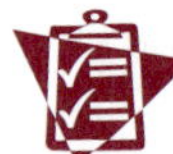

CLINICAL FINDINGS

SYMPTOMS AND SIGNS

- Pain in the affected bone
- Alteration in hearing and vision
- Loosening of teeth (if jaw involvement)
- Headaches
- Damage to cartilage, with resultant arthritis
- Nephrolithiasis
- High output heart failure (from AV shunting in bone marrow)
- Kyphosis
- Frontal bossing
- Leonine facies

LABORATORY FINDINGS

- Elevated serum calcium
- Elevated serum alkaline phosphatase
- Elevated urine calcium
- Elevated urinary pyridinoline

IMAGING FINDINGS

- Soft-tissue masses and cortical breakthrough on plain x-rays suggest malignant transformation
- Radiographs include both early lytic lesions and late sclerotic findings

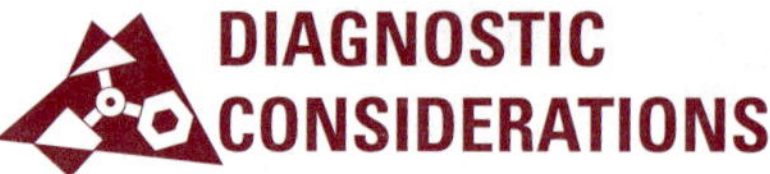

DIAGNOSTIC CONSIDERATIONS

- Always consider metastatic disease to bone

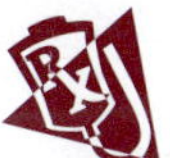

WORK-UP

- Complete history (including family) and physical exam
- Appropriate x-rays
- Serum calcium, alkaline phosphatase, and urinary pyridinoline

TREATMENT AND MANAGEMENT

- Treatment does not cure but prolongs periods of remission
- Goals should include aggressive pain control

SURGERY

Indications

- Progressive bowing of the tibia or femur
- Delayed union of fractures
- Unstable fractures
- Arthritis refractory to medical treatment
- Focal nerve compression of the spine or cranium

MEDICATIONS

- Bisphosphonates inhibit osteoclast resorption
- Injectable calcitonin

TREATMENT MONITORING

- Repeat radiographs, especially of weight bearing joints, to monitor degeneration
- Serum alkaline phosphatase (from every 3 to 12 months)

COMPLICATIONS

- Malignant degeneration into osteosarcomas, fibrosarcomas, or undifferentiated spindle cell sarcomas

RESOURCES

REFERENCES

- Schneider D et al. Diagnosis and treatment of Paget's disease of bone. *Am Fam Physician.* 2002;65:2069.
- Hullar TE, Lustig LR. Paget's disease and fibrous dysplasia. *Otolaryngol Clin North Am.* 2003;36:707.

Paget Disease of Breast

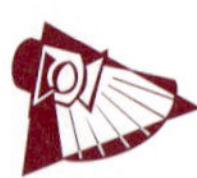

ESSENTIAL FEATURES

- Infiltrating ductal carcinoma involving the nipple epithelium

EPIDEMIOLOGY

- 1% of all breast cancers
- No age group predilection
- Changes may be limited to the nipple, extend to the areola, or to the skin around the areola
- 50–60% have a palpable tumor
- If lesion is confined to nipple only, axillary metastases present in only 5% of patients
- Paget disease of the breast has been associated with breast carcinoma developing in males who had Klinefelter syndrome

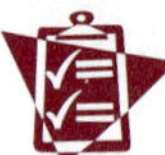

CLINICAL FINDINGS

SYMPTOMS AND SIGNS

- Burning and pruritus of the nipple
- Superficial erosion or ulceration of the nipple
- Serous or bloody nipple discharge
- Nipple retraction

IMAGING FINDINGS

- Mammography may show thickening of the nipple, calcifications, or lesion anywhere in the breast

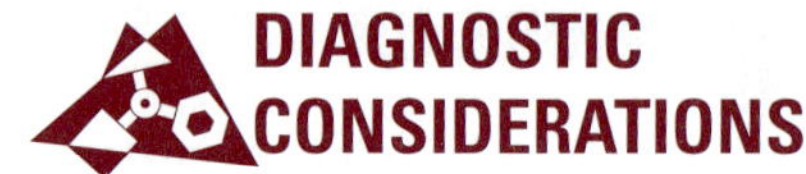

DIAGNOSTIC CONSIDERATIONS

RULE OUT

- Inflammatory breast carcinoma

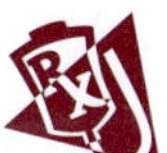

WORK-UP

- Complete history and physical exam
- Bilateral mammogram
- Biopsy of the nipple erosion

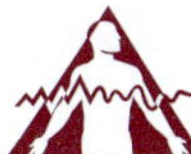

TREATMENT AND MANAGEMENT

- Multimodality treatment is the same as for carcinoma of the female breast

SURGERY

Indications

- May consider excision of nipple-areola complex alone if no palpable tumor and no extensive disease visualized on mammogram

TREATMENT MONITORING

- Self breast exams
- Semiannual clinical breast exam
- Annual mammogram

COMPLICATIONS

- Edema of the arm
- Metastatic spread

PROGNOSIS

- Disease is manifestation of mammary carcinoma, and thus prognosis is determined by extent of associated carcinoma
- No underlying mass and treated by modified radical mastectomy, 10-year survival is 82–100%
- Palpable invasive tumor, but node negative, treated with modified radical mastectomy, 10-year survival is 70%

RESOURCES

REFERENCES

- Chaudry MA et al. Paget's disease of the nipple: a ten-year review including clinical, pathological, and immunohistochemical findings. *Breast Cancer Res Treat.* 1986;8:139.
- Dixon AR et al. Paget's disease of the nipple. *Br J Surg.* 1991;78:722.

PRACTICE GUIDELINES

- The National Comprehensive Cancer Network
  http://www.nccn.org

CANCER STAGING

- See Breast Staging Table on page 744.

STAGE GROUPING

Stage 0	Tis	N0	M0
Stage I	T1*	N0	M0
Stage IIA	T0	N1	M0
	T1*	N1	M0
	T2	N0	M0
Stage IIB	T2	N1	M0
	T3	N0	M0
Stage IIIA	T0	N2	M0
	T1*	N2	M0
	T2	N2	M0
	T3	N1	M0
	T3	N2	M0
Stage IIIB	T4	N0	M0
	T4	N1	M0
	T4	N2	M0
Stage IIIC	Any T	N3	M0
Stage IV	Any T	Any N	M1

*T1 includes T1mic

Note: Stage designation may be changed if post-surgical imaging studies reveal the presence of distant metastases, provided that the studies are carried out within 4 months of diagnosis in the absence of disease progression and provided that the patient has not received neoadjuvant therapy.

Pain, Abdominal, Nonspecific

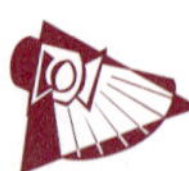

ESSENTIAL FEATURES

- Nonspecific abdominal pain is a diagnosis of exclusion characterized by abdominal pain without identifiable organic pathology
- Mild, fleeting abdominal pain
- Abdominal pain short-lived (< 6hrs)
- Improvement or no change in abdominal pain since onset of symptoms
- Patients frequently complain of nausea and/or diarrhea
- Lack of associated serious signs or symptoms

EPIDEMIOLOGY

- Most common diagnosis among children complaining of abdominal pain
  - Accounts for up to 33% of all cases
- Adults with the symptoms of nonspecific abdominal pain are often diagnosed with irritable bowel syndrome
- Nonspecific abdominal pain is a diagnosis of exclusion
  - Extreme care should be taken before diagnosing this disorder in the very young or old and immunocompromised

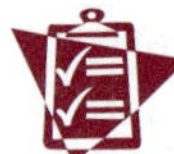

CLINICAL FINDINGS

SYMPTOMS AND SIGNS

- Patient appears comfortable
- No documented fever
- Vital signs normal
- No evidence of peritoneal irritation

LABORATORY FINDINGS

- Normal WBC count
- Normal serum chemistries, amylase, lipase, and UA

IMAGING FINDINGS

- **Abdominal x-ray:** Reveal no free air and a normal bowel gas distribution
- **CT scan:** Although expensive, it is quite specific in ruling out surgical etiologies of abdominal pain

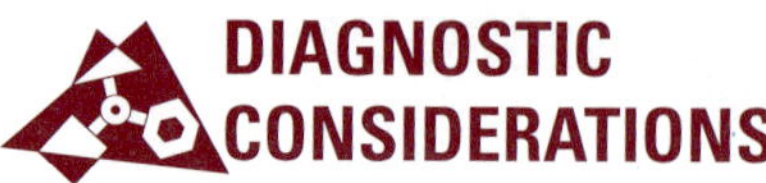

DIAGNOSTIC CONSIDERATIONS

- Irritable bowel syndrome
- Viral gastroenteritis
- Dysmenorrhea
- Psychosomatic pain
- Abdominal wall pain
- Causalgia
- Acute hip bursitis
- Hip joint dislocation
- Thoracolumbar spinal nerve root compression
- Constipation
- Mesenteric adenitis

RULE OUT

- Surgical etiology of abdominal pain
  - Acute appendicitis
  - Acute cholecystitis
  - Bowel obstruction
  - Perforated peptic ulcer
  - Incarcerated hernia
  - Diverticulitis
- Inflammatory bowel disease
- Acute salpingitis/pelvic inflammatory disease

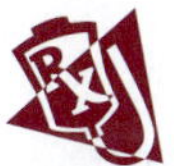

WORK-UP

- CBC count
- Basic chemistries
- UA
- Amylase and lipase
- Abdominal x-ray
- Abdominal/pelvic CT may be indicated when diagnosis is in doubt

WHEN TO ADMIT

- Admission for 24-hour observation may be indicated if a surgical etiology is contemplated (most commonly "rule out appendicitis")
- Most patients can be sent home and asked to come to the emergency department if their symptoms recur or worsen

WHEN TO REFER

- Patients with recurrent abdominal symptoms may benefit from a gastroenterology consult
- Young female patients with cyclical pain that correlates with their menstrual cycle benefit from a thorough gynecologic evaluation

TREATMENT AND MANAGEMENT

- Educate patients regarding significant signs and symptoms that should prompt them to return to the emergency department
- Arrange outpatient follow-up as indicated

SURGERY

Indications

- None

MEDICATIONS

- Avoid narcotics
- NSAIDs may be beneficial and nonaddictive

COMPLICATIONS

- Misdiagnosis

PROGNOSIS

- Excellent

RESOURCES

- Doherty GM, Boey JH. The Acute Abdomen. In: Way LW, Doherty GM (editors). *Current Surgical Diagnosis & Treatment,* 11e. New York: McGraw-Hill; 2003:503–516.

Pancreatic Abscess

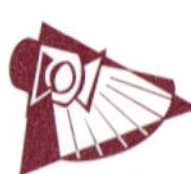

ESSENTIAL FEATURES

- Acute pancreatitis that clinically fails to improve, worsens or improves transiently followed by worsening of signs and symptoms
- Fever
- Leukocytosis
- CT scan showing pancreatic necrosis and fluid collection; sometimes gas bubbles
- Percutaneous aspiration of pancreatic fluid showing organisms on Gram stain and culture

EPIDEMIOLOGY

- Pancreatic abscess complicates about 5% of cases of acute pancreatitis and carries a high mortality
- It tends to develop in severe cases accompanied by hypovolemic shock and pancreatic necrosis and is an especially frequent complication of postoperative pancreatitis
- Abscess formation follows secondary bacterial contamination of necrotic pancreatic debris and hemorrhagic exudates; the organisms may spread to the pancreas hematogenously as well as directly through the wall of the transverse colon

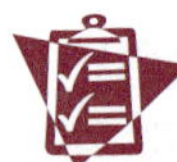

CLINICAL FINDINGS

SYMPTOMS AND SIGNS

- Epigastric pain
- Palpable tender mass
- Fever
- Jaundice (if biliary obstruction from inflammation)

LABORATORY FINDINGS

- Leukocytosis
- Elevated bilirubin
- Aspirated fluid collection
  - Gram stain and culture demonstrating microbial organisms

IMAGING FINDINGS

- **Chest film:** Pleural fluid and diaphragmatic paralysis
- **CT scan:** Fluid collection in the area of the pancreas; gas in the collection suggests infection
- Percutaneous CT scan-guided aspiration: To obtain a specimen for Gram stain and culture

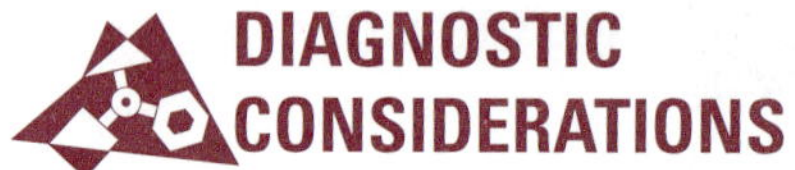

DIAGNOSTIC CONSIDERATIONS

- An abscess should be suspected when a patient with severe acute pancreatitis does not improve and rising fever develops or when symptoms return after a period of recovery
- Distinguishing uninfected pancreatic necrosis from infected abscess may be difficult
  - CT findings and aspiration of fluid collection may aid in making the diagnosis

RULE OUT

- Uninfected pancreatic necrosis, which may not require surgical treatment

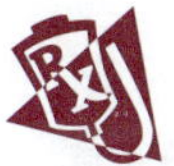

WORK-UP

- CBC count
- Abdominal CT scan with aspiration of fluid collection for Gram stain and culture

WHEN TO ADMIT

- All cases

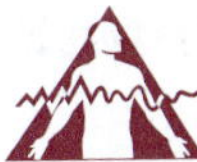

TREATMENT AND MANAGEMENT

- Percutaneous drainage is inadequate
- Surgical drainage and debridement of necrotic pancreatic debris and external drainage is required

SURGERY

Indications

- All cases of infected pancreatic abscess
- An indication for operation in sterile pancreatic necrosis is controversial

MEDICATIONS

- Broad-spectrum antibiotics

COMPLICATIONS

- Postoperative hemorrhage (immediate or delayed)
- Pancreatic fistula

PROGNOSIS

- Mortality rate is 20%, a consequence of the severity of the condition, incomplete surgical drainage, and delayed diagnosis

PREVENTION

- Controversial whether antibiotic administration in severe acute pancreatitis reduces risk of infected pancreatic abscess

RESOURCES

REFERENCES

- Baril NB et al. Does an infected peripancreatic fluid collection or abscess mandate operation? *Ann Surg.* 2000;231:361.
- Tsiotos GG, Sarr MG. Management of fluid collections and necrosis in acute pancreatitis. *Curr Gastroenterol Rep.* 1999;1:139.

Pancreatic Adenocarcinoma

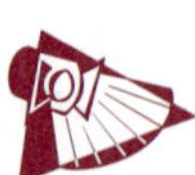

ESSENTIAL FEATURES

- Marked weight loss, abdominal pain and jaundice are common presenting symptoms
- Pancreatic mass often visible on CT scan
- Biliary and duodenal obstruction from tumor growth may occur if located in the pancreatic head

EPIDEMIOLOGY

- Incidence and mortality rates are roughly the same, underscoring the abysmal prognosis—5-year survival, < 3%
- Third leading cause of cancer in men between ages 35 and 54
- Risk factors include:
  - Cigarette smoking
  - Dietary consumption of meat (especially fried meat) and fat
  - Previous gastrectomy (> 20 years earlier)
  - Race (In the United States, but not in Africa, blacks are more susceptible than whites.)
- The peak incidence is in the fifth and sixth decades
- In 67% of cases, the tumor is located in the head of the gland; the remainder occurs in the body or tail
- Early local extension to contiguous structures; metastases to regional lymph nodes and the liver; and later, metastases to lungs, peritoneum, and distant lymph nodes

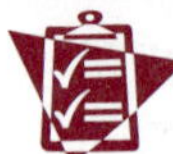

CLINICAL FINDINGS

SYMPTOMS AND SIGNS

- Weight loss
- Abdominal pain
- Back pain (worse prognosis)
- Nausea/vomiting
- Migratory thrombophlebitis
- Palpable epigastric mass
- Obstructive jaundice, often with pruritus and/or cholangitis
- Palpable, nontender gallbladder in the right upper quadrant (Courvoisier sign)
- Sudden onset of diabetes mellitus in 25% of patients

LABORATORY FINDINGS

- Elevated alkaline phosphatase
- Elevated serum bilirubin
- Elevated serum levels of the tumor marker CA 19-9; sensitivity is too low to use as a screening tool

IMAGING FINDINGS

- **CT scan**
  - Pancreatic mass
  - Dilated pancreatic duct and/or bile duct
  - Allows determination of resectability in most cases
- **ERCP**
  - In patients with a typical clinical history and a pancreatic mass on CT, ERCP is unnecessary
  - Stenosis or obstruction of the pancreatic duct and/or bile duct ("double-duct sign")
- **Upper GI series**
  - Determines patency of the duodenum
  - Useful in deciding whether a gastrojejunostomy will have to be performed

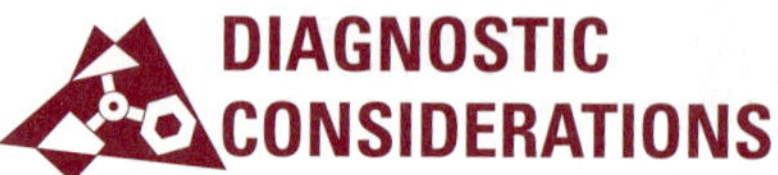

DIAGNOSTIC CONSIDERATIONS

- Tumors of the body and tail cause biliary and duodenal obstruction less commonly than tumors in the head
- Percutaneous aspiration of pancreatic mass risks tumor spread; contraindicated in surgical candidates
- CA 19-9 useful to follow the results of treatments; after complete resection, levels rise again with recurrence.
- CT findings suggesting unresectability:
  - Local tumor extension
  - Contiguous organ invasion
  - Distant metastases
  - Involvement of the superior mesenteric or portal vessels
  - Ascites

RULE OUT

- Chronic pancreatitis
- Other periampullary neoplasms:
  - Carcinoma of the ampulla of Vater, distal common bile duct, or duodenum
- Retroperitoneal lymphoma
- Retroperitoneal sarcoma

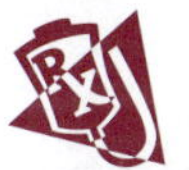

WORK-UP

- CT scan
- ERCP or endoscopic US if pancreatic cancer suspected but mass not visualized on CT scan
- If mass determined unresectable by CT scan, percutaneous or endoscopic US–guided needle aspiration for cytologic confirmation of diagnosis

WHEN TO ADMIT

- Severe abdominal pain
- Duodenal obstruction prohibiting adequate enteral nutrition

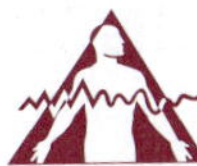

TREATMENT AND MANAGEMENT

- For curable lesions of the head, pancreaticoduodenectomy (Whipple operation) is indicated
- Laparoscopy may be useful for staging

SURGERY

Indications

- Pancreatic mass suspicious for pancreatic adenocarcinoma
- If unresectable, biliary-enteric anastomosis or endoscopic biliary stent and gastrojejunostomy

Contraindications

- Tumor involvement of mesenteric vessels
- Local spread
- Distant metastases

MEDICATIONS

- Radiation therapy combined with chemotherapy (gemcitabine): Neoadjuvant, adjuvant or palliative
- Celiac plexus block for pain

TREATMENT MONITORING

- If neoadjuvant chemoradiation given, interval CT or endoscopic US to determine whether unresectable tumor has been made resectable

COMPLICATIONS

- Biliary obstruction
- Duodenal obstruction
- Severe abdominal pain

PROGNOSIS

- Mean survival: Palliative therapy, 7 months; potentially curative resection, 18 months
- With clear margins, 20% of patients live longer than 5 years

RESOURCES

REFERENCES

- Molinari M et al. Palliative strategies for locally advanced unresectable and metastatic pancreatic cancer. *Surg Clin North Am.* 2001;81:651.
- Farnell MB et al. The Mayo clinic approach to the surgical treatment of adenocarcinoma of the pancreas. *Surg Clin North Am.* 2001;81:611.

PRACTICE GUIDELINES

- The National Comprehensive Cancer Network http://www.nccn.org

CANCER STAGING

- See Exocrine Pancreas Staging Table on page 748.

STAGE GROUPING

Stage 0	Tis	N0	M0
Stage IA	T1	N0	M0
Stage IB	T2	N0	M0
Stage IIA	T3	N0	M0
Stage IIB	T1	N1	M0
	T2	N1	M0
	T3	N1	M0
Stage III	T4	Any N	M0
Stage IV	Any T	Any N	M1

Pancreatic Ascites & Pancreatic Pleural Effusion

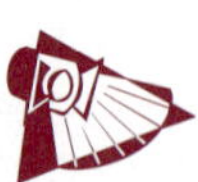

ESSENTIAL FEATURES

- History of chronic pancreatitis, recurrent acute pancreatitis, or pancreatic trauma
- ERCP demonstrating disruption of pancreatic duct
- Chemical analysis of ascites or pleural fluid demonstrating elevated amylase level

EPIDEMIOLOGY

- Pancreatic ascites or pleural effusion consists of accumulated pancreatic fluid in the abdomen or chest, originating from a pancreatic fistula, without peritonitis or severe pain
- Most often due to chronic leakage of a pseudocyst; a few cases are due to disruption of a pancreatic duct (trauma)
- The principal causative factors are alcoholic pancreatitis in adults and traumatic pancreatitis in children

CLINICAL FINDINGS

SYMPTOMS AND SIGNS

- Marked weight loss
- Abdominal distention (ascites)
- Respiratory difficulty (effusion)

LABORATORY FINDINGS

- The fluid ranges in appearance from straw-colored to blood-tinged; contains elevated protein (> 2.9 g/dL) and amylase levels (usually > 3000 IU/dL)

IMAGING FINDINGS

- **ERCP:** Demonstrates the point of fluid leak
- **CT scan**
  - Small leaks not detected by ERCP may be imaged by CT scan performed immediately after ERCP while contrast media is still in the pancreatic duct
  - Associated pseudocysts can also be imaged by CT scan
- **US:** Allows monitoring of treatment

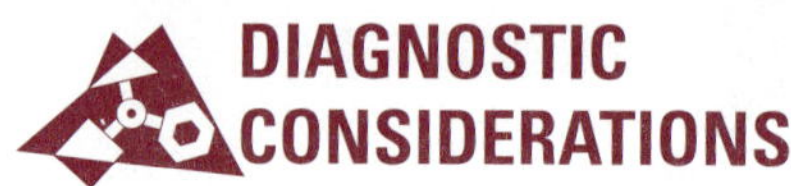

DIAGNOSTIC CONSIDERATIONS

- Once this condition is suspected, definitive diagnosis is based on chemical analysis of the ascitic fluid and ERCP

RULE OUT

- Ascites from underlying hepatic disease
- Pleural effusion from underlying pulmonary disease

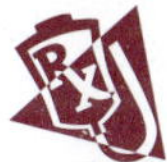

WORK-UP

- Aspiration of fluid (chest or abdomen) and analysis for amylase concentration
- ERCP
- CT scan (if ERCP fails to identify source or if associated with pseudocyst)

WHEN TO ADMIT

- Respiratory difficulty

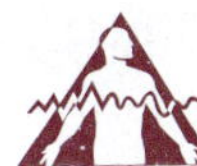

TREATMENT AND MANAGEMENT

- Drain fluid and chest tube (effusion); no oral intake, total parenteral nutrition, somatostatin
- Surgery: Internal drainage
- Endoscopic stenting of the pancreatic duct and may be successful

SURGERY

Indications

- No improvement after 2–3 weeks of medical treatment
- Recurrence after removal of chest tube

MEDICATIONS

- Somatostatin
- Total parenteral nutrition

TREATMENT MONITORING

- US or CT scan to assess fluid accumulation

PROGNOSIS

- Excellent with therapy
- The death rate is low in patients treated before debilitation becomes severe

RESOURCES

REFERENCES

- Kaman L et al. Internal pancreatic fistulas with pancreatic ascites and pancreatic pleural effusions: recognition and management. *Aust N Z J Surg.* 2001;71:221.

Pancreatic Insufficiency

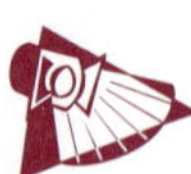

ESSENTIAL FEATURES

- Associated with chronic pancreatitis and extensive pancreatic resections
- Fat malabsorption and steatorrhea are the principal symptoms

EPIDEMIOLOGY

- Pancreatic insufficiency may be a sequelae of pancreatectomy or pancreatic disease, particularly chronic pancreatitis
- The principal problems in otherwise uncomplicated pancreatic insufficiency is fat malabsorption, steatorrhea, and accompanying caloric malnutrition, which do not appear until loss of > 90% of pancreatic exocrine function
- Total pancreatectomy causes about 70% fat malabsorption; if the pancreatic remnant is normal, subtotal resections may have little effect on absorption
- Pancreatic insufficiency affects fat absorption more than protein or carbohydrate
- Malabsorption of vitamins is rarely a significant problem; fat-soluble vitamins do not require pancreatic enzymes for absorption

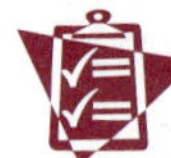

CLINICAL FINDINGS

SYMPTOMS AND SIGNS

- Fat malabsorption and steatorrhea
- Diarrhea may or may not be present
- Weight loss may occur from caloric malnutrition
- Signs and symptoms of underlying disease process (chronic pancreatitis)

LABORATORY FINDINGS

- Exam of a stool specimen for fat globules is specific and relatively sensitive for fat malabsorption

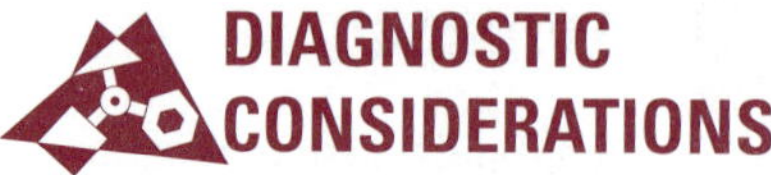

DIAGNOSTIC CONSIDERATIONS

- **Secretin or cholecystokinin test:** Measures HCO_3 concentration in pancreatic juice following administration of either secretin or cholecystokinin
- **Pancreolauryl test:** Fluorescein, release and absorption of which is dependent on pancreatic esterase, is given and urinary excretion is measured
- **PABA excretion (bentiromide) test:** Bentiromide, cleaved by chymotrypsin to release PABA, is administered and urinary excretion of PABA is measured
- **Fecal fat balance test:** After ingesting a diet containing 75–100 g of fat, the amount of dietary fat is measured

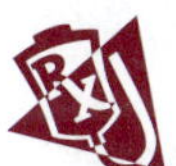

WORK-UP

- Fecal fat determination
- Other tests of pancreatic exocrine function if diagnosis remains unclear
- Appropriate diagnosis of underlying disease process

WHEN TO ADMIT

- Severe malnutrition

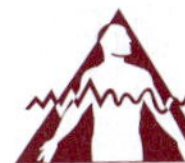

TREATMENT AND MANAGEMENT

- The diet should aim for 3000–6000 kcal/d, emphasizing carbohydrate (400 g or more) and protein (100–150 g); dietary restriction of fat is important mainly to control diarrhea

SURGERY

Indications

- No surgical intervention indicated

MEDICATIONS

- Pancrelipase replacement
- H_2 receptor blockers to retard gastric acid destruction of lipase
- Medium-chain triglycerides (MCT)

COMPLICATIONS

- Fat malnutrition

PROGNOSIS

- Symptoms often improve with pancreatic enzyme replacement

RESOURCES

REFERENCES

- DiMagno EP. Gastric acid suppression and treatment of severe exocrine pancreatic insufficiency. *Best Pract Res Clin Gastroenterol.* 2001;15:477.
- Layer P, Keller J. Pancreatic enzymes: secretion and luminal nutrient digestion in health and disease. *J Clin Gastroenterol.* 1999;28:3.

Pancreatic Neoplasms, Cystic

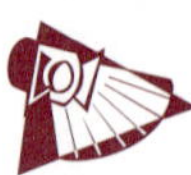

ESSENTIAL FEATURES

- Abdominal pain
- Imaging findings consistent with cystic pancreatic mass
- May be incidental finding on CT scan
- Overall better prognosis than pancreatic adenocarcinoma
- 4 major types:
  1. Mucinous cystic neoplasm (MCN)
  2. Serous cystic neoplasm (SCN)
  3. Intraductal papillary mucinous neoplasm (IPMN)
  4. Solid pseudopapillary tumor (SPT)
- All have malignant potential except SCN, which is very seldom invasive or metastatic.

EPIDEMIOLOGY

- **MCN (1–2% of pancreatic tumors)**
  - 2:1 female predominance
  - Most in body or tail of pancreas
  - Usual age at diagnosis fourth or fifth decade
  - High malignant potential to develop mucinous cystadenocarcinoma
- **SCN (1–2% of pancreatic tumors)**
  - 2:1 female predominance
  - Usual age at diagnosis seventh decade
  - Rarely behave malignantly
- **IPMN (< 5% of pancreatic tumors)**
  - Usual age at diagnosis eighth decade
  - Most in head of pancreas
  - 35% with invasive adenocarcinoma
- **SPT (< 1% of pancreatic tumors)**
  - Commonly in women < 25 years old
  - Most in tail of pancreas
  - Metastases in 10–15% of patients at presentation
  - Seldom invasive

CLINICAL FINDINGS

SYMPTOMS AND SIGNS

- Epigastric mass
- Abdominal pain
- Jaundice if tumor obstructs biliary tract.
- IPMN may be associated with acute pancreatitis

IMAGING FINDINGS

- **CT scan**
  - MCN: Unilocular or multilocular cyst
  - SCN: Honeycomb pattern of microcysts
  - IPMN: Cyst communicates with often dilated pancreatic duct
  - SPT: Sharply circumscribed with thick pericystic fibrous capsule

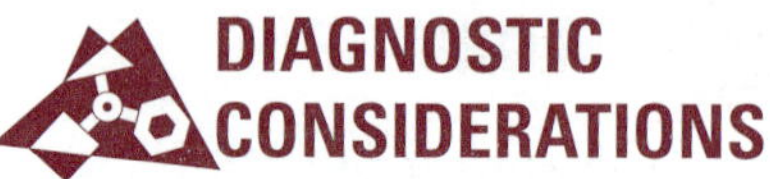

DIAGNOSTIC CONSIDERATIONS

- Cystic tumor of the pancreas apparent on CT scan

RULE OUT

- Pancreatic pseudocyst if associated with acute or chronic pancreatitis

WORK-UP

- CT scan for diagnosis and assessment of resectability
- ERCP for biliary decompression if associated with symptomatic jaundice
- Pancreatic biopsy indicated prior to neoadjuvant or palliative therapy if tumor unresectable

WHEN TO ADMIT

- Severe symptoms or cholangitis associated with biliary obstruction

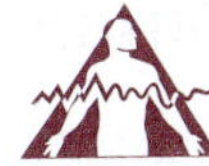

TREATMENT AND MANAGEMENT

SURGERY

- Pancreatic resection if resectable
- Pancreaticoduodenectomy for tumors in pancreatic head
- Distal pancreatectomy for lesions in pancreatic body or tail

Indications

- All cystic neoplasms should be resected

Contraindications

- Unresectable lesions: Vascular encasement or occlusion on CT scan

COMPLICATIONS

- Malignant degeneration
- Biliary obstruction

PROGNOSIS

- MCN: 70% at 5 years
- SCN: Resection curative
- IPMN: > 60% at 5 years
- SPT: 95% cured with resection

RESOURCES

REFERENCES

- Balcom JH et al. Cystic lesions in the pancreas: when to watch, when to resect. *Curr Gastroenterol Rep.* 2000;2:152.
- Sarr MG et al. Cystic neoplasms of the pancreas: benign to malignant epithelial neoplasms. *Surg Clin North Am.* 2001;81:497.

Pancreatic Pseudocyst

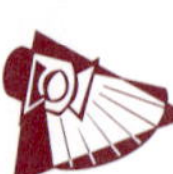

ESSENTIAL FEATURES

- Recent history of acute pancreatitis, pancreatic trauma, or known chronic pancreatitis
- Epigastric mass and pain
- Mild fever and leukocytosis
- Persistent serum amylase elevation
- Pancreatic cyst demonstrated by US or CT scan

EPIDEMIOLOGY

- Pancreatic pseudocysts are encapsulated collections of pancreatic secretions
  - They arise following acute pancreatitis or from chronic ductal obstruction (chronic pancreatitis) or acute ductal disruption (trauma)
- The walls of a pseudocyst are formed by inflammatory fibrosis of the peritoneal, mesenteric, and serosal membranes, which limits spread of the pancreatic juice as the lesion develops
- Pseudocysts develop in about 2% of cases of acute pancreatitis
  - The cysts are single in 85% of cases
- A pseudocyst should be suspected when a patient with acute pancreatitis does not recover after 1 week of treatment or when, after improving for a time, symptoms return
- Pseudocysts can contain collections of sterile or infected material

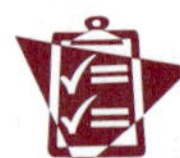

CLINICAL FINDINGS

SYMPTOMS AND SIGNS

- Abdominal pain is most common
- Fever
- Weight loss
- Jaundice, due to obstruction of the intrapancreatic segment of the bile duct
- Palpable, tender mass in the epigastrium

LABORATORY FINDINGS

- Elevated serum amylase
- Leukocytosis
- Elevated bilirubin levels reflect biliary obstruction

IMAGING FINDINGS

- **CT scan**
  - Diagnostic study of choice
  - Size and shape of the cyst and its relationship to other viscera can be seen
  - A pancreatic duct obstruction may be found with chronic pancreatitis
  - A dilated common bile duct suggests biliary obstruction
- **US:** May be useful to follow changes in size of an acute pseudocyst already imaged by CT scans
- **ERCP:** Should be performed if there is obstruction or disruption of the pancreatic duct as these findings would require endoscopic or surgical treatment

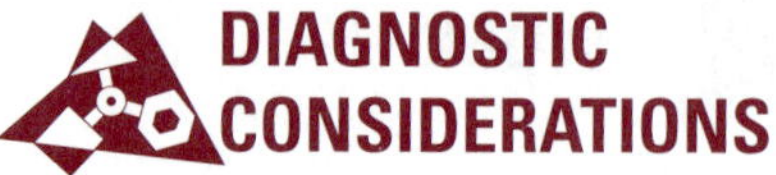

DIAGNOSTIC CONSIDERATIONS

- With wide use of sensitive imaging studies in the diagnosis of pancreatic disease, small asymptomatic pseudocysts are often demonstrated
  - The natural history of these subclinical lesions is benign
  - There is no indication for prophylactic surgical treatment
- Pancreatic pseudocyst associated with ductal obstruction (chronic pancreatitis) or disruption (trauma) is unlikely to resolve without correction of the underlying defect

RULE OUT

- Pancreatic abscess
- Acute pancreatic phlegmon
- Pancreatic adenocarcinoma
- Pancreatic neoplastic cysts
  - Account for about 5% of all cases of cystic pancreatic masses
  - May be indistinguishable preoperatively from pseudocyst
  - Cyst wall must be biopsied to exclude neoplasia

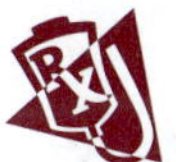

WORK-UP

- Serum amylase
- Serum bilirubin
- CBC count
- Abdominal CT
- ERCP if indicated

WHEN TO ADMIT

- Severe symptoms
- Infection

TREATMENT AND MANAGEMENT

- Asymptomatic cysts may be observed; 40% will resolve within 8–12 weeks
- Drainage options:
  - Internal (cystgastrostomy or jejunostomy)
  - External
  - Percutaneous (infected)

SURGERY

Indications

- All symptomatic pseudocysts
- Cysts > 5 cm that have not resolved by 8–12 weeks after acute pancreatitis
- Infected pseudocysts (external surgical or percutaneous)

Contraindications

- Cysts < 8–12 weeks after acute pancreatitis

TREATMENT MONITORING

- If expectant management, interval CT or US to monitor resolution; if no resolution or symptoms develop, drainage indicated

COMPLICATIONS

- Infection
- Sudden perforation with peritonitis
- Bleeding into the cyst cavity or a viscus into which the cyst has eroded

PROGNOSIS

- The recurrence rate is about 10%; more frequent after external drainage
- In most cases, surgical treatment is uncomplicated and definitive

RESOURCES

REFERENCES

- Cooperman AM. Surgical treatment of pancreatic pseudocysts. *Surg Clin North Am.* 2001;81:411.
- Heider R et al. Percutaneous drainage of pancreatic pseudocysts is associated with a higher failure rate than surgical treatment in unselected patients. *Ann Surg.* 1999;229:781.

Pancreatitis, Acute

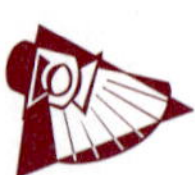

ESSENTIAL FEATURES

- Abrupt onset of epigastric pain, frequently with back pain
- Nausea and vomiting
- Elevated serum or urinary amylase
- Cholelithiasis or excessive alcohol consumption

EPIDEMIOLOGY

- A nonbacterial inflammatory disease caused by activation, interstitial liberation, and autodigestion of the pancreas by its own enzymes
- **Biliary:** 40% of cases; if untreated, high risk of additional acute attacks
- **Alcoholic:** 40% of cases
- **Hypercalcemia**
- **Hyperlipidemia**
- **Familial:** Usually begins in childhood; chronic pancreatitis often develops
- **Iatrogenic:** Postoperative; cardiopulmonary bypass, ERCP
- **Drug-induced:** Corticosteroids, estrogen contraceptives, azathioprine, thiazide diuretics, tetracyclines
- **Obstructive:** Congenital (pancreas divisum) or after injury or inflammation
- **Idiopathic:** 15% of patients; there is no identifiable cause of the condition

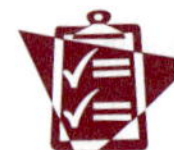

CLINICAL FINDINGS

SYMPTOMS AND SIGNS

- Severe epigastric pain that radiates through to the back
- Nausea and vomiting
- Tachycardia and postural hypotension
- Normal or slightly elevated temperature
- Distention and generalized or epigastric tenderness
- Decreased or absent bowel sounds
- Abdominal mass due to pancreatic phlegmon, pseudocyst, or abscess
- Bluish discoloration in the flank (Grey Turner sign) or periumbilical area (Cullen sign), indicating retroperitoneal dissection of blood

LABORATORY FINDINGS

- Either elevated Hct (dehydration) or decreased (hemorrhagic pancreatitis)
- Moderate leukocytosis
- Mild elevation of serum bilirubin; greater with choledocholithiasis
- Elevated serum amylase
- Elevated serum lipase
- Increased urine amylase excretion (> 5000 U/24 h)
- Decreased serum calcium

IMAGING FINDINGS

- **Abdominal x-ray**
  - Isolated dilation of a segment of gut (sentinel loop) adjacent to the pancreas
  - Distended right colon that abruptly stops in the mid or left transverse colon (colon cutoff sign) due to colonic spasm adjacent to the pancreatic inflammation
  - Calcification suggesting chronic pancreatitis
- **Chest film:** Left-sided pleural effusion
- **CT scan**
  - Perform if no improvement after 48–72 hours
  - May demonstrate phlegmon, necrosis, pseudocyst or abscess formation
- **Abdominal US:** Gallstones, dilated common bile duct or choledocholithiasis (biliary pancreatitis)

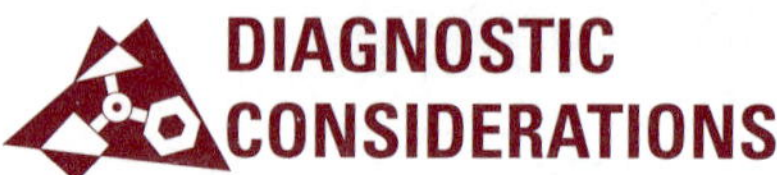

DIAGNOSTIC CONSIDERATIONS

- Elevated amylase levels may occur with gangrenous cholecystitis, small bowel obstruction, mesenteric infarction, and perforated ulcer (rarely > 500 IU/dL)
- Leukocytosis > 12,000/μL is unusual in the absence of abscess
- Hemorrhagic pancreatitis: Bleeding into the parenchyma and retroperitoneal structures with extensive necrosis
- Severe acute pancreatitis
  - Shock
  - Multiple organ failure
  - Acute respiratory distress syndrome
  - Myocardial depression
  - Renal insufficiency
  - Gastric stress ulceration

RULE OUT

- Acute cholecystitis
- Penetrating or perforated duodenal ulcer
- High small bowel obstruction
- Acute appendicitis
- Mesenteric infarction
- Chronic hyperamylasemia
- Necrotizing pancreatitis
- Infected necrotizing pancreatitis
- Pancreatic abscess

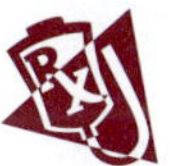

WORK-UP

- Serum amylase
- Serum lipase
- Aspartate transaminase (AST), alanine transaminase (ALT), bilirubin
- Serum electrolytes
- CBC count
- Abdominal x-ray
- Chest film
- Abdominal US (if biliary source suspected)
- Abdominal CT scan if no improvement within 48–72 hrs

WHEN TO ADMIT

- All cases should be admitted

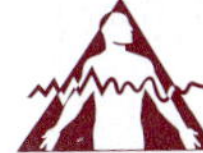

TREATMENT AND MANAGEMENT

- No enteral intake/NG suction
- Fluid replacement
- Correction of electrolyte derangements
- Treatment of underlying etiology

SURGERY

Indications

- **Biliary pancreatitis:** Cholecystectomy after resolution but prior to discharge
- Infected necrotizing pancreatitis
- Pancreatic abscess

Contraindications

- Mild pancreatitis

MEDICATIONS

- No role for routine use of antibiotics; reserved for necrotizing pancreatitis and pancreatic abscess

TREATMENT MONITORING

- Abdominal CT if no improvement within 48–72 hrs

COMPLICATIONS

- Necrotizing pancreatitis/abscess
- GI bleeding
- Intraperitoneal bleeding
- Pseudocyst

PROGNOSIS

- **Acute pancreatitis:** 10% mortality
- **Necrotizing pancreatitis:** 50% mortality
- Respiratory insufficiency and hypocalcemia indicate a poor prognosis

Ranson's criteria of severity of acute pancreatitis.[1]

Criteria present initially

Age > 55 years
WBC > 16,000/μL
Blood glucose > 200 mg/dL
Serum lactic dehydrogenase > 350 IU/L
AST > 250 IU/dL

Criteria developing during first 24 hours

Hct fall > 10%
Blood urea nitrogen rise > 8 mg/dL
Serum Ca^{2+} < 8 mg/dL
Arterial Po_2 < 60 mm Hg
Base deficit > 4 mEq/L
Estimated fluid sequestration > 6000 mL

[1]Morbidity and mortality rates correlate with the number of criteria present. Mortality rates correlate as follows: 0–2 criteria present = 2%; 3 or 4 = 15%; 5 or 6 = 40%; 7 or 8 = 100%.

RESOURCES

REFERENCES

- Dervenis C, Bassi C. Evidence-based assessment of severity and management of acute pancreatitis. *Br J Surg.* 2000;87:257.
- Uhl W et al. Acute gallstone pancreatitis: timing of laparoscopic cholecystectomy in mild and severe disease. *Surg Endosc.* 1999;13:1070.

Pancreatitis, Chronic

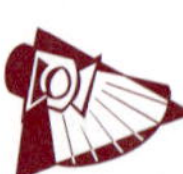

ESSENTIAL FEATURES

- Persistent or recurrent abdominal pain
- Pancreatic calcification on x-ray in 50%
- Pancreatic insufficiency in 30%; malabsorption and diabetes mellitus
- Most often due to alcoholism

EPIDEMIOLOGY

- May be familial (familial pancreatitis) or due to chronic partial obstruction of the pancreatic duct which is either congenital (pancreas divisium) or following healing after injury (trauma) or inflammation (alcoholic chronic pancreatitis)
- Over time, the parenchyma drained by the obstructed duct is replaced by fibrous tissue, and chronic pancreatitis develops
- Pathologic changes in the gland include:
  - Destruction of parenchyma
  - Fibrosis
  - Dedifferentiation of acini
  - Calculi
  - Ductal dilation
- A dilated ductal system reflects obstruction, and when dilation is present, procedures to improve ductal drainage usually relieve pain

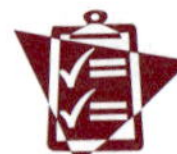

CLINICAL FINDINGS

SYMPTOMS AND SIGNS

- Severe pain that is typically felt deep in the upper abdomen and radiating through to the back; it waxes and wanes from day to day
- Malabsorption and steatorrhea

LABORATORY FINDINGS

- Serum amylase may or may not be elevated in acute exacerbations
- Secretin and cholecystokinin stimulation tests detect exocrine malfunction
- High glucose and/or low insulin levels
- Elevated serum bilirubin and alkaline phosphatase levels resulting from entrapment of the bile duct
- Thrombocytopenia due to hypersplenism secondary to splenic vein thrombosis

IMAGING FINDINGS

- **Abdominal x-ray:** Calcification of the pancreas
- **CT scan:** Pancreatic calcification, stones in and dilation of the pancreatic duct and dilated bile duct if obstructed
- **ERCP:** Pancreatic ductal stones and irregularity, with dilation and stenoses, and occasionally ductal occlusion; bile duct dilation

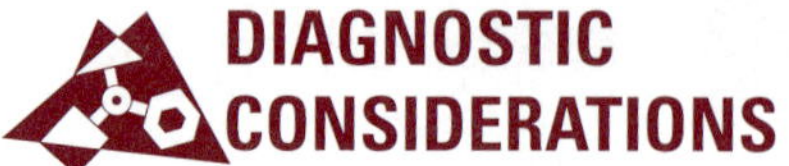

DIAGNOSTIC CONSIDERATIONS

- Chronic pancreatitis may be asymptomatic, may present with signs and symptoms stemming from a complications, or it may produce abdominal pain, malabsorption, diabetes mellitus, or any combination
- Splenic vein thrombosis, a complication of chronic pancreatitis, may present with secondary hypersplenism or gastric varices
- Biliary obstruction, another complication of chronic pancreatitis, may present with jaundice

RULE OUT

- Pancreatic pseudocyst
- Pancreatic adenocarcinoma

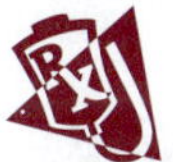

WORK-UP

- Serum amylase
- Blood glucose
- CT scan
- ERCP

WHEN TO ADMIT

- Acute exacerbation with severe abdominal pain

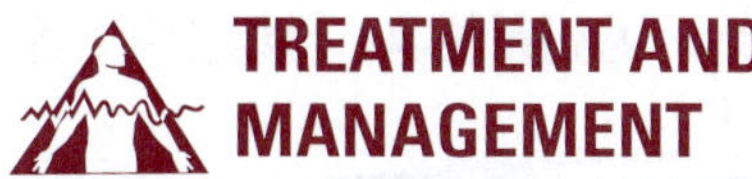

TREATMENT AND MANAGEMENT

SURGERY

- Facilitates pancreatic drainage:
  - Longitudinal pancreaticojejunostomy (dilated duct)
  - Pancreaticoduodenectomy (nondilated duct)
  - Total pancreatectomy (failure of other procedures)

Indications

- Chronic intractable pain
- Relief of pain with endoscopic stenting of the pancreatic duct may predict those patients who will benefit from an operation

MEDICATIONS

- Celiac plexus block
- Pancreatic enzymes
- Insulin

TREATMENT MONITORING

- Patients with chronic pancreatitis have an increased risk of pancreatic adenocarcinoma and should be monitored for early symptoms

COMPLICATIONS

- Pancreatic pseudocyst
- Diabetes mellitus
- Pancreatic exocrine deficiency
- Biliary obstruction

PROGNOSIS

- **Pain relief:** Longitudinal pancreatico-jejunostomy and pancreatico-duodenectomy, 80% of patients; celiac plexus block, < 30% of patients

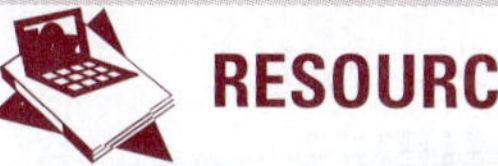

RESOURCES

REFERENCES

- Apte MV et al. Chronic pancreatitis: complications and management. *J Clin Gastroenterol.* 1999;29:225.
- Pitchumoni CS. Chronic pancreatitis: pathogenesis and management of pain. *J Clin Gastroenterol.* 1998;27:101.

Paraesophageal Hiatal Hernia

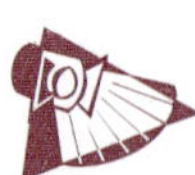

ESSENTIAL FEATURES

- Often asymptomatic
- Symptoms of mechanical obstruction include:
  - Dysphagia
  - Incarceration
  - Stasis gastric ulcer

EPIDEMIOLOGY

- Acquired diaphragmatic defect containing variable amounts of stomach with or without other abdominal viscera
- Type II: Rolling; upper dislocation of fundus of the stomach alongside a normally positioned intra-abdominal gastroesophageal junction (GEJ)
  - Since the GEJ functions normally in type II hernias, reflux is uncommon
- Type III: Mixed; upper displacement of the fundus and the GEJ
- Type IV: Hernia contains other abdominal vicera (colon, small intestine)
- Herniation caused by combined effects of age, stress, and other degenerative factors on the diaphragm
- Always at risk for strangulation, necrosis or gastric perforation
- Type III more common than type II
- More common in women than in men; incidence increases with age

CLINICAL FINDINGS

SYMPTOMS AND SIGNS

- Often asymptomatic
- Pain or pressure in the lower chest after eating
- Vomiting
- Early satiety
- Hematemesis
- Dyspnea and pain on inspiration
- Decreased breath sounds in the left chest
- Bowel sounds in the left chest
- Palpitations due to cardiac dysrhythmias

LABORATORY FINDINGS

- Anemia in 30% of patients

IMAGING FINDINGS

- **Chest film**: Gastric air-fluid level behind cardiac shadow
- **Upper GI contrast radiography**: Cephalad displacement of the stomach and possibly other abdominal viscera above the diaphragm
- **Endoscopy**: On retroversion, orifice of the herniated portion of the stomach adjacent to the GEJ (type II) or pouch with gastric rugal folds above the diaphragm with GEJ entering side of pouch (type III)

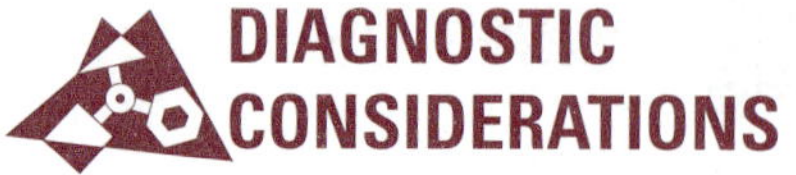

DIAGNOSTIC CONSIDERATIONS

- Preoperative manometry or pH testing is unreliable predictor of true reflux since distorted anatomy may give rise to abnormal findings that may be corrected by reduction of hernia
- Upper GI contrast radiography most reliable means of diagnosis

RULE OUT

- Gastric volvulus
- Strangulated viscera
- Gastric necrosis

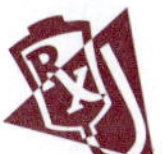

WORK-UP

- Upper GI contrast radiography

WHEN TO ADMIT

- Suspected strangulation
- Upper GI bleeding
- Complete gastric obstruction

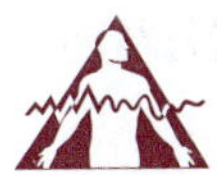

TREATMENT AND MANAGEMENT

SURGERY

- The herniated viscera is returned to the abdomen and the enlarged hiatus is closed snugly around the GEJ
- A fundoplication may be performed to anchor the stomach or prevent reflux

Indications

- Since complications are frequent even in the absence of symptoms, operative repair is indicated

COMPLICATIONS

- Upper GI hemorrhage
- Incarceration
- Obstruction
- Strangulation

PROGNOSIS

- Excellent

RESOURCES

REFERENCES

- Hashemi M et al. Current concepts in the management of paraesophageal hiatal hernia. *J Clin Gastroenterol.* 1999;29:8.
- Luketich JD et al. Laparoscopic repair of giant paraesophageal hernia: 100 consecutive cases. *Ann Surg.* 2000;232:608.

Parathyroid Carcinoma

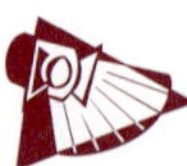

ESSENTIAL FEATURES

- Associated with profound hypercalcemia

EPIDEMIOLOGY

- Found in 0.5–1% of patients with hyperparathyroidism
- Cancer is palpable in 50% of the patients
- 5% of parathyroid cancers are nonfunctional
- Patients with parathyroid cancer are on average younger at the time of diagnosis than patients with benign hyperparathyroidism
- Equal distribution among men and women

CLINICAL FINDINGS

SYMPTOMS AND SIGNS

- Palpable neck mass
- Hoarseness
- Fatigue, depression, nausea, vomiting, dehydration, polydipsia, polyuria
- Pathologic fractures
- Nephrolithiasis (70% of patients)
- Nephrocalcinosis
- Severe renal dysfunction (20–50% of patients)
- Pancreatitis and peptic ulceration (10–15% of patients)

LABORATORY FINDINGS

- Profound hypercalcemia
- Elevated intact parathyroid hormone (PTH)

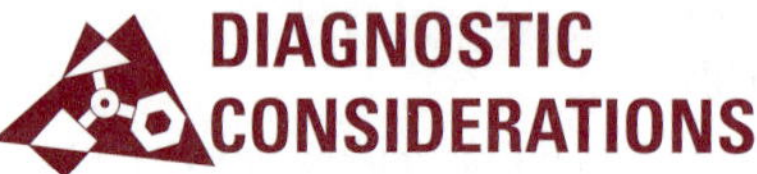

DIAGNOSTIC CONSIDERATIONS

- Parathyroid carcinoma is suspected at operation if parathyroid is hard, whitish, has an irregular capsule, or is invasive
- Rarely diagnosed preoperatively

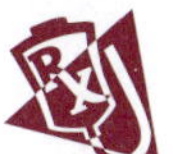

WORK-UP

- Physical exam
- Measure PTH levels
- Chest and neck CT scan

TREATMENT AND MANAGEMENT

- Anecdotal evidence for role of radiation therapy in local control of disease

SURGERY

- Surgical resection is mainstay of treatment
- En bloc resection should be carried out where possible (including ipsilateral thyroid lobe and central compartment lymph nodes)
- Resection of local recurrent or metastatic disease is recommended if possible

Indications

- All parathyroid carcinomas should be resected

MEDICATIONS

- Palliative drug: IV bisphosphonate to maintain eucalcemia

TREATMENT MONITORING

- Physical exam
- Serum calcium and intact PTH levels

PROGNOSIS

- Indolent malignancy, with local and distant metastases occurring over many years
- 5-year survival rates range from 40% to 69%

RESOURCES

REFERENCES

- Rosen IB et al. Parathyroid cancer: clinical variations and relationship to autotransplantation. *Can J Surg.* 1994;37:465.
- Sandelin K et al. Dilemmas in management of parathyroid carcinoma. *Surgery.* 1991;110:978.
- Obara T, Fujimoto Y. Diagnosis and treatment of patients with parathyroid carcinoma: an update and review. *World J Surg.* 1991;15:738.

Patent Ductus Arteriosus (PDA)

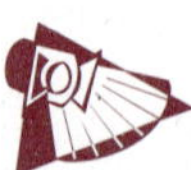

ESSENTIAL FEATURES

- A congenital heart lesion that increases pulmonary artery (PA) blood flow
- Results in left-to-right shunt, results in lung infection, pulmonary vascular congestion, PA hypertension, right heart failure, pulmonary vasoconstriction, pulmonary vascular obstructive disease
- **Eisenmenger syndrome:** Increased pulmonary hypertension such that left-to-right shunt ceases and shunt becomes right-to-left, requiring heart-lung transplant
- Inhaled nitric oxide, oxygen, or IV tolazoline reverses PA vasoconstriction
- PA band is palliative and can reduce PA flow to alleviate RV failure and progression of pulmonary hypertension
- Ductus arteriosus normal component of fetal circulation connecting main PA to aorta distal to left subclavian artery
- In utero, ductus carries 60% of ventricular output, patency maintained by high flow, prostaglandins (from placenta), low oxygen tension
- At birth, increased pulmonary resistance, prostaglandin level decrease, increased oxygen tension causes duct closure
- Closure occurs between 1 and 3 days
- Closure does not always occur
- Causes left-to-right shunt, heart failure, and pulmonary hypertension
- Associated with other anomalies
- May limit flow to systemic organs

EPIDEMIOLOGY

- Incidence of PDA: 2–3% of live births
- Increases with prematurity, > 50% in infants born at 30 wks gestation
- 5% of untreated PDA die of heart and pulmonary failure by age 1

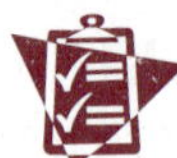

CLINICAL FINDINGS

SYMPTOMS AND SIGNS

- **Older patients:**
  - Often asymptomatic
  - Continuous murmur over pulmonary area
  - Loud S_2
  - Bounding peripheral pulses
- **Infants:**
  - Poor feeding
  - Respiratory distress
  - Frequent respiratory infection
  - Heart failure
- **Diagnosis by physical exam:**
  - Wide pulse pressure
  - To-and fro-murmur (usually systolic, occasionally continuous)
- **Large shunts (5%):** Develop pulmonary vascular disease
- Usually asymptomatic, found during routine exam
- **Premature infant:** Distinguish heart failure from pulmonary dysfunction of prematurity
- Inability to wean from ventilator is common presentation

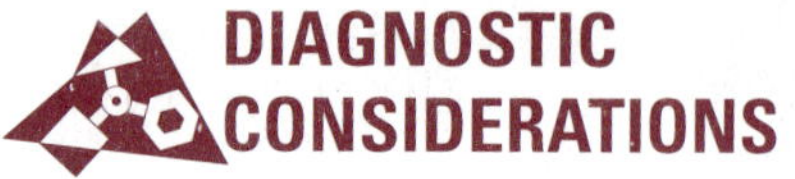

DIAGNOSTIC CONSIDERATIONS

- Echocardiography done on high-risk patients

RULE OUT

- Primary pulmonary dysfunction from prematurity

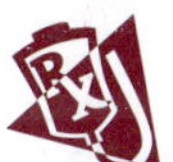

WORK-UP

- Echocardiography diagnostic

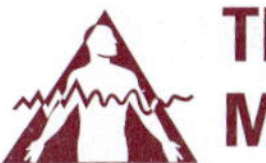

TREATMENT AND MANAGEMENT

- Treatment varies with age
- **Premature infant:** Medical therapy with indomethacin (50% success)

SURGERY

- **Term infant or child:** Surgical obliteration by ligation, clipping, or division
- **Larger infants/children:** Video thoracoscopy
- Transcatheter technique for larger patient may have fewer complications

Indications

- Term infant/older child
- Failed medical therapy in premature infant

MEDICATIONS

- Indomethacin (prostaglandin inhibitor) 50% success, efficacy decreases with age

COMPLICATIONS

- Injury to recurrent laryngeal nerve, hemorrhage, chylothorax uncommon

PROGNOSIS

- Operative mortality near 0%
- Recurrence < 1% among patients who are treated surgically

RESOURCES

REFERENCES

- Backer CL et al. Congenital Heart Surgery Nomenclature and Database Project: patent ductus arteriosus, coarctation of the aorta, interrupted aortic arch. *Ann Thorac Surg.* 2000;69:S298.
- Hawkins JA et al. Cost and efficacy of surgical ligation versus transcatheter coil occlusion of patent ductus arteriosus. *J Thorac Cardiovasc Surg.* 1996;112:1634.

Pectus Excavatum/Carinatum

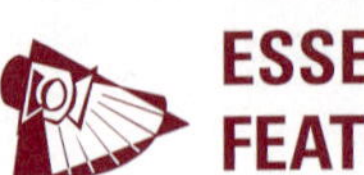

ESSENTIAL FEATURES

- Often present at birth but becomes more pronounced as adolescence progresses
- Excavatum can be associated with Marfan syndrome and scoliosis

EPIDEMIOLOGY

- Males more commonly affected than females

CLINICAL FINDINGS

SYMPTOMS AND SIGNS

- Excavatum: Posterior curve of sternum with right side usually more curved
- Carinatum: Protruding sternum

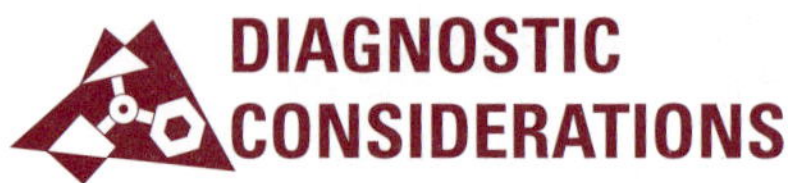

DIAGNOSTIC CONSIDERATIONS

- Evaluate for underlying pulmonary or cardiac dysfunction

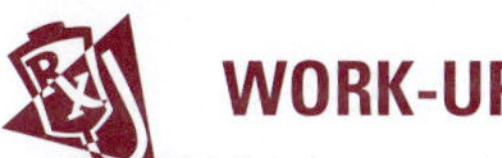

WORK-UP

- Physical exam

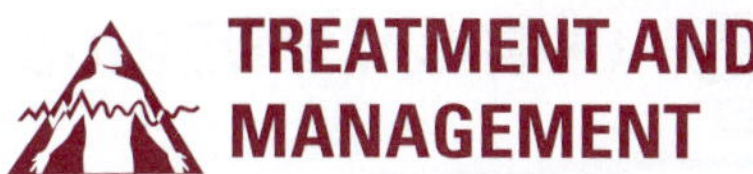

TREATMENT AND MANAGEMENT

SURGERY

- **Excavatum:** Early and middle teenage years (osteotomy or Nuss bar placement)
- **Carinatum:** Osteotomy and sternal fracture

Indications

- Severity of deformity and psychosocial impact

COMPLICATIONS

- Pneumothorax
- Injury to great vessels or heart (rare)
- Recurrence (5–15% with osteotomy repair)

PROGNOSIS

- Recurrence rate of 5–15%

RESOURCES

REFERENCES

- Nuss D et al. A 10-year review of a minimally invasive technique for the correction of pectus excavatum. *J Pediatr Surg.* 1998;33:545.

Pediatric Abdominal Wall Defects

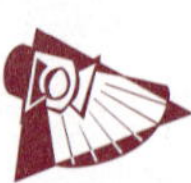

ESSENTIAL FEATURES

- Gastroschisis: Associated with other abnormalities 10% of time, most often intestinal atresia, associated with preterm infants
- Omphalocele: Associated with other abnormalities 50% of time, nearly always full-term infants

EPIDEMIOLOGY

- Gastroschisis: 1/3000–1/8000 births
- Omphalocele 1/6000–1/10,000 births

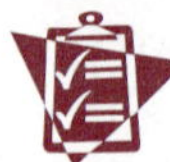

CLINICAL FINDINGS

SYMPTOMS AND SIGNS

- Gastroschisis nearly always located to right of umbilicus, inflamed bowel and foreshortened mesentery secondary to exposure to amniotic fluid
- Umbilical cord part of sac in omphalocele along with peritoneum

IMAGING FINDINGS

- Abdominal wall defect often noted with prenatal US

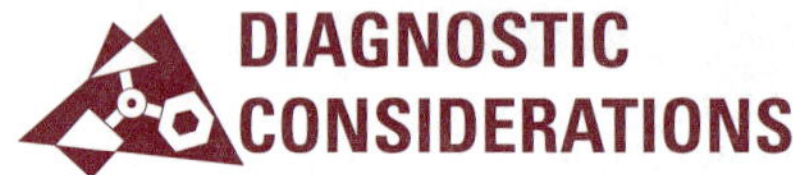

DIAGNOSTIC CONSIDERATIONS

- Associated congenital abnormalities, especially intestinal atresia with gastroschisis

RULE OUT

- Intestinal atresia with gastroschisis

WORK-UP

- History and physical exam
- Chest film
- Echocardiogram (for omphalocele)
- Renal US (for omphalocele)
- CBC count
- Metabolic panel

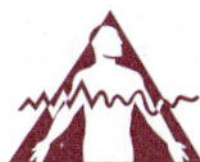

TREATMENT AND MANAGEMENT

SURGERY

- Primary repair possible in 60–70%
- Silastic pouch or silo construction followed by gradual reefing and eventual closure
- Giant omphaloceles: Nonoperative initial therapy, gradual epithelialization, and closure months to years later

MEDICATIONS

- Total parenteral nutrition during resolution of ileus

COMPLICATIONS

- Abdominal compartment syndrome
- Necrotizing enterocolitis (15% in gastroschisis)
- Delayed ileus or intestinal dysmotility (especially in gastroschisis)

RESOURCES

REFERENCES

- Albanese CT et al. Pediatric Surgery. In: Way LW, Doherty GM (editors). *Current Surgical Diagnosis & Treatment,* 11e. New York: McGraw-Hill; 2003: 1339–1341.

Pediatric Airway Obstruction

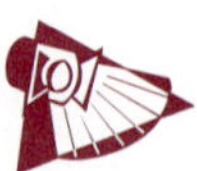

ESSENTIAL FEATURES

- Nasal etiologies include:
  - Choanal atresia
  - Teratoma
  - Encephalocele
- Oral cavity etiologies include:
  - Macroglossia
  - Micrognathia
  - Hypoplastic mandible with cleft palate
- Pharyngeal and laryngeal etiologies include cysts or tumors
  - Hemangiomas, lymphangiomas, cystic hygromas, and teratomas are most common
- Acquired etiologies include:
  - Foreign body aspiration
  - Acute epiglottitis

EPIDEMIOLOGY

- Epiglottitis occurs most commonly at age 4
- Congenital lesions usually apparent at birth

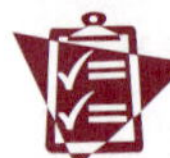

CLINICAL FINDINGS

SYMPTOMS AND SIGNS

- Restlessness
- Tachypnea
- Dyspnea
- Chest wall retractions
- Inspiratory stridor
- Respiratory arrest
- Drooling
- Dysphagia
- Fever (with epiglottitis)

LABORATORY FINDINGS

- Leukocytosis with epiglottitis
- Blood gas showing respiratory acidosis

IMAGING FINDINGS

- Lateral cervical plain film showing edema of epiglottis and ballooning of pharynx
- Chest film showing aspirated foreign body

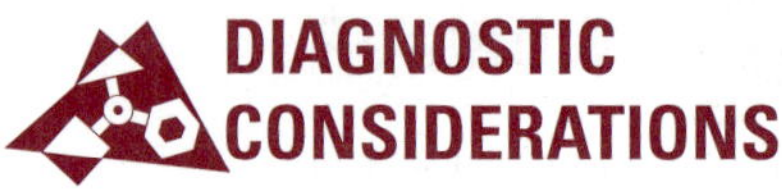

DIAGNOSTIC CONSIDERATIONS

- Age of presentation
- Severity of respiratory distress

RULE OUT

- Epiglottitis

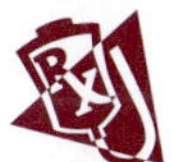

WORK-UP

- History and physical exam
- Chest film
- Lateral cervical film (for suspected epiglottitis)
- Laryngoscopy (in operating room under anesthesia for suspected epiglottitis)
- Bronchoscopy (usually for aspirated foreign body)

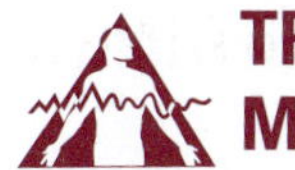

TREATMENT AND MANAGEMENT

SURGERY

- Tracheostomy for some obstructions
- Resection of tumors or cysts causing airway obstruction
- Bronchoscopy with foreign body extraction or treatment of other congenital endobronchial lesions

MEDICATIONS

- Third-generation cephalosporin for epiglottitis
- Intralesional or systemic corticosteroids for obstructing hemangioma
- Mechanical ventilation for extreme cases
- Oropharyngeal suctioning and NG decompression

COMPLICATIONS

- Recurrent airway obstruction
- Aspiration pneumonia

PREVENTION

- *Haemophilus influenza* type B vaccine

RESOURCES

REFERENCES

- Albanese CT et al. Pediatric Surgery. In: Way LW, Doherty GM (editors). *Current Surgical Diagnosis & Treatment,* 11e. New York: McGraw-Hill; 2003; 1306–1308.

Pediatric Intestinal Obstruction (Nonpyloric Stenosis)

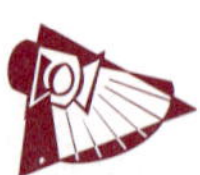

ESSENTIAL FEATURES

- Other etiologies:
  - Intestinal atresia
  - Intestinal duplication
  - Mesenteric or omental cyst
  - Meckel diverticulum
  - Foreign body
  - Meconium ileus
  - Annular pancreas
- 10–20% of patients with abdominal wall defects have intestinal atresia
- 90–95% of duodenal atresia is distal to ampulla
- 90% of jejunoileal atresias have complete atresia
- Distal ileum most common site of atresia
- 3.6–20% of patients have multiple areas of intestinal atresia
- Patent accessory pancreatic duct common with annular pancreas
- 50% of duodenal atresia with complete atresia and 50% with webs or diaphragm
- Trisomy 21 associated with duodenal atresia
- 10–20% of patients with cystic fibrosis develop meconium ileus (concretions of meconium usually found just proximal to ileocecal valve secondary to decreased pancreatic exocrine activity)
- 33–50% of patients with meconium ileus undergo proximal volvulus, perforation, or atresia that occurs in utero
- Cardiac anomalies associated with duodenal atresia
- 5–10% of patients with Meckel diverticulum will present with obstruction secondary to volvulus or intussusception
- 95% of foreign bodies that pass beyond the gastroesophageal junction pass through remainder of GI tract uneventfully
- Mesenteric cysts 2-fold more common than omental cysts
- Omental and mesenteric cysts diagnosed before 10 years of age

EPIDEMIOLOGY

- Intestinal atresia: 3.5/10,000 births
- All congenital duodenal obstructions: 1/6000–1/10,000 births

CLINICAL FINDINGS

SYMPTOMS AND SIGNS

- Bilious emesis
- Abdominal distention
- Irritability
- Maternal polyhydramnios
- Failure to pass meconium
- Umbilical cord ulceration (rarely with intestinal atresia)
- Abdominal mass if mesenteric/omental cyst or duplication

LABORATORY FINDINGS

- Test for CFTR mutations or sweat chloride analysis in patients with meconium ileus to diagnose cystic fibrosis

IMAGING FINDINGS

- **Abdominal x-ray:** Shows transition point of gas (soap bubble appearance intraluminal in meconium ileus)
- **Upper or lower GI series:** Demonstrates transition point of obstruction (concretions in meconium ileus)
- **CT scan or US:** May demonstrate cystic mass with mesenteric or omental cysts

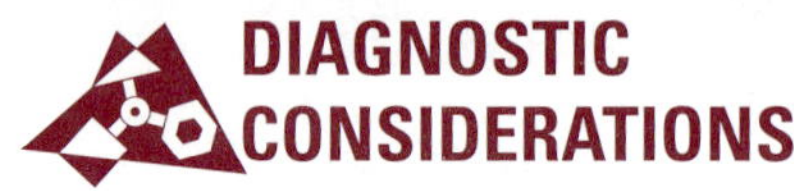

DIAGNOSTIC CONSIDERATIONS

RULE OUT

- Malrotation

Pediatric Intestinal Obstruction (Nonpyloric Stenosis)

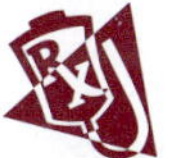

WORK-UP

- History and physical exam
- Abdominal x-ray
- Upper and/or lower GI series
- CFTR or sweat chloride (to document cystic fibrosis in patients with meconium ileus)
- Echocardiogram in patients with duodenal atresia

TREATMENT AND MANAGEMENT

SURGERY

- Primary anastomosis following short segmental resection (if web associated) after careful exam for other sites of obstruction or atresia
- Duodenoduodenostomy for annular pancreas and duodenal atresia (possible excision of web for atresia)
- Operative retrieval of foreign body if symptomatic, or an alkaline battery, or if persists in 1 location (no transition) for 1 week or more or several weeks in stomach

MEDICATIONS

- Nonoperative management possible in 65% cases of meconium ileus, enemas using gastrograffin, tween-80, or N-acetylcysteine are beneficial

COMPLICATIONS

- Short bowel syndrome if left with < 40 cm
- Damage to ampulla during excision of duodenal web (in cases of atresia)
- Delayed gastric emptying, gastroesophageal reflux disease, or impaired duodenal motility following correction of duodenal obstruction

PROGNOSIS

- 93% 5-year survival following repair after intestinal atresia

PREVENTION

- Exocrine pancreatic enzyme replacement to avoid meconium ileus

RESOURCES

- Albanese CT et al. Pediatric Surgery. In: Way LW, Doherty GM (editors). *Current Surgical Diagnosis & Treatment,* 11e. New York: McGraw-Hill; 2003; 1315–1327.

Pediatric Neck Masses

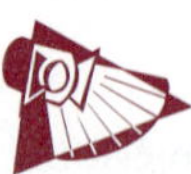

ESSENTIAL FEATURES

- Etiologies include:
  - Branchial cleft remnants
  - Thyroglossal duct cyst
  - Lymphadenopathy
  - Vascular malformations and cystic hygroma
  - Dermoid inclusion cysts
  - Cervical thymic cysts
- Branchial cleft remnants
  - Present most commonly as cysts later in childhood
  - Sinuses, fistulae, and cartilage remnants present at birth
  - Second branchial cleft remnants most common
- Thyroglossal duct cyst presents later in childhood
- Benign lymphadenopathy most common neck mass of childhood
  - Usually secondary to upper respiratory tract infections
  - Occasionally accompanied by suppurative lymphangitis
- 65% of lymphangioma and cystic hygroma are present at birth and 80% are present by age 1

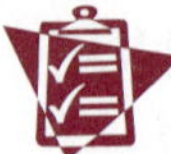

CLINICAL FINDINGS

SYMPTOMS AND SIGNS

- **Branchial cleft cysts**
  - Present later in childhood when secretions build up, occasionally with erythema and tenderness due to infection
  - Present from angle of mandible (first cleft) down to lower third of sternocleidomastoid (second cleft) with fistulas being present to external auditory meatus (first), tonsillar fossa (second), pyriform sinus (third and fourth)
  - Masses or cysts can present anywhere between fistula openings and internal cleft sites
- **Thyroglossal duct cyst**
  - Presents as midline cystic neck mass usually overlying hyoid
  - Often moves during swallowing or draining sinus in early childhood
  - Occasionally presents as painful draining mass if infected
- **Suppurative lymphangitis:** Presents as painful, erythematous, draining mass following an upper respiratory tract infection
- **Hemangiomas:** Become apparent after first few weeks of life usually as blue, spongy, rubbery, and sometimes extensive in cutaneous regions or airway
- **Lymphangioma and cystic hygroma:** Typically present as asymptomatic mass anywhere in body but have a high tendency to become infected

IMAGING FINDINGS

- Barium injection or CT often required to demonstrate fistula tract for branchial cleft remnants

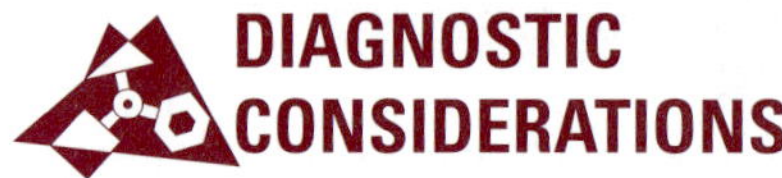

DIAGNOSTIC CONSIDERATIONS

- Malignant degeneration (rare) or infection in branchial cleft remnants
- Malignancy in lymph nodes

RULE OUT

- Malignant lymph nodes and infection with atypical bacteria such as mycobacterium

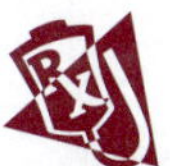

WORK-UP

- History and physical exam
- Barium injection of fistula tract for branchial cleft fistula
- CT for suspected branchial cleft remnants
- US with duplex for some masses difficult to diagnose

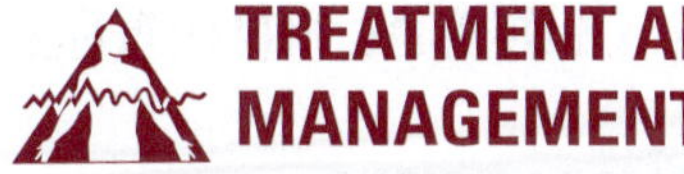

TREATMENT AND MANAGEMENT

SURGERY

- Incision and drainage of branchial cleft cyst if infected
- Dissection and excision of branchial cleft cyst or fistula once infection resolved
- Thyroglossal duct cyst excision including midpoint of hyoid and tract up to base of foramen cecum
- Incision and drainage of suppurative lymphangitis if initially unresponsive to antibiotics
- Excisional biopsy for enlarged lymph node present > 8 wks, larger than 2 cm, firm, immobile
- Excision or sclerotherapy of lymphangioma or cystic hygroma

Contraindications

- Definitive excision contraindicated in presence of active infection

MEDICATIONS

- Intralesional corticosteroid or systemic corticosteroid for hemangioma that can compress airway or obstruct eyes

COMPLICATIONS

- Injury to other structures of neck for branchial cleft remnants such as facial nerve, hypoglossal nerve, vagus, recurrent laryngeal, superior laryngeal, or carotid artery

PROGNOSIS

- Hemangiomas usually grow between 6 and 12 months and resolve spontaneously by the time the patient is 5 years of age
- < 5% recurrence rate for excision of branchial cleft remnants or thyroglossal duct cysts

RESOURCES

- Brown RL, Azizkhan RG. Pediatric head and neck lesions. *Pediatr Clin North Am.* 1998;45:899.

Pediatric Thoracic Masses

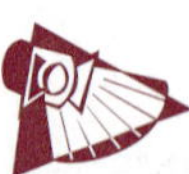

ESSENTIAL FEATURES

- Resectable lung metastases
  - Osteogenic sarcoma
  - Soft-tissue sarcoma
  - Wilms tumor
- Primary lung tumors
  - Bronchial "adenoma": Malignant (most common)
  - Bronchogenic carcinoma (90% mortality rate)
  - Pulmonary blastoma, sarcomas, inflammatory pseudotumor (benign)
  - Hamartoma (benign)
- Mediastinal tumors
  - Neurogenic (posterior mediastinum, include neuroblastoma, ganglioneuroblastoma, and ganglioneuroma)
  - Neurofibroma, lymphoma, teratoma (anterior mediastinum)
- Chest wall
  - Ewing sarcoma
  - Chondrosarcoma
  - Liposarcoma

CLINICAL FINDINGS

SYMPTOMS AND SIGNS

- Cough with sputum
- Hemoptysis
- Chest pain
- Dyspnea
- Fever
- Postobstructive pneumonia

LABORATORY FINDINGS

- Leukocytosis

IMAGING FINDINGS

- **Chest film:** Can identify mass
- **Chest CT:** Can identify various etiologies of chest mass and relative location

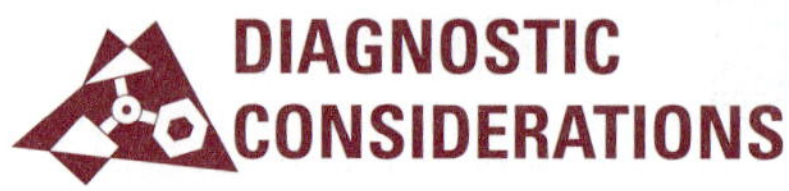

DIAGNOSTIC CONSIDERATIONS

- Evaluate for sites of primary disease

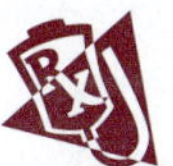

WORK-UP

- History and physical exam
- Chest film
- Chest CT
- Bronchoscopy for central lesions
- Thoracoscopy and possible biopsy

TREATMENT AND MANAGEMENT

SURGERY

- Formal resection (wedge or lobectomy) indicated for nearly all of above etiologies or excision of mediastinal lesions

PROGNOSIS

- Excellent for most pulmonary neoplasms
  - Outcome better for neuroblastomas in chest than for those in abdomen
  - Bronchogenic carcinoma, 80% mortality

RESOURCES

- Albanese CT et al. Pediatric Surgery. In: Way LW, Doherty GM (editors). *Current Surgical Diagnosis & Treatment,* 11e. New York: McGraw-Hill; 2003: 1311–1312.

Pelvic Inflammatory Disease (PID)

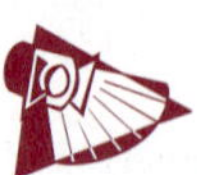

ESSENTIAL FEATURES

- Lower abdominal pain
- Fever and chills
- Menstrual disturbances
- Purulent cervical discharge
- Cervical and adnexal tenderness

EPIDEMIOLOGY

- Also referred to as salpingitis or endometritis
- PID is a polymicrobial infection of the upper genital tract
- Associated with the sexually transmitted organisms *Neisseria gonorrhoeae* or *Chlamydia trachomatis*, as well as endogenous organisms including anaerobes, *Haemophilus influenza*, enteric gram-negative rods, and streptococci
- Most common in young, nulliparous, sexually active women with multiple partners
- PID is more likely to occur when there is a history of PID, recent sexual contact, sexual contact with a partner who has a sexually transmitted disease, recent onset of menses, or when an intrauterine device is used for contraception
- Other risk markers include nonwhite race, frequent douching, and smoking
- The use of oral contraceptives or barrier methods of contraception are protective

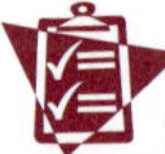

CLINICAL FINDINGS

SYMPTOMS AND SIGNS

- Lower abdominal pain
- Cervical motion tenderness
- Adnexal discomfort
- Temperature > 38.3 °C
- Purulent cervical discharge
- Menstrual disturbances
- Right upper quadrant pain (perihepatitis seen in Fitz-Hugh and Curtis syndromes)

LABORATORY FINDINGS

- Elevated ESR or C-reactive protein
- Cervical infection with *N gonorrhoeae* or *C trachomatis*
- Histopathologic evidence of endometritis on endometrial biopsy
- β-hCG negative
- Urine microscopic exam will frequently show a few RBCs and WBCs but is culture negative

IMAGING FINDINGS

- Transvaginal US demonstrates fluid-filled tubes often with free pelvic fluid in the cul-de-sac and tubo-ovarian complex

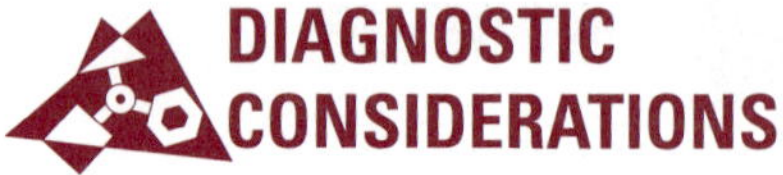

DIAGNOSTIC CONSIDERATIONS

- Acute appendicitis
- Ectopic pregnancy
- Septic abortion
- Hemorrhagic ovarian cysts or tumors
- Ruptured ovarian cysts or tumors
- Torsed ovarian cyst or tumor
- Myoma degeneration
- Acute enteritis

RULE OUT

- Ectopic pregnancy
- Septic abortion
- Torsed or hemorrhagic ovarian cyst

WORK-UP

- Thorough pelvic exam
- Endocervical culture for *N gonorrhoeae* and *C trachomatis*
- CBC count
- Basic chemistries
- β-hCG
- Transvaginal US
- Endometrial biopsy

WHEN TO ADMIT

- Patient clinically toxic
- When surgical emergencies such as acute appendicitis cannot be ruled out
- Presence of tubo-ovarian abscess
- Patient is pregnant
- Unable to follow or tolerate outpatient antibiotic regimen
- Failure to clinically respond to outpatient oral antibiotic therapy
- Patient is immunodeficient

WHEN TO REFER

- Patient clinically toxic
- When surgical emergencies such as acute appendicitis cannot be ruled out
- Presence of tubo-ovarian abscess
- Patient is pregnant
- Patient is immunodeficient
- Failure to respond to conservative IV antibiotic therapy

TREATMENT AND MANAGEMENT

- Early antibiotic therapy against *N gonorrhoeae, C trachomatis,* and enteric organisms is essential to prevent long-term sequelae
- Sexual partner should be examined and treated appropriately
- Outpatient antibiotic therapy is acceptable for uncomplicated cases

SURGERY

Indications

- Diagnostic laparoscopy used to confirm PID if diagnosis is uncertain, or in cases without a clinical response to antibiotics within 48 hours
- Tubo-ovarian abscesses may require surgical excision or percutaneous/transvaginal drainage if inadequate response to antibiotics within 48 hours
- Unilateral adnexectomy in the presence of isolated unilateral disease
- Hysterectomy with bilateral salpingo-oophorectomy may be necessary for overwhelming infection or intractable pelvic pain

MEDICATIONS

- IV antibiotic regimens:
  - Cefoxitin or cefotetan + doxycycline
  - Clindamycin + gentamycin
- Outpatient antibiotic regimens:
  - Single dose IV cefoxitin or ceftriaxone + doxycycline PO
  - Ofloxacin + metronidazole

TREATMENT MONITORING

- Resolution of fever and chills
- Amelioration of abdominal pain
- WBC normalization
- Shrinkage of tubo-ovarian abscess on transvaginal US

COMPLICATIONS

- Infertility
- Ectopic pregnancy
- Dyspareunia
- Chronic pelvic pain

PROGNOSIS

- 25% of women develop long-term sequelae
- Risk of infertility increases with repeated episodes of infection, estimated at 10% with first, 25% with second, and 50% with third episode
- Patients are more susceptible to repeated bouts of PID

RESOURCES

REFERENCES

- Monif GRG. Pelvic inflammatory disease redefined. *Infect Med.* 2001;18:190.

Peptic Ulcer Hemorrhage

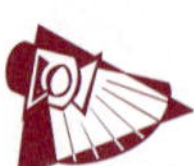

ESSENTIAL FEATURES

- History of—or risk factors for—peptic ulcer disease (PUD)
- **Acute hemorrhage:** Hematemesis or hematochezia perhaps with shock
- **Chronic hemorrhage:** Anemia with melena or trace amounts of blood in stool

EPIDEMIOLOGY

- Most common cause of massive upper GI hemorrhage
- 20% of patients with PUD will have a bleeding episode, accounting for 40% of deaths from PUD
- Chronic gastric and duodenal ulcers have about the same tendency to bleed, more severe bleeding with gastric ulcers
- Bleeding duodenal ulcers are usually located on the posterior surface of the duodenal bulb and erode into the gastroduodenal artery
- Rebleeding in the hospital has been attended by a death rate of about 30%
- Gastric ulcer rebleed 3 times more commonly than duodenal ulcers
- Most instances of rebleeding occur within 2 days from the time the first episode has stopped

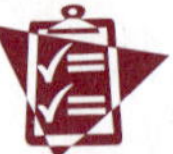

CLINICAL FINDINGS

SYMPTOMS AND SIGNS

- Epigastric pain
- Abdominal tenderness
- **Acute hemorrhage:**
  - Hematemesis or hematochezia
  - Hypotension or shock
- **Chronic hemorrhage:**
  - Weakness
  - Anemia
  - Fecal occult blood

LABORATORY FINDINGS

- **Acute hemorrhage:** Hct may not be reflective of blood lost
- **Chronic hemorrhage:** Anemia
- Obtain blood for type and cross
- Prothrombin time (PT), partial thromboplastin time (PTT), international normalized ratio (INR) to evaluate for coagulopathy
- Platelet count to evaluate for thrombocytopenia
- Serial Hct to follow adequacy of transfusion and ongoing requirements

IMAGING FINDINGS

- **Upper GI endoscopy:** Bleeding ulcer, visible vessel, ulcer with adherent clot

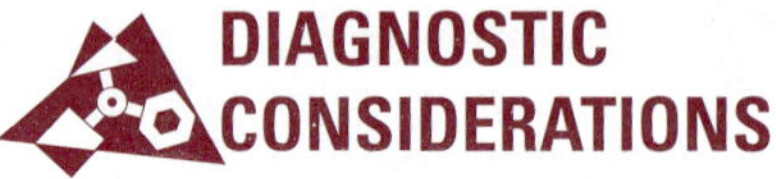

DIAGNOSTIC CONSIDERATIONS

- Diagnosis and treatment should be simultaneous
- Upper GI endoscopy should be performed immediately in cases of acute hemorrhage for diagnosis and possible treatment

RULE OUT

- Other causes of upper GI bleeding than PUD:
  - Esophageal varices
  - Gastritis
  - Mallory-Weiss syndrome
  - Gastric cancer

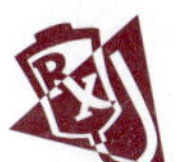

WORK-UP

- **Acute hemorrhage:**
  - Admission to ICU
  - NG lavage
  - Laboratory tests (CBC, type and cross, PT, PTT, INR)
  - Upper GI endoscopy
- **Chronic hemorrhage:**
- Laboratory tests (CBC, PT, PTT, INR)
- Urgent endoscopy (upper and lower if source unclear)

WHEN TO ADMIT

- All patients with obvious GI bleeding should be admitted

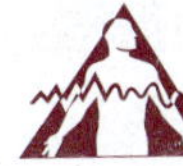

TREATMENT AND MANAGEMENT

- Replace blood loss with crystalloid and blood products
- NG lavage
- Endoscopy for localization and possible treatment

SURGERY

Indications

- Massive hemorrhage with shock
- Ongoing transfusion requirements
- Recurrent hemorrhage
- Excise ulcer (gastric) or oversew vessel (duodenal) and vagotomy

MEDICATIONS

- H_2 blockers, proton pump inhibitors (may reduce risk of rebleed)

TREATMENT MONITORING

- Twice-daily CBC
- Treatment of PUD after bleeding episode

COMPLICATIONS

- Rebleeding: Repeat endoscopic therapy for first rebleeding episode if patient is stable

PROGNOSIS

- 75% managed by endoscopic means alone
- Surgery required in < 10% of cases
- 15% mortality for massive hemorrhage

PREVENTION

- Adequate treatment of PUD

RESOURCES

REFERENCES

- Rockall TA. Management and outcome of patients undergoing surgery after acute upper gastrointestinal hemorrhage. Steering Group for the National Audit of Acute Upper Gastrointestinal Hemorrhage. *J R Soc Med.* 1998;91:518.

Peptic Ulcer Perforation

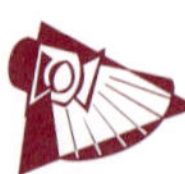

ESSENTIAL FEATURES

- Acute onset of severe upper abdominal pain
- Immediate chemical peritonitis from gastroduodenal secretions followed by bacterial peritonitis in 12–24 hours
- Free air on abdominal x-ray

EPIDEMIOLOGY

- The patient may or may not have had preceding chronic symptoms of peptic ulcer disease
- Perforation complicates peptic ulcer about half as often as hemorrhage
- Most perforated ulcers are located anteriorly
- 15% mortality rate correlates with increased age, female sex, and gastric perforations
- The diagnosis is overlooked in about 5% of patients
- In < 10% of cases, acute bleeding from a posterior "kissing" ulcer complicates the anterior perforation
- Severity of illness and occurrence of death are directly related to the interval between perforation and surgical closure

CLINICAL FINDINGS

SYMPTOMS AND SIGNS

- Perforation usually elicits a sudden, severe upper abdominal pain
- The patient appears severely distressed, lying quietly with the knees drawn up and breathing shallowly to minimize abdominal motion
- Fever is absent at the start but spikes within 12–24 hours
- Rebound tenderness and abdominal rigidity
- Reduced or absent bowel sounds
- Free air in the abdomen with abdominal distention and diffuse tympany

LABORATORY FINDINGS

- A mild leukocytosis in the range of 12,000/μL in the early stages followed by rise to 20,000/μL within 12–24 hours
- Mild rise in the serum amylase caused by absorption of the enzyme from duodenal secretions within the peritoneal cavity
- Infection with *Helicobacter pylori*

IMAGING FINDINGS

- **Abdominal x-rays:** Reveal free subdiaphragmatic air in 85% of patients
- If no free air is demonstrated and the clinical picture suggests perforated ulcer, an emergency upper GI contrast radiographic series should be performed

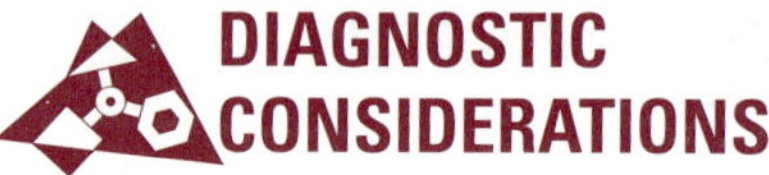

DIAGNOSTIC CONSIDERATIONS

- Pain may be localized to the right lower quadrant if gastroduodenal contents collect in the right lateral peritoneal gutter
- Atypical perforations occur in patients already hospitalized for some unrelated illness, and the significance of the new symptom of abdominal pain is not appreciated
- Free air in the abdomen in a patient with sudden upper abdominal pain should clinch the diagnosis

RULE OUT

- Acute pancreatitis and acute cholecystitis
- The simultaneous onset of pain and free air in the abdomen in the absence of trauma usually means perforated peptic ulcer
  - Free perforation of colonic diverticulitis and acute appendicitis are other rare causes

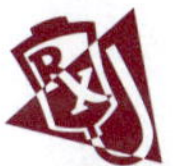

WORK-UP

- Diagnosis and treatment should be simultaneous
- Whenever a perforated ulcer is considered, an NG tube should be inserted to reduce further contamination of the peritoneal cavity
- Blood should be drawn for CBC, electrolyte and amylase, and IV antibiotics (eg, cefazolin, cefoxitin) should be started
- Fluid resuscitation should precede diagnostic measures
- X-rays should be obtained as soon as the clinical status will permit

WHEN TO ADMIT

- All cases of free perforation require surgical intervention and necessitate admission

TREATMENT AND MANAGEMENT

SURGERY

- All free perforations should be repaired by secure closure of the hole with omentum (Graham-Steele closure) sutured into place rather than bringing together the 2 edges with sutures

Indications

- Perforation usually associated with peptic ulcer disease; addition of parietal cell vagotomy or truncal vagotomy and pyloroplasty vs treatment of *H pylori* is controversial

MEDICATIONS

- Treatment of *H pylori* infection
- H_2 blockers, proton pump inhibitors
- Antibiotics (cefazolin, cefoxitin)

TREATMENT MONITORING

- Clinical improvement

COMPLICATIONS

- Other complications of peptic ulcer disease (bleeding, obstruction, intractability)

PROGNOSIS

- 15% mortality, most accounted for by delay in treatment, advanced age, and comorbid diseases

RESOURCES

REFERENCES

- Millat B et al. Surgical treatment of complicated duodenal ulcers: controlled trials. *World J Surg.* 2000;24:299.
- Svanes C. Trends in perforated peptic ulcer: incidence, etiology, treatment, and prognosis. *World J Surg.* 2000;24:277.

Peritoneal Neoplasms

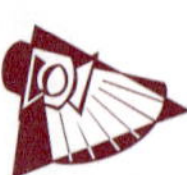

ESSENTIAL FEATURES

- Most tumors affecting the peritoneum are secondary implants from intraperitoneal cancers (ovarian, gastric, pancreatic, etc)
- Primary peritoneal tumors are derived from the mesodermal lining of the peritoneum
- Patients usually present with advanced stages of disease
- History of asbestos exposure in the case of malignant mesothelioma

EPIDEMIOLOGY

- The most common peritoneal neoplasms include peritoneal mesothelioma and pseudomyxoma peritonei
- Malignant mesothelioma occurs most commonly in men, with a long latent period (averaging 40 years) after prolonged asbestos exposure
- Pleural malignant mesotheliomas outnumber peritoneal by 3:1
- Pseudomyxoma peritonei is caused by a low-grade mucinous cystadenocarcinoma of the appendix or ovary that secretes large amounts of mucus-containing epithelial cells

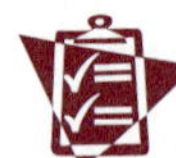

CLINICAL FINDINGS

SYMPTOMS AND SIGNS

- Weight loss
- Crampy abdominal pain
- Large abdominal mass or distention due to ascites
- Frequently intermittent or chronic small bowel obstruction

LABORATORY FINDINGS

- Ascites cytologic studies for peritoneal mesothelioma rarely positive
- Ascites cytologic studies for pseudomyxoma peritonei may demonstrate diagnostic mucus-containing epithelial cells

IMAGING FINDINGS

- **CT scans of the lower thorax and abdomen:** Demonstrate pleural effusions, ascites, peritoneal and mesenteric thickening, and low-density soft-tissue masses involving the omentum and peritoneum
- Malignant mesothelioma may have evidence of asbestos exposure on chest film as well pleural plaques on thoracic CT
- In pseudomyxoma peritonei, US and CT scans show distinctive peritoneal scalloping of the liver margin and intra-abdominal calcified plaques

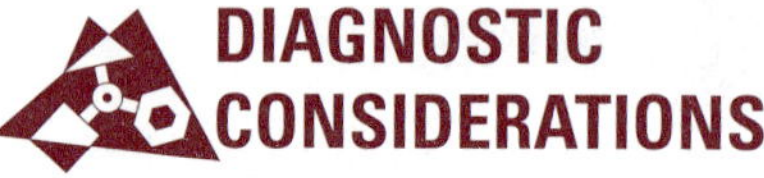

DIAGNOSTIC CONSIDERATIONS

- Chronic inflammatory peritonitis
- Peritoneal mesothelioma
- Cystic mesotheliomas
- Well-differentiated papillary mesotheliomas
- Pseudomyxoma peritonei
- Benign appendiceal mucocele
- Mesenteric cyst
- Mesenteric lipodystrophy
- Carcinomatosis
- Abdominal lymphoma

RULE OUT

- Carcinomatosis
- Chronic inflammatory peritonitis

WORK-UP

- Thorough history (including asbestos exposure) and physical exam
- Abdominal pelvic CT scan to evaluate extent of lesion(s)
- Chest film or thoracic CT scan to evaluate for metastatic disease
- Diagnostic paracentesis: Lactic dehydrogenase (LDH) level, albumin, amylase, triglyceride level, WBC count, cytologic studies, Gram stain, and culture
- Percutaneous biopsy of accessible peritoneal thickening vs diagnostic laparoscopy with biopsy

WHEN TO ADMIT

- Symptoms seldom develop until advanced stages of disease, at which time patients have abdominal pain, distention, and frequently small bowel obstruction requiring admission

WHEN TO REFER

- General surgeons instrumental in establishing the diagnosis, performing cytoreductive surgery, and administering intraperitoneal chemotherapy in conjunction with medical oncology

TREATMENT AND MANAGEMENT

- Palliative cytoreductive surgery: Gross tumor debulking and omentectomy (plus appendectomy and bilateral salpingo-oopherectomy in pseudomyxoma peritonei)
- Intraperitoneal chemotherapy
- Adjuvant intracavitary radiation

SURGERY

Indications

- Bowel obstruction
- Malignant fistula formation
- Palliation

MEDICATIONS

- Cisplatin/doxorubicin-based adjuvant chemotherapy for malignant mesothelioma
- Fluorouracil-based adjuvant chemotherapy for pseudomyxoma peritonei

TREATMENT MONITORING

- Therapy is palliative thus gross tumor recurrence is expected and usually heralded by ascites formation

COMPLICATIONS

- Bowel obstruction
- Malignant intestinal fistula formation
- Tumor recurrence
- Symptomatic ascites

PROGNOSIS

- **Malignant mesothelioma:** Long-term survivors (beyond 1 year) have been reported with cytoreductive surgery combined with intraperitoneal chemotherapy
- **Pseudomyxoma peritonei:** Survival rate 50% at 5 years and 30% at 10 years

RESOURCES

REFERENCES

- Sebbag G et al. Results of treatment of 33 patients with peritoneal mesothelioma. *Br J Surg.* 2000;87:1587.
- Sugarbaker PH. Management of peritoneal-surface malignancy: the surgeon's role. *Langenbecks Arch Surg.* 1999;384:576.

Peritonitis, Bacterial

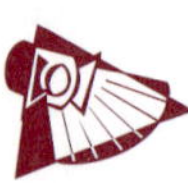

ESSENTIAL FEATURES

- Bacterial peritonitis is a suppurative response of the peritoneal lining to direct bacterial contamination
- Clinical manifestations include:
  - Fever and chills
  - Tachycardia
  - Acute abdomen
  - Free air on plain films

EPIDEMIOLOGY

- Primary bacterial peritonitis is caused mainly by hematogenous spread or transluminal invasion in patients with advanced liver disease and reduced ascitic fluid protein concentration
- Surgical causes are classified as secondary bacterial peritonitis resulting from bacterial contamination originating from within the viscera
- Secondary bacterial peritonitis most commonly follows disruption of a hollow viscus
- Most common etiology in young patients is perforated appendicitis
- Most common etiology in elderly patients is complicated diverticulitis or perforated peptic ulcer

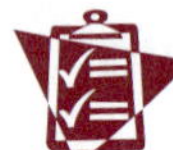

CLINICAL FINDINGS

SYMPTOMS AND SIGNS

- Fever and chills
- Tachycardia
- Oliguria
- Severe abdominal pain with rebound tenderness, guarding, and rigidity ("acute abdomen")
- Diminished bowel sounds
- Physical signs of peritonitis may be subtle in the very young or old and in patients who are immunosuppressed

LABORATORY FINDINGS

- Leukocytosis
- Abnormal liver profile or renal function test
- Mild elevation in amylase
- Elevated ESR and C-reactive protein
- Bacteremia

IMAGING FINDINGS

- **Abdominal x-ray:** Demonstrates free air and ileus pattern and may suggest the primary etiology
- **Water soluble contrast study:** Demonstrates the location of the perforated viscus
- **Abdominal pelvic CT scan with IV and PO contrast:** Best exam for characterizing source of bacterial peritonitis, although an operation should not be delayed to obtain this test in patients with an acute abdomen

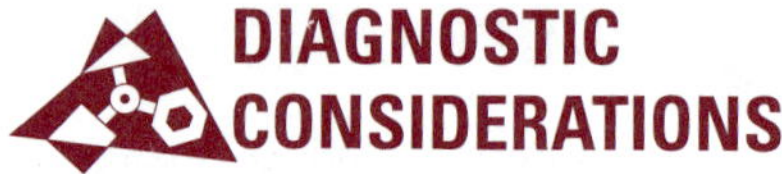

DIAGNOSTIC CONSIDERATIONS

- Primary bacterial peritonitis
- Etiology of secondary bacterial peritonitis:
  - Appendicitis
  - Perforated gastroduodenal ulcers
  - Diverticulitis
  - Gangrenous cholecystitis
  - Acute salpingitis
  - Nonvascular small bowel perforation
  - Large bowel perforation
  - Mesenteric ischemia
  - Acute necrotizing pancreatitis
  - Postoperative complications
  - Others
- Familial Mediterranean fever

RULE OUT

- Primary bacterial peritonitis in patients with advanced liver disease (high operative mortality)
- Nonoperative causes of peritonitis
  - Pancreatitis
  - Pyelonephritis
  - Acute salpingitis

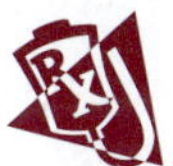

WORK-UP

- Thorough history and physical exam
- CBC count
- Basic chemistries
- Amylase and lipase
- UA
- Liver profile
- Coagulation studies
- Abdominal x-rays

WHEN TO ADMIT

- All patients with bacterial peritonitis should be admitted for appropriate surgical and medical management

WHEN TO REFER

- Primary bacterial peritonitis is ideally cared for nonoperatively by gastroenterologists
- Secondary bacterial peritonitis should be managed by a general surgeon

TREATMENT AND MANAGEMENT

- Resuscitation with IV fluids and electrolyte replacement
- Operative control of the abdominal sepsis
- Systemic antibiotics
- Cardiorespiratory ICU support as indicated

SURGERY

Indications

- Operative goal is to correct the underlying cause of abdominal sepsis:
  - Perforated viscus
  - Ruptured appendix
  - Infected necrotizing pancreatitis
  - Gangrenous cholecystitis
  - Abscess drainage

MEDICATIONS

- Systemic empiric antibiotics that cover aerobic and anaerobic enteric organisms
- Directed antibiotic therapy based on operative cultures

TREATMENT MONITORING

- Good urinary output
- Resolution of tachycardia
- Amelioration of fever and leukocytosis
- Resolution of ileus

COMPLICATIONS

- Uncontrolled abdominal sepsis and death
- Abscess formation
- Deep wound infections
- Anastomotic dehiscence
- Fistula formation

PROGNOSIS

- Overall mortality for generalized peritonitis is 40%
- Factors contributing to mortality include:
  - Type/duration of underlying disease
  - Associated comorbidities
  - Reduced cardiac status
  - Low preoperative albumin

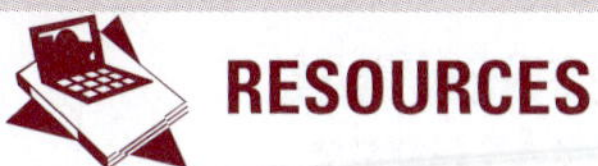

RESOURCES

REFERENCES

- Troidle L et al. Differing outcomes of gram-positive and gram-negative peritonitis. *Am J Kidney Dis.* 1998;32:623.

Peutz-Jeghers Syndrome

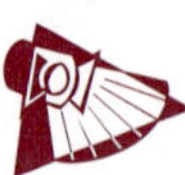

ESSENTIAL FEATURES

- Autosomal dominant syndrome
- Multiple GI non-neoplastic hamartomas
- Predisposition to cancers
- **Characteristic mucocutaneous pigmentation:** Dark, macular lesions on mouth, buccal mucosa, lips, anus
- Polyps occur primarily in jejunum and ileum
- Can act as lead point for intussusception due to obstruction

EPIDEMIOLOGY

- Familial autosomal dominant
- Mapped to chromosome 19p13.3, encodes serine/threonine kinase
- Carriers of the gene predisposed to a number of early-onset cancers
- Increased risk of GI and gonadal, breast, pancreas, and biliary cancers

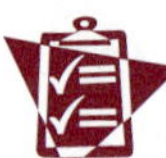

CLINICAL FINDINGS

SYMPTOMS AND SIGNS

- Mucocutaneous lesions present from birth
- Cutaneous lesions may involve buccal mucosa and may extend beyond vermilion border of the lips

LABORATORY FINDINGS

- **Polyps:** Hamartomas consist of supportive framework of smooth muscle tissue covered by hyperplastic epithelium

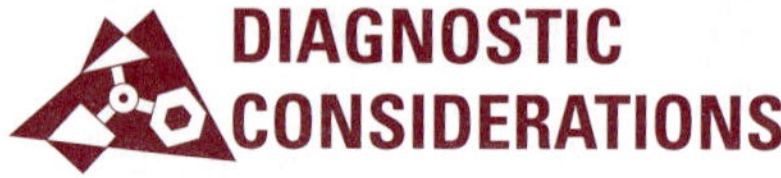

DIAGNOSTIC CONSIDERATIONS

- Neoplasms of small bowel:
  - Adenocarcinoma
  - Carcinoid tumor
  - Leiomyoma/leiomyosarcoma

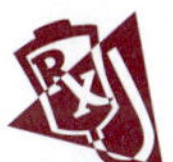

WORK-UP

WHEN TO ADMIT

- Complications from polyps:
  - Intussusception
  - Obstruction
  - Bleeding

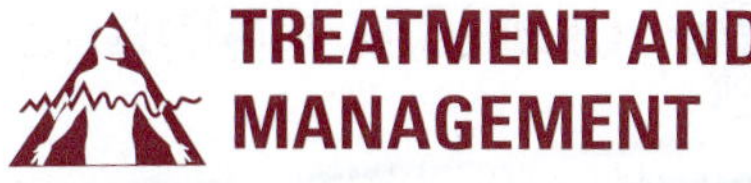

TREATMENT AND MANAGEMENT

SURGERY

- Removal of polyps
  - Endoscopic techniques should be used when possible

Indications

- Complete bowel obstruction
- Intractable GI bleeding
- Development of malignancy
- Surgery may be required for intussusception caused by small-intestinal polyps

TREATMENT MONITORING

- Screening for gonadal tumors and breast cancer

COMPLICATIONS

- Intestinal obstruction
- GI bleeding
- Cancer of small bowel/colon (uncommon)

RESOURCES

REFERENCES

- Bond JH. Polyp guideline: diagnosis, treatment, and surveillance for patients with colorectal polyps. Practice Parameters Committee of the American College of Gastroenterology. *Am J Gastroenterol.* 2000;95:3053.

Pharyngoesophageal (Zenker) Diverticulum

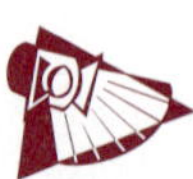

ESSENTIAL FEATURES

- Dysphagia, pressure symptoms, and gurgling sounds in the neck
- Regurgitation of undigested food, halitosis
- Manual emptying of the diverticulum by the patient

EPIDEMIOLOGY

- Diverticula are acquired lesions that result from the protrusion of mucosa and submucosa through a defect in the musculature due to high pressures generated during swallowing (pulsion type, most common) or from the pulling outward of the esophagus from inflamed peribronchial mediastinal lymph nodes (traction type)
- Diverticula arise posteriorly in the midline—above the cricopharyngeus muscle and below the inferior constrictor of the pharynx; the sac projects laterally
- Pulsion diverticula are 3 times more common in men than in women; most patients are over age 60
- The body of the esophagus often shows abnormal motility; an associated hiatal hernia is common and abnormal reflux is present in about 33% of patients

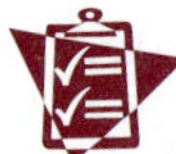

CLINICAL FINDINGS

SYMPTOMS AND SIGNS

- **Dysphagia:** Related to the size of the diverticulum
- Undigested food is regurgitated into the mouth, especially when the patient is in the recumbent position
- The patient may manually massage the neck after eating to empty the sac
- Swelling of the neck
- Gurgling noises after eating
- Halitosis and a sour metallic taste in the mouth

IMAGING FINDINGS

- A smoothly rounded blind pouch is visible on fluoroscopic exam
- Esophagoscopy is hazardous because the instrument may enter the ostium of the diverticulum and lead to perforation

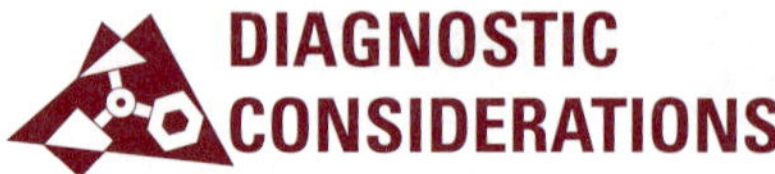

DIAGNOSTIC CONSIDERATIONS

- Esophageal manometry and pH measurements will show if the diverticulum is associated with an abnormal response of the cricopharyngeus muscle to swallowing (delayed opening of the sphincter) and the amount of gastroesophageal reflux

RULE OUT

- Malignant lesions
- Achalasia of the cricopharyngeus muscle
- Cervical esophageal webs (may also occur along with diverticula)

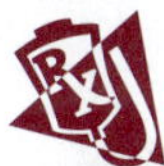

WORK-UP

- Radiographic contrast fluoroscopic esophagogram
- Manometry
- pH testing

WHEN TO ADMIT

- Diverticular perforation with mediastinitis or abscess
- Aspiration pneumonitis or pneumonia
- Severe dysphagia prohibiting enteral intake

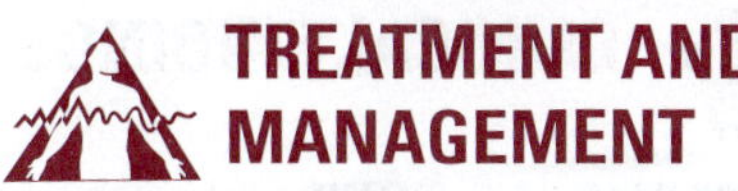

TREATMENT AND MANAGEMENT

SURGERY

- Excision of the diverticulum and division of the cricopharyngeal muscle
- Other options:
  - Diverticulopexy
  - Oropharyngeally placed ligating and dividing stapler

Indications

- All cases
- If the patient also has significant gastroesophageal reflux, this should be corrected before the upper sphincter is divided, in order to avoid aspiration

COMPLICATIONS

- Aspiration leading to pneumonitis
- Diverticular perforation with mediastinitis or paraesophageal abscess
- Mucosal ulceration and bleeding

PROGNOSIS

- Excellent

RESOURCES

REFERENCES

- Feeley MA et al. Zenker's diverticulum: analysis of surgical complications from diverticulectomy and cricopharyngeal myotomy. *Laryngoscope.* 1999;109:858.

Pheochromocytoma

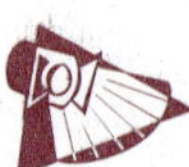

ESSENTIAL FEATURES

- Episodic headache, excessive sweating, palpitations, and visual blurring
- Hypertension, frequently sustained, with or without paroxysms
- Postural tachycardia and hypotension
- Elevated urinary catecholamines or their metabolites, hypermetabolism, hyperglycemia

EPIDEMIOLOGY

- Found in < 0.1% of patients with hypertension
- 5% of tumors discovered incidentally on CT scan
- Most occur sporadically
- Associated with familial syndromes, such as:
  - Multiple endocrine neoplasia type 2A (MEN 2A)
  - MEN 2B
  - Recklinghausen disease
  - von Hippel-Lindau disease
- Pheochromocytomas are present in 40% of patients with MEN 2
- 90% of patients with pheochromocytoma are hypertensive
- Rule of 10s:
  - 10% malignant
  - 10% familial
  - 10% bilateral
  - 10% multiple tumors
  - 10% extra-adrenal
- Hypertension less common in children
- In children, 50% of patients have multiple or extra-adrenal tumors
- Extra-adrenal pheochromocytomas:
  - Abdomen (75%)
  - Bladder (10%)
  - Chest (10%)
  - Pelvis (2%)
  - Head and neck (3%)

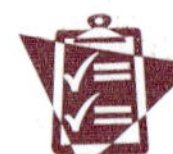

CLINICAL FINDINGS

SYMPTOMS AND SIGNS

- Clinical findings are variable
- Episodic or sustained hypertension
- Triad of palpitation, headache, and diaphoresis
- Anxiety, tremors
- Weight loss
- Dizziness, nausea, and vomiting
- Abdominal discomfort, constipation, diarrhea
- Visual blurring
- Tachycardia, postural hypotension
- Hypertensive retinopathy

LABORATORY FINDINGS

- Hyperglycemia
- Elevated plasma metanephrines
- Elevated 24-hour urine metanephrines and free catecholamines
- Elevated urinary vanillylmandelic acid (VMA)
- Elevated plasma catecholamines

IMAGING FINDINGS

- Adrenal mass seen on CT or MRI
- Characteristic bright appearance on T2-weighted MRI
- Asymmetric uptake on MIBG scan (particularly useful for extra-adrenal, multiple, or malignant pheochromocytomas)

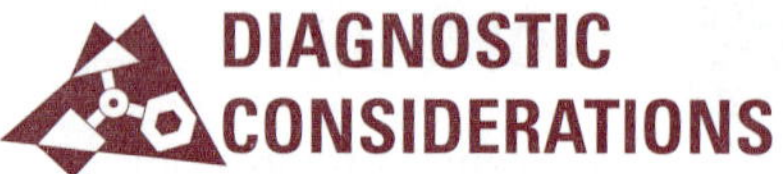

DIAGNOSTIC CONSIDERATIONS

- Avoid arteriography or fine-needle aspiration as they can precipitate a hypertensive crisis
- Early recognition during pregnancy is key because if left untreated, half of fetuses and nearly half of the mothers will die

RULE OUT

- Other causes of hypertension
- Hyperthyroidism
- Anxiety disorder
- Carcinoid syndrome

WORK-UP

- History and physical exam
  - Suspect pheochromocytoma based on symptoms
- CT, MRI, or other scans
- Plasma and urine studies (metanephrines, catecholamines, VMA)
- Begin treatment with a-blockers
- Possible MIBG scan
- Operative excision of tumor

WHEN TO ADMIT

- Hypertensive crisis (can develop multisystem organ failure, mimicking severe sepsis)

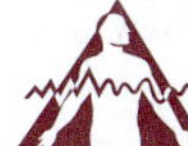

TREATMENT AND MANAGEMENT

- a-Adrenergic blocking agents should be started as soon as the biochemical diagnosis is established to restore blood volume, to prevent a severe crisis, and to allow recovery from the cardiomyopathy

SURGERY

Indications

- All pheochromocytomas should be excised

Contraindications

- Metastatic disease
- Inadequate medical preparation (α blockade)

MEDICATIONS

- α-Adrenergic blocking agents, such as phenoxybenzamine
- Other agents include metyrosine, prazosin, and calcium channel blockers
- β-Adrenergic blocking agents can be used only after full a blockade has been achieved
- Avoid opioids as they stimulate histamine release

TREATMENT MONITORING

- Blood pressure
- Plasma metanephrines

COMPLICATIONS

- Long-term complications of hypertension (stroke, renal failure, myocardial infarction, congestive heart failure)
- Arrhythmia
- Sudden death

PROGNOSIS

- Operative mortality is 1–2%
- Mild to moderate essential hypertension may persist after surgery
- Treatment with ^{131}I-MIBG may help patients with metastatic or recurrent malignant pheochromocytomas

RESOURCES

REFERENCES

- Duh Q-Y. Editorial: Evolving surgical management for patients with pheochromocytoma. *J Clin Endocrinol Metab.* 2001;86:1477.
- Kebebew E et al. Benign and malignant pheochromocytoma: diagnosis, treatment, and follow up. *Surg Oncol Clin North Am.* 1998;7:765.
- Prys-Roberts C. Phaeochromocytoma-recent progress in its management. *Br J Anaesth.* 2000:85:44.

PRACTICE GUIDELINES

- The National Comprehensive Cancer Network http://www.nccn.org

Pilonidal Disease

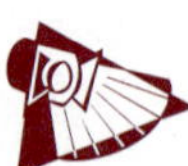

ESSENTIAL FEATURES

- Acute, chronic, recurring abscess or chronic draining sinus over the sacrococcygeal or perianal region
- An acquired infection of natal cleft hair follicles that become distended and obstructed and rupture into the subcutaneous tissues to form a pilonidal abscess
- Hair from the surrounding skin is pulled into the abscess cavity by the friction generated by the gluteal muscles during walking

EPIDEMIOLOGY

- Incidence of pilonidal disease is highest in white males (3:1 male:female ratio) between ages 15 and 40 with a peak incidence between 16 and 20 years
- Most common in the hirsute, moderately obese patient

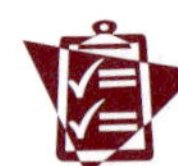

CLINICAL FINDINGS

SYMPTOMS AND SIGNS

- Pain, fluctuant mass
- Tenderness
- Purulent drainage
- Inspissated hair
- Induration
- Patients may present with small midline pits or abscesses on or off the midline near the coccyx or sacrum
- Physical exam may reveal a spectrum of disease from acute suppuration and an undrained abscess or chronic draining sinuses with multiple mature tracts with hairs protruding from the pit-like openings
- Most sinus tracts run cephalad

LABORATORY FINDINGS

- No specific findings

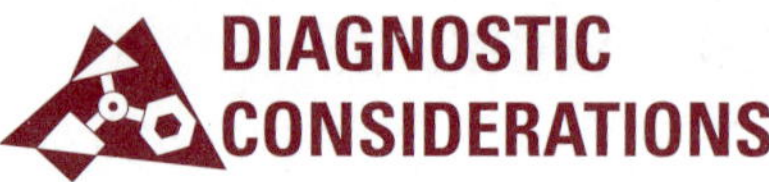

DIAGNOSTIC CONSIDERATIONS

- Cryptoglandular abscess
- Fistula-in-ano
- Hidradenitis suppurativa
- Furuncle
- Actinomycosis
- Tuberculous granuloma
- Osteomyelitis with draining sinuses

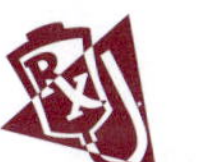

WORK-UP

- History and physical exam

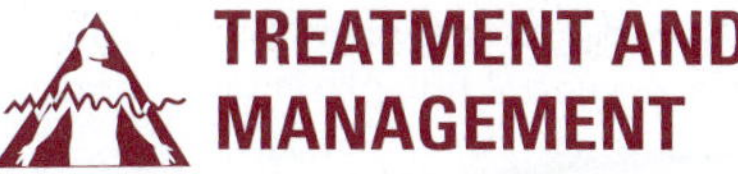

TREATMENT AND MANAGEMENT

SURGERY

- Pilonidal abscesses may be drained under local anesthesia
- Probe may be inserted into the primary opening and the abscess unroofed
- Granulation tissue and inspissated hair are pulled out
- Excision of midline pits with removal of hair from lateral tract
- Excision with open packing, marsupialization, or primary closure with or without flaps

MEDICATIONS

- Antibiotics usually not indicated

COMPLICATIONS

- Untreated pilonidal disease may result in multiple draining sinuses with chronic recurrent abscess, drainage, soiling of clothing, and, rarely, necrotizing wound infections or malignant degeneration
- Carcinoma arising from chronic pilonidal sinus is rare, usually well-differentiated squamous cell carcinoma
  - Treatment is wide excision

PROGNOSIS

- Cure rates of 60–80% have been reported after primary unroofing and extraction of hair
- Conservative excision of midline pits with removal of hair from lateral tracts and postoperative weekly shaving has 90% success rate

PREVENTION

- Meticulous skin care (shaving of natal cleft)
- Perineal hygiene, wound cleansing

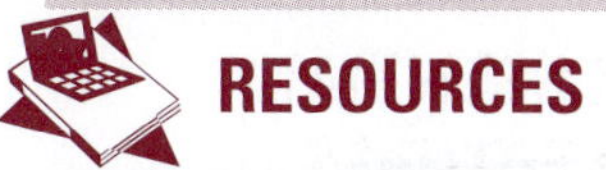

RESOURCES

REFERENCES

- Abu Galala KH et al. Treatment of pilonidal sinus by primary closure with a transposed rhomboid flap compared with deep suturing: a prospective randomized clinical trial. *Eur J Surg.* 1999;165:468.
- Spivak H et al. Treatment of chronic pilonidal disease. *Dis Colon Rectum.* 1996;39:1136.

Pleural Effusion

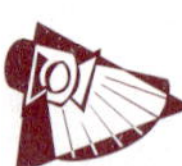

ESSENTIAL FEATURES

- Presence of fluid within pleural space
- Etiology includes:
  - Increased pulmonary hydrostatic pressure
  - Decreased intravascular oncotic pressure
  - Increased capillary permeability
  - Decreased intrapleural pressure (atelectasis)
  - Decreased lymphatic drainage (carcinomatosis)
  - Rupture of vascular or lymphatic structure (trauma)
- When nature of fluid of known, more specific terms may be used:
  - Pyothorax: Pus in pleural cavity (empyema)
  - Hemothorax: Blood in thorax
  - Chylothorax: Chyle in thorax
  - Hydrothorax: Collection of serous fluid (transudative or exudative)
- Etiology for hydrothorax:
  - Tuberculosis: History of exposure, can be sanguineous; > 1000 lymphocytes, positive for acid-fast bacilli, positive tuberculin skin test, positive pleural biopsy, glucose < 60 mg/dL
  - Cancer: 67% bloody, cytology positive in 50%, glucose rarely < 60 mg/dL
  - Congestive heart failure (CHF): Presence of CHF, serous, < 10,000 RBCs, right-sided in up to 70%, may be bilateral; interlobal fissure fluid collection called "pseudotumors"
  - Pneumonia: Respiratory infection, serous, neutrophils predominate in fluid, culture and stain positive for organisms, infiltrate on chest film
  - Rheumatoid arthritis: Joint involvement, turbid or yellow-green color, lymphocytes predominate, glucose < 20 mg/dL, rapid clotting time, eosinophils present
  - Pulmonary embolism: Risk for embolism, often sanguineous
  - Other causes: Nephrotic syndrome, rupture of hydronephrosis into pleural space (elevated creatinine in fluid), pancreatitis (left-sided, elevated amylase), cirrhosis (5% of patients with ascites)
- Etiology for chylothorax:
  - Most often due to surgical procedures
  - Other causes include trauma, malignancy, central line placement, thoracic aortic aneurysms, filariasis
  - Blunt trauma: Thoracic duct shearing at diaphragm

EPIDEMIOLOGY

- > 25% of pleural effusions are secondary to malignancy
- Malignant effusions occur in patients with lung cancer (35%), breast cancer (23%), lymphoma (10%)
- 10% of malignant effusions secondary to primary pleural tumors (mesothelioma most common)

CLINICAL FINDINGS

SYMPTOMS AND SIGNS

- Decreased respiratory excursions
- Diminished breath sounds
- Dullness to percussion
- Decreased vocal/tactile fremitus
- Pleural friction rub
- Long-standing disease: Contraction of hemithorax

LABORATORY FINDINGS

- Fluid: Acid-fast bacilli: TB
- Send fluid for total protein, lactic dehydrogenase (LDH), glucose, specific gravity, amylase, creatinine, pH, cytology

IMAGING FINDINGS

- **Chest film:** Blunting of costophrenic angle = 250–500 mL of fluid; entire hemithorax effusion: > 2 L

DIAGNOSTIC CONSIDERATIONS

- Criteria for diagnosing transudates by thoracentesis fluid:
  - LDH < 200 U/dL (fluid:serum ratio < 0.6
  - Total protein < 3 g/dL (fluid:serum < 0.5)
  - Specific gravity < 1.016
- Malignant effusions:
  - Serous, serosanguineous, bloody
  - Cytology positive in 50–75% with repeated thoracentesis
- Closed pleural biopsy positive thoracentesis cytology: 80% diagnostic yield
- Thoracoscopy with pleural biopsy: 97% diagnostic yield

RULE OUT

- TB
- Cancer
- CHF
- Pneumonia
- Rheumatoid arthritis/collagen disease
- Pulmonary embolism

WORK-UP

- Chest film
- Thoracentesis

TREATMENT AND MANAGEMENT

- Malignant effusions
  - Goal is palliation plus lung reexpansion
  - Chest tube (drains 1 L initially, allow 200 mL drainage every hour until completely drained)
  - Chemical pleurodesis (talc, doxycycline)
  - Bilateral pleurodesis contraindication due to risk of acute respiratory distress syndrome
- CHF
  - Treat underlying failure
  - Diuresis
- Chylothorax
  - Closed chest tube drainage
  - Low fat diet
  - Chyle typically causes pleurodesis; however, drainage > 7 days may need intervention (significant protein losses)
  - Video-assisted thoracoscopic technique: Ligation of thoracic duct at diaphragm between aorta and azygous vein

SURGERY

Indications

- Recurrent malignant effusions
- Chylothorax: Drainage > 7 days

COMPLICATIONS

- Drainage of pleural effusion: Bleeding, pneumothorax, reexpansion pulmonary edema

PROGNOSIS

- Varies with etiology

RESOURCES

REFERENCES

- Alfageme I et al. Empyema of the thorax in adults: etiology, microbiologic findings, and management. *Chest.* 1993;103:839.
- Therapy of pleural effusion: A statement by the Committee on Therapy of the American Thoracic Society. *Am Rev Respir Dis.* 1968;97:479.

Pleural Space Trauma

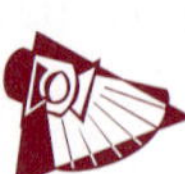

ESSENTIAL FEATURES

- Hemothorax is classified by the amount of blood
  - Minimal < 350 mL
  - Moderate 350–1500 mL
  - Massive > 1500 mL
- The rate of bleeding after evacuation of the hemothorax is more important than the initial return of blood on placement of the chest tube
- Hemothorax should be suspected with penetrating or severe blunt thoracic injury
- In 85% of cases, tube thoracostomy is all the treatment necessary
- Pneumothorax occurs with laceration of the lung or chest wall following penetrating or blunt trauma
- Tension pneumothorax develops when a flap-valve leak allows air to enter the pleural space but not exit
- Increasing intrapleural pressure interferes with venous return and must be immediately relieved

EPIDEMIOLOGY

- Trauma patients

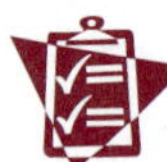

CLINICAL FINDINGS

SYMPTOMS AND SIGNS

- **Hemothorax:** Decreased breath sounds, dullness to percussion
- **Pneumothorax:** Possibly tympany to percussion, decreased breath sounds
- **Tension pneumothorax:** Tracheal deviation away from affected side, tympany to percussion, decreased breath sounds, hypotension, distended neck veins
- **Sucking chest wound:** Obvious chest wall defect
- Hypoxia
- Dyspnea

LABORATORY FINDINGS

- Hypoxemia

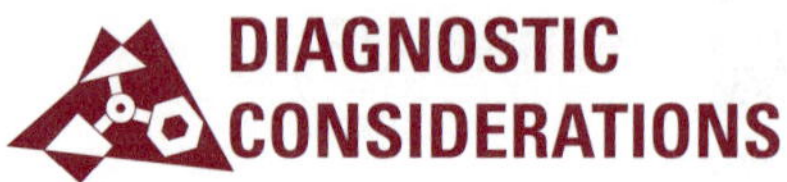

DIAGNOSTIC CONSIDERATIONS

- Mechanism and physical exam often pinpoint problem
- Underlying and abdominal injuries can often dictate course of therapy

WORK-UP

- Physical exam
- Chest film (upright or semi-upright)

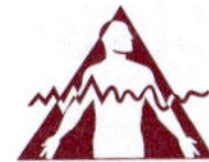

TREATMENT AND MANAGEMENT

- Initial resuscitation and stabilization

SURGERY

- **Hemothorax**
  - Tube thoracostomy (chest tube) NOT needle aspiration
  - Thoracotomy or thoracoscopy are rarely indicated
- **Pneumothorax:** Tube thoracostomy
- **Tension pneumothorax:** Needle thoracostomy followed by tube thoracostomy
- **Sucking chest wound:** Occlusive dressing and tube thoracostomy followed by operative reconstruction of chest wall

Indications

- Initial chest tube output > 1000 mL
- Chest tube output > 100–200 mL/h

RESOURCES

REFERENCES

- Brasel KJ et al. Treatment of occult pneumothoraces from blunt trauma. *J Trauma.* 1999;46:987.
- Etoch S et al. Tube thoracostomy. *Arch Surg.* 1995;130:521.
- Pape HC et al. Appraisal of early evaluation of chest trauma: development of a standardized scoring system for initial clinical decision-making. *J Trauma.* 2000;49:496.
- Feliciano DV et al. Advances in the diagnosis and treatment of thoracic trauma. *Surg Clin North Am.* 1999;79:1417.

Pleural Tumors

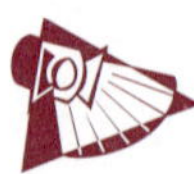

ESSENTIAL FEATURES

Localized Fibrous Tumors of Pleura

- Previously called "localized mesotheliomas"
- Arise from subpleural fibroblasts
- Cause pulmonary nodules to pleural masses
- Involvement of visceral pleura more common than parietal
- Benign (70%) patterns
  - Fibrous
  - Cellular
  - Mixed
- Malignant (30%) patterns
  - Tubulopapillary
  - Fibrous
  - Dimorphic
- Behave as sarcomas

Diffuse Malignant Pleural Mesothelioma

- Most common primary tumor of pleura
- 4 histologic variants
  - Epithelial or rubopapillary (35–40%): Associated with pleural effusions, better prognosis
  - Fibrosarcomatous/mesenchymal (20%) "dry" mesotheliomas
  - Mixed (35–40%)
  - Undifferentiated (5–10%)

EPIDEMIOLOGY

Diffuse Malignant Pleural Mesothelioma

- Strong link to asbestos exposure: 300 × increased risk
- Amphibole fibers (crocidolite, amosite, etc) and soil silicate zeolite lodge in terminal airways migrate to pleura
- Latency after asbestos exposure: 15–50 years
- Right hemithorax (60%) affected more than left (35%), bilateral (5%)

CLINICAL FINDINGS

SYMPTOMS AND SIGNS

Localized Fibrous Tumors of Pleura

- Most asymptomatic
- Large tumors may produce symptoms of bronchial compression
  - Dyspnea
  - Cough
  - Chest heaviness
- Rarely, hypoglycemia from production of insulin-like peptide (4%)
- Clubbing, hypertrophic pulmonary osteoarthropathy (20–35%)

Diffuse Malignant Pleural Mesothelioma

- Dyspnea on exertion common
- Chest wall discomfort common
- Cough, fever, malaise, weight loss, dysphagia
- Advanced disease:
  - Pain
  - Abdominal distention
  - Pericardial tamponade
  - Superior vena cava (SVC) syndrome

IMAGING FINDINGS

Localized Fibrous Tumors of Pleura

- **Chest film:** Well circumscribed mass, may move with changes in position
- Pleural effusion in 15%

Diffuse Malignant Pleural Mesothelioma

- **Chest film:** Pleural thickening, effusion (75%), narrowing of intercostals spaces
- **CT scan:** Diffuse irregular pleural thickening

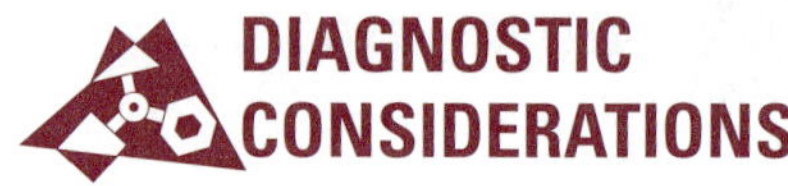

DIAGNOSTIC CONSIDERATIONS

Localized Fibrous Tumors of Pleura

- Fine-needle aspiration (FNA) may be suggestive
- Surgical excision often necessary for diagnosis

Diffuse Malignant Pleural Mesothelioma

- FNA usually inadequate
- Biopsy via small incision or video-assisted thoracoscopic surgery (VATS)
- Immunohistochemistry stains for carcinoembryonic antigen (CEA), LeuM1, B72.3, BerEP4, negative; vimentin and keratin stains positive
- Calretinin stain (specific for mesothelial cells) usually positive

WORK-UP

- Chest film
- Chest CT scan
- Fluorodeoxyglucose positron emission tomography (FDG-PET) scan sometimes useful

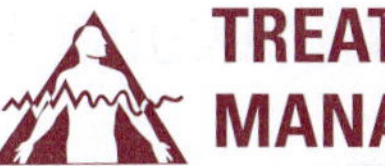

TREATMENT AND MANAGEMENT

Localized Fibrous Tumors of Pleura

- Complete resection; lobectomy usually not required, wedge resection recommended if visceral pleural involved
- If arises from parietal pleura, chest wall resection necessary
- After excision, no further therapy needed

Diffuse Malignant Pleural Mesothelioma

- Radiation and chemotherapy alone have no impact on survival
- Surgery: 2 approaches
  1. Radical pleuropneumonectomy
  2. Parietal pleurectomy with decortication: Better outcome and lower morbidity when combined with radiation therapy
- Chemotherapy, photodynamic therapy, immunotherapy, gene therapy, intraoperative chemoradiation therapy being done at some centers under clinical trials

TREATMENT MONITORING

Localized Fibrous Tumors of Pleura

- Incomplete resection generally requires postoperative radiation therapy

PROGNOSIS

Localized Fibrous Tumors of Pleura

- Good, if resection is complete
- If resection is incomplete, median survival is 7 months

Diffuse Malignant Pleural Mesothelioma

- Median survival: 7–16 months
- With surgical treatment and radiation: Median survival up to 25 months

RESOURCES

REFERENCES

- Cheng AY. Neoplasms in the mediastinum, chest wall, and pleura. *Curr Opin Oncol.* 1999;6:17.

Pneumatosis Intestinalis

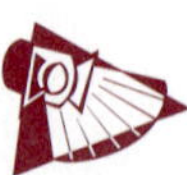

ESSENTIAL FEATURES

- Gas filled cysts in the wall of the intestine and mesentery
- May be primary and idiopathic; an incidental finding; or secondary to chronic obstructive pulmonary disease, infectious gastroenteritis, or connective tissue disorders
- Fulminant pneumatosis is associated with bacterial infection and necrosis of the bowel wall.

EPIDEMIOLOGY

- Characterized by gas-filled cysts in the wall of the gut and mesentery
- 15% of cases are primary and idiopathic
- Secondary pneumatosis comprises 85% of cases; cysts may be located anywhere in the GI tract
- Conditions that underlie secondary pneumatosis intestinalis include:
  - Inflammatory bowel disease
  - Infectious gastroenteritis
  - Corticosteroid therapy
  - Connective tissue disorders
  - Intestinal obstruction
  - Diverticulitis
  - Chronic obstructive pulmonary disease
  - Acute leukemia
  - Lymphoma
  - AIDS
  - Organ transplantation
- Fulminant pneumatosis is associated with acute bacterial infection and necrosis of the bowel wall, usually associated with intestinal infarction; pneumoperitoneum is sometimes present

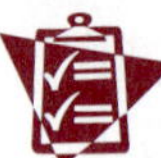

CLINICAL FINDINGS

SYMPTOMS AND SIGNS

- Abdominal discomfort
- Diarrhea
- Passing of excessive amounts of gas
- Abdominal distention
- Abdominal tenderness

LABORATORY FINDINGS

- Nonspecific in most cases
- When associated with intestinal necrosis:
  - Leukocytosis
  - Metabolic acidosis
  - Increased serum lactate

IMAGING FINDINGS

- **Abdominal x-rays and CT scan:** Linear gas deposits in the intestinal wall; if perforation is present, free air may be visualized

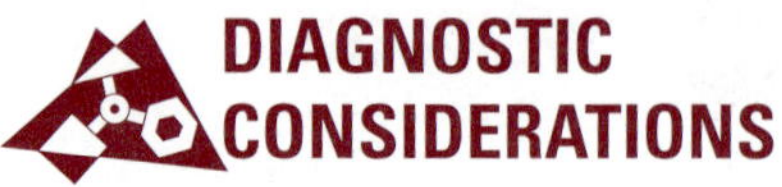

DIAGNOSTIC CONSIDERATIONS

- Pneumatosis intestinalis may be an incidental finding (primary and most cases of secondary pneumatosis) or indicative of bowel wall necrosis with gas produced by invading bacteria

RULE OUT

- Intestinal ischemia
- Strangulation obstruction

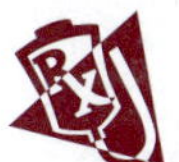

WORK-UP

- Abdominal x-ray or CT scan

WHEN TO ADMIT

- Suspected intestinal necrosis

TREATMENT AND MANAGEMENT

- Primary and secondary pneumatosis: No specific treatment; oxygen administration may lead to resolution
- Fulminant pneumatosis: Bowel resection

SURGERY

Indications

- Intestinal necrosis
- Intestinal ischemia
- Strangulation obstruction

Contraindications

- Idiopathic pneumatosis
- Secondary pneumatosis associated with systemic disease without bowel necrosis

MEDICATIONS

- Oxygen administration

COMPLICATIONS

- Perforation if associated with necrosis
- Sepsis

PROGNOSIS

- **Primary and secondary:** Excellent
- **Fulminant:** High mortality related to intestinal necrosis

RESOURCES

REFERENCES

- Christl SU et al. Impaired hydrogen metabolism in pneumatosis cystoides intestinalis. *Gastroenterology.* 1993;104:392.
- Hoover EL et al. Avoiding laparotomy in nonsurgical pneumoperitoneum. *Am J Surg.* 1992;164:99.

Pneumonia

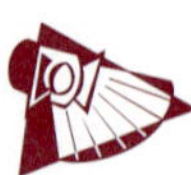

ESSENTIAL FEATURES

- Leading cause of death from nosocomial infection
- Aspiration of gastric contents in patients with impaired airway protective defenses, due to intubation or level of consciousness, plays central role in pathogenesis
- Diagnosis can be difficult to distinguish from other likely causes of postoperative or post-injury infection

EPIDEMIOLOGY

- Majority of cases occur outside of ICU
- Incidence 4–7/1000 admissions
- 13–18% of all nosocomial infections
- 25% of ICU patients will develop pneumonia
- 75% of critically ill patients have oropharynx colonized with pathogenic bacteria within 48 hours
- Gram-negative bacilli predominate (*Pseudomonas, E coli, Serratia, H influenzae, Enterobacter, Klebsiella,* etc)
- Risk factors include:
  - Old age
  - **Mechanical ventilation**
  - Head injury
  - H_2-receptor antagonists or proton pump inhibitors
  - Frequent ventilator setting changes
  - Winter months
  - Large volume aspiration of gastric contents
  - Thoracic surgery
  - Chronic lung disease
- Intubation increases risk by 6- to 20-fold

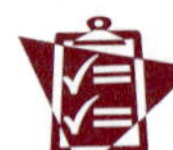

CLINICAL FINDINGS

SYMPTOMS AND SIGNS

- Fever
- Increase and change in character of sputum
- Hypoxia
- Decreased breath sounds over affected region of lung
- Tachypnea

LABORATORY FINDINGS

- Leukocytosis
- Hypoxemia

IMAGING FINDINGS

- Pulmonary infiltrate on chest film or CT scan

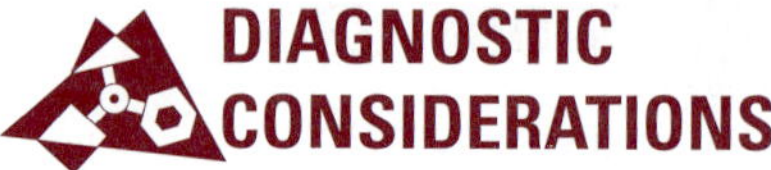

DIAGNOSTIC CONSIDERATIONS

- Chest film infiltrate has positive predictive value (PPV) of 64% at best
- Sputum Gram stain is unreliable
- Protected brush specimen (PBS) has sensitivity of 64–100% when > 1000 CFU/mL detected on culture
- Bronchoalveolar lavage (BAL) has sensitivity of 72–100% when > 10,000 CFU/mL detected
- BAL cell count with < 50% polymorphonuclear leukocytes (PMNs) nearly excludes pneumonia
- Atelectasis
- Pulmonary embolus
- Other likely causes of fever in patient's clinical situation
- Lung tumor, in appropriate clinical circumstance

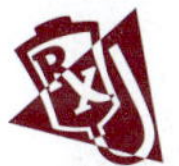

WORK-UP

- Chest film
- CBC count
- Sputum Gram stain and culture
- Blood culture
- Consider BAL or PBS to improve sensitivity and specificity
- Serial imaging exams may be helpful to reveal evolution of infiltrate

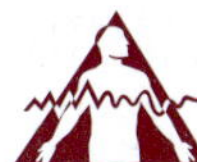

TREATMENT AND MANAGEMENT

- Consider prior antibiotic exposure when choosing therapy
- Empiric coverage must be appropriate for patient and unit endogenous flora
- Early and appropriate antibiotic coverage is essential
- Duration of treatment is 10–14 days with some recommending longer courses for *Pseudomonas, S aureus,* and *Acinetobacter*
- Respiratory therapy to assist patient to clear secretions essential

MEDICATIONS

- Antibiotics

TREATMENT MONITORING

- Clinical improvement
- Resolution of tachypnea, hypoxemia and leukocytosis; radiographic changes often lag behind clinical improvement

COMPLICATIONS

- Empyema
- Lung abscess

PROGNOSIS

- Associated mortality, 20–50%
- Excess risk of death, 33%

PREVENTION

- Avoid supine positioning
- Prompt extubation
- Vigorous respiratory therapy and early ambulation to preserve pulmonary clearance mechanisms

RESOURCES

REFERENCES

- Kozlow AH et al. Epidemiology and impact of aspiration pneumonia in patients undergoing surgery in Maryland, 1999-2000. *Crit Care Med.* 2003;31:1930.
- Montravers P et al. Diagnostic and therapeutic management of nosocomial pneumonia in surgical patients: results of the Eole study. *Crit Care Med.* 2002;30:368.

Pneumothorax

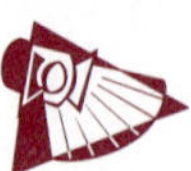

ESSENTIAL FEATURES

- Air in pleural space
- Breach in parietal or visceral pleura
- Described as percentage of chest cavity involved
- Open pneumothorax is associated with open sucking chest wound
- Tension pneumothorax causes shift in mediastinum toward contralateral lung
- 5–10% small pleural effusion present, may be hemorrhagic

EPIDEMIOLOGY

- Etiologies of spontaneous pneumothorax include:
  - Secondary to some pathologic process
  - Rupture of bleb is most common
  - Male:female ratio 6:1
  - Age 16 to 24 years, tall, thin, smoking are risk factors
  - Apical bullae (patients with chronic obstructive pulmonary disease [COPD])
  - Pneumocystic pneumonia
  - Metastatic cancer
  - Rupture of esophagus
  - Lung abscess
  - Cystic fibrosis

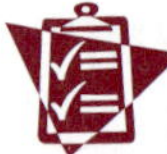

CLINICAL FINDINGS

SYMPTOMS AND SIGNS

- Pleuritic chest pain
- Dyspnea, hypoxia, hypocapnia
- Diaphoresis, cyanosis, weakness, hypotension, cardiovascular collapse
- Tachypnea, tachycardia, deviation of trachea away (tension)
- Decreased breath sounds, hyperresonance, diminished local fremitus

LABORATORY FINDINGS

- ECG: May show nonspecific axis deviation, ST changes, T wave inversion

IMAGING FINDINGS

- **Chest film:** Diagnostic
- **CT scan:** May help differentiate pneumothorax from apical pleural bleb

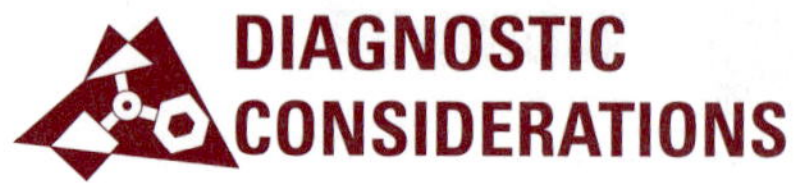

DIAGNOSTIC CONSIDERATIONS

- 1 cm pneumothorax correlates with 25% loss of lung volume

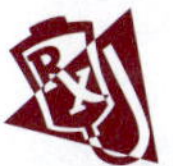

WORK-UP

- 1% of pneumothorax reabsorbed daily

WHEN TO REFER

- Patients with cystic fibrosis
- Patients with AIDS and pneumocystis pneumonia

TREATMENT AND MANAGEMENT

- **Small (< 25%), minimal symptoms:** Can be monitored conservatively
- **Larger asymptomatic, symptomatic, increasing pneumothorax, or associated with effusion:**
  - Insert chest tube
  - Underwater suction drainage or Heimlich (can treat as outpatient)
- Select patients can get aspiration without chest tube, but 20–50% have recurrence
- Patients with AIDS and pneumocystis pneumonia has high failure rate and mortality

SURGERY

- Pleurodesis with doxycycline or talc
- Axillary thoracotomy with apical bullectomy, parietal pleurectomy, and pleurodesis (preferred technique)
- Complete parietal pleurectomy
- Transplantation: Patients with cystic fibrosis or severe COPD; pleurodesis may be contraindicated in these patients

Indications

- Pleurodesis:
  - Air leaks > 7 days
  - Lung does not fully expand
  - High-risk occupation (scuba divers, pilots)

Contraindications

- Pleurodesis:
  - Cystic fibrosis, severe COPD (relative)

TREATMENT MONITORING

- Repeat chest film mandatory within 24 hours of chest tube removal due to recurrence

COMPLICATIONS

- Recurrence
  - Spontaneous, 50%
  - After 2 episodes, 75%
  - After 3 episodes, > 80%

RESOURCES

REFERENCES

- Brasel KJ et al. Treatment of occult pneumothoraces from blunt trauma. *J Trauma.* 1999;46:987.
- Etoch S et al. Tube thoracostomy. *Arch Surg.* 1995;130:521.

Polyposis Syndromes

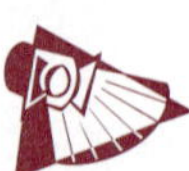

ESSENTIAL FEATURES

- Familial adenomatous polyposis (FAP) (adenomatous polyposis coli) is a rare but important disease because colorectal cancer develops before age 40 in nearly all untreated patients
- FAP: Autosomal dominant
- APC gene localized to chromosome 5q21
- Thousands of polyps (occasionally fewer) of varying size and configuration are present in the colon and rectum
- Extracolonic manifestations are associated with FAP:
  - Endocrine adenoma
  - Osteoma
  - Epidermoid cyst
  - Small bowel adenoma
  - Visceral malignancy
  - Desmoid tumor
  - Thyroid carcinoma
  - Hepatoblastoma
- **Gardner syndrome:** Variant of FAP with polyposis, desmoid tumors, osteomas of mandible or skull, and sebaceous cysts
- **Turcot syndrome:** Variant of FAP with polyposis and a medulloblastoma or glioma
- Congenital hypertrophy of retinal pigment epithelium (always bilateral, more than 4 lesions on each side) predicts FAP with 97% sensitivity
  - This abnormality is present as early as 3 months of age in affected members
- Polyps begin to appear at puberty
- Cancer develops in these patients at a mean age of 35 years

EPIDEMIOLOGY

- Autosomal dominant pattern of inheritance
- Colorectal cancer develops before age 40 years
- In a family with FAP, each first-degree relative of an affected patient has a 50% likelihood of inheriting the mutated gene
- By age 16, about 50% of affected patients have polyps
- With each passing year, a negative sigmoidoscopic exam result reduces further the likelihood that a patient carries the gene

CLINICAL FINDINGS

SYMPTOMS AND SIGNS

- Most patients are asymptomatic
- Lower GI bleeding
- Alteration in bowel habit
- Crampy abdominal pain

IMAGING FINDINGS

- Lower endoscopy (sigmoidoscopy or colonoscopy) reveals numerous colonic/rectal polyps

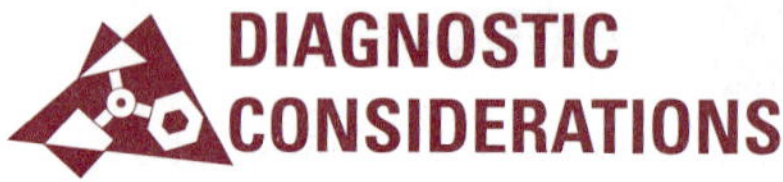

DIAGNOSTIC CONSIDERATIONS

- Sporadic polyps
- Sporadic colorectal adenocarcinoma

RULE OUT

- Colorectal adenocarcinoma

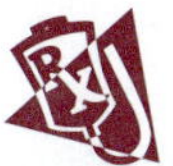

WORK-UP

- History and physical exam
- Flexible sigmoidoscopy/colonoscopy will need to be done from puberty until age 40 or 50 to be certain the family members do not have polyposis
- Upper endoscopy to look for gastroduodenal lesions

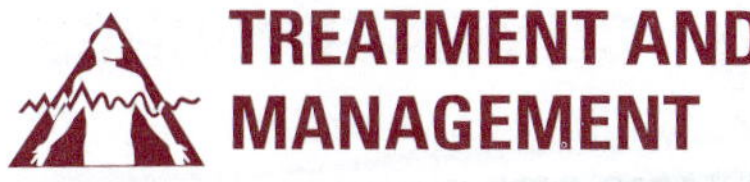

TREATMENT AND MANAGEMENT

SURGERY

- Once polyposis is diagnosed, colectomy should be done

Indications

- FAP: 100% penetrance develop colorectal carcinoma
- Abdominal colectomy ("subtotal colectomy") with ileorectal anastomosis: Leaves risk of rectal carcinoma
- Total colectomy and the ileoanal pouch procedure is preferred for most patients, especially if there are numerous adenomas in the rectum

MEDICATIONS

- Sulindac has been reported to induce regression of rectal polyps after ileorectal anastomosis

TREATMENT MONITORING

- When FAP is known in a family, the relatives at risk should undergo surveillance endoscopy annually beginning in their middle teens

COMPLICATIONS

- Recurrence, development of malignancy in unresected tissue (rectal)
- Extracolonic manifestations
- Increased risk of visceral malignancy
- Development of desmoid tumors in mesentery or abdominal wall

PROGNOSIS

- If the rectal mucosa is excised completely, the risk of subsequent rectal neoplasia is essentially nil
- Desmoid tumors grow slowly and capriciously, but they prove fatal in 10% of patients with FAP

PREVENTION

- Prophylactic colectomy does not alter the extracolonic manifestations

RESOURCES

REFERENCES

- Lal G, Gallinger S. Familial adenomatous polyposis. *Semin Surg Oncol.* 2000;18:314.
- Spagnesi MT et al. Rectal proliferation and polyp occurrence in patients with familial adenomatous polyposis after sulindac treatment. *Gastroenterology.* 1994;106:362.
- Calland JF et al. Genetic syndromes and genetic tests in colorectal cancer. *Semin Gastrointest Dis.* 2000;11:207.

Polyps, Colorectal

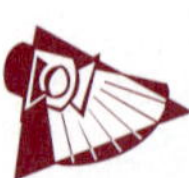

ESSENTIAL FEATURES

- Colorectal polyps are masses of tissue that project into the lumen
- Heterogeneous group of sessile or pedunculated; benign or malignant; mucosal, submucosal, or muscular lesions
- Types include:
  - Neoplastic (adenomas/carcinomas)
  - Hamartomas
  - Inflammatory
  - Hyperplastic
- Most adenomas are tubular, tubulovillous, or villous
- Hyperplastic polyps are diminutive lesions most often found in the left colon
- Hamartomas are uncommon (rarely malignant)
- Adenomas are a premalignant lesion
- Vast majority of adenocarcinomas of the large bowel in North America and Europe are believed to evolve from adenomas

EPIDEMIOLOGY

- Estimates of the incidence of colonic and rectal polyps in the general population range from 9% to 60%
- Polypoid adenomas are found in about 25% of asymptomatic adults who undergo screening colonoscopy
- Prevalence of adenomas is 30% at age 50 years, 40% at age 60, 50% at age 70, and 55% at age 80
- Mean age is 55 years
- 50% of polyps occur in the sigmoid or rectum
- 50% of patients with adenoma have more than 1 lesion, and 15% have more than 2 lesions
- Increased incidence of adenomas in breast cancer patients has been reported
- Inflammatory polyps have no malignant potential
- Cancer developing in association with hamartomas is rare
- 25% of patients who have 5 or more adenomatous polyps have a synchronous colon cancer at the initial colonoscopy

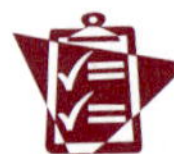

CLINICAL FINDINGS

SYMPTOMS AND SIGNS

- Most polyps are asymptomatic but the larger the lesion, the more likely it is to cause symptoms
- Rectal bleeding most common symptom
- Blood is bright red or dark red depending on the location of the polyp
- Bleeding is usually intermittent
- Altered bowel habits (constipation, increased frequency)
- Crampy abdominal pain
- Physical exam yields little information about the colonic polyps themselves
- Polyp may be palpable by digital rectal exam

LABORATORY FINDINGS

- Anemia may be present with rectal bleeding

IMAGING FINDINGS

- **Barium enema:** Rounded filling defect with smooth, sharply defined margins
- **Colonoscopy:** Most reliable means of diagnosis with biopsy; treatment with polypectomy

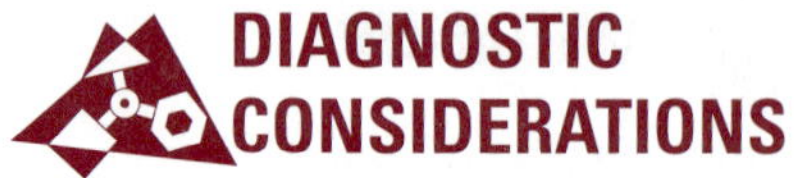

DIAGNOSTIC CONSIDERATIONS

- Malignant neoplasm
- Artifacts seen on barium enema (such as fecal matter, air bubbles, appendices epiploicae, lymph nodes) may be confused with polyps
- Diverticula

RULE OUT

- Malignant neoplasm

WORK-UP

- History and physical exam
- Digital rectal exam
- Proctoscopy
- Colonoscopy with biopsy/polypectomy
- Barium enema

WHEN TO ADMIT

- Bleeding or other complications such as perforation, severe abdominal pain, obstruction

TREATMENT AND MANAGEMENT

- Polyps of the colon and rectum are treated because they produce symptoms, because they may be malignant when first discovered, or because they may become malignant later
- Small polyps can be removed with an electrocautery snare

SURGERY

Indications

- Large, sessile, soft, velvety lesions in the rectum are usually villous adenomas; these tumors have high malignant potential and must be excised completely
- Open or laparoscopic-assisted colonic resection should be considered if colonoscopy is unsuccessful, if the lesion is large and sessile, or if there are many polyps
- Patients with hereditary nonpolyposis colon cancer (HNPCC) and others with multiple polyps may require total abdominal colectomy with ileorectal anastomosis
- Guidelines for resection include:
  - Gross margin is not clear at endoscopy
  - Microscopic margin is not clear
  - Cancer is not well-differentiated
  - There is lymphatic or venous invasion
  - Cancer does invade the stalk

TREATMENT MONITORING

- Repeat/surveillance endoscopy

COMPLICATIONS

- Bleeding
- Obstruction
- Progression to malignancy

PROGNOSIS

- Malignant potential of an adenoma depends on size, growth pattern, and the degree of epithelial atypia
- Cancer is found in 1% of adenomas under 1 cm in diameter, 10% of adenomas 1–2 cm in size, and up to 45% of adenomas > 2 cm
- Sessile adenomas only a few millimeters in diameter may become malignant
- 5% of tubular adenomas, 22% of tubulovillous adenomas, and 40% of villous adenomas become malignant
- Potential for cancerous transformation rises with increasing degrees of epithelial dysplasia
- Cumulative risk of eventual cancer at the polyp site was 2.5% at 5 years, 8% at 10 years, and 24% at 20 years
- Villous adenomas recur at the excision site in about 15% of cases after local removal
- Tubular adenomas seldom recur
- Risk of metachronous neoplasms following excision of a colorectal adenoma is greatest if there were multiple index lesions or if an adenoma was sessile, villous, or over 2 cm in diameter
- If the colon is cleared by total colonoscopy at the time of excision of the index polyp, follow-up colonoscopy at 3 years is just as effective as colonoscopy at 1 and 3 years in preventing development of ominous neoplasms

RESOURCES

REFERENCES

- Management of colonic polyps and adenomas. Patient Care Committee of the Society for Surgery of the Alimentary Tract (SSAT). *J Gastrointest Surg.* 1999;3:220.
- Macrae F. Wheat bran fiber and development of adenomatous polyps: evidence from randomized, controlled clinical trials. *Am J Med.* 1999;106(Supply 1A):38S.
- Lal G, Gallinger S. Familial adenomatous polyposis. *Semin Surg Oncol.* 2000;18:314.
- Bond JH. Polyp guideline: diagnosis, treatment and surveillance for patients with colorectal polyps. Practice Parameters Committee of the American College of Gastroenterology. *Am J Gastroenterol.* 2000;95:3053.

WEB SITES

- http://digestive.niddk.nih.gov/ddiseases/pubs/colonpolyps_ez/index.htm

Polyps, Gastric

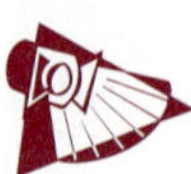

ESSENTIAL FEATURES

- Evidence of polyp in the stomach on upper GI endoscopy
- May be associated with gastric outlet obstruction if located in the distal stomach

EPIDEMIOLOGY

- **Hyperplastic polyps** (> 80%)
  - Represent overgrowth of normal epithelium
  - Not true neoplasms
  - No relationship to gastric cancer
- **Adenomatous polyps**
  - 30% contain a focus of adenocarcinoma
  - The incidence of cancer in an adenomatous polyp rises with increasing size; those with a stalk and those < 2 cm are usually not malignant
  - About 10% of benign adenomatous polyps undergo malignant change during prolonged follow-up
  - Adenocarcinoma found elsewhere in the stomach in 20% of patients with a benign adenomatous polyp
- Polyps located in distal stomach are more apt to cause symptoms
- Occur predominantly in the elderly

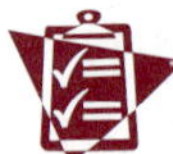

CLINICAL FINDINGS

SYMPTOMS AND SIGNS

- Most asymptomatic
- Vague epigastric discomfort
- Dyspepsia
- Occult GI bleeding
- Gastric outlet obstruction with nausea and vomiting if polyp is located in the distal stomach

LABORATORY FINDINGS

- Anemia may develop from chronic blood loss or deficient iron absorption
- Over 90% of patients are achlorhydric after maximal stimulation
- Vitamin B_{12} absorption is deficient in 25%, although megaloblastic anemia is present in only a few

IMAGING FINDINGS

- **Upper GI endoscopy:** Reveals presence of gastric polyp
- Gastric polyp may also be visible on upper GI contrast radiographic study
- In all cases, histologic diagnosis is required by endoscopy and polypectomy or biopsy

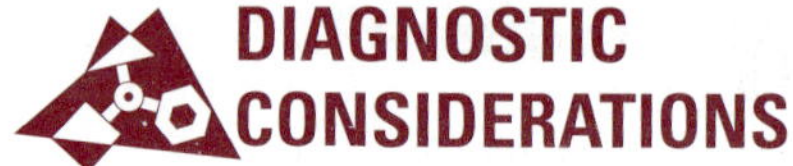

DIAGNOSTIC CONSIDERATIONS

- Most gastric polyps are discovered incidentally on upper GI radiographic or endoscopic studies

RULE OUT

- Gastric cancer

WORK-UP

- Upper GI endoscopy or contrast radiography will detect the lesion
- Endoscopy should be performed in all cases for histologic diagnosis and to exclude cancer
- Endoscopy may be diagnostic and therapeutic

WHEN TO ADMIT

- High-grade gastric outlet obstruction preventing adequate enteral nutrition
- Severe bleeding from polyp

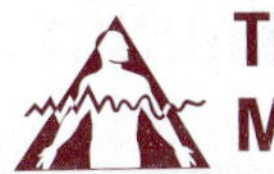

TREATMENT AND MANAGEMENT

SURGERY

- Endoscopic removal can be performed successfully in most cases
- Laparotomy and gastrotomy if endoscopy is unsuccessful

Indications

- Failure of endoscopic polypectomy
- Cancer found in polyp
- Gastrectomy may be required for multiple polyps

TREATMENT MONITORING

- Surveillance endoscopy for patients with gastric adenomas

COMPLICATIONS

- Occult GI bleeding
- Gastric outlet obstruction

PROGNOSIS

- Recurrent polyps are uncommon

RESOURCES

REFERENCES

- Abraham SC et al. Hyperplastic polyps of the stomach: associations with histologic patterns of gastritis and gastric atrophy. *Am J Surg Pathol.* 2001;25:500.

Popliteal Artery Diseases

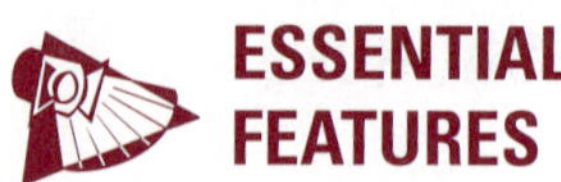

ESSENTIAL FEATURES

Popliteal Entrapment

- Rare cause of stenosis or occlusion
- Occurs because of anomalous course of popliteal artery
- Popliteal artery passes medial to medial head of gastrocnemius muscle (normally passes lateral)
  - Causes compression of popliteal artery when knee extended
- 5 anatomic variations
- Fibrous thickening progresses to occlusion, with poststenotic dilation which may be source for mural embolus

Cystic Degeneration of Popliteal Artery

- Arterial stenosis produced by mucoid cyst in adventitia
- Located in middle third of artery

EPIDEMIOLOGY

Popliteal Entrapment

- Occurs more often in young, healthy persons

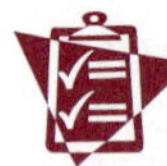

CLINICAL FINDINGS

SYMPTOMS AND SIGNS

Popliteal Entrapment

- Symptoms range from calf claudication to severe ischemia
- Diminished pedal pulses with foot dorsiflexion and plantar flexion
- Atherosclerotic changes absent

Cystic Degeneration of Popliteal Artery

- Calf claudication most common
- Decreased pedal pulse strength
- Mass may be palpated (rarely)

IMAGING FINDINGS

Popliteal Artery Entrapment

- MRI often useful to diagnose

Cystic Degeneration of Popliteal Artery

- **Arteriography:** Sharply localized zone of politeal stenosis with smooth concentric tapering, having hourglass appearance
- **US/CT scan:** Can demonstrate cyst in artery wall

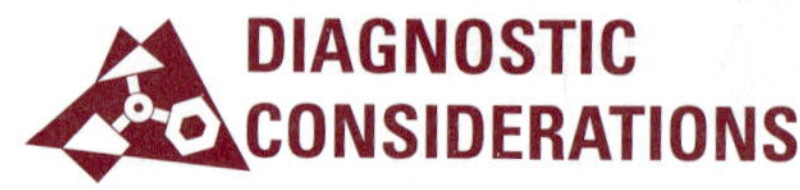

DIAGNOSTIC CONSIDERATIONS

- Atherosclerotic changes absent

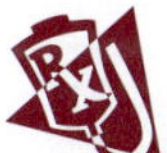

WORK-UP

- Complete history and physical exam
  - Consider diagnosis in young healthy patient with calf claudication or ischemia

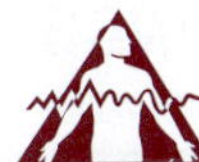

TREATMENT AND MANAGEMENT

SURGERY

Popliteal Entrapment

- Division of medial head of gastrocnemius muscle, graft replacement of diseased artery; lumbar sympathectomy performed as well

Cystic Degeneration of Popliteal Artery

- Cyst excision, may recur
- Arterial excision and graft replacement may be necessary in some patients

RESOURCES

REFERENCES

- Ring DH Jr et al. Popliteal artery entrapment syndrome: arteriographic findings and thrombolytic therapy. *J Vasc Interv Radiol.* 1999:10:713.
- O'Hara N et al. Surgical treatment for popliteal artery entrapment syndrome. *Cardiovasc Surg.* 2001;9:141.

Porphyria, Acute

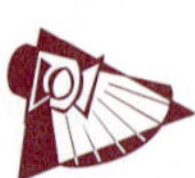

ESSENTIAL FEATURES

- Acute porphyrias are a group of inherited diseased that arise from errors in heme biosynthesis leading to overproduction of a porphyrin species
- Acute intermittent porphyria has the most serious consequences and is the form in which patients commonly manifest an acute abdomen
- Classic patient is a young women (teens to early 20s) with an unexplained abdominal crisis
- Abdominal symptoms are thought to be due to acute (abdominal visceral) autonomic dysfunction
- Acute peripheral or CNS dysfunction
- Recurrent psychiatric illnesses
- Hyponatremia
- Porphobilinogen in the urine during acute attacks

EPIDEMIOLOGY

- Acute intermittent porphyria is inherited in an autosomal dominant fashion, although the trait remains clinically silent in the majority of carriers
- Acquired forms of porphyria disorders may be caused by chemicals, drugs, or heavy metals such as lead
- Acute porphyria may be precipitated by starvation or certain drugs, classically the barbiturates, anticonvulsants, and sulfonamides

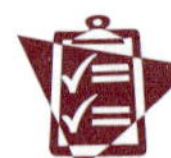

CLINICAL FINDINGS

SYMPTOMS AND SIGNS

- Absence of fever
- Intermittent abdominal pain of varying severity, from mild colic to an acute abdomen
- Central, peripheral, or autonomic neuropathy which can be profound including: respiratory paralysis, quadriplegia, or seizures
- Recurrent psychiatric illness

LABORATORY FINDINGS

- Absence of leukocytosis
- Often a profound hyponatremia secondary to syndrome of inappropriate antidiuretic hormone (SIADH)
- Increased amount of porphobilinogen in the urine (freshly voided specimen may turn dark when exposed to bright light and room air)

IMAGING FINDINGS

- No radiographic abnormalities

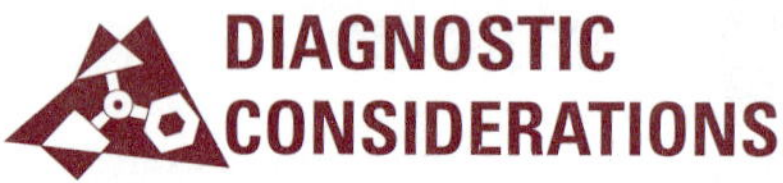

DIAGNOSTIC CONSIDERATIONS

- The differential diagnosis is that of an acute abdomen:
  - Appendicitis
  - Perforated gastroduodenal ulcers
  - Diverticulitis
  - Gangrenous cholecystitis
  - Acute salpingitis
  - Nonvascular small bowel perforation
  - Large bowel perforation
  - Mesenteric ischemia
  - Acute necrotizing pancreatitis
  - Bowel obstruction
  - Incarcerated hernia
  - Ureteral or renal colic
  - Others

RULE OUT

- Surgical abdomen

WORK-UP

- CBC count
- Basic chemistries
- Amylase and lipase
- UA
- Urine porphobilinogen
- Abdominal pelvic CT scan with IV and PO contrast helpful in ruling out surgical etiology

WHEN TO ADMIT

- Patients with an episode of acute intermittent porphyria should be admitted for supportive medical management until attack resolves

WHEN TO REFER

- Acute porphyria attacks are best managed by hematologists
- ICU care may be indicated based on severity of attack and associated neuropathy

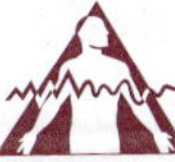

TREATMENT AND MANAGEMENT

- IV glucose (a minimum of 300 g carbohydrate per day)
- Hematin administration
- Analgesics
- Correction of hyponatremia
- Treatment as indicated for associated neuropathy

SURGERY

- Laparoscopy

Indications

- In confusing cases, a diagnostic laparoscopy may exclude an abdominal surgical catastrophe

MEDICATIONS

- Carbohydrates
- Hematin

COMPLICATIONS

- Most common complications are related to the associated neuropathy

PROGNOSIS

- 3-fold increase in mortality in patients recognized to have acute intermittent porphyria

PREVENTION

- Avoidance of drugs known to precipitate attacks, especially barbiturates and sulfonamides
- Avoidance of starvation
- High carbohydrate diet

RESOURCES

- Hambleton J, Toy P. Special Medical Problems in Surgical Patients. In: Way LW, Doherty GM (editors). *Current Surgical Diagnosis & Treatment,* 11e. New York: McGraw-Hill; 2003:53.

Portal Hypertension

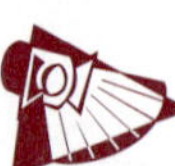

ESSENTIAL FEATURES

- Etiologies include:
  - Cirrhosis
  - Congenital hepatic fibrotic disorders
  - Acute liver failure
  - Budd-Chiari syndrome
  - Heart failure
  - Congenital atresia
  - Portal or splanchnic vein thrombosis
- Bleeding gastroesophageal varices most important complication
- 30% will bleed
- 50% mortality for those who bleed
- 30% re-bleed in 6 weeks
- 70% re-bleed in 1 year
- Bleeding most commonly from esophageal varices
- 10–15% have associated gastric varices
- Presence of varices related to degree of liver dysfunction
- Portal vein-hepatic vein gradient invariably > 12 mm Hg

EPIDEMIOLOGY

- Most patients with history of cirrhosis
- Presenting symptom of cirrhosis in many patients

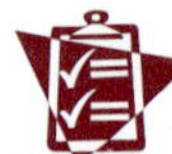

CLINICAL FINDINGS

SYMPTOMS AND SIGNS

- Hematemesis
- Melena
- Jaundice
- Encephalopathy
- Distended abdominal wall veins (caput medusa)
- Ascites
- Edema
- Shock
- Palmar erythema

LABORATORY FINDINGS

- Hyperbilirubinemia
- Elevated international normalized ratio (INR)
- Anemia
- Azotemia

IMAGING FINDINGS

- **CT scan:** Dilated venous collaterals, possible venous thrombosis (hepatic, portal, superior mesenteric vein, splenic, etc.)
- **US:** Dilated portal vein, possible thrombosis of portal vein or hepatic veins
- **Mesenteric venography:** Dilated collaterals, thrombi, or blush from bleeding
- **Hepato-portal venography:** Wedge pressure generally > 12 mm Hg in presence of varices
- Esophagogastroscopy for diagnosis of varices and possible sclerotherapy

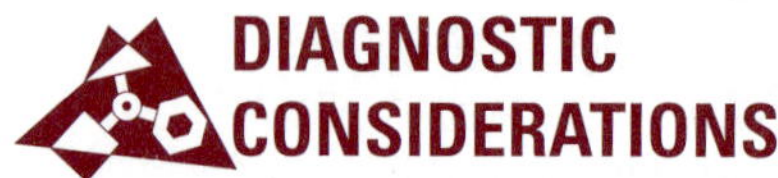

DIAGNOSTIC CONSIDERATIONS

- Presence of thrombi
- Childs classification or Model of End-Stage Liver Disease (MELD) to determine transjugular intrahepatic portosystemic shunt (TIPS) vs surgical shunt
- Mesenteric venography if diagnoses other than cirrhosis being considered (eg, Budd-Chiari syndrome or portal vein thrombosis)

RULE OUT

- Other sources of upper GI bleeding using esophagogastroscopy

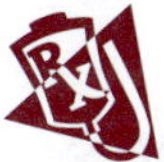

WORK-UP

- ABCs if patient has upper GI bleeding
- Assessment of MELD or Child class
- Assessment of underlying etiology
- Early gastroesophagoscopy for banding or sclerotherapy
- Octreotide to control bleeding
- Blood products as necessary
- Invasive monitoring as necessary
- Sengstaken-Blakemore tube if necessary
- Portal venography if diagnosis in doubt or patient is a candidate for surgical shunt

WHEN TO ADMIT

- All patients with bleeding varices

TREATMENT AND MANAGEMENT

- Sclerotherapy or banding of varices
- TIPS
- Sengstaken-Blakemore tube placement

SURGERY

- Liver transplantation
- Surgical portosystemic shunt (TIPS vs total vs partial vs selective)
- Gastric devascularization (Segura)

Indications

- **Liver transplantation:** Availability of donor, no medical comorbidities, not currently drinking alcohol
- **Surgical shunt:** Childs A failed endoscopic therapy elective (selective) or emergent (partial)
- **Gastric devascularization:** Gastric varices and failed endoscopic therapy

MEDICATIONS

- β-Blockers
- Nitrates
- Vasopressin (during bleeding)
- Octreotide (during bleeding)

TREATMENT MONITORING

- Repeat gastroesophagoscopy for suspicion of bleeding
- Duplex US for suspicion of shunt thrombosis

COMPLICATIONS

- Encephalopathy (for shunts)
- Hemorrhage
- Shunt thrombosis
- Of liver transplantation:
  - Primary nonfunction
  - Rejection
  - Biliary leak or stricture
  - Hemorrhage
  - Hepatic artery thrombosis

PROGNOSIS

- Survival related to MELD or Child class
- Variceal ligation or sclerotherapy 80% success rate; rebleed rate 70% at 1 year
- TIPS 90–100% success rate; 40–60% mortality at 6–7 weeks; 25% encephalopathy; thrombosis in 50%

RESOURCES

REFERENCES

- Krige JE, Beckingham IJ. ABC of diseases of liver, pancreas, and biliary system. Portal hypertension—1: varices. *BMJ.* 2001;322:348.
- Krige JE, Beckingham IJ. ABC of diseases of liver, pancreas, and biliary system: portal hypertension—2. Ascites, encephalopathy, and other conditions. *BMJ.* 2001;322:416.

Postsplenectomy Sepsis

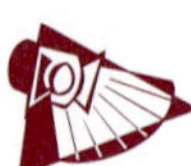

ESSENTIAL FEATURES

- Increased risk of bacteremia and sepsis following splenectomy because of failure to clear encapsulated bacteria
- Risk is greatest in children (especially in the first 2 years after surgery) and those undergoing splenectomy for hematologic disorders

EPIDEMIOLOGY

- Persons are more susceptible to fulminant bacteremia after splenectomy as a result of:
  - Decreased clearance of encapsulated bacteria from the blood
  - Decreased levels of IgM
  - Decreased opsonic activity
- The risk of fatal sepsis is lower when splenectomy performed for trauma than for hematologic disorders, probably due to autotransplantation
- There is a low risk of infection even in otherwise normal adults
- Most of these infections occur after the first year, and nearly 50% occur more than 5 years after splenectomy
- *S pneumoniae, H influenzae,* and meningococci are the most common pathogens

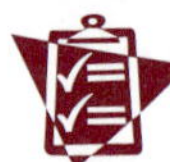

CLINICAL FINDINGS

SYMPTOMS AND SIGNS

- Mild, nonspecific symptoms are followed by high fever and shock from sepsis, which may rapidly lead to death

LABORATORY FINDINGS

- Leukocytosis

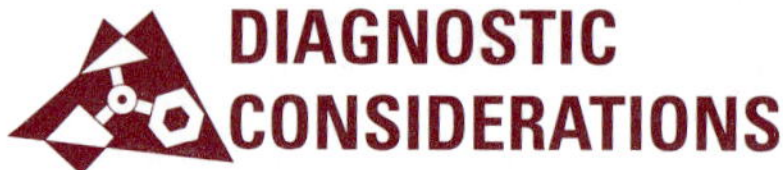

DIAGNOSTIC CONSIDERATIONS

- Awareness of this fatal complication has led to efforts to avoid splenectomy or to perform partial splenectomy or splenic repair for ruptured spleens to maintain adequate splenic function
- Splenic autotransplantation may also achieve partial restoration of splenic function after splenectomy

RULE OUT

- Other causes of sepsis

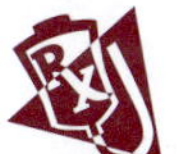

WORK-UP

- WBC count
- Blood cultures

WHEN TO ADMIT

- All confirmed or suspected cases

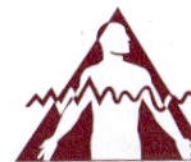

TREATMENT AND MANAGEMENT

- Antibiotics
- Splenectomy should be deferred until age 6 unless the hematologic problem is especially severe

SURGERY

Indications

- None

MEDICATIONS

- Antibiotics

COMPLICATIONS

- Disseminated intravascular coagulation

PROGNOSIS

- Improved with early recognition and aggressive treatment

PREVENTION

- Preoperative vaccination against *Pneumococcae* and *H influenzae* type b
- Prophylactic ampicillin (< age 6)

RESOURCES

REFERENCES

- Brigden ML et al. Prevention and management of overwhelming postsplenectomy infection—an update. *Crit Care Med.* 1999; 27:836.

Proctitis & Anusitis, Infectious

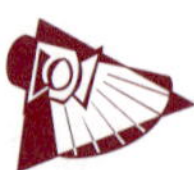

ESSENTIAL FEATURES

- Proctitis and anusitis are nonspecific terms for varying degrees of inflammation due to infectious or inflammatory diseases
- Causative agent or event determines the symptoms, signs, and appropriate management
- Attention should be paid to sexual practices and sexually transmitted diseases

Herpes Proctitis

- Lesions appear as vesicles, which rupture to form ulcers
- Ulcers that may become secondarily infected
- Commonly caused by herpes simplex virus type 2 (HSV-2)
- Transmitted by sexual contact

Anorectal Syphilis

- Chancre is an indurated, nontender perianal ulcer at the site of inoculation
- Proctitis, pseudotumors, and condylomata lata may also be present

Gonococcal Proctitis

- The gram-negative diplococcus *Neisseria gonorrhoeae* is the causative agent
- Commonly symptomatic in men, less often in women

Chlamydial Proctitis and Lymphogranuloma Venereum

- Causative agent is *Chlamydia trachomatis*

Chancroid: *Haemophilus ducreyi*

- Soft ulcer and local lymphadenitis

EPIDEMIOLOGY

Herpes Proctitis

- No history of anoreceptive intercourse is required because the disease may spread by extension from the vagina
- Number of HSV-2 infections rising

Anorectal Syphilis

- Transmitted from spirochete-containing lesions of skin or mucous membranes
- Marked increase in incidence of disease in homosexual men in recent years

Gonococcal Proctitis

- More common in women and homosexual men

Chlamydial Proctitis and Lymphogranuloma Venereum

- Spread by anal intercourse or direct extension through the lymphatics of the rectovaginal septum

Chancroid: *H ducreyi*

- Autoinoculation is common
- More common in tropical countries, rare in United States

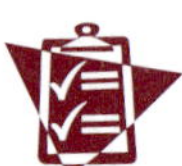

CLINICAL FINDINGS

SYMPTOMS AND SIGNS

Herpes Proctitis

- Patients may present early with anal pain and vesicles or later with ulcerations, discharge, rectal bleeding, tenesmus, and even fear of defecation because of severe pain
- Fever and generalized malaise
- Inguinal adenopathy

Anorectal Syphilis

- Patients present with chancre, a nontender ulcer at the site of inoculation and proctitis

Gonococcal Proctitis

- Symptoms range from none to painful defecation
- Rectal bleeding and discharge, perianal excoriation, and fistulas may develop
- Mucosa may appear friable and edematous

Chlamydial Proctitis and Lymphogranuloma Venereum

- Symptoms of chlamydial proctitis range from none to rectal pain, bleeding, and discharge
- Small shallow ulcer
- Inguinal adenopathy may be quite marked
- Late findings include hemorrhagic proctitis and rectal stricture

Chancroid: *H ducreyi*

- Soft perianal ulcer that is painful, often multiple, and bleeds easily
- Inguinal lymph nodes become fluctuant, rupture, and drain
- Associated painful penile lesions

LABORATORY FINDINGS

Herpes Proctitis

- Viral culture of the vesicle or biopsy of the ulcer is diagnostic
- Diagnosis from skin lesion can be made using Tzanck smear
- Multinucleated giant cells suggest herpesvirus infection

Anorectal Syphilis

- Darkfield microscopy of exudate and serologic testing are the preferred methods of diagnosis
- Serologic tests (VDRL and rapid plasmin reagin [RPR]) may initially be negative and should be repeated several months later
- Specific treponemal antigen tests (FTA-ABS)

Gonococcal Proctitis

- Culture on Thayer-Martin medium reveals gram-negative diplococci
- ELISA and DNA probe assays are available

Chlamydial Proctitis and Lymphogranuloma Venereum

- The diagnosis is made with the LGV complement fixation test; tissue cultures are also used
- *Chlamydiae* form cytoplasmic inclusions seen in Giemsa stain and immunofluorescence

Chancroid: *H ducreyi*

- Culture on heated blood agar supplemented with factor X is diagnostic

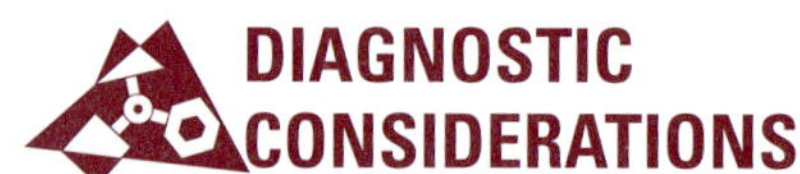

- Concomitant/multiple concurrent infections

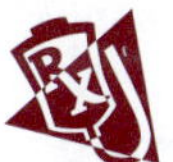

WORK-UP

- History and physical exam
  - Particular attention should be paid to sexual practices and sexually transmitted diseases
- Cultures of the anus, vagina, urethra, and pharynx should be obtained

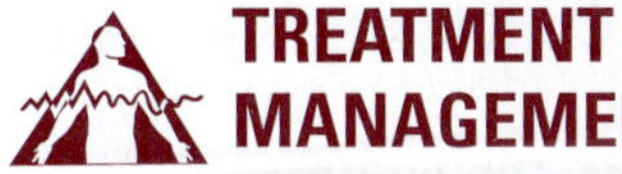

TREATMENT AND MANAGEMENT

Herpes Proctitis

- Oral acyclovir is the treatment of choice but is not curative

Anorectal Syphilis

- Penicillin is the treatment of choice (tetracycline or erthyromycin are alternatives)

Gonococcal Proctitis

- Intramuscular procaine penicillin G and oral probenecid; resistant strains should be treated with spectinomycin

Chlamydial Proctitis and Lymphogranuloma Venereum

- Treatment with 21 days of tetracycline is recommended, but erythromycin is an acceptable alternative

Chancroid: *H ducreyi*

- Azithromycin, erythromycin, ciprofloxacin, or ceftriaxone

SURGERY

Indications

- Strictures may require dilation
- Although uncommon, strictures may cause bowel obstruction and require colostomy

TREATMENT MONITORING

- Follow-up exam and cultures should be performed to confirm adequate therapy

COMPLICATIONS

Anorectal Syphilis

- Progression to tertiary syphilis with nervous system and cardiovascular organ involvement

Chlamydial Proctitis and Lymphogranuloma Venereum

- May progress to urethritis, cervicitis, salpingitis, pelvic inflammatory disease (PID)

Gonococcal Proctitis

- Ascending infection, urethritis, PID, cervicitis, septic arthritis

PROGNOSIS

Herpes Proctitis

- No drug treatment prevents recurrences

Anorectal Syphilis

- Good

Gonococcal Proctitis

- Excellent

PREVENTION

- Contacts must be sought, tested, and treated
- Avoidance of contact with lesions and ulcers

RESOURCES

REFERENCES

- Rompalo AM. Diagnosis and treatment of sexually acquired proctitis and proctocolitis: an update. *Clin Infect Dis.* 1999;28(Suppl 1):S84.
- Tabet SR et al. Incidence of HIV and sexually transmitted diseases (STD) in a cohort of HIV-negative men who have sex with men (MSM). *AIDS.* 1998;12:2041.

Proctitis, Inflammatory & Radiation

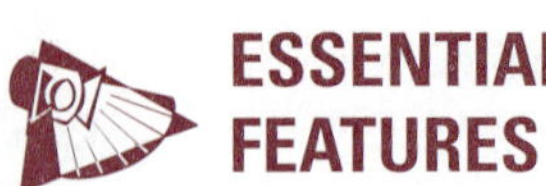

ESSENTIAL FEATURES

Inflammatory Proctitis

- A mild form of ulcerative colitis that is limited to the rectum
- The disease course is often self-limited

Radiation Proctitis

- Occurs in a patient with a history of radiation to the rectum
- Disease may develop months to years after the injury

EPIDEMIOLOGY

Inflammatory Proctitis

- Colonic manifestations of ulcerative colitis develop in 10% of patients

Radiation Proctitis

- Follows radiation injury

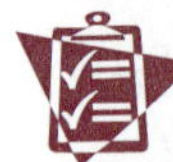

CLINICAL FINDINGS

SYMPTOMS AND SIGNS

Inflammatory Proctitis

- Rectal bleeding, discharge, diarrhea, and tenesmus

Radiation Proctitis

- Diarrhea, rectal bleeding, discharge, tenesmus, pain, and incontinence
- Symptoms of late disease are secondary to strictures, fistulas, and telangiectasias
- Patients with late disease present with the following:
  - Recurrent urinary tract infections
  - Vaginal discharge
  - Fecal incontinence
  - Rectal bleeding
  - Changes in stool caliber
  - Constipation

IMAGING FINDINGS

Inflammatory Proctitis

- **Sigmoidoscopy:** Rectal mucosa is inflamed and friable, but the remainder of the colon appears normal on exam

Radiation Proctitis

- Endoscopy may reveal friable edematous mucosa, telangiectasias, or strictures and may show internal openings of fistulas

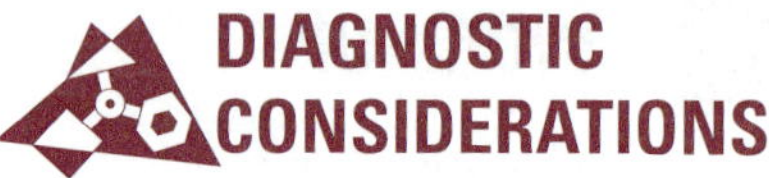

DIAGNOSTIC CONSIDERATIONS

- Infectious proctitis
- Crohn disease
- Malignancy

RULE OUT

- An infectious process must be ruled out before initiating corticosteroid therapy
- Malignancy

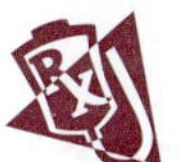

WORK-UP

- History and physical exam
- Sigmoidoscopy/colonoscopy
- Biopsies are taken at endoscopy to rule out infectious processes and Crohn disease

WHEN TO ADMIT

- Severe bleeding
- Bowel obstruction
- Bowel perforation

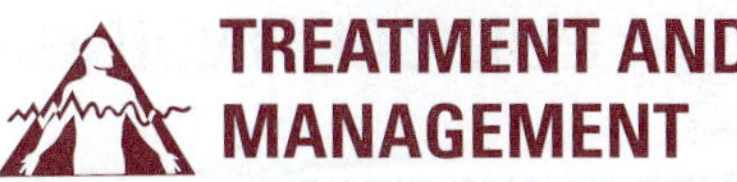

TREATMENT AND MANAGEMENT

Inflammatory Proctitis

- Corticosteroid retention enemas are given for 2 weeks
- If there is no response, a short course of oral corticosteroids may be given
- Mesalamine (5-aminosalicylic acid) may be given orally or rectally in an enema or suppository

Radiation Proctitis

- Initial therapy includes bulk-forming agents, antidiarrheals, and antispasmodics
- Topical corticosteroids, mesalamine preparations, misoprostol suppositories, and short-chain fatty acids have all been used

SURGERY

Indications

- **Radiation proctitis**
  - Treat late complications of radiation injury: Dilatation of strictures and laser coagulation of telangiectasias
  - Surgical success in treating fistulas to the bladder or vagina is interposition or transposition of healthy nonirradiated tissue into the field
  - Infrequently is the rectum so badly damaged that it must be removed

MEDICATIONS

- Corticosteroid enema
- Oral steroids
- Mesalamine, oral or rectal

TREATMENT MONITORING

- Lack of response to appropriate therapy calls for reassessment of the patient

COMPLICATIONS

- Obstruction
- Perforation
- Hemorrhage
- Colonic involvement in inflammatory proctitis
- Fistula
- Stricture

PROGNOSIS

- The disease usually responds to conservative measures and resolves rapidly
- Good for radiation proctitis

RESOURCES

REFERENCES

- Babb RR. Radiation proctitis: a review. *Am J Gastroenterol.* 1996;91:1309.
- Fantin AC et al. Argon beam coagulation for treatment of symptomatic radiation-induced proctitis. *Gastrointest Endosc.* 1999;49(4 Part 1):515.
- Taylor JG et al. KTP laser therapy for bleeding from chronic radiation proctopathy. *Gastrointest Endosc.* 2000;52:353.

Pruritus Ani

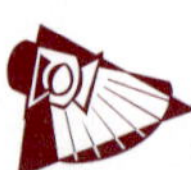

ESSENTIAL FEATURES

- Severe perianal itching, often at night
- When chronic, skin becomes white, leathery, and thickened
- Usually idiopathic
- Most patients have tried many over-the-counter preparations without relief
- Agents may exacerbate the problem by keeping the perineum moist, causing further irritation, or by creating a contact dermatitis
- Poor cleansing of the perineum may lead to irritation
- Frequent washing with soaps and detergents dries the skin, also leading to pruritus
- Pinworms *(Enterobius vermicularis)* are the most common cause of perianal itching in children
- Pruritus may result from tight clothing, obesity, and living in a hot climate
- When a specific cause cannot be found, it is considered idiopathic

EPIDEMIOLOGY

- Pinworms *(E vermicularis)* are the most common cause of perianal itching in children under 12 years of age
- Enterobius (pinworm) is an intestinal roundworm (nematode) transmitted by ingestion of eggs
- Adult male and female worms live in the colon
  - At night the female migrates from the anus and releases thousands of fertilized eggs on the perianal skin
  - Eggs develop into larvae and become infectious
- Reinfection occurs if eggs are carried into the mouth after scratching the perianal skin

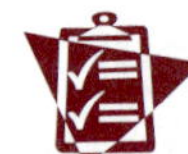

CLINICAL FINDINGS

SYMPTOMS AND SIGNS

- Severe perianal itching, often worse at night
- Skin is thickened, white, and leathery in the chronic state
- Skin is normal to weeping in the acute stage
- In children with pinworms, perianal itching is most severe at night when the pinworm deposits its eggs on the perianal skin

LABORATORY FINDINGS

- Scotch tape test: Diagnosis of pinworms is made by applying cellophane tape to the perianal skin, which collects the eggs
- Scrapings of the perianal skin viewed microscopically may reveal fungi or parasites

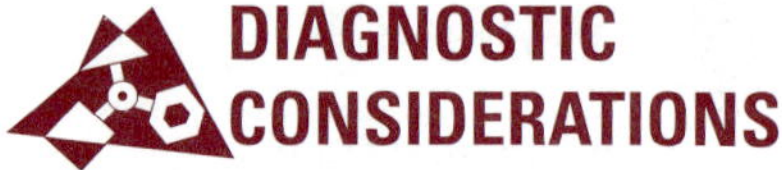

DIAGNOSTIC CONSIDERATIONS

- Associated with other perianal lesions that distort normal anal anatomy such as hemorrhoids, fistulas, fissures, tumors of the anorectum, previous surgery, and radiation therapy
- Primary dermatologic diseases:
  - Lichen planus
  - Atopic eczema
  - Psoriasis
  - Seborrheic dermatitis
- Infectious etiology:
  - Fungal (dermatophytosis, candidiasis)
  - Parasitic (*E vermicularis,* scabies, or pediculosis)
  - Bacterial superinfection
- Contact dermatitis from local anesthetic creams or soaps
- Systemic diseases (diabetes, liver disease)
- Perianal neoplasms (Bowen disease and extramammary Paget disease)

RULE OUT

- Perianal neoplasms (Bowen disease and extramammary Paget disease)

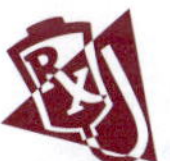

WORK-UP

- History and physical exam
- Biopsy and histologic evaluation may be necessary in refractory cases to rule out underlying malignancy
- Scotch tape test

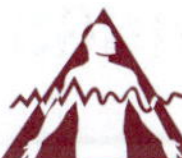

TREATMENT AND MANAGEMENT

- Treat identifiable causes of pruritus ani (infection, hemorrhoids, contact dermatitis)
- Patients should be educated about proper perineal care, and the use of soaps and topical ointments should be discouraged
- The perineum should be kept dry
- Alteration in dietary habits may be necessary
  - Coffee, tea, cola drinks, beer, chocolate, and tomatoes can cause perianal itching and should be excluded from the diet for at least 2 weeks

SURGERY

MEDICATIONS

- For *Enterobius* infection: Mebendazole or pyrantel pamoate

COMPLICATIONS

- Severe excoriation
- Ulceration
- Secondary infection of the perineum

PROGNOSIS

- Symptoms should resolve with alterations in dietary and cleaning habits
- Relapse is common, and reeducation is often effective

PREVENTION

- Keep perineum dry
- Strict perineal hygiene

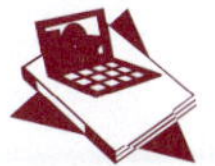

RESOURCES

REFERENCES

- Welton ML. Anorectum. In: Way LW, Doherty GM (editors). *Current Surgical Diagnosis & Treatment,* 11e. New York: McGraw-Hill; 2003:775–776.

Pulmonary Atresia

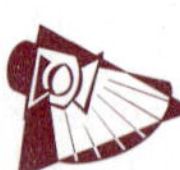

ESSENTIAL FEATURES

- A congenital heart lesion that decreases pulmonary arterial blood flow resulting in a right-to-left shunt
- Cyanosis and decreased oxygen delivery causes compensatory polycythemia (Hct > 70%) and spontaneous thrombosis
- Exercise, acidosis, pain worsens cyanosis, can cause hypoxic spells
- Squatting increases systemic resistance, causing increased pulmonary flow and oxygen
- β-Blockers (decreases spasm), fluid intake, HCO_3 administration, norepinephrine (increases systemic resistance) may help decrease hypoxia
- Clubbing due to proliferation of capillaries and AV fistulas in extremities
- Bronchial and mediastinal arteries enlarge
- Ductus arteriosus maintains flow to lungs during fetal development
- Alprostadil early can allow time for optimization before definitive treatment
- Operative options to increase pulmonary flow:
  - **Blalock-Taussig shunt:** Subclavian artery to ipsilateral pulmonary artery (PA) end to side fashion
  - Modified Blalock-Taussig shunt: Subclavian to PA using PTFE
  - **Glenn:** Superior vena cava (SVC) to PA shunt
  - **Fontan:** SVC and inferior vena cava (IVC) rerouted to PA
  - Excision of obstructive muscle, patch enlargement of infundibulum, and valve replacement
- Pulmonary valve replaced by diaphragm of tissue, causing obstruction
- PA normal size
- Atrial septal defect (ASD) or patent ductus arteriosus (PDA) necessary for survival after first few hours of birth
- RV and tricuspid annulus typically small
- RV: Coronary artery fistulas and coronary artery stenoses are common
- Some coronary flow dependent on increased pressures in RV

CLINICAL FINDINGS

SYMPTOMS AND SIGNS

- Cyanosis present at birth
- Duct closure: Profound hypoxia, acidosis

LABORATORY FINDINGS

- ECG: Lack of normal RV dominance

IMAGING FINDINGS

- **Chest film:** Diminished flow into lungs
- **Echocardiography:** Diagnostic
- **Catheterization:** Define coronary anatomy, RV-dependent coronary circulation

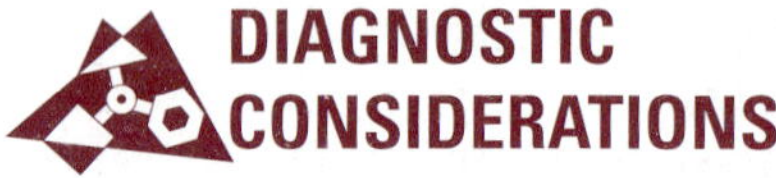

DIAGNOSTIC CONSIDERATIONS

- Echocardiography, catheterization needed

WORK-UP

- Chest film
- ECG
- Echocardiography
- Catheterization

TREATMENT AND MANAGEMENT

- ASD creation or ductus maintenance (alprostadil) necessary for early survival
- Surgical treatment depends on RV development and right heart dependent coronary circulation
- Systemic-PA shunt + patch reconstruction of right heart outlow tract (not performed if poor RV development or right-dependent coronary circulation)
- With further ventricle development, may close shunt and ASD
- If ventricles do not develop, consider Fontan

SURGERY

Indications

- Indicated if diagnosed

PROGNOSIS

- 1-year mortality, 10–20%
- Prognosis improving

RESOURCES

REFERENCES

- Jahangiri M et al. Improved results with selective management in pulmonary atresia with intact ventricular septum. *J Thorac Cardiovasc Surg.* 1999;118:1046.
- Rychik J et al. Outcome after operations for pulmonary atresia with intact ventricular septum. *J Thorac Cardiovasc Surg.* 1998;116:924.

Pulmonary Contusion

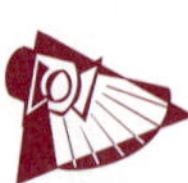

ESSENTIAL FEATURES

- Pulmonary contusion is due to sudden parenchymal concussion and occurs after blunt trauma or wounding with a high-velocity missile
- Most lung lacerations are caused by penetrating injuries and hemopneumothorax is usually present
- Lung hematomas are the result of local parenchymal destruction and hemorrhage

EPIDEMIOLOGY

- Pulmonary contusion occurs in 75% of patients with flail chest but can occur without associated rib fracture
- 35% of patients with pulmonary contusion have an associated myocardial contusion

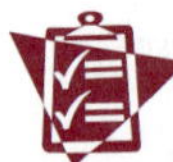

CLINICAL FINDINGS

SYMPTOMS AND SIGNS

- Pulmonary contusion: Thin, blood-tinged secretions, chest pain, restlessness, apprehensiveness, and labored respirations
- Eventually, dyspnea, cyanosis, tachypnea, and tachycardia develop

LABORATORY FINDINGS

- Hypoxemia

IMAGING FINDINGS

- Chest film findings of pulmonary contusion include patchy parenchymal opacification or diffuse linear peribronchial densities; overlying evidence of chest trauma including skeletal injuries
- Lung hematoma: Initially a poorly defined density that becomes more circumscribed a few days to 2 weeks after injury

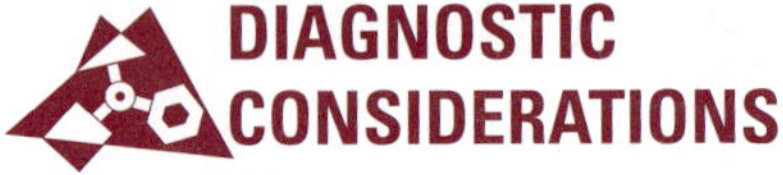

DIAGNOSTIC CONSIDERATIONS

- Treatment of pulmonary contusion is often delayed because clinical and radiologic findings may not appear for 12–48 hours after injury
- Associated abdominal injuries may dictate course of care

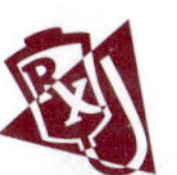

WORK-UP

- Physical exam
- Chest film
- ABG measurements

TREATMENT AND MANAGEMENT

- Initial resuscitation and stabilization
- Pulmonary contusion: Supplemental oxygen, intubation and mechanical ventilation, avoid excessive hydration
- Pulmonary laceration: Tube thoracostomy; most do not need surgery
- Pulmonary hematoma: Expectant management is usually adequate
- Supplemental oxygen
- Intubation and mechanical ventilation if necessary for ventilatory support
- Fluid resuscitation
- Chest wall splinting
- Analgesia

TREATMENT MONITORING

- Serial ABG measurements
- Serial chest films

COMPLICATIONS

- Pneumonia
- Acute respiratory distress syndrome

PROGNOSIS

- Pulmonary contusion has 15% overall mortality

RESOURCES

REFERENCES

- Brasel KJ et al. Treatment of occult pneumothoraces from blunt trauma. *J Trauma.* 1999;46:987.
- Cohn SM. Pulmonary contusion: review of a clinical entity. *J Trauma.* 1997;42:973.

Pulmonary Edema, Cardiogenic

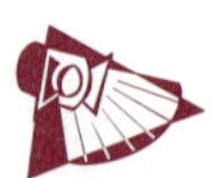

ESSENTIAL FEATURES

- Hypoxemia
- Rales

EPIDEMIOLOGY

- Post–myocardial infarction patients can present with pulmonary edema
- Surgical stress or fluid shifts in patients with underlying coronary artery disease
- Fluid overload

CLINICAL FINDINGS

SYMPTOMS AND SIGNS

- Hypoxemia
- Shortness of breath
- Rales
- Presence of third heart sound

LABORATORY FINDINGS

- Elevated pulmonary arterial wedge pressures on pulmonary artery catheterization

IMAGING FINDINGS

- **Chest film**
  - Cephalization of blood flow
  - Kerley B lines
  - Perihilar infiltrates

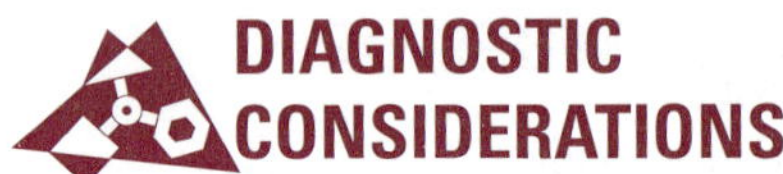

DIAGNOSTIC CONSIDERATIONS

- Diagnosis often requires the combination of physical exam and invasive monitoring findings
- Causes can include arrhythmia or muscle failure as the underlying cause of the cardiac dysfunction

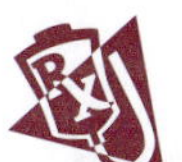

WORK-UP

- Physical exam
- ABG measurements
- Chest film

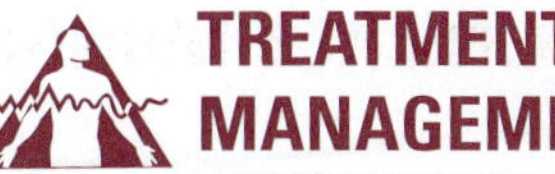

TREATMENT AND MANAGEMENT

- Minimize fluid intake
- Minimize salt intake
- Diuresis
- Supplemental oxygen
- Intubation and mechanical ventilation

MEDICATIONS

- Diuretics
- Inotropes (rarely indicated)

TREATMENT MONITORING

- Fluid balance
- Serial ABG measurements
- Symptomatic improvement
- Monitor pulmonary capillary wedge pressure (PCWP)
- Serial chest films

COMPLICATIONS

- Pneumonia

PROGNOSIS

- Determined by etiology of cardiac insufficiency

PREVENTION

- Careful attention to fluid balance

RESOURCES

REFERENCES

- Chang MC et al. Redefining cardiovascular performance during resuscitation: ventricular stroke work, power, and the pressure-volume diagram. *J Trauma.* 1998;45:470.

Pulmonary Edema, Neurogenic

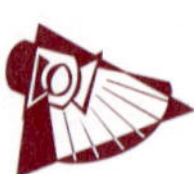

ESSENTIAL FEATURES

- Head injury
- Increased intracranial pressure
- Caused by pooling of blood in denervated autonomic venules and small veins
- Usually due to spinal cord injury
- Not caused by isolated head injury

EPIDEMIOLOGY

- Post-traumatic

CLINICAL FINDINGS

SYMPTOMS AND SIGNS

- Hypotension after trauma
- Warm extremities—sometimes with hyperemia
- No other evident causes of shock, such as hypovolemic or cardiogenic

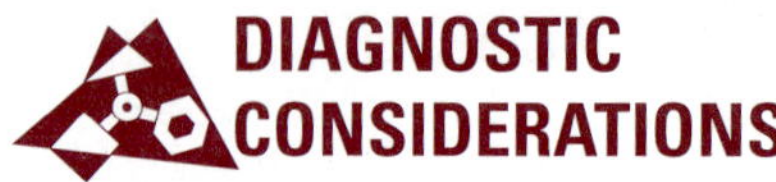

DIAGNOSTIC CONSIDERATIONS

- Hypovolemic shock
- Cardiogenic shock
- Septic shock

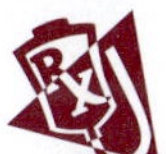

WORK-UP

- Therapeutic test: Trendelenburg followed by 2 L IV fluid bolus
- If shock persists, consider phenylephrine infusion and other causes
- Radiographic evaluation of spinal column

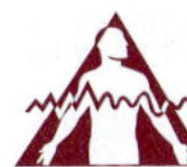

TREATMENT AND MANAGEMENT

- Supportive care of blood pressure to maintain perfusion
- Stabilize and protect spine from further injury

RESOURCES

REFERENCES

- Irish JC et al. Penetrating and blunt neck trauma: 10-year review of a Canadian experience. *Can J Surg.* 1997;40:33.

Pulmonary Stenosis, Congenital

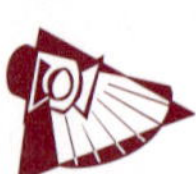

ESSENTIAL FEATURES

- An obstructive congenital heart lesion
- Pulmonary stenosis (PS) impedes forward blood flow and increases ventricular afterload
- Without ventricular septal defect (VSD), obstructive lesion causes hypertrophy of corresponding ventricle
- Ventricular hypertrophy can cause dysrhythmias, ischemia, and fibrosis
- In most, commissures are fused causing a dome like structure
- Most patients have patent foramen ovale
- Few patients have atrial septal defect (ASD)
- May be associated with poorly developed right ventricle, may require urgent intervention
- Isolated infundibular stenosis (below pulmonary valve) is extremely rare and often less severe

EPIDEMIOLOGY

- 5–8% of cardiac anomalies: PS with intact ventricular septum and normal aortic root
- 50% of deaths from PS occur in infants

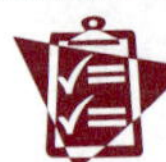

CLINICAL FINDINGS

SYMPTOMS AND SIGNS

- Poor feeding, hypoxic spells
- Occasionally sudden death
- Older children may be asymptomatic
- Fatigue, dyspnea on exertion, dizziness, angina
- Murmur easily detected

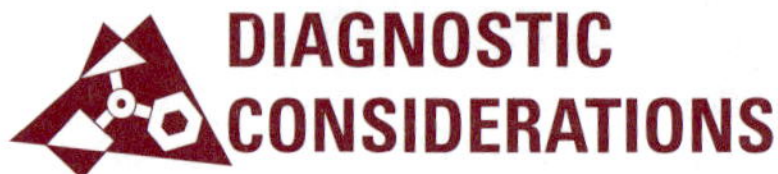

DIAGNOSTIC CONSIDERATIONS

- Evaluate for other cardiac or extracardiac anomalies

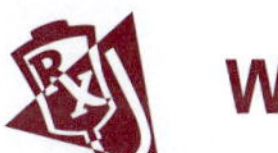

WORK-UP

- Physical exam
- Echocardiography

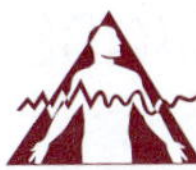

TREATMENT AND MANAGEMENT

- Neonates: PGE_1 (alprostadil) maintain patent ductus arteriosus until pulmonary valve obstruction relieved

SURGERY

- Isolated pulmonary stenosis: Catheter balloon dilation > 90% successful
- Surgical valvotomy (may need transannular patch, or systemic to pulmonary shunt) if catheter intervention unsuccessful

Indications

- Pulmonary valve gradient > 50 mm Hg
- Severe RV failure
- Cyanotic spells
- Systemic RV pressure

PROGNOSIS

- > 90% respond well to catheter or surgical therapy
- **Critical PS:** Mortality is 3–10% after treatment
- Restenosis 10–25%
- RV hypertrophy: Regresses after stenosis relieved

RESOURCES

REFERENCES

- Hanley FL et al. Outcomes in critically ill neonates with pulmonary stenosis and intact ventricular septum: a multiinstitutional study. Congenital Heart Surgeons Society. *J Am Coll Cardiol.* 1993;22:183.

Pulmonary Thromboembolism

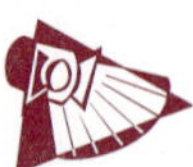

ESSENTIAL FEATURES

- Deep venous thrombosis (DVT) most common source of pulmonary embolism (PE)
- Uncommon causes of embolism include:
  - Air (complications from central lines)
  - Fat (long bone fractures, respiratory insufficiency, coagulopathy, encephalopathy, petechiae)
  - Amniotic (during active labor)
  - Tumor emboli from RA or inferior vena cava (IVC)
- < 10% of PE cause pulmonary infarction
- Size and frequency of PE determines disease and outcome
- PE obstructing large pulmonary artery: RV failure
- PE causes release of vasoactive amines causing severe pulmonary vasoconstriction, increased dead space and hypoxia from right-to-left shunt
- Reflex bronchial vasoconstriction common

EPIDEMIOLOGY

- 50,000 deaths yearly in United States
- Third leading cause of death in hospital patients
- Only 30–40% have suspected DVT
- PE develops in 60% of untreated proximal lower extremity DVT

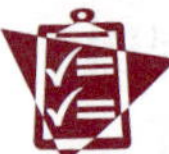

CLINICAL FINDINGS

SYMPTOMS AND SIGNS

- Dyspnea and chest pain (present in 75%)
- Tachycardia, tachypnea, altered mental status
- Classic triad: Dyspnea, chest pain, hemoptysis (15%)
- Pleural rub and S1Q3T3 rarely found

LABORATORY FINDINGS

- **ABG measurement:** Hypoxia with respiratory alkalosis
- **ECG:** New onset atrial fibrillation, ST/T wave changes, sinus tachycardia
- Elevated D-dimer levels

IMAGING FINDINGS

- **Chest film:** Often normal, may show pulmonary cap
- **ECG:** May show atrial fibrillation, ischemic changes, or RV strain (S1Q3T3), but usually only sinus tachycardia.
- **$\dot{V}/\dot{Q}$scan:** Sensitivity & specificity of 90%, however, 67% of studies are inconclusive
- **Spiral CT:** More accurate than $\dot{V}/\dot{Q}$scan
- **Magnetic resonance angiography:** Excellent sensitivity and specificity
- **Pulmonary angiogram:** Invasive but gold standard

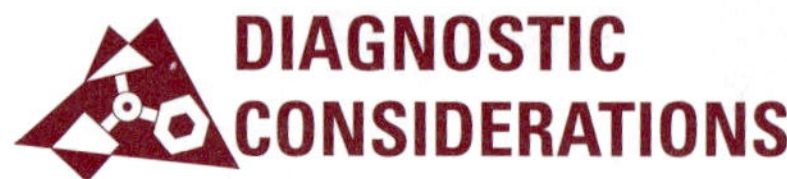

DIAGNOSTIC CONSIDERATIONS

- Evaluate for other causes of chest pain and hypoxia, such as pneumonia
- Evaluation may be clouded by other possibilities including postoperative pneumonia, which can make $\dot{V}/\dot{Q}$ scan nondiagnostic
- Spiral CT of chest most sensitive and efficient in postoperative patient

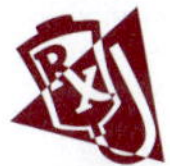

WORK-UP

- ABG measurement
- Chest film
- Duplex Doppler of lower extremity
- $\dot{V}/\dot{Q}$ scan (often inconclusive), cannot be interpreted in face of abnormal chest film
- Spiral CT of chest accuracy better than $\dot{V}/\dot{Q}$ and does not need clinical correlation
- Magnetic resonance pulmonary angiogram
- Pulmonary angiogram gold standard
  - Used less often now that CT is sensitive

TREATMENT AND MANAGEMENT

- Initial stabilization with pressors and ventilatory support
- Start heparin/low-molecular-weight heparin expediently
- Consider thrombolytics if large clot burden, sever respiratory compromise, hemodynamic instability

SURGERY

- IVC filter
- Open surgical thrombectomy: High mortality (Trendelenburg procedure)
- Catheter-based suction embolectomy: only in experienced operators
- Extracorporeal membrane oxygenation (ECMO) can be a last resort in a critical situation

Indications

- IVC filter
  - Contraindication to anticoagulation
  - Venous thrombosis extension on anticoagulation
- Open pulmonary embolectomy
  - Intractable hemodynamic instability
  - Thrombolytics inadequate or not available
  - Rarely indicated or useful

PROGNOSIS

- Preventable cause of hospital death

PREVENTION

- DVT prophylaxis in perioperative period

RESOURCES

REFERENCES

- Cross JJ et al. A randomized trial of spiral CT and ventilation perfusion scintigraphy for the diagnosis of pulmonary embolism. *Clin Radiol.* 1998;53:177.
- Hull RD. Low-molecular-weight heparin vs. heparin in the treatment of patients with pulmonary embolism: American-Canadian Thrombosis Study Group. *Arch Intern Med.* 2000;160:229.

Pulmonary Venous Connection, Total Anomalous

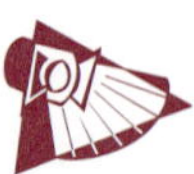

ESSENTIAL FEATURES

- A congenital heart lesion that increases pulmonary arterial blood flow
- Results in left-to-right shunt, results in lung infection, pulmonary vascular congestion, pulmonary artery (PA) hypertension, right heart failure, pulmonary vasoconstriction, pulmonary vascular obstructive disease
- **Eisenmenger syndrome:** Increased pulmonary hypertension such that left-to-right shunt ceases and shunt becomes right-to-left, requiring heart-lung transplant
- Inhaled nitric oxide, oxygen, or IV tolazoline reverses PA vasoconstriction
- PA band is palliative and can reduce PA flow to alleviate RV failure and progression of pulmonary hypertension
- Pulmonary veins do not make direct connection with LA, instead confluence connects to central systemic veins, draining into RA
- Blood gets to LA atrium via atrial septal defect (ASD) or patent ductus arteriosus (PDA)
- Similar oxygen saturation in PA and aorta
- 3 types (depends on site of connection):
  - **Type I, Supracardiac:** Left-sided vertical vein drains into innominate vein (45%)
  - **Type II, cardiac:** Connection to RA or coronary sinus (25%)
  - **Type III, infracardiac:** Connection to infradiaphgragmatic inferior vena cava (IVC) or portal vein (25%) 5% have mixed venous drainage
- Pulmonary venous obstruction occurs in nearly all with infracardiac connection, < 25% with supracardiac connection
- Obstruction leads to increased pulmonary vascular resistance
- Associated anomalies rare

CLINICAL FINDINGS

SYMPTOMS AND SIGNS

- **No obstruction:** Symptoms relate to pulmonary overcirculation and hypertension (poor feeding, failure to thrive, tachypnea, diaphoresis)
- **Obstruction:** Profound cyanosis, respiratory failure, hypotension within first few hours of life
- **Infants:** Severe heart failure, cyanosis poor pulses, acidosis
- Pulmonary midsystolic murmur, some with fixed split, loud S_2
- Oxygen saturation similar in aorta and PA
- PA and wedge pressures elevated
- Degree of obstruction determines clinical presentation
- Enlarged RA and RV with severe pulmonary vascular congestion

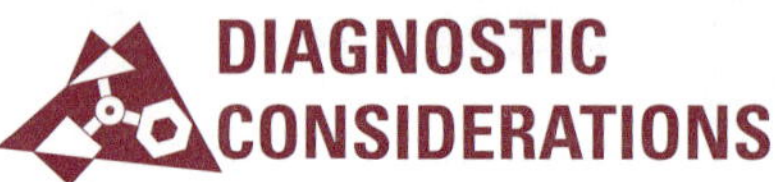

DIAGNOSTIC CONSIDERATIONS

- Must distinguish type (I, II, III) in order to plan repair
- Presence of other associated cardiac anomalies uncommon but high mortality

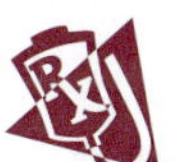

WORK-UP

- Echocardiography
- Cardiac catheterization if diagnosis unclear or if balloon septostomy necessary

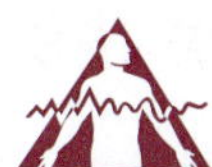

TREATMENT AND MANAGEMENT

- All should be surgically repaired
- Timing dictated by degree of obstruction
- Intubation, resuscitation
- No medical therapy

SURGERY

- Supracardiac and infracardiac: Anastomosis of pulmonary venous confluence to LA, legate anomalous connection
- Cardiac drainage: Unroofing coronary sinus and patch closure of atrial septum (coronary sinus drains into LA)
- Critically ill neonates with obstruction may need hypothermic circulatory arrest to repair lesion

Indications

- All should be surgically repaired
- Obstructed total anomalous pulmonary venous connection: Surgical emergency

TREATMENT MONITORING

- Postoperatively after cardiac connection repair: Alkalosis, increased oxygen tension, sedation, deep analgesia to prevent PA hypertensive crisis

PROGNOSIS

- Mortality limited to patients with severe obstruction (10–15%) due to pulmonary hypertension
- Patients with associated anomalies have high mortality (> 30%)
- Recurrence of pulmonary obstruction: 5–10%
- Good long-term prognosis for patients who survive without recurrence

RESOURCES

REFERENCES

- Calderone CA et al. Surgical management of total anomalous pulmonary venous drainage: impact of coexisting cardiac anomalies. *Ann Thorac Surg.* 1998;66:1521.
- Lacour-Gayet F et al. Surgical management of progressive pulmonary venous obstruction after repair of total anomalous pulmonary venous connection. *J Thorac Cardiovasc Surg.* 1999;117:679.

Pyelonephritis, Acute

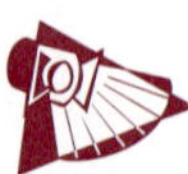

ESSENTIAL FEATURES

- High fever and chills
- Dysuria
- Pyuria
- Bacturia

EPIDEMIOLOGY

- Common in women
- Usually ascending infection
- Often incompetent ureterovesical junction
- In men, frequently due to obstructive uropathy
- Associated with vesicoureteral reflux in children younger than 1 year

CLINICAL FINDINGS

SYMPTOMS AND SIGNS

- Flank, abdominal, or back pain
- Fever and chills
- Frequency of urination
- Urgency of urination
- Constitutional symptoms

LABORATORY FINDINGS

- Leukocytosis
- Pyuria
- Bacturia
- Microscopic hematuria
- Bacteremia

IMAGING FINDINGS

- **Abdominal x-ray:** Loss of psoas stripe
- **Intravenous pyelography (IVP):** Delayed visualization and poor concentrating ability
- **CT scan:** Zones of decreased renal contrast enhancement and perinephric fat stranding

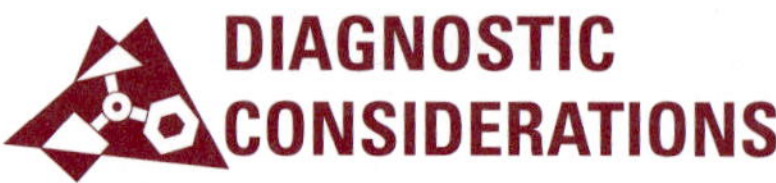

DIAGNOSTIC CONSIDERATIONS

- Acute cystitis
- Ureteral colic
- Renal colic
- Renal infarct
- Pancreatitis
- Ruptured abdominal aortic aneurysm (AAA)
- Psoas abscess
- Pelvic abscess
- Acute salpingitis
- Pneumonia
- Acute cholecystitis
- Diverticulitis
- Intestinal angina
- Acute appendicitis

RULE OUT

- Pancreatitis
- Ruptured AAA
- Obstruction in males
- Vesicoureteral-reflux in children younger than 1year

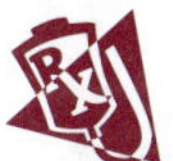

WORK-UP

- CBC count
- Basic chemistries
- UA
- Urine culture and sensitivity
- Amylase and lipase
- Abdominal x-ray
- Evaluate males for obstruction with US
- Children younger than 1year should have a voiding cysto-urethrogram (VCU)

WHEN TO ADMIT

- Constitutional symptoms
- Nausea and vomiting
- Failure to tolerate PO fluids and medications
- Bacteremia

WHEN TO REFER

- Presence of obstructive uropathy
- Radiographic abnormality
- Presence of vesicoureteral reflux
- Recurrent episodes

TREATMENT AND MANAGEMENT

- IV hydration to ensure good urine production
- Symptomatic therapy for flank pain and irritative voiding symptoms
- Specific IV antibiotic therapy
- Evaluate for obstructive uropathy if no clinical improvement in 48 hours
- Empiric antibiotic therapy until culture results available
- Substitute PO antibiotics after fever and other constitutional symptoms have resolved

SURGERY

Indications

- Obstructive uropathy
- Perinephric abscess
- Vesicoureteral reflux

MEDICATIONS

- Outpatient: 1 week fluoroquinolone
- Inpatient: IV penicillin and aminoglycoside
- Narrow antibiotic therapy to culture results

TREATMENT MONITORING

- Resolution of constitutional symptoms
- Relieve of dysuria

COMPLICATIONS

- Perinephric or psoas abscess
- Chronic pyelonephritis
- Acute renal failure
- Chronic renal insufficiency

PROGNOSIS

- Typically excellent

PREVENTION

- Empiric antibiotics for some patients with mild forms of vesicoureteral reflux

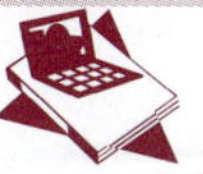

RESOURCES

REFERENCES

- Williams RD et al. Urology. In: Way LW, Doherty GM (editors). *Current Surgical Diagnosis & Treatment,* 11. New York: McGraw-Hill; 2003: 1037–1038.

Pyloric Obstruction

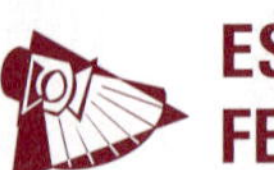

ESSENTIAL FEATURES

- History of symptomatic peptic ulcer disease
- Anorexia, vomiting, and failure to gain relief from antacids
- Vomitus contains undigested food

EPIDEMIOLOGY

- Duodenal ulcer is a more common cause of obstruction than gastric ulcer
- Gastric ulcers that cause obstruction are close to the pylorus
- Obstruction is less common than either bleeding or perforation

CLINICAL FINDINGS

SYMPTOMS AND SIGNS

- History of symptomatic peptic ulcer disease
- Increasing ulcer pain with anorexia, vomiting of undigested food, and failure to gain relief from antacids
- Absence of bile pigment in vomitus reflects level of duodenal obstruction
- Weight loss, dehydration, and malnutrition may be marked
- Peristalsis of the distended stomach may be visible
- Upper abdominal distention and tenderness are usually apparent
- Tetany with advanced alkalosis

LABORATORY FINDINGS

- Serum studies show hypochloremia, hypokalemia, hyponatremia, and increased HCO_3
- Anemia in about 25% of patients
- Prolonged vomiting leads to metabolic alkalosis with dehydration, which may lead to prerenal azotemia
- Large amounts of sodium and HCO_3^- are excreted in the urine
- Test for infection with *Helicobacter pylori*

IMAGING FINDINGS

- **Abdominal x-rays:** May show a large gastric fluid level
- **Contrast radiographic upper GI series:** Shows retention of contrast proximal to the obstruction, with luminal narrowing at the level of the obstruction
- **Gastroscopy:** Demonstrates luminal narrowing and is indicated to rule out an obstructing neoplasm

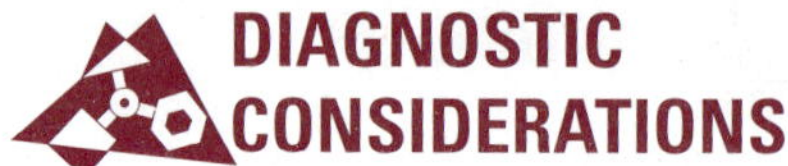

DIAGNOSTIC CONSIDERATIONS

- Consider obstruction in any patient with a history of peptic ulcer disease and prolonged vomiting, abdominal distention, and pain

RULE OUT

- Obstruction due to peptic ulcer must be differentiated from that caused by a malignant tumor of the antrum, the duodenum, or the pancreas

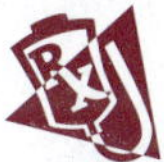

WORK-UP

- Contrast radiographic upper GI series to confirm the diagnosis
- Upper GI endoscopy to rule out malignancy as the cause of obstruction
- CBC count and serum electrolytes
- Evaluation for *H pylori* infection

WHEN TO ADMIT

- High-grade obstruction with ongoing vomiting, inability to tolerate oral intake, severe dehydration, or derangement of serum electrolytes

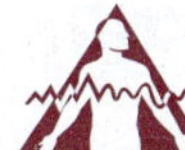

TREATMENT AND MANAGEMENT

- Replacement of fluid and electrolytes
- NG tube for decompression

SURGERY

- If conservative management fails, truncal or parietal cell vagotomy and drainage procedure is indicated

Indications

- Failure of the obstruction to resolve completely within 5–7 days
- Recurrent obstruction of any degree

Contraindications

- Inadequate trial of conservative treatment

MEDICATIONS

- H_2 blockers, proton pump inhibitors
- Treatment of *H pylori* infection
- Total parenteral nutrition if patient is malnourished

TREATMENT MONITORING

- **Saline load test:** 700 mL of saline is infused; 30 minutes later, the stomach is aspirated; if > 350 mL is aspirated, obstruction remains
- Technetium gastric emptying study

COMPLICATIONS

- Recurrence
- Other complication of peptic ulcer disease (bleeding, perforation, intractability)

PROGNOSIS

- About 67% of patients with acute obstruction fail to improve sufficiently on medical therapy and require an operation

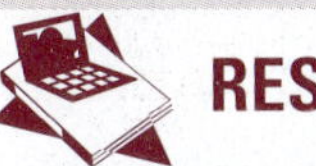

RESOURCES

REFERENCES

- Jamieson GG. Current status of indications for surgery in peptic ulcer disease. *World J Surg.* 2000;24:256.

Pyloric Stenosis

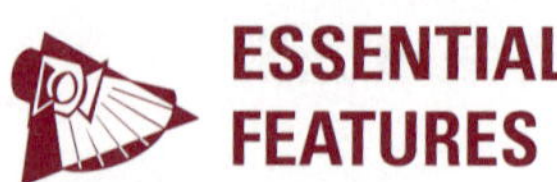

ESSENTIAL FEATURES

EPIDEMIOLOGY

- 0.1–0.4% incidence
- 7% incidence among children of affected parent
- 4-fold higher incidence in males
- Higher incidence in first born

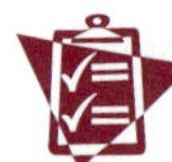

CLINICAL FINDINGS

SYMPTOMS AND SIGNS

- Nonbilious postprandial emesis 2–12 weeks of life becoming progressively projectile
- Palpable pylorus in right upper quadrant or epigastric region ("olive")
- Visible or palpable gastric peristaltic waves

LABORATORY FINDINGS

- Transient unconjugated hyperbilirubinemia in 1–2% of cases
- Hypokalemic, hypochloremic, metabolic alkalosis

IMAGING FINDINGS

- **US:** Shows hypertrophic pylorus, 95% sensitive
- **Upper GI:** Shows narrowed and elongated pylorus, 95% sensitive

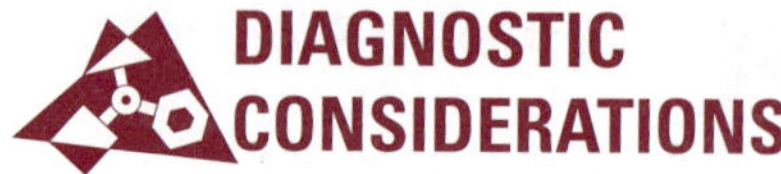

DIAGNOSTIC CONSIDERATIONS

- Repeated nonbilious vomiting in early infancy may be due to the following:
  - Overfeeding
  - Intracranial lesions
  - Pylorospasm
  - Antral web
  - Gastroesophageal reflux
  - Pyloric duplication
  - Duodenal stenosis
  - Malrotation of the bowel
  - Adrenal insufficiency

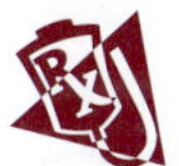

WORK-UP

- History and physical exam
- Serum electrolytes
- Abdominal x-ray
- US of abdomen if diagnosis in doubt
- Upper GI if diagnosis still in doubt

TREATMENT AND MANAGEMENT

SURGERY

- Laparoscopic or open pyloromyotomy

Indications

- Normalization of serum electrolytes
- Persistent vomiting

MEDICATIONS

- Volume resuscitation and correction of chloride to at least 90 mEq/L and CO_2 to less than 30 mEq/L

TREATMENT MONITORING

- Serum electrolytes before surgery

COMPLICATIONS

- Duodenal or gastric injury
- Incomplete myotomy (recurrent gastric outlet obstruction)

PROGNOSIS

- Excellent

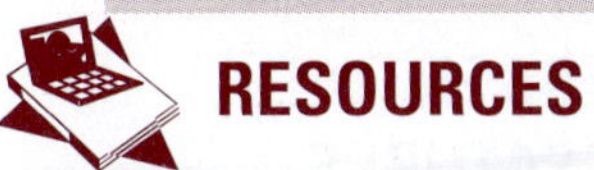

RESOURCES

REFERENCES

- Albanese CT et al. Pediatric Surgery. In: Way LW, Doherty GM (editors). *Current Surgical Diagnosis & Treatment,* 11e. New York: McGraw-Hill; 2003: 1315–1316.

Rabies

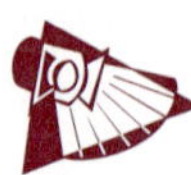

ESSENTIAL FEATURES

- Viral (ssRNA rhabdovirus) encephalitis of mammals transmitted through the saliva of an infected animal
- Humans are usually inoculated by the bite of a rabid bat, raccoon, skunk, fox, or other wild animal
- Modes of transmission include mucous membranes (eyes, nose, mouth), aerosolization, and corneal transplantation
- After local (primary) infection, the virus enters peripheral nerves and is transported to the CNS, making it difficult to detect (eclipse phase)
- Subsequent incubation period varies in humans from several days to typically 1–3 months

EPIDEMIOLOGY

- 30% of victims have no memory or evidence of a bite
- Only 4 of 8513 reported cases were in humans (1997)
- Death rate: 1–4 deaths per year

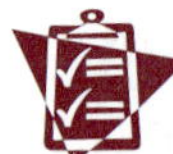

CLINICAL FINDINGS

SYMPTOMS AND SIGNS

- Clinical symptoms begin with pain and numbness around the site of the wound
- Nonspecific flu-like symptoms of fever, irritability, malaise, and progressive cerebral dysfunction
- Delirium, hallucinations, insomnia, paralysis, and convulsions occur terminally

LABORATORY FINDINGS

- Direct fluorescent antibody (dFA) test on brain tissue is used most frequently to diagnose rabies in animals
- No single test can rule out rabies absolutely
- Serum and cerebrospinal fluid (CSF) are tested for antibodies
- Skin biopsy is examined by dFA
- Saliva can be tested by nested reverse transcription polymerase chain reaction (RT-PCR)

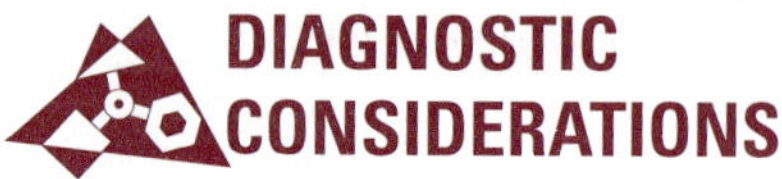

DIAGNOSTIC CONSIDERATIONS

- Rabies virus has distinctive bullet shape and nonsegmented, negative-stranded RNA genome
- After local (primary) infection, the virus enters peripheral nerves and is transported to the CNS, making it difficult to detect (eclipse phase)
- Subsequent incubation period varies in humans from several days to typically 1–3 months

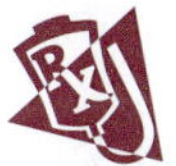

WORK-UP

- Information useful in determining the risk of potential rabies infection includes:
  - Geographic location of the incident
  - Type of animal involved
  - How the exposure occurred
  - Vaccination status of the animal
  - Whether the animal can be safely captured and tested for rabies
- Test serum and CSF for antibodies
- Skin biopsy
- Saliva tested with RT-PCR
- Suspected cases of rabies: Contact public health department
- Any animal suspected of being rabid should be killed and its brain studied with a rabies-specific fluorescent antibody

TREATMENT AND MANAGEMENT

- Since the established disease is almost invariably fatal, early preventive measures are essential
- Wound should be washed thoroughly with soap and water
- Before exposure, rabies vaccine prophylaxis
- After exposure, vaccine plus immune globin

SURGERY

MEDICATIONS

- Human rabies immune globulin
- Human diploid cell vaccine

COMPLICATIONS

- Established disease is almost invariably fatal

PROGNOSIS

- Most human deaths occur in people who fail to seek medical assistance

PREVENTION

- Wound should be washed thoroughly with soap and water
- Rabies prophylaxis has proved nearly 100% successful

RESOURCES

WEB SITE

- http://www.cdc.gov/ncidod/dvrd/rabies

Rectal Fixation, Abnormal

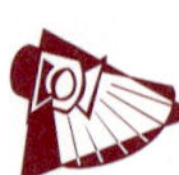

ESSENTIAL FEATURES

- Group of diseases in which the attachment of the rectum to the sacrum has lengthened, allowing the rectum to block the act of defecation, to protrude into the vagina, or to prolapse through the anus
- Increased mobility related to chronic straining
- May be secondary to colonic dysmotility
- Includes internal intussusception, rectal prolapse

EPIDEMIOLOGY

- Cause of rectal prolapse poorly understood; considered a form of intussusception
- High incidence of rectal prolapse noted in patients affected by mental retardation
- Female:male ratio is 5:1
- 50% of patients with rectal prolapse are male or nulliparous women

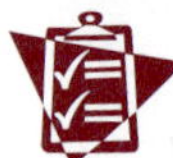

CLINICAL FINDINGS

SYMPTOMS AND SIGNS

- **Internal intussusception:** Sense of rectal fullness, urge to defecate, mass
  - Mass may be ulcerated, located anterior, 4–12 cm from the anal verge
- **Rectal prolapse:** Rectal bleeding, mucus discharge, tenesmus, incontinence, pain, feeling of incomplete evacuation
  - Large external mass of prolapse tissue with concentric mucosal rings
- Rectal exam may reveal decreased or absent sphincter tone

LABORATORY FINDINGS

- Histologic exam reveals diffuse submucosal cysts with a characteristic fibrosis pattern distinguishing it from colorectal malignancy
- Anal manometry may reveal diminished luminal pressure

IMAGING FINDINGS

- Sigmoidoscopy may reveal the circumferential intussusceptum or an ulcerated mass that appears malignant
- Defecography may demonstrate rectal prolapse or intussusception
- Evaluation of the entire colon with colonoscopy is necessary to rule out a malignancy

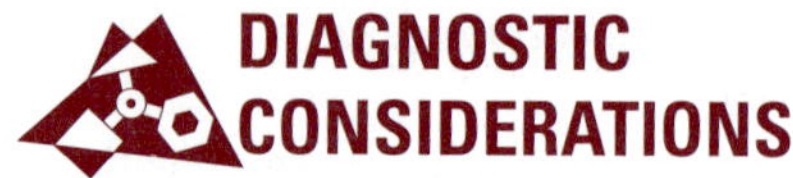

DIAGNOSTIC CONSIDERATIONS

- Anorectal malignancy
- Hemorrhoids (prolapsed)

RULE OUT

- Colorectal malignancy

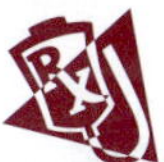

WORK-UP

- Patients with internal intussusception and rectal prolapse need anorectal manometry, pudendal nerve latency studies, defecography, and barium enema or colonoscopy
- Defecography will show the intussusception or prolapse and may reveal the cause
- Evaluation of the entire colon with either barium enema or colonoscopy is necessary to rule out a malignancy
- For patients without active prolapse, it may be necessary to give an enema, allow the patient to defecate, and then examine the perineum
  - This often induces a prolapse, allowing the diagnosis to be made in the office

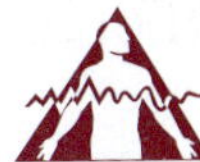

TREATMENT AND MANAGEMENT

- Mild to moderate intussusception is treated with bulk agents, modification of bowel habits, and reassurance
- The patient is instructed to stimulate a bowel movement in the morning and avoid the urge to defecate the remainder of the day because the fullness they sense is the proximal rectum intussuscepting into the distal rectum
  - With time, the urge to defecate resolves and so does the intussusception

SURGERY

- Two classes of operations for rectal prolapse: abdominal and perineal
  - Abdominal procedures have a lower recurrence rate and preserve the reservoir capacity of the rectum but carry more risk
  - Perineal procedures avoid an intra-abdominal anastomosis but remove the rectum, eliminate the rectal reservoir, and have higher recurrence rates
  - The abdominal procedures are generally preferred in low-risk active patients under age 50 and in those who are require other abdominal procedures simultaneously
- Abdominal procedures for patients with severe intussusception or rectal prolapse with normal sphincter function are sigmoid resection with or without rectopexy and rectopexy alone
- Rectopexy may be performed with sutures or prosthetic materials
- Perineal operations for rectal prolapse consist of perineal rectosigmoidectomy and modified Delorme procedure

Indications

- Severe rectal intussusception and/or failure of conservative measures

Contraindications

- Severe medical comorbidities
  - Perineal approach (which may be performed using perineal nerve block or epidural anesthesia) may be favored over abdominal approach (which requires general anesthesia

MEDICATIONS

- Bulking agents

COMPLICATIONS

- Nerve injury from prolapse or chronic straining
- Descending perineum syndrome
- Bleeding
- Incontinence
- Severe rectal prolapse may become so edematous that it cannot be reduced, and it may progress to ischemia and gangrene

PROGNOSIS

- Addition of a sigmoid resection at the time of rectopexy lowers recurrence and incidence of postoperative constipation without increasing the morbidity
- Rectopexy corrects the mobility of the rectum but does not correct the underlying disorder for patients with pelvic floor dysfunction or chronic constipation
- Sigmoid resection removes the intussusceptum and the mobile portion of colon
  - Thus, in the constipated patient or the patient with a redundant sigmoid colon, resection is preferable to fixation alone
- Sphincter function returns and incontinence resolves in 65% of patients who were incontinent preoperatively, but there is no way to predict who will respond
- The prognosis for patients with mild to moderate intussusception who are treated with bulking agents is excellent
- Persons with severe intussusception and those who have rectal prolapse without sphincter dysfunction should do well; those with sphincter dysfunction have a 60–70% chance of regaining function

RESOURCES

REFERENCES

- Jacobs LK et al. The best operation for rectal prolapse. *Surg Clin North Am.* 1997;77:49.

Rectal Ulcer, Solitary

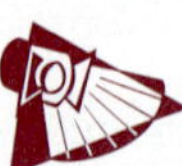

ESSENTIAL FEATURES

- Obliteration of rectal lamina propria by fibroblasts
- Term "solitary rectal ulcer" misnomer as patients may present with no ulcer, single or multiple ulcers, or polypoid lesions
- May be clinically associated and caused by pelvic floor abnormalities such as rectal prolapse, intussusception
- Results in defecation disorder with intense straining
- Possible etiology: Ischemic insult or trauma to rectal mucosa

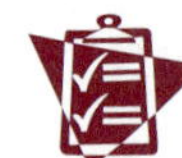

CLINICAL FINDINGS

SYMPTOMS AND SIGNS

- Difficulty in initiating bowel movements
- May be associated with rectal prolapse
- Fecal incontinence
- Sense of rectal fullness
- Tenesmus
- Sense of incomplete evacuation
- Patients may resort to regular to extensive use of enemas, suppositories
- Pain on defecation
- Passage of mucus and blood per rectum

IMAGING FINDINGS

- **Proctoscopy**
  - Most lesions located anterior and anterolateral quadrants of rectal wall 10–12 cm above anal verge
  - Ulcers may solitary, multiple, circumferential, usually shallow
  - Mucosa erythematous, edematous
- **Defecography:** May reveal inappropriate puborectalis contraction during straining
- **Electromyography:** Evidence of pudendal neuropathy
- **Anal manometry:** Decreased resting and squeezing pressure; increased rectal sensitivity and reaction to balloon distention
- **Endorectal US:** Increased diameter of internal anal sphincter; rectal wall muscle hypertrophy

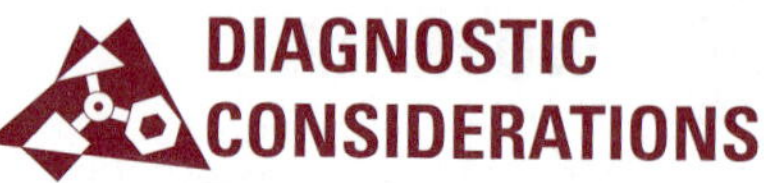

DIAGNOSTIC CONSIDERATIONS

- Neoplasm
- Stricture
- Rectal prolapse
- Rectal intussusception
- Nonrelaxing puborectalis muscle
- Diverticular disease
- Colitis cystica profunda
- Crohn colitis

RULE OUT

- Neoplasm

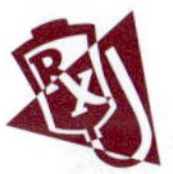

WORK-UP

- History and physical exam (patient should be observed while straining on commode to evaluate for rectal prolapse)
- Rule out malignancy
- Sigmoidoscopy or colonoscopy
- Defecography
- Electromyography
- Anal manometry

TREATMENT AND MANAGEMENT

- After ruling out malignancy, patients should be reassured
- Treatment options range from dietary modification to biofeedback, rectopexy, coloanal anastomosis, diverting colostomy
- Therapy based on severity of symptoms and associated diseases
- Asymptomatic patients in whom solitary rectal ulcer was found during screening or work-up for an unrelated disease, should be monitored expectantly with dietary fiber and bulking agents
- Dietary modification
  - Increase daily fiber intake to 30–40 g
  - Increase fluid intake
  - Avoid caffeine and alcoholic beverages
- Bowel habit modifications
  - Spend less time on commode
  - Avoid excessive straining
- Pelvic floor retraining: Biofeedback techniques (balloon expulsion exercises) and psychological counseling

SURGERY

Indications

- Pelvic floor pathologies (evidence on defecography) such as rectal prolapse should undergo repair of prolapse (perineal proctectomy or rectopexy)

Contraindications

- Lack of anatomic pelvic floor pathology (prolapse/intussusception)

MEDICATIONS

- Dietary fiber, bulking agents

COMPLICATIONS

- Rarely, life-threatening hemorrhage

PROGNOSIS

- Combination of dietary and bowel habit modification results in reasonable relief in 60–70%
- After operation, recurrence of prolapse and solitary rectal ulcer over 20 years is ~ 13%

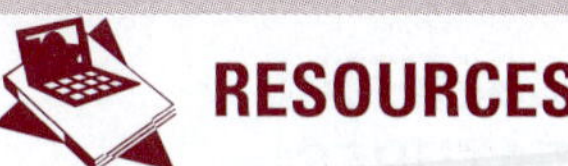

RESOURCES

REFERENCES

- Welton ML. Anorectum. In: Way LW, Doherty GM (editors). *Current Surgical Diagnosis & Treatment,* 11e. New York: McGraw-Hill; 2003:768–771.

Rectovaginal Fistula

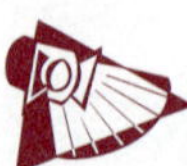

ESSENTIAL FEATURES

- Passing stool and flatus through the vagina
- Communication between the anterior wall of the rectum and posterior wall of the vagina
- Tract generally visible or palpable
- Etiologies include:
  - Obstetric injury
  - Crohn disease
  - Diverticulitis
  - Radiation
  - Undrained cryptoglandular disease
  - Foreign body trauma
  - Surgical extirpation of anterior rectal tumors
  - Malignancies of the rectum, cervix, or vagina
- Classified as low, middle, or high
- Considered low if can be repaired from a perineal approach
- Considered high if must be repaired transabdominally

EPIDEMIOLOGY

- Obstetric injury accounts for the majority of rectovaginal fistulae

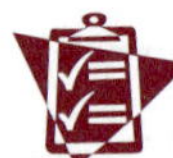

CLINICAL FINDINGS

SYMPTOMS AND SIGNS

- Passing stool and flatus through the vagina is characteristic
- There may be varying degrees of incontinence
- With low or small fistula, passage of flatus through vagina most common complaint
- Large fistula
  - Vaginal discharge with fecal odor
  - Passage of flatus and stool per vagina
  - Vaginitis
- An opening in the vagina or rectum may be seen or felt on physical exam
- Anoscopy may detect opening in anal canal

LABORATORY FINDINGS

- No specific findings

IMAGING FINDINGS

- A vaginogram or barium enema may identify the fistula
- If the fistula is not demonstrated on radiographic or physical exam, a dilute methylene blue enema may be administered with a tampon in the vagina
  - If a fistula is present, it should be confirmed by methylene blue staining of the tampon
- Proctoscopy may be required to visualize opening in mid to high fistula

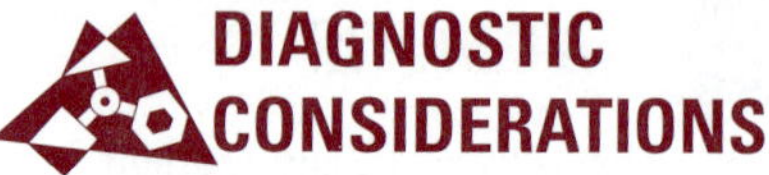

DIAGNOSTIC CONSIDERATIONS

- The signs and symptoms of a rectovaginal fistula are fairly unmistakable
  - The important differential is the cause of the fistula, as this affects management

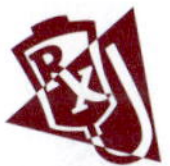

WORK-UP

- Complete history and physical exam
- History of obstetric trauma, foreign body, inflammatory bowel disease, radiation injury
- Bimanual exam
- Methylene blue enema
- Anoscopy or proctoscopy

WHEN TO ADMIT

- Signs of perineal sepsis

TREATMENT AND MANAGEMENT

- The cause and location of the fistula determine the treatment
  - Involvement of surrounding tissue by the disease process that leads to the fistula may limit the surgical options
- Inciting event (injury, inflammation, radiation injury) should be allowed to heal or subside prior to undertaking repair
- About 50% of small rectovaginal fistulae secondary to obstetric trauma heal spontaneously
- Fistulas secondary to cryptoglandular disease may close spontaneously once the primary process is drained
- Fistulas secondary to Crohn disease rarely heal spontaneously
  - Require aggressive medical therapy
  - Once in remission, local advancement flap procedures may be performed
- Temporary diverting colostomy may be necessary in patients with severe disease or complex rectovaginal fistulae that do not respond to local measures

SURGERY

Indications

- Fistulas secondary to radiation injury are not amenable to local procedures
  - Transabdominal resection and coloanal anastomosis is preferred
- High rectovaginal fistulas are best treated via a transabdominal approach allowing for resection of diseased bowel involved in the creation of the fistula
- For a low, simple fistula and some mid-rectovaginal fistulae, perform endorectal advancement of an anorectal flap

Contraindications

- For elderly or medically unfit patients, a permanent colostomy may be the procedure of choice

COMPLICATIONS

- The major complication of a rectovaginal fistula is impaired hygiene and incontinence

PROGNOSIS

- Determined by the cause of the fistula

RESOURCES

REFERENCES

- Hyman N. Endoanal advancement flap repair for complex anorectal fistula. *Am J Surg.* 1999;178:337.
- Tsang CB et al. Anal sphincter integrity and function influences outcome in rectovaginal fistula repair. *Dis Colon Rectum.* 1998;41:1141.

Renal Artery Aneurysms

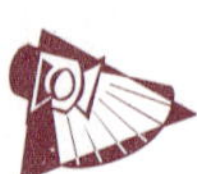

ESSENTIAL FEATURES

- Uncommon
- Usually saccular located at primary or secondary bifurcation
- 4 categories:
  1. True aneurysm
  2. Dissecting aneurysm
  3. Aneurysms associated with fibrodysplastic disease
  4. Arteritis-related microaneurysms
- Renovascular hypertension can be due to:
  - Associated arterial stenosis
  - Dissection
  - AV fistula
  - Thromboembolism
  - Compression of adjacent arterial branches
- Rupture is rare except during pregnancy, results in loss of kidney; death is rare
- Emboli from aneurysm to distal vessels occur rarely

EPIDEMIOLOGY

- < 0.1% of population
- Associated with hypertension
- Occurs slightly more often in women than in men
- Rupture rate, 3%

CLINICAL FINDINGS

SYMPTOMS AND SIGNS

- Most asymptomatic
- Discovered incidentally or during work-up for hypertension
- 30% of patients present with renovascular hypertension
- Rupture (during pregnancy)

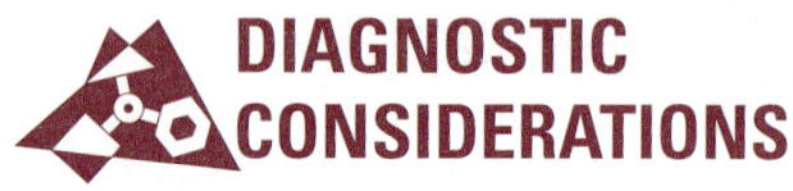

DIAGNOSTIC CONSIDERATIONS

- Must consider arteritis
- Evaluation of other sites of aneurysm formation (visceral and peripheral)

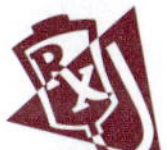

WORK-UP

- Angiography or magnetic resonance imaging for definition
- CT scan can be useful for follow-up

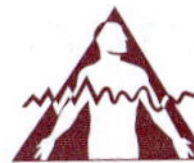

TREATMENT AND MANAGEMENT

- Small renal aneurysms managed conservatively with CT scans, angiography every 2 years

SURGERY

- Repair when indicated: repair in situ, ligate and bypass
- Nephrectomy if ruptured

Indications

- Women of childbearing age
- Patients with associated renal artery disease
- Large aneurysms (increased rate of rupture with larger aneurysms not proven)

RESOURCES

REFERENCES

- Messina LM et al. Visceral artery aneurysms. *Surg Clin North Am.* 1997;77:425.

Renal Failure

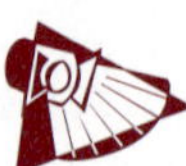

ESSENTIAL FEATURES

- Oliguric (urinary output < 400 mL/d) and nonoliguric
- Mortality in surgical ICU of 50–90%
- Etiologies of parenchymal disease include:
  - Acute tubular necrosis
  - Pigment nephropathy
  - Nephrotoxic agents
  - Acute rejection following transplantation
  - Prerenal and postrenal causes

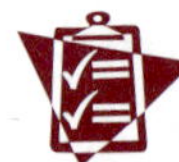

CLINICAL FINDINGS

SYMPTOMS AND SIGNS

- Diminished urinary output
- Altered mental status
- Abdominal pain
- Edema
- Prolonged bleeding time secondary to platelet dysfunction
- Tenderness over transplant allograft
- Hypertension

LABORATORY FINDINGS

- Elevated creatinine
- Hyperkalemia
- Hyperphosphatemia
- Elevated blood urea nitrogen
- Urine osmolarity isotonic with serum levels
- Urine sodium > 40
- Fractional excretion of sodium > 3%
- Hyponatremia
- Hypocalcemia
- Metabolic acidosis
- Anemia

IMAGING FINDINGS

- **Renal US:** Shows dampened waveform in arterial thrombosis or diastolic reversal of flow in venous obstruction or allograft rejection post-transplantation

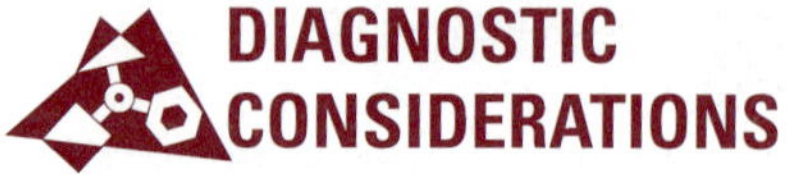

DIAGNOSTIC CONSIDERATIONS

- Duration since transplantation
- Underlying critical illness in acute renal failure

RULE OUT

- Renal artery or vein thrombosis immediately post-transplant
- Ureter obstruction or leak post-transplant

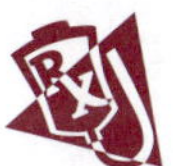

WORK-UP

- History and physical exam
- Serum and urine creatinine
- Serum and urine sodium
- Serum potassium
- Serum phosphate
- Renal US

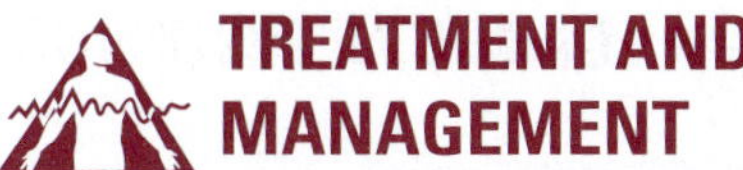

TREATMENT AND MANAGEMENT

SURGERY

Indications

- Removal of allograft if hyperacute rejection

MEDICATIONS

- Optimization of cardiac output
- Diuresis and renal replacement therapy (intermittent hemodialysis, continuous venovenous hemofiltration and dialysis if hemodynamically unstable)
- Adequate nutrition
- Treatment of underlying disease
- Pulse corticosteroids and/or OKT3 for acute allograft rejection

PROGNOSIS

- 50–90% mortality (highest if oliguric)
- 90% recover renal function if survive underlying inciting illness (recovery unlikely if > 6 weeks postresolution of illness)

PREVENTION

- Avoidance of nephrotoxic agents and maintain organ perfusion in critically ill
- Adequate immunosuppression and compliance post-renal transplant

RESOURCES

- Brennan DC. Special Medical Problems in Surgical Patients. In: Way LW, Doherty GM (editors). *Current Surgical Diagnosis & Treatment,* 11e. McGraw-Hill; 2003:48–51.

Renovascular Hypertension

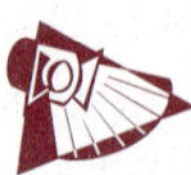

ESSENTIAL FEATURES

- Caused most often by renal artery stenosis (RAS)
  - 67% caused by atherosclerosis
  - 33% fibromuscular dysplasia
- Rare causes of renovascular hypertension
  - Renal artery aneurysms
  - Emboli
  - Dissections
  - Hypoplastic renal arteries and stenotic proximal aorta
- Juxtaglomerular complex secrete increased renin resulting in increased angiotensin II, aldosterone levels; leads to chronic changes in kidneys

Atherosclerosis

- Stenosis at orifice of main renal artery
- Usually starts in aorta extends into renal artery, rarely originates in renal artery

Fibromuscular Dysplasia

- Involves middle to distal 33% of renal artery
- Medial dysplasia most common (85%)

EPIDEMIOLOGY

- 23% of Americans have hypertension
- 2–7% of hypertension is caused by renovascular disease

Atherosclerosis

- More common in males older than 45 years, bilateral in 95%

Fibromuscular Dysplasia

- Bilateral in 50%
- Primarily in women
- Hypertension often occurs before age 45

CLINICAL FINDINGS

SYMPTOMS AND SIGNS

- Most asymptomatic
- Irritability, headache, depression
- Persistent elevation of diastolic blood pressure
- Bruit frequently present in abdomen

IMAGING FINDINGS

- **Intravenous pyelography (IVP)**
  - Common screening test to compare 2 kidneys
  - Atrophic kidney suggests diagnosis
- **Renal arteriography**
  - Most precise for delineating obstructive lesion
  - Perform for high clinical suspiscion, worsening renal function
  - Collateral renal vessels suggest > 10 mm Hg pressure gradient across stenoses
  - Minimize contrast to avoid contrast nephropathy

DIAGNOSTIC CONSIDERATIONS

- Consider this diagnoses for early-onset hypertension, antihypertensive drug resistance, deterioration of renal function, diastolic blood pressure > 115 mm Hg, deterioration of renal function with ACE inhibitors
- Selective renal vein blood renin levels
  - Renal vein renin ratio (RVRR): Involved kidney to uninvolved kidney; > 1.5 is diagnostic
- RVRR not accurate if bilateral RAS
- Captopril stimulation test causes drop in blood pressure in renin-dependent hypertension
- Captopril renal scintigraphy: Preferred study to establish diagnosis
- Duplex US
  - Up to 90% sensitive
  - Peak systolic velocities in renal artery > 180 cm/s suggests diagnosis
- Magnetic resonance angiography (MRA) with gadolinium avoids nephrotoxicity, overestimates stenosis

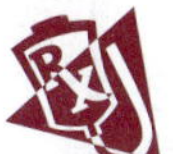

WORK-UP

- IVP, duplex may be used for screening
- Arteriogram or MRA should be performed prior to any surgical intervention

TREATMENT AND MANAGEMENT

- Primarily treated with medical therapy

SURGERY

- **Endarterectomy:** If lesion focal and close to aorta
- **Arterial replacement**
  - Preferred for fibromuscular dysplasia
  - Saphenous vein or hypogastric artery are preferred
- Splenorenal, iliorenal, hepatorenal bypasses are nonanatomic bypasses with good results
- Nephrectomy should be considered if unilateral and atrophic kidney
- Percutaneous angioplasty/stent best for focal lesions distant from aorta; patients with fibromuscular dystrophy preferred

Indications

- Extent of disease in renal arteries
- Poor response to medical therapy
- Associated arterial disease
- Patient's life expectancy

PROGNOSIS

- Percutaneous transluminal angioplasty (PTA)
  - 90% immediate success in patients with fibromuscular dysplasia
  - 60% remain cured at 1 year
  - Not as good for patients with atherosclerosis
- Operations for fibromuscular dysplasia: 90% success
- Operations for atherosclerosis: 60% success
- Surgical mortality in adults: 2–8%

RESOURCES

REFERENCES

- Helin KH et al. Predicting the outcome of invasive treatment of renal artery disease. *J Intern Med.* 2000;247:105.
- Giroux MF et al. Percutaneous revascularization of the renal arteries: predictors of outcome. *J Vasc Interv Radiol.* 2000;11:713.
- van Rooden CJ et al. Long-term outcome of surgical revascularization in ischemic nephropathy: normalization of average decline in renal function. *J Vasc Surg.* 1999;29:1037.

Retroperitoneal Abscess

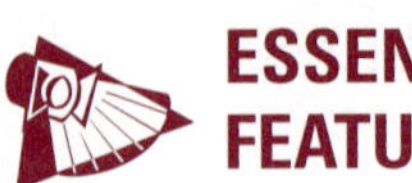

ESSENTIAL FEATURES

- Fever
- Flank, abdominal, back, or thigh pain
- Leukocytosis

EPIDEMIOLOGY

- Retroperitoneal abscesses are less common than intraperitoneal abscesses
- Primary abscesses are caused by hematogenous bacterial spread, most commonly *S aureus*
- Primary abscesses are more common in underdeveloped countries
- Secondary abscesses result from spread of infection from adjacent organs, principally from the intestine
- Most common cause of retroperitoneal abscesses in developed countries is complicated Crohn disease

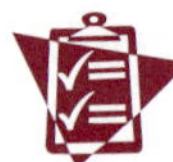

CLINICAL FINDINGS

SYMPTOMS AND SIGNS

- Fever
- Flank, abdominal, back, or thigh pain
- Anorexia
- Weight loss
- Nausea and vomiting
- Positive iliopsoas sign
- Hip pain on extension

LABORATORY FINDINGS

- Leukocytosis
- Evidence of inflammation: Elevated C-reactive protein and ESR levels
- Common to have mild hematuria and pyuria when abscess adjacent to ureter or bladder

IMAGING FINDINGS

- **CT scan**
  - Most accurately delineates these lesions and can differentiate between retroperitoneal hematomas or tumors
  - Gas bubbles are diagnostic of a retroperitoneal abscess
  - Helpful in diagnosing the underlying etiology in patients with secondary retroperitoneal abscesses
- Abscesses are confined to specific compartments whereas neoplasms frequently violate fascial barriers

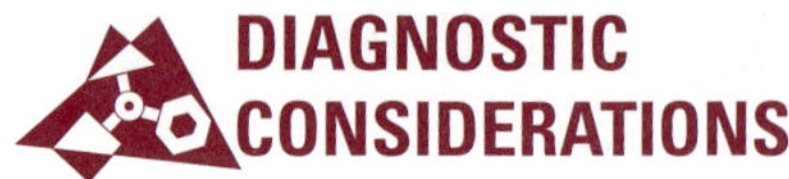

DIAGNOSTIC CONSIDERATIONS

- Etiology of retroperitoneal abscess:
  - Crohn disease
  - Ruptured appendicitis
  - Pancreatitis
  - Perforated diverticulitis
  - Posterior penetrating duodenal ulcer
  - Regional enteritis
  - Retroperitoneal trauma
  - Pyelonephritis
  - Osteomyelitis

RULE OUT

- Retroperitoneal hematoma
- Retroperitoneal tumors
- Intra-abdominal process with retroperitoneal extension

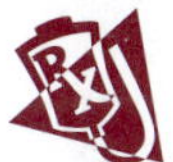

WORK-UP

- CBC count
- Basic chemistries
- Amylase and lipase
- UA, culture, and sensitivity
- Blood cultures
- Most retroperitoneal abscesses are discovered radiographically during the work-up for another diagnostic consideration (ie, appendicitis)
- Abdominal/pelvic CT scan with IV and PO contrast essential to characterize

WHEN TO ADMIT

- All patients should be admitted for definitive therapy and treatment monitoring

WHEN TO REFER

- Most patients should be managed by general surgeons
- Subspecialty referral depends on underlying diagnosis (eg, Crohn disease)

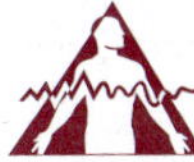

TREATMENT AND MANAGEMENT

- Percutaneous drainage may be attempted in well-defined uniloculated abscesses
- Percutaneous catheter-based drainage has a lower success in retroperitoneal abscesses than with intra-abdominal abscesses

SURGERY

- Most patients will require open surgical debridement and drainage, ideally via an extraperitoneal flank approach

Indications

- Multiloculated abscesses
- No clinical improvement within 2 days of percutaneous drainage
- Involvement of psoas muscle or significant amount of necrotic debris present (catheters provide poor drainage for thick liquid or solid debris)
- Large stellate-shaped abscesses that dissect along fascial planes

MEDICATIONS

- Systemic empiric antibiotics that cover aerobic and anaerobic enteric organisms
- Directed antibiotic therapy based on operative cultures

TREATMENT MONITORING

- Failure of fever or sepsis to subside within 3 days indicates inadequate drainage

COMPLICATIONS

- Osteomyelitis caused by invasion of vertebral bodies of the hip
- Abscess crossing the midline causing a contralateral retroperitoneal abscess
- Abscess tracking down the ipsilateral thigh compartments

PROGNOSIS

- Retroperitoneal abscesses are difficult to drain completely thus residual or recurrent abscess formation is common
- Mortality approaches 25%
- Failure of clinical septic picture to improve within 2–3 days heralds poor prognosis
- Bacteremia a poor prognostic indicator

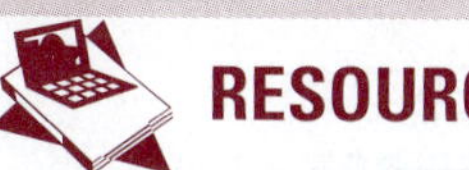

RESOURCES

REFERENCES

- Farthmann EH et al. Epidemiology and pathophysiology of intraabdominal infections (IA). *Infection.* 1998;25:329.

Retroperitoneal Fibrosis

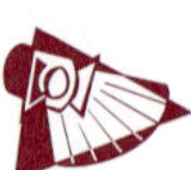

ESSENTIAL FEATURES

- Retroperitoneal fibrosis is characterized by extensive fibrotic encasement of the retroperitoneal tissues
- Most common in men over age 50 who have renal failure secondary to obstructive uropathy
- Diffuse desmoplastic involvement of the retroperitoneum may alternatively give rise to obstructive jaundice or small or large bowel obstruction
- Classic diagnostic triad includes:
  - Bilateral hydronephrosis/hydroureter
  - Medial deviation of the ureters
  - Extrinsic ureteric compression at the L4–5 level
- Over 67% of cases are idiopathic
- Known etiologies include:
  - Drugs
  - Inflammatory disorders
  - Retroperitoneal hemorrhage
  - Peri-aneurysmal (abdominal aortic aneurysm [AAA]) inflammation
  - Irradiation
  - Urinary extravasation
  - Cancer
- Most common drugs associated with retroperitoneal fibrosis are methsergide and β-blockers
- Most common inflammatory condition associated with retroperitoneal fibrosis is Sjögren syndrome

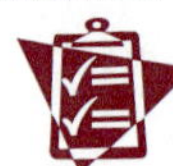

CLINICAL FINDINGS

SYMPTOMS AND SIGNS

- Low back or flank pain
- Symptoms of bowel obstruction
- Jaundice (occasionally)

LABORATORY FINDINGS

- Uremia
- Elevated creatinine
- Pyuria
- Microscopic hematuria
- Elevated ESR and C-reactive protein levels
- Elevated bilirubin (occasionally)

IMAGING FINDINGS

- **US:** Demonstrates hydronephrosis
- **CT scan or MRI:** Demonstrates the classic findings that suggest the diagnosis:
  - Fibrotic process
  - Bilateral hydronephrosis/ hydroureter
  - Medial deviation of the ureters
  - Extrinsic ureter compression
- MRI more sensitive in differentiating between fibrosis and lymphoma or metastatic carcinoma

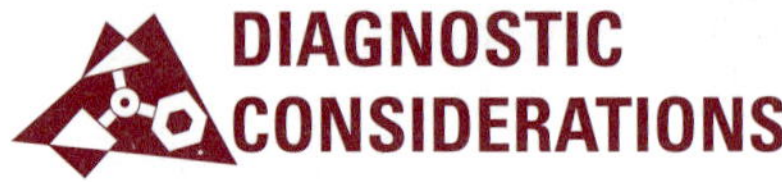

DIAGNOSTIC CONSIDERATIONS

- Retroperitoneal hematoma
- Retroperitoneal abscess
- Retroperitoneal sarcoma
- Retroperitoneal teratoma
- Metastatic disease
- Lymphoma
- Mesenteric lipodystrophy
- Peritoneal mesothelioma

RULE OUT

- AAA
- Medication-induced fibrosis
- Underlying malignancy, most commonly metastatic carcinoma or lymphoma

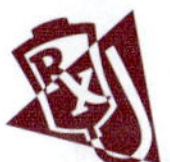

WORK-UP

- Complete history including risk factors and symptoms of systemic inflammatory diseases, such as Sjögren syndrome
- Physical exam with thorough musculoskeletal evaluation
- Radiographic characterization to evaluate for neoplasm and AAA
- Percutaneous or operative biopsy of fibrotic mass for evidence of malignancy

WHEN TO ADMIT

- Most patients will have an obstructive uropathy that will require inpatient urinary decompression

WHEN TO REFER

- Urology for urinary decompression

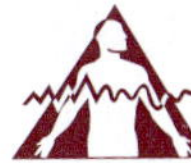

TREATMENT AND MANAGEMENT

- Urinary decompression via ureteric stents or percutaneous nephrostomy
- Repair of AAA if present
- Discontinuation of suspect medications
- Initiate anti-inflammatory medications

SURGERY

Indications

- Diagnostic laparoscopy with biopsy to rule out neoplasm and definitively establish the diagnosis of retroperitoneal fibrosis
- Ureterolysis in select patients

MEDICATIONS

- Prednisone and other immunosuppresants have been used with varying success

TREATMENT MONITORING

- Clinical resolution of urinary obstruction
- Repeat imaging study

COMPLICATIONS

- Renal insufficiency/failure
- Bowel obstruction
- Failure of fibrosis to resolve requiring lifelong ureteral stents or percutaneous nephrostomy tubes

PROGNOSIS

- Prognosis for gradual resolution is good as long as there is no underlying cancer

RESOURCES

REFERENCES

- Marzano A et al. Treatment of idiopathic retroperitoneal fibrosis using cyclosporine. *Ann Rheum Dis.* 2001;60:427.

Retroperitoneal Hemorrhage

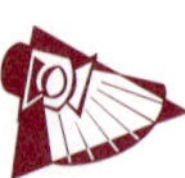

ESSENTIAL FEATURES

- Nonlocalizing abdominal, flank, or low back discomfort
- Dropping Hct with or without clinical evidence of hemorrhagic shock
- Occurs in patients with a history of trauma, femoral vascular access, or anticoagulation/antiplatelet medications

EPIDEMIOLOGY

- Spontaneous retroperitoneal hemorrhage occurs in critically ill patients who are taking anticoagulant or antiplatelet medications, or both
- Femoral vascular access common etiology of clinically silent large retroperitoneal hematoma formation
- Traumatic retroperitoneal hematoma can occur after either blunt or penetrating trauma
- Traumatic retroperitoneal hematomas divided into 3 anatomic zones:
  - Zone 1: Centrally located, associated with pancreaticoduodenal injuries or major abdominal vascular injury
  - Zone 2: Flank or perinephric regions, associated with injuries to the genitourinary system or colon
  - Zone 3: Pelvic location, frequently associated with pelvic fractures or ileal-femoral vascular injury

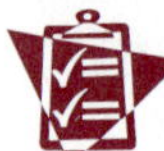

CLINICAL FINDINGS

SYMPTOMS AND SIGNS

- Symptoms depend on anatomic location of the retroperitoneal hemorrhage
- Nonlocalizing abdominal, flank, or low back discomfort
- Subtle increasing abdominal girth with more cephalad located hemorrhage
- Pelvic hematomas may compress the bladder causing urinary symptoms
- Pancreaticoduodenal hematomas may cause gastric outlet obstruction
- Perinephric hematomas may manifest in hematuria
- Femoral nerve palsy
- Flank and groin ecchymosis are a late sign of retroperitoneal hemorrhage

LABORATORY FINDINGS

- Cardinal laboratory finding is a falling Hct
- Ancillary laboratory findings are depend on associated organ injury such as elevated amylase/lipase with pancreatic injury

IMAGING FINDINGS

- **Abdominal/pelvic CT with IV and PO contrast:** Demonstrates the retroperitoneal hematoma as well as associated vascular or organ injury
- **CT scan:** Reliably differentiates between hematoma, tumor, and abscess
- **US:** Useful as an initial study to verify the presence of a hematoma
- US bladder scanner frequently will diagnose pelvic hematoma in patients with urinary symptoms following femoral vessel catheterization

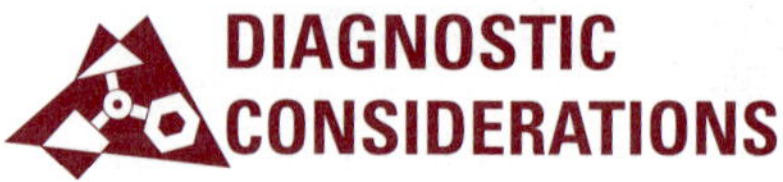

DIAGNOSTIC CONSIDERATIONS

- Retroperitoneal tumors
- Retroperitoneal abscess
- Intraperitoneal process with retroperitoneal extension

RULE OUT

- Associated vascular or adjacent organ injury:
  - Pancreaticoduodenal injury
  - Abdominal or pelvic vascular injury
  - Renal laceration
  - Ureter disruption
  - Bladder injury
  - Ascending/descending colon injury
  - Pelvic fracture
  - Femoral pseudoaneurysm formation

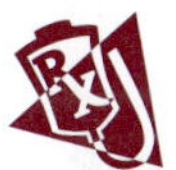

WORK-UP

- Serial Hct evaluation
- Coagulation assessment
- Amylase and lipase
- UA
- Trauma work-up as indicated
- Abdominal/pelvic CT scan with IV and PO contrast
- Angiogram
- Obtain IV urogram (sometimes)

WHEN TO ADMIT

- All patients should be admitted and closely monitored in the acute setting

WHEN TO REFER

- Referral depends on etiology and/or anatomic location of injury:
  - Trauma
  - Vascular
  - Orthopedic
- Spontaneous retroperitoneal hemorrhage as well as many blunt pelvic vascular injuries can be successfully managed in interventional radiology with percutaneous embolization techniques

TREATMENT AND MANAGEMENT

- Large bore IV access
- Type and cross 6 U packed RBCs
- Normalization of coagulation factors
- Serial Hct evaluation
- Patients with spontaneous retroperitoneal hemorrhage as well as blunt zone 3 injuries with falling Hct should have an angiogram with focal embolization

SURGERY

Indications

- All Zone 1 injuries
- Penetrating zone 2 injuries as well as blunt zone 2 injuries associated with an expanding hematoma
- Penetrating zone 3 injuries
- Evidence of femoral nerve palsy

Contraindications

- Relative contraindications include patients receiving anticoagulation therapy
- Blunt zone 3 injury

MEDICATIONS

- Erythropoietin and iron to correct anemia in select patients

TREATMENT MONITORING

- Serial Hct evaluation
- Repeat CT scan or US in selected patients with falling Hct

COMPLICATIONS

- Uncontrolled hemorrhage and death
- Hemorrhagic shock
- Gastric outlet obstruction with duodenal hematomas
- Urinoma development
- Femoral nerve palsy

PROGNOSIS

- Depends on location and severity of injury

RESOURCES

REFERENCES

- Sartorelli KH et al. Nonoperative management of hepatic, splenic, and renal injuries in adults with multiple injuries. *J Trauma.* 2000;49:56.

Retroperitoneal Sarcoma

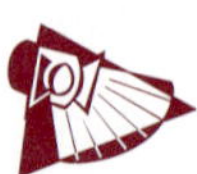

ESSENTIAL FEATURES

- Mesenchymal-derived soft-tissue neoplasms
- Metastasize via the hematogenous route with the majority of metastases to the liver or lung
- Behavior tends to be dictated by tumor grade rather than cell type of origin
- Rarely cause symptoms until they grow to a large size
- Vague abdominal symptoms are the most common presenting complaint

EPIDEMIOLOGY

- Account for 15% of all sarcomas and 55% of all retroperitoneal tumors
- Most common variant is a liposarcoma

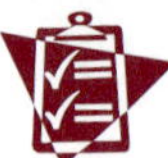

CLINICAL FINDINGS

SYMPTOMS AND SIGNS

- Nonspecific vague abdominal symptoms most common complaint
- Abdominal discomfort
- Early satiety
- Nausea and vomiting
- Weight loss
- Palpable abdominal mass

LABORATORY FINDINGS

- A small percentage of patients present with hypoglycemia simulating an insulinoma

IMAGING FINDINGS

- **Chest film or thoracic CT scan:** May demonstrate pulmonary metastases
- **Abdominal CT scan or MRI**
  - Demonstrates the soft-tissue neoplasm and its relationship to adjacent retroperitoneal structures
  - MRI is typically more accurate than CT scan in defining the extent of tumor and invasion of surrounding structures

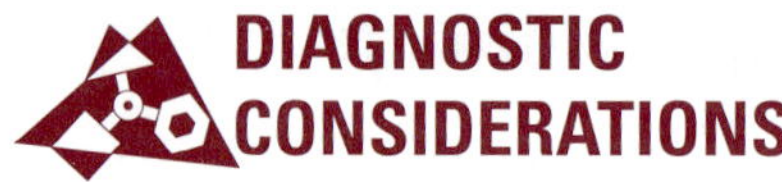

DIAGNOSTIC CONSIDERATIONS

- Retroperitoneal sarcoma
- Retroperitoneal teratoma
- Retroperitoneal cyst
- Retroperitoneal abscess
- Retroperitoneal hematoma
- Mesenteric cyst
- Mesenteric lipodystrophy
- Pseudomyxoma peritonei
- Malignant peritoneal mesothelioma
- Adrenal mass
- Renal cell carcinoma
- Intra-abdominal process with retroperitoneal extension

RULE OUT

- Retroperitoneal abscess
- Retroperitoneal hematoma
- Adrenal mass
- Renal cell carcinoma
- Intra-abdominal process with retroperitoneal extension

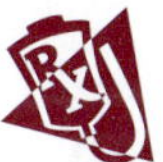

WORK-UP

- Thorough history and physical exam
- Abdominal pelvic CT scan or MRI (preferred) to evaluate extent of lesion
- Chest film or thoracic CT scan to evaluate for metastatic disease
- Image-guided core needle biopsy vs open/laparoscopic incisional biopsy to establish diagnosis

WHEN TO ADMIT

- Work-up of these lesions can usually be performed as an outpatient
- Admission for bowel obstruction or other tumor-related complications

WHEN TO REFER

- Multidisciplinary management of retroperitoneal tumors essential to ensure accurate diagnosis and appropriate treatment:
  - Surgeon
  - Medical oncologist
  - Radiation oncologist
  - Pathologist
  - Radiologist

TREATMENT AND MANAGEMENT

- Neoadjuvant chemoradiation

SURGERY

- Complete surgical extirpation with in-bloc resection of involved structures

Indications

- Operative excision in all patients without evidence of metastases and where all gross tumor can be removed (approximately 50% of cases)
- Resection of pulmonary metastases should be considered in patients who have achieved local control and who have less than 4 pulmonary lesions

Contraindications

- Widespread metastatic disease
- Inability to resect all grossly evident tumor
- Tumor involvement of adjacent retroperitoneal structures is not a contraindication as long as they can be resected in continuity with the primary lesion

MEDICATIONS

- Chemotherapy (most recently doxorubicin or "radiation sensitizers" such as IUdR have gained favor)
- No definitive evidence from adjuvant therapy

TREATMENT MONITORING

- Serial radiographic imaging including the chest for evidence of metastatic disease and the tumor bed for local recurrence

COMPLICATIONS

- Due to the magnitude of the procedure and frequent adjacent organ resection, standard postoperative complications are common
- Postoperative recovery not uncommonly prolonged

PROGNOSIS

- Retroperitoneal sarcomas have a worse clinical prognosis than trunk or extremity sarcomas
- Most patients with retroperitoneal sarcoma eventually die of the disease, frequently with locally recurrent tumor
- Majority of recurrences occur in the first 2 years following initial resection

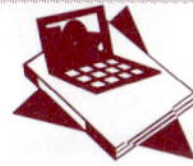

RESOURCES

PRACTICE GUIDELINES

- The National Comprehensive Cancer Network
  http://www.nccn.org

CANCER STAGING

- See Soft Tissue Sarcoma Staging Table on page 755.

STAGE GROUPING

Stage I	T1a, 1b, 2a, 2b	N0	M0
	G1-2	G1	Low
Stage II	T1a, 1b, 2a	N0	M0
	G3-4	G2-3	High
Stage III	T2b	N0	M0
	G3-4	G2-3	High
Stage IV	Any T	N1	M0
	Any G	Any G	High or Low
	Any T	N0	M1
	Any G	Any G	High or Low

Salivary Gland Infections

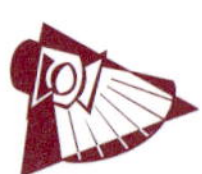

ESSENTIAL FEATURES

- Paired major salivary glands include parotid, submandibular, and sublingual glands
- Minor salivary glands are distributed in the mucosa of the lips, cheeks, hard and soft palate, uvula, floor of mouth, tongue, and peritonsillar region
- Few salivary glands in the nasopharynx, paranasal sinuses, larynx, trachea, bronchi, and lacrimal glands
- Infectious and inflammatory diseases of the salivary glands are common, and frequently involve the major salivary glands, especially the parotids
- Tend to occur in those patients whose overall health is compromised (by poor nutrition, dehydration, altered fluid and electrolyte balance, or immunocompromise)
- Etiologies include:
  - Actinomycosis
  - Acute bacterial sialoadenitis
  - Cat scratch disease
  - Mumps
  - TB

EPIDEMIOLOGY

- *S aureus* is the most common bacteria in acute bacterial sialoadenitis
- Mumps is the most common viral etiology of sialoadenitis; other etiologies include coxsackievirus A and echovirus
- Mumps primarily affects children and young adults
- Fungal sialoadenitis (usually with actinomycosis) usually follows dental manipulations

CLINICAL FINDINGS

SYMPTOMS AND SIGNS

- Parapharyngeal edema
- Pain
- Fever
- Indurated, enlarged, tender gland
- External pressure on the gland release purulent material from gland opening
- Fluctuance
- Bilateral swelling and clear salivary secretions suggest viral etiology
- Trismus

LABORATORY FINDINGS

- Leukocytosis

IMAGING FINDINGS

- X-ray for sialolith
- CT scan if suspect abscess
- Sialogram
- Radionuclide scanning

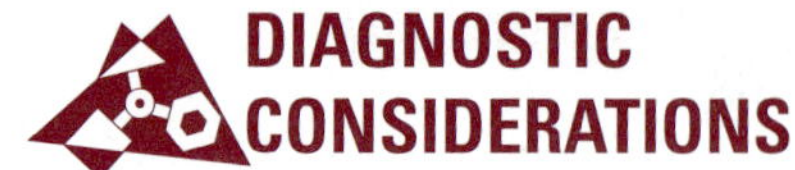

DIAGNOSTIC CONSIDERATIONS

- Abscess and fluctuance easily palpated in submandibular glands; septations in parotid gland lead to formation of multiple, small, nonpalpable abscesses

RULE OUT

- Salivary gland tumor

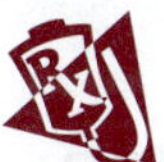

WORK-UP

- History and physical exam
- Cultures of salivary secretions; possibly blood cultures (depending on degree of systemic illness)

TREATMENT AND MANAGEMENT

- Antibiotic therapy and fluid management is the mainstay of treatment of acute bacterial sialoadenitis
- No specific treatment for viral sialoadenitis

SURGERY

Indications

- Lack of clinical improvement with antibiotics alone; aim of surgical intervention is formal abscess drainage
- Gland excision for chronic/recurrent sialoadenitis or sialolithiasis

MEDICATIONS

- Antibiotics, antifungals, antituberculous chemotherapy

COMPLICATIONS

- Chronic sialoadentis
- Altered salivary flow
- Sialolithiasis
- Tooth damage due to reduced salivary flow

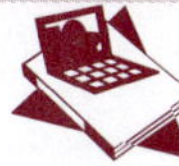

RESOURCES

REFERENCES

- Baldwin AJ, Foster ME. Tuberculous parotitis. *Br J Oral Maxillofacial Surg.* 2002;40:444.
- Brook I. Acute bacterial suppurative parotitis: microbiology and management. *J Craniofacial Surg.* 2003;14:37.
- Steyer TE. Peritonsillar abscess: diagnosis and treatment. *Am Fam Physician.* 2002;65:93.

Salivary Gland Tumors

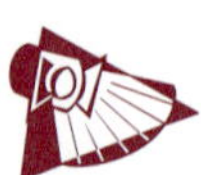

ESSENTIAL FEATURES

- Paired major salivary glands include parotid, submandibular, and sublingual glands
- Minor salivary glands are distributed in the mucosa of the lips, cheeks, hard and soft palate, uvula, floor of mouth, tongue, and peritonsillar region
- Few salivary glands in the nasopharynx, paranasal sinuses, larynx, trachea, bronchi, and lacrimal glands

EPIDEMIOLOGY

- About 5% of head and neck tumors are in the salivary glands
- 5 times more prevalent in major than minor salivary glands (70% in parotids)
- Malignancy rates by gland:
  - 15% of parotid tumors
  - 50% of submandibular tumors
  - 90% of minor salivary gland tumors
- 70% of parotid tumors are pleomorphic adenomas (50% of all salivary gland tumors)
- Mixed tumors are more common in women, with peak incidence in fifth decade
- Warthin tumor accounts for 5% of parotid tumors
  - Typically occur in men in sixth and seventh decade of life
  - 10% bilateral
- Monomorphic tumors are rare and seen most commonly in the minor salivary glands of the lip
- Mucoepidermoid carcinoma is the most common parotid cancer
- Acinic cell carcinomas are found almost exclusively in the parotid
- **Descending frequency of minor salivary gland carcinomas:** Adenoid cystic, adenocarcinoma, mucoepidermoid
- 70% of minor salivary gland carcinomas occur in the oral cavity, principally hard palate

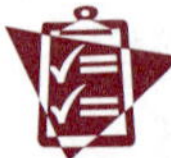

CLINICAL FINDINGS

SYMPTOMS AND SIGNS

- Nodule in the parapharyngeal space
- Enlarged cervical lymph nodes
- Pain
- Weakness in the muscles of facial expression
- Trismus
- Cranial nerve palsies

IMAGING FINDINGS

- **CT or MRI:** Can identify extent of salivary gland mass, extension in surrounding nerves, and local nodal spread

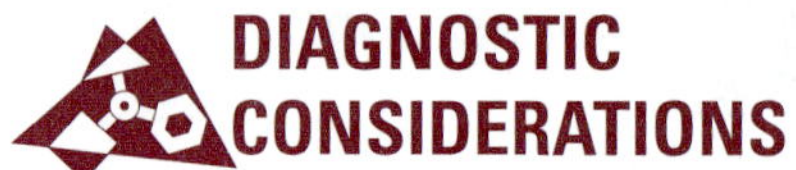

DIAGNOSTIC CONSIDERATIONS

- Majority of tumors derived from intercalated and excretory duct cells; rarely, myoepithelial cells
- Benign neoplasms of the salivary gland:
  - Pleomorphic adenoma
  - Mixed tumor
  - Monomorphic adenomas
  - Oncocytoma
  - Warthin tumor (papillary cystadenoma lymphomatosum)
- Malignant neoplasm of the salivary gland:
  - Acinic cell carcinoma
  - Adenocarcinoma
  - Adenoidcystic carcinoma
  - Malignant mixed tumor
  - Mucoepidermoid carcinoma
  - Squamous cell carcinoma
  - Undifferentiated carcinoma
- In parotid region, presence of pain, rapid enlargement of preexisting nodule, skin involvement or facial nerve paralysis suggests cancer
- Enlarged cervical lymph nodes in association with salivary gland tumors are considered manifestations of cancer until proven otherwise

RULE OUT

- For swelling in the parotid gland:
  - Parotitis
  - Primary parotid tumor
  - Upper jugular chain lymph node enlargement
  - Tumor of the tail of the submandibular gland
  - An enlarged preauricular or parotid lymph node
  - A branchial cleft cyst
  - An epithelial inclusion cyst
  - Mesenchymal tumor

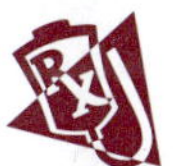

WORK-UP

- Complete history and physical exam
- Biopsy
  - Either fine-needle aspiration or local excisional biopsy with margin of normal tissue
- For minor salivary gland, often perform incisional biopsy to plan for definitive treatment (as these are more often malignant)

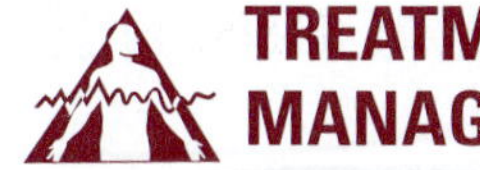

TREATMENT AND MANAGEMENT

SURGERY

- Benign tumors are removed with margin of normal tissue
- For low-grade salivary gland cancers, complete excision is sufficient
- High-grade salivary gland cancers usually require postoperative radiation therapy; clinically involved lymph nodes are removed by radical or modified radical neck dissection

Indications

- All benign and malignant salivary gland tumors are excised; extent of operation depends on location of tumor (ie, superficial or deep to the facial nerve in the parotid gland, in the submandibular gland, or minor salivary gland) and whether preoperative diagnosis of malignancy was made

TREATMENT MONITORING

- Routine physical exam of head and neck region, including testing of facial nerve function

COMPLICATIONS

- Facial nerve paralysis

PROGNOSIS

- Depends on stage, histologic grade, cancer site, patient's age, and adequacy of surgical removal
- Mixed tumors are slow growing, lobular and benign; will often leave facial nerve function intact; will grow back unless completely resected
- Recurrences of adenoidcystic carcinoma can appear 15 years or more after initial treatment
- Stage I and II: 10-year survival rate, about 80%
- Stage III and IV: 10-year survival rate, about 30%

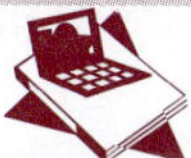

RESOURCES

REFERENCES

- Anderson J et al. Prognostic factors in minor salivary gland cancer. *Head Neck.* 1995;17:1.
- Carrau RL et al. Management of tumors of the parapharyngeal space. *Oncology.* 1997;11:633.
- Kelley DJ et al. Management of the neck in parotid carcinoma. *Am J Surg.* 1996;172:695.
- Spiro RH. Management of malignant tumors of the salivary glands. *Oncology.* 1998;12:671.

PRACTICE GUIDELINES

- The National Comprehensive Cancer Network http://www.nccn.org

CANCER STAGING

- See Major Salivary Glands Staging Table on page 751.

STAGE GROUPING

Stage I	T1	N0	M0
Stage II	T2	N0	M0
Stage III	T3	N0	M0
	T1	N1	M0
	T2	N1	M0
	T3	N1	M0
Stage IVA	T4a	N0	M0
	T4a	N1	M0
	T1	N2	M0
	T2	N2	M0
	T3	N2	M0
	T4a	N2	M0
Stage IVB	T4b	Any N	M0
	Any T	N3	M0
Stage IVC	Any T	Any N	M1

Sarcoidosis

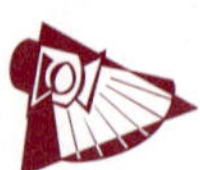

ESSENTIAL FEATURES

- Also known as Boeck sarcoid, benign lymphogranulomatosis
- Noncaseating granulomatous disease involving lungs, liver, spleen, lymph, skin, and bones
- Cause is unknown
- 20% have myocardial involvement
- 30% have cutaneous involvement
- 70% have hepatic and splenic involvement
- Mediastinal and scalene lymph nodes microscopically involved in 90% and 80%, respectively

EPIDEMIOLOGY

- Highest incidence: Scandinavia, England, United States
- Incidence in blacks 15 times more than in whites
- 50% between ages 20 and 40 years
- Women affected more often than men

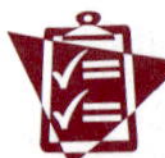

CLINICAL FINDINGS

SYMPTOMS AND SIGNS

- May present with nonspecific pulmonary symptoms (20–30%), including fever (15%) and cough
- Erythema nodosum may herald onset
- Weight loss, fatigue, weakness, malaise, enlarged lymph nodes (75%)
- Migratory or persistent polyarthritis
- CNS symptoms (rarely)

LABORATORY FINDINGS

- Elevated serum and bronchoalveolar ACE levels
- Elevated lysozyme levels

IMAGING FINDINGS

- Chest film: 5 stages
  - Stage 0: No abnormality
  - Stage 1: Hilar/mediastinal adenopathy alone
  - Stage 2: Hilar adenopathy with pulmonary abnormalities
  - Stage 3: Diffuse pulmonary disease without adenopathy
  - Stage 4: Pulmonary fibrosis
- Mediastinal lymph node involvement characteristically bilateral and symmetric
- Asymmetric hilar adenopathy: Consider lymphoma or other disease
- Pleural effusions/cavitation rare: Consider TB, pneumonia

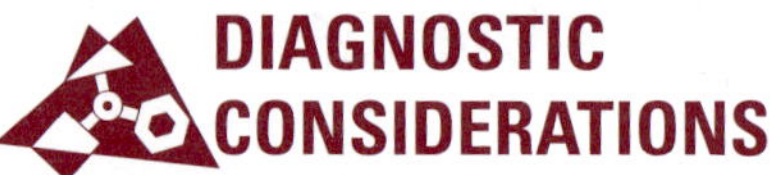

DIAGNOSTIC CONSIDERATIONS

- Diagnosis of exclusion
- Suggested by chest film, gallium 67 scanning, elevated serum and bronchoalveolar ACE and lysozyme levels
- Pathologic documentation of noncaseating granulomas via transbronchial or mediastinoscopy

RULE OUT

- Hodgkin disease
- Non-Hodgkin lymphoma

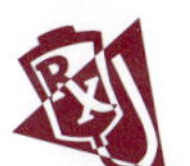

WORK-UP

- Chest film
- Chest CT scan
- Bronchoscopy and biopsy if pulmonary compromise

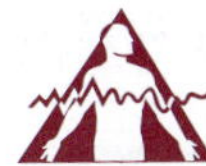

TREATMENT AND MANAGEMENT

- No therapy needed for asymptomatic patients
- Corticosteroids for patients with pulmonary impairment or are symptomatic

COMPLICATIONS

- Corticosteroid side effects

PROGNOSIS

- Long-term mortality as high as 10%

RESOURCES

REFERENCES

- Paramothayan S et al. Immunosuppressive and cytotoxic therapy for pulmonary sarcoidosis. *Cochrane Database Syst Rev.* 2003;(3):CD003536.
- Kruithoff KL et al. Giant splenomegaly and refractory hypercalcemia due to extrapulmonary sarcoidosis. *Arch Intern Med.* 1993;153:2793.

Septic Shock

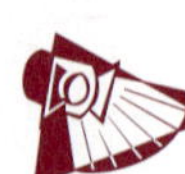

ESSENTIAL FEATURES

- Infection
- Either high or low cardiac output
- Hypotension
- Low systemic vascular resistance

EPIDEMIOLOGY

- ICU patients

CLINICAL FINDINGS

SYMPTOMS AND SIGNS

- Fever and chills
- Hypotension
- Evidence of infection or perforation
- Warm, flushed skin
- Tachycardia
- Anxiety and confusion

LABORATORY FINDINGS

- Elevated WBC count
- Acidemia

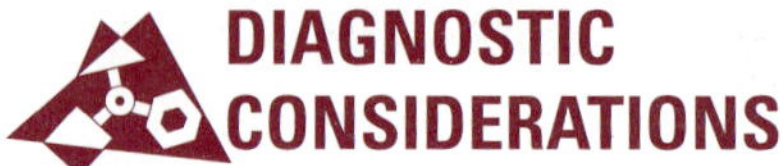

DIAGNOSTIC CONSIDERATIONS

- High-output septic shock can be produced by bowel perforation, necrotic intestine, abscesses, gangrene, and soft-tissue infections
- Cardiovascular findings of low-output sepsis are identical to those of hypovolemic shock
  - Diagnosis usually clear from clinical circumstances

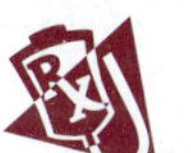

WORK-UP

- Physical exam
- CBC count

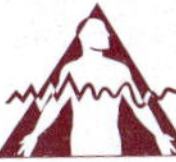

TREATMENT AND MANAGEMENT

- Invasive monitoring (pulmonary artery catheter)
- IV fluid resuscitation
- Inotropes
- Antibiotics
- Correction of GI leaks
- Debridement of necrotic tissue
- Drainage of pus

SURGERY

- Remove necrotic tissue or debride or drain infection

Indications

- GI leaks or bowel necrosis
- Necrotic tissue
- Drainable pus collections

MEDICATIONS

- Inotropes
- Antibiotics
- Vasopressors (rarely)

TREATMENT MONITORING

- Pulmonary artery catheter
- Arterial line

COMPLICATIONS

- Multiorgan system failure

PROGNOSIS

- Determined by underlying etiology

RESOURCES

REFERENCES

- Holcroft JW, Wisner DH. Shock & Acute Pulmonary Failure in Surgical Patients. In: Way LW, Doherty GM (editors). *Current Surgical Diagnosis & Treatment,* 11e. New York: McGraw-Hill; 2003:209–210.

Short Bowel Syndrome

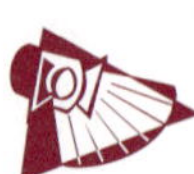

ESSENTIAL FEATURES

- Extensive small bowel resection
- Diarrhea
- Steatorrhea
- Malnutrition

EPIDEMIOLOGY

- May develop after extensive resection of the small intestine
- When 3 m or less of the small intestine remain, serious nutritional abnormalities develop; with 2 m or less remaining, function is clinically impaired in most patients, and many patients with 1 m or less of normal bowel require parenteral nutrition at home indefinitely
- If the jejunum is resected, the ileum is able to take over most of its absorptive function
- Because transport of bile salts, vitamin B_{12}, and cholesterol is localized to the ileum, resection of this region is poorly tolerated
  - Bile salt malabsorption causes diarrhea, and steatorrhea occurs if 100 cm or more of distal ileum is resected
- Steatorrhea and diarrhea are more pronounced if the ileocecal valve is removed

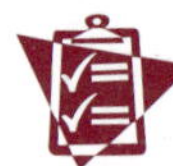

CLINICAL FINDINGS

SYMPTOMS AND SIGNS

- Diarrhea (> 2 L of daily fluid and electrolyte losses)

LABORATORY FINDINGS

- Hemoconcentration
- Metabolic acidosis
- Hypokalemia
- Hypocalcemia

IMAGING FINDINGS

- **GI contrast radiographic studies:** Show decreased intestinal length and decreased transit time

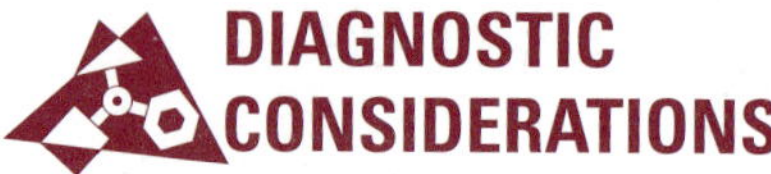

DIAGNOSTIC CONSIDERATIONS

- The progression from strict dependence on IV feeding to oral intake is possible because of intestinal adaptation, a compensatory increase of absorptive capacity in the intestinal remnant; food in the lumen of the intestine is required for full adaptation, which may require up to 2 years
- Calcium oxalate urinary tract calculi form in 7–10% of patients who have extensive ileal resection (or disease) and an intact colon; this results from excessive absorption of oxalate from the colon

RULE OUT

- Other causes of steatorrhea and diarrhea
  - Blind loop syndrome
  - Small intestinal lymphoma
  - Pancreatic exocrine insufficiency
  - Inflammatory bowel disease

WORK-UP

- Quantification and electrolyte analysis of diarrheal fluid
- Serum electrolytes
- GI contrast radiography

WHEN TO ADMIT

- Severe malnutrition

TREATMENT AND MANAGEMENT

- Initially, no enteral intake and total parenteral nutrition (TPN)
- Oral feedings should be initiated when diarrhea subsides to < 2.5 L/d while continuing IV nutrition

MEDICATIONS

- Vitamin B_{12}
- H_2 blockers
- Antidiarrheal agents
- Supplemental electrolytes as indicated

COMPLICATIONS

- Oxalate urinary calculi
- Cholelithiasis
- Catheter sepsis

PROGNOSIS

- In most patients, intestinal adaptation and oral intake can be achieved

RESOURCES

REFERENCES

- Chris Anderson-Hill D, Heimburger DC. Medical management of the difficult patient with short-bowel syndrome. *Nutrition.* 1993;9:536.
- Thompson JS. Surgical considerations in the short bowel syndrome. *Surg Gynecol Obstet.* 1993;176:89.

Sialolithiasis

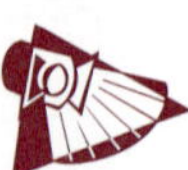

ESSENTIAL FEATURES

- Both a cause and a consequence of chronic sialadenitis
- May produce suppurative sialadenitis
- Stones are composed of inorganic calcium and sodium phosphate deposited on an organic nidus or cellular debris

EPIDEMIOLOGY

- 80–90% occur in the ducts of the submandibular glands
- 20–40% of stones are radiolucent

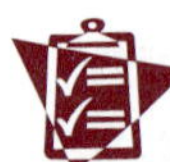

CLINICAL FINDINGS

SYMPTOMS AND SIGNS

- Painful swelling
- Patients may complain of extrusion of gravel from the ducts
- Symptoms worse with eating

IMAGING FINDINGS

- Soft-tissue films reveal radiodense stone
- CT may show sialoliths

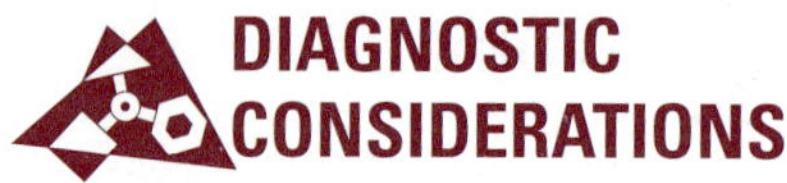

DIAGNOSTIC CONSIDERATIONS

- Diagnosis confirmed by palpation of stone or demonstration of decreased salivary flow

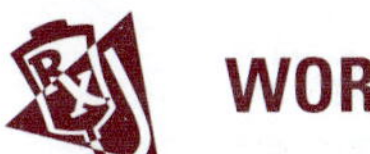

WORK-UP

- Physical exam
- CT scan

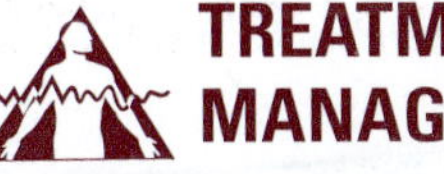

TREATMENT AND MANAGEMENT

- Intraoral removal of stones by ductal dilation and massage

SURGERY

- Operation involves excision of the gland

Indications

- For stones in the hilum of the gland that cause chronic pain and swelling

RESOURCES

REFERENCES

- Rowe LD. Otolaryngology—Head & Neck Surgery. In: Way LW, Doherty GM (editors). *Current Surgical Diagnosis & Treatment,* 11e. McGraw-Hill; 2003:987.

Sjögren Syndrome

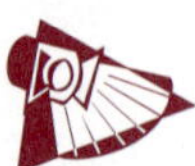

ESSENTIAL FEATURES

- Chronic, systemic inflammatory disorder of unknown etiology
- Dry mouth, eyes, and other mucous membranes
- Associated with rheumatic disorders such as rheumatoid arthritis, scleroderma, and systemic lupus erythematosus (SLE) (all have lymphocytic infiltration into affected tissues)
- Association with HLA-DR3
- Primary Sjögren involves just the eyes, mouth, and mucous membranes (sicca syndrome or complex); secondary Sjögren has an associated generalized collagen-vascular disease

EPIDEMIOLOGY

- More common than SLE, but less common than rheumatoid arthritis
- Arthritis occurs in about 33% of patients

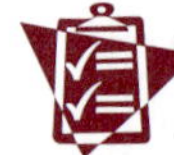

CLINICAL FINDINGS

SYMPTOMS AND SIGNS

- Dessicated cornea and conjunctiva
- 33% of patients have enlarged parotid glands—usually firm, smooth, mildly tender, and fluctuate in size
- Taste and smell sensations can be diminished
- May have dry skin
- Dry mucous membranes throughout the body
- Alopecia
- Joint inflammation

LABORATORY FINDINGS

- Schirmer test: Measures quantity of tears secreted in 5 minutes in response to irritation stimuli; decreased in Sjögren
- Evaluate salivary glands by salivary flow, sialography, salivary scintiscan, or biopsy
- Elevated levels of serum antibodies to gamma globulin, nuclear protein, and many tissue constituents
- Elevated rheumatoid factor (70% of cases)
- Negative VDRL
- Elevated ESR (70% of cases)
- Proteinuria (in presence of interstitial nephritis)

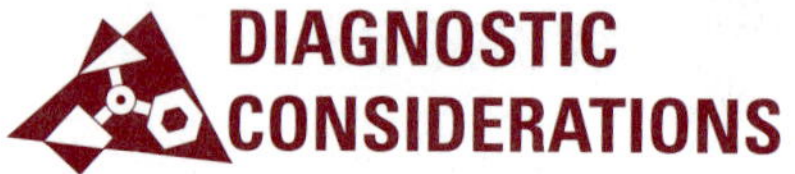

DIAGNOSTIC CONSIDERATIONS

- Dryness of the respiratory tract may lead to lung infections
- Associated with chronic hepatobiliary disease and pancreatitis
- May develop fibrinus pericarditis, sensory neuropathy, and renal insufficiency (due to interstitial nephritis)
- Patients are also at risk for Waldenstrom macroglobulinemia
- Slit lamp exam is useful to evaluate for Sjögren

RULE OUT

- Lymphoma (44-fold increased risk for lymphoma in patients with Sjögren syndrome)

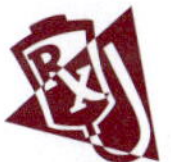

WORK-UP

- History and physical exam suggests diagnosis

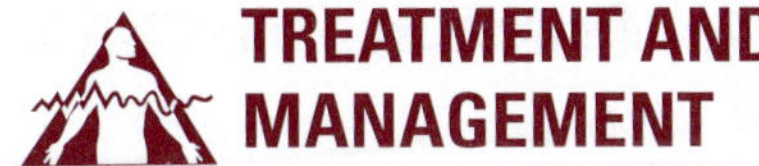

TREATMENT AND MANAGEMENT

SURGERY

Indications

- Tarsorrhaphy if artificial tears fail

MEDICATIONS

- Artificial tears
- Saliva substitute, chewing sugar-free gum, and sipping fluids throughout the day
- Oral corticosteroids or immunosuppressants are rarely indicated as connective tissue involvement is usually mild and chronic

PROGNOSIS

- Related to the underlying connective tissue disorder
- Death rarely occurs from pulmonary failure, renal failure, or lymphoma

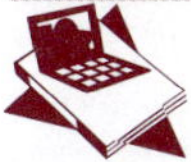

RESOURCES

- Belafsky PC, Postma GN. The laryngeal and esophageal manifestations of Sjögren's syndrome. *Curr Rheumatol Rep.* 2003;5:297.
- Borchers AT et al. Immunopathogenesis of Sjögren's syndrome. *Clin Rev Allergy Immunol.* 2003;25:89.

Small Intestine Carcinoid

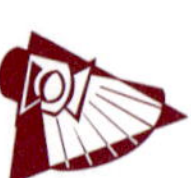

ESSENTIAL FEATURES

- Arise from neuroendocrine cells throughout the gut and produce endocrine and vasocative substances
- Metastases more likely in tumors > 2 cm
- Most are small and asymptomatic
- Hepatic metastases produce the carcinoid syndrome—cutaneous flushing, diarrhea, bronchoconstriction
- Resection of primary and isolated hepatic metastases indicated for cure or palliation

EPIDEMIOLOGY

- Arise from gut enterochromaffin cells
- Part of amine precursor uptake decarboxylase (APUD) system: Describes related neuroendocrine cells
- Midgut carcinoids produce serotonin, substance P, neuromedin A, bradykinin, dopamine, and histamine
- 85% of GI carcinoid tumors are in the appendix; 15% are in the small intestine, 90% of which are in the ileum
- Multiple synchronous tumors are present in 40% of cases
- At the time of surgical diagnosis, 40% of tumors have invaded the muscularis and 45% have metastasized to lymph nodes or liver
  - Of primary tumors < 1 cm in diameter, fewer than 2% metastasize, but 80% of those > 2 cm have spread at the time of operation
- 20% of patients have a second noncarcinoid tumor—breast, lung, and colon

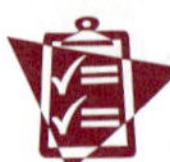

CLINICAL FINDINGS

SYMPTOMS AND SIGNS

- Small tumors are usually asymptomatic
- Obstruction due to mesenteric desmoplastic reaction
- Abdominal pain
- GI bleeding
- Intestinal ischemia
- Abdominal tenderness
- **Carcinoid syndrome**
  - Cutaneous flushing
  - Diarrhea
  - Bronchoconstriction
  - Right-sided cardiac valvular disease

LABORATORY FINDINGS

- Elevated urinary levels of 5-hydroxyindoleacetic acid (5-HIAA)

IMAGING FINDINGS

- **GI contrast radiography**
  - Tethering of bowel loops
  - Abrupt transitions between tumor involved and normal small bowel
- **CT scan**
  - Mesenteric nodal or hepatic metastases
  - Hypervascular lesions
- Somatostatin receptor scintigraphy (octreoscan)

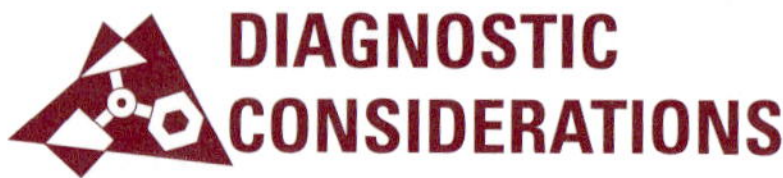

DIAGNOSTIC CONSIDERATIONS

- Mesenteric desmoplastic reaction and mesenteric vascular sclerosis is thought to be secondary to serotonin secretion and results in obstruction, bowel ischemia, and obstruction
- Biologically active substances secreted by carcinoids are usually inactivated in the liver, but hepatic metastases or primary ovarian or bronchial carcinoids release these compounds directly into the systemic circulation, where they produce symptoms

RULE OUT

- Other neuroendocrine tumors
- Benign and malignant small intestinal tumors

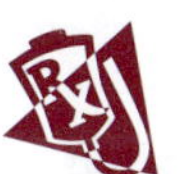

WORK-UP

- Urinary 5-HIAA
- CT scan
- Somatostatin receptor scintigraphy (octreoscan)

WHEN TO ADMIT

- High-grade obstruction
- Intestinal ischemia or infarction
- GI bleeding
- Severe symptomatic carcinoid syndrome

TREATMENT AND MANAGEMENT

SURGERY

- All accessible carcinoid tumors should be resected for cure or palliation
- Localized hepatic metastases should be resected

Indications

- All tumors

MEDICATIONS

- Chemotherapy (streptozocin, 5-fluorouracil, doxorubicin) may be beneficial for metastatic disease if progressive
- Octreotide and histamine antagonists for carcinoid syndrome

COMPLICATIONS

- Obstruction
- Intestinal ischemia
- Carcinoid syndrome

PROGNOSIS

- 70% overall 5-year survival rate
- 14-year median survival from time of diagnosis
- 8-year median survival from onset of the carcinoid syndrome

RESOURCES

REFERENCES

- Basson MD et al. Biology and management of the midgut carcinoid. *Am J Surg.* 1993;165:288.
- Søoreide O et al. Surgical treatment as a principle in patients with advanced abdominal carcinoid tumors. *Surgery.* 1992;111:48.

PRACTICE GUIDELINES

- The National Comprehensive Cancer Network http://www.nccn.org

Small Intestine Diverticula

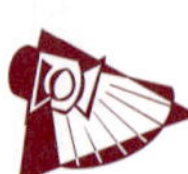

ESSENTIAL FEATURES

- Most jejunoileal diverticula are acquired true diverticula
  - Meckel diverticulum is congenital
- May be asymptomatic or associated with obstruction, bleeding, or inflammation (diverticulitis)

EPIDEMIOLOGY

- **Acquired diverticula** are found in 1.3% of the population
- Most contain all layers of the intestinal wall (true diverticula)
- Often multiple, they diminish in frequency from the ligament of Treitz to the ileocecal valve
- **Meckel diverticulum** is a congenital, true diverticulum that results from persistence of the vitelline duct and occurs on the antimesenteric border of the ileum
- Heterotrophic gastric or pancreatic tissue may be present in the diverticulum
- Follow the rule of 2:
  - Occur in males twice as often as females
  - Occur in 2% of the population
  - Become symptomatic in 2% of cases
  - Occur 2 ft proximal to the ileocecal valve
  - May extend over 2 inches in length
  - Can cause 2 symptoms: Bleeding and obstruction

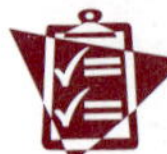

CLINICAL FINDINGS

SYMPTOMS AND SIGNS

- Most are asymptomatic
- Symptoms may be due to obstruction, inflammation, bleeding, or bacterial overgrowth
- Abdominal pain
- GI hemorrhage
- Diarrhea and malabsorption

LABORATORY FINDINGS

- Elevated WBC count (inflammation)
- Anemia (bleeding)

IMAGING FINDINGS

- **Upper GI contrast radiography:** May outline the diverticula and any associated obstruction
- **CT scan:** May reveal the diverticula as well as associated inflammation or obstruction
- **Meckel diverticulum:** ^{99}technetium-pertechnate scan can identify ectopic gastric mucosa in the diverticulum

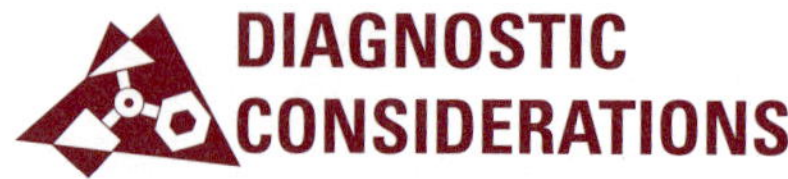

DIAGNOSTIC CONSIDERATIONS

- Jejunoileal diverticula may be associated with disturbed motility
- Blind loop syndrome is caused by chronic partial obstruction or bacterial overgrowth in large diverticula
- Obstruction in Meckel diverticulum may be due to volvulus around a persistent omphalomesenteric band or intussusception
- Bleeding in Meckel diverticulum is due to ulceration from acid secreted by heterotopic gastric mucosa

RULE OUT

- Other causes of GI bleeding, small bowel obstruction, or small bowel inflammation

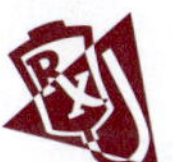

WORK-UP

- Upper GI contrast radiography or CT scan
- ^{99}Technetium-pertechnate scan in suspected cases of Meckel diverticulum

WHEN TO ADMIT

- Complications
  - Obstruction
  - Bleeding
  - Inflammation

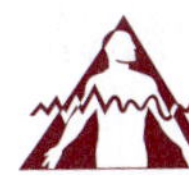

TREATMENT AND MANAGEMENT

- Asymptomatic diverticula require no treatment

SURGERY

- Small bowel resection and anastomosis required for complications

Indications

- Inflammation (diverticulitis)
- Bleeding
- Obstruction
- Perforation

COMPLICATIONS

- Inflammation (diverticulitis)
- Perforation
- Bleeding
- Obstruction

PROGNOSIS

- Diverticula are treated completely by segmental small bowel resection

RESOURCES

REFERENCES

- Akhrass R et al. Small-bowel diverticulosis: perceptions and reality. *J Am Coll Surg.* 1997;184:383.
- Longo WE, Vernava AD. Clinical implications of jejunoileal diverticular disease. *Dis Colon Rectum.* 1992;35:381.

Small Intestine Enteropathies, Noninfectious

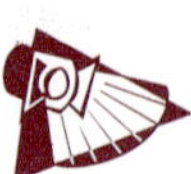

ESSENTIAL FEATURES

- Damage to the small intestinal mucosa due to NSAIDs or radiation exposure
- Ensuing inflammation can result in mucosal ulceration, diarrhea, and GI bleeding
- Late complications of NSAID and radiation enteropathy include stricture and obstruction

EPIDEMIOLOGY

NSAID Enteropathy

- NSAIDs increase intestinal permeability, leading to mucosal inflammation
- Enteropathy, with subclinical intestinal inflammation and occult blood loss, develops in 70% of patients who have taken NSAIDs for > 6 months
- Mucosal ulceration or transmural inflammation and fibrosis with circumferential strictures develop in < 1%

Radiation Enteropathy

- Injury to blood vessels in the bowel wall leads to endothelial proliferation and fibrosis that obliterates the vessel lumen producing chronic intestinal ischemia
- Incidence of bowel injury is dose-related
  - 5% after 4500 cGy
  - 30% after 6000 cGy
- Fixed loops of small bowel in the radiation field increases the risk of intestinal complications

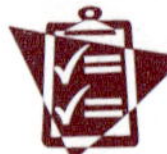

CLINICAL FINDINGS

SYMPTOMS AND SIGNS

- Nausea and vomiting
- Abdominal pain
- GI bleeding
- Diarrhea, which may be bloody
- Abdominal tenderness

LABORATORY FINDINGS

- Anemia

IMAGING FINDINGS

- **Abdominal x-ray**
  - If obstruction is present, dilated loops of bowel proximal to the obstruction with air-fluid levels and thickened bowel wall
  - Free air suggests perforation
- **Upper GI contrast radiography:** Narrowed, stenotic segment of bowel
- **CT scan**
  - Dilated bowel with bowel wall edema proximal to the obstruction with narrowed, stenotic bowel at the site of obstruction
  - Free air suggests perforation
- **Endoscopy**
  - Inflamed mucosa
  - May identify the strictured segment of bowel

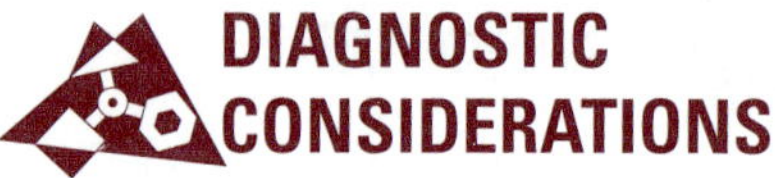

DIAGNOSTIC CONSIDERATIONS

- Strictures, either inflammatory (NSAID enteropathy) or ischemic (radiation enteropathy) can present as a late complication and result in obstruction or perforation

RULE OUT

- Crohn disease
- Ischemia
- TB
- Lymphoma
- Primary or recurrent carcinoma

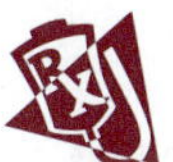

WORK-UP

- Abdominal x-ray
- GI contrast radiography
- CT scan
- Endoscopy

WHEN TO ADMIT

- Obstruction
- Perforation
- Bleeding

TREATMENT AND MANAGEMENT

NSAID Enteropathy

- Discontinue drug

Radiation Enteropathy

- Symptoms may appear as early as 1 month or as late as 30 years after completion of therapy

SURGERY

- Resection indicated for complications

Indications

- Obstruction
- Perforation
- Bleeding
- Abscess
- Fistula

COMPLICATIONS

- Obstruction
- Perforation
- Bleeding
- Abscess

PROGNOSIS

- Good for NSAID enteropathy after medication is discontinued
- Symptoms are usually minor and transient with radiation enteropathy

RESOURCES

REFERENCES

- Allison MC et al. Gastrointestinal damage associated with the use of nonsteroidal anti-inflammatory drugs. *N Engl J Med.* 1992;327:749.
- Cross MJ, Frazee RC. Surgical treatment of radiation enteritis. *Am Surg.* 1992;58:132.

Small Intestine Fistulas

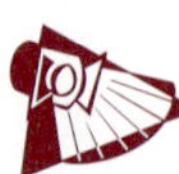

ESSENTIAL FEATURES

- Fever and sepsis
- Abdominal pain
- Localized abdominal tenderness
- External drainage of small bowel contents
- Dehydration and malnutrition

EPIDEMIOLOGY

- May form spontaneously as a result of disease (Crohn disease), but > 95% are surgical complications
- A high-output fistula produces > 500 mL/24 h
- Most associated with abscesses, which often drain incompletely so that persistent sepsis is a common feature
- Intestinal fluid escaping through the fistula may excoriate the skin
- Fluid and electrolyte losses may be severe, especially if it is located in the upper tract or if there is partial or complete distal intestinal obstruction
- 30% of fistulas close spontaneously
  - Crohn disease, irradiated bowel, cancer, foreign body, distal obstruction, extensive disruption of intestinal continuity, and a short (< 2 cm) fistula tract are associated with failure of fistulas to heal

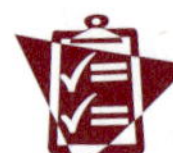

CLINICAL FINDINGS

SYMPTOMS AND SIGNS

- Fever
- Abdominal pain until bowel contents discharge
- Rapid weight loss
- Abdominal tenderness

LABORATORY FINDINGS

- Leukocytosis
- Hemoconcentration
- Electrolyte abnormalities based on loss through fistula output
- Metabolic acidosis

IMAGING FINDINGS

- Contrast medium administered orally, per rectum, or through the fistula (fistulogram) delineates the abnormal anatomy (including intrinsic bowel disease) and demonstrates the location and number of fistulas, the length and course of fistula tracts, associated abscess cavities, and the presence of distal obstruction
- **CT scan:** May identify associated abscesses and allow for percutaneous drainage

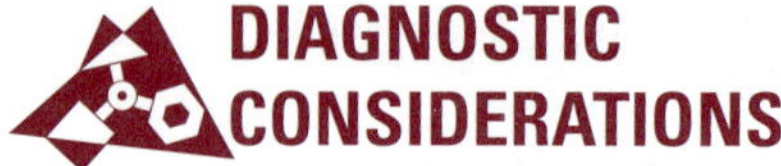

DIAGNOSTIC CONSIDERATIONS

- Fluid should be collected from fistula output for measurement of volume and electrolyte composition; subsequent maintenance of homeostasis depends on accurately measuring losses and replacing them
- In many cases, an incompletely drained abscess can be managed by an interventional radiologist, who passes a catheter through a fistula tract into the associated abscess cavity
  - Drainage is accomplished, and the fistula may close as the sump tube is gradually withdrawn over a period of weeks.

RULE OUT

- Associated carcinoma
- Inflammatory bowel disease
- Anastomotic disruption
- GI perforation
- Distal GI obstruction

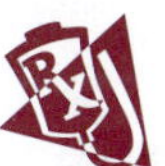

WORK-UP

- GI contrast radiography (upper GI, barium enema, fistulogram)
- CT scan
- Serum electrolytes
- CBC count

WHEN TO ADMIT

- In all acute cases for fluid and electrolyte replacement, delineation of tract, drainage of associated abscesses, and nutrition

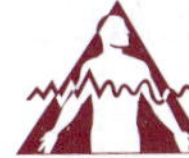

TREATMENT AND MANAGEMENT

- Fluid, electrolyte, and nutritional replacement
- Protection of skin from excoriation
- Abscess drainage
- No enteral intake and NG suction

SURGERY

- The fistulous segment should be resected, associated obstruction relieved, and continuity reestablished by end-to-end anastomosis

Indications

- Persistence > 1 month

Contraindications

- The operation should be postponed until intra-abdominal inflammation has resolved—typically 2–3 months after the last operation

MEDICATIONS

- H_2 receptor antagonists
- Somatostatin
- Total parenteral nutrition

COMPLICATIONS

- Fluid and electrolyte losses
- Malnutrition
- Sepsis
- Abscess

PROGNOSIS

- With proper management, survival rates are 80–95%
- Uncontrolled sepsis is the chief cause of death

RESOURCES

REFERENCES

- Borison DI et al. Treatment of enterocutaneous and colocutaneous fistulas with early surgery or somatostatin analog. *Dis Colon Rectum.* 1992;35:635.

Small Intestine Tumors, Benign

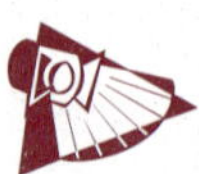

ESSENTIAL FEATURES

- Often asymptomatic or subtly symptomatic
  - Symptomatic tumors are more likely to be malignant
- Benign tumors are more likely pedunculated and more commonly cause intussusception
- May be a cause of GI bleeding

EPIDEMIOLOGY

Adenoma

- Tubular
  - Low malignant potential
  - Can cause obstruction or intussusception
- Villous
  - Significant malignant potential, associated with inherited colonic polyposis syndromes
  - Brunner gland: No malignant potential

Stromal Tumors

- Mesenchymal neoplasms
- The most common symptomatic benign neoplasm
- Most in the jejunum
- Associated with ulceration, bleeding, and obstruction

Lipomas

- Most in the ileum, may cause obstruction
- No malignant potential

Hamartomas

- Part of Peutz-Jeghers syndrome
- Polypoid and may cause intermittent intussusception and bleeding
- Rare malignant potential

Hemangiomas

- Small and diffuse or large and isolated, can be a source of recurrent GI hemorrhage

CLINICAL FINDINGS

SYMPTOMS AND SIGNS

- Often asymptomatic
- Abdominal pain
- GI bleeding
- Abdominal distention
- Abdominal tenderness

LABORATORY FINDINGS

- Anemia

IMAGING FINDINGS

- **Contrast radiography or enteroclysis:** May visualize tumor as a filling defect or mass lesion.
- **CT scan:** Mass may be visualized after administration of contrast
- **Endoscopy**
  - Most lesions are inaccessible
  - Allows direct visualization as well as biopsy for diagnosis

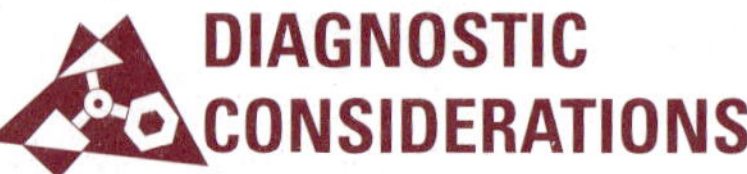

DIAGNOSTIC CONSIDERATIONS

- Most benign tumors of the small intestine are asymptomatic
  - When symptoms occur, they are often related to obstruction, intussusception, or bleeding
- Differentiating benign from malignant stromal tumors may be difficult

RULE OUT

- Malignant tumors

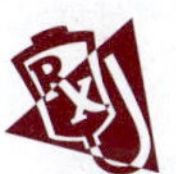

WORK-UP

- Contrast radiography
- CT scan
- Endoscopy if feasible

WHEN TO ADMIT

- High-grade obstruction
- Bleeding

TREATMENT AND MANAGEMENT

- Many benign tumors require no specific treatment if asymptomatic

SURGERY

- Symptomatic lesions require either resection or endoscopic excision

Indications

- Symptoms (obstruction, bleeding)
- Tubular or villous adenomas
- All stromal tumors
- Large or extensive hemangiomas
- Large hamartomas

COMPLICATIONS

- Obstruction
- Bleeding
- Intussusception

PROGNOSIS

- Good after resection of benign lesions

RESOURCES

REFERENCES

- Blanchard DK et al. Tumors of the small intestine. *World J Surg.* 2000;24:421.
- Miettinen M et al. Gastrointestinal stromal tumors: recent advances in understanding their biology. *Hum Pathol.* 1999;30:1213.

Small Intestine Tumors, Malignant

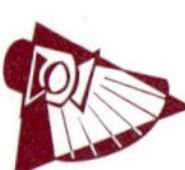

ESSENTIAL FEATURES

- Often symptomatic
  - Abdominal pain most common presenting complaint
- Circumferential luminal growth results in progressive obstruction
- Bleeding is a feature of ulcerated tumors
- Besides primary neoplasms, the small bowel may be a site of metastatic disease
- Diagnosis usually radiographic by contrast study or CT scan
- Resection indicated for cure and palliation

EPIDEMIOLOGY

Adenocarcinoma

- 50% of cases
- Risk factors include:
  - Crohn disease
  - Polyposis syndromes
  - Villous adenomas
  - Family history of nonpolyposis colorectal cancer

Lymphoma

- 15–20% of cases
- Most common extranodal lymphoma
- May be primary or part of disseminated disease
- Most are non-Hodgkin B-cell
- More common in the ileum
- Risk factors include:
  - Malabsorption
  - Inflammatory intestinal disease
  - Immunosuppression

Stromal Tumors

- 10–20% of cases
- Distinction between benign and malignant difficult
- Tumors are extraluminal and subserosal
- Metastases present in 30% at presentation

Metastatic Tumors

- Affect small bowel by direct extension, carcinomatosis, or hematogenous spread

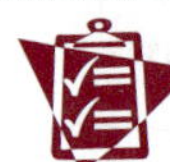

CLINICAL FINDINGS

SYMPTOMS AND SIGNS

- Abdominal pain
- GI bleeding
- Malabsorption (lymphoma)
- Weight loss
- Abdominal distention
- Abdominal tenderness
- Palpable abdominal mass (stromal tumor)

LABORATORY FINDINGS

- Anemia

IMAGING FINDINGS

Adenocarcinoma

- **Radiographic contrast study**
  - Annular with ulcerated mucosa
  - "Apple core" appearance
- **CT scan:** Detection of metastases and staging

Lymphoma

- **Radiographic contrast study:** Thickened mucosa, ulceration, submucosal nodules
- **CT scan**
  - Diffuse bowel wall thickening, mesenteric adenopathy, mass lesion
  - Detection of metastases and staging

Stromal Tumors

- **Radiographic contrast study**
  - Extraluminal mass
  - Central necrosis with contrast filling
- **CT scan**
  - Extraluminal mass with vascularity and central necrosis
  - Detection of metastases and staging

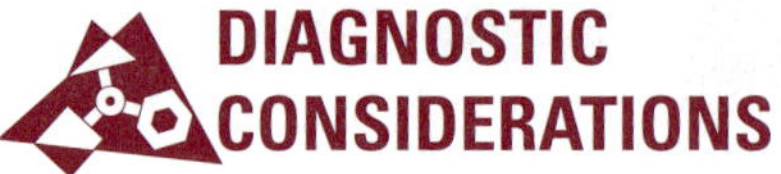

DIAGNOSTIC CONSIDERATIONS

- Most small intestinal tumors are not accessible by endoscopy and diagnosis relies on symptoms, radiographic appearance, and clinical suspicion
- Differentiating benign and malignant stromal tumors based on mitotic frequency, nuclear atypia, cellularity, size of tumor, and central necrosis

RULE OUT

- Benign tumors of the small intestine

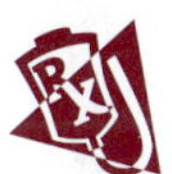

WORK-UP

- CBC count
- GI contrast radiograph study
- CT scan
- Endoscopy and biopsy (if lesion is accessible)

WHEN TO ADMIT

- High-grade obstruction
- Bleeding

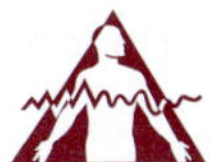

TREATMENT AND MANAGEMENT

SURGERY

- All malignant tumors require wide segmental resection
- Even if not curative, resection may palliate obstruction and bleeding

Indications

- All malignant tumors

MEDICATIONS

- Chemotherapy and radiation therapy have proved beneficial for lymphoma
- Imatinib mesylate for stromal tumors

COMPLICATIONS

- Obstruction
- Perforation
- Bleeding

PROGNOSIS

Adenocarcinoma

- 80% survival if localized
- 10–15% with positive nodes

Lymphoma

- 5-year survival is 20–40%

Stromal Tumors

- 20% survival if high-grade

RESOURCES

REFERENCES

- Cunningham JD et al. Malignant small bowel neoplasms: histopathologic determinants of recurrence and survival. *Ann Surg.* 1997;225:300.
- North JH et al. Malignant tumors of the small intestine. *Am Surg.* 2000;66:46.

PRACTICE GUIDELINES

- The National Comprehensive Cancer Network http://www.nccn.org

CANCER STAGING

- See Small Intestine Staging Table on page 755.

STAGE GROUPING

Stage 0	Tis	N0	M0
Stage I	T1	N0	M0
	T2	N0	M0
Stage II	T3	N0	M0
	T4	N0	M0
Stage III	Any T	N1	M0
Stage IV	Any T	Any N	M1

Small Intestine, Infectious Diseases

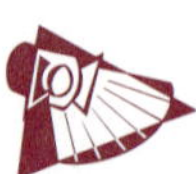

ESSENTIAL FEATURES

- Infection leads to acute enteritis (acute inflammation of the small intestine) and mesenteric lymphadenitis (inflammation of regional small intestinal lymph nodes)
- Small intestinal infections often mimic surgical conditions of the abdomen such as acute appendicitis
- May also cause complications (such as perforation or bleeding) that require surgical intervention

EPIDEMIOLOGY

- **HIV-associated enteropathy**
  - Associated with opportunistic GI infections
  - Intestinal perforation is a known complication
- ***Yersinia* enteritis:** Associated with acute gastroenteritis, terminal ileitis, mesenteric lymphadenitis, hepatic and splenic abscesses
- ***Campylobacter jejuni:*** Raw milk, untreated drinking water, and undercooked poultry are recognized vehicles of transmission
- **TB**
  - Most infections due to swallowing the human tubercle bacillus
  - About 1% of patients with pulmonary TB have intestinal involvement
  - Recent immigration from endemic areas and infection with HIV are risk factors
  - Often affects the distal ileum
- ***Salmonella typhi:*** May cause ulcers in the distal ileum or cecum

CLINICAL FINDINGS

SYMPTOMS AND SIGNS

- Fever
- Diarrhea
- Chronic or relapsing bloody diarrhea in severe cases
- Nausea and vomiting
- Abdominal pain
- Abdominal tenderness

LABORATORY FINDINGS

- Elevated WBC count with eosinophilia
- Culture of stool or tissue obtained by biopsy may allow isolation and identification of the pathogen
- Organisms may be visualized by microscopic exam of stool or biopsy specimens

IMAGING FINDINGS

- **Plain film radiography or CT scan:**
  - Findings are nonspecific
  - Intestinal dilation, bowel wall thickening, and fat stranding in the mesentery may be observed
- **Endoscopy:** May reveal mucosal lesions, inflammation, and ulcerations and allow biopsy for potential isolation and identification of the infectious pathogen

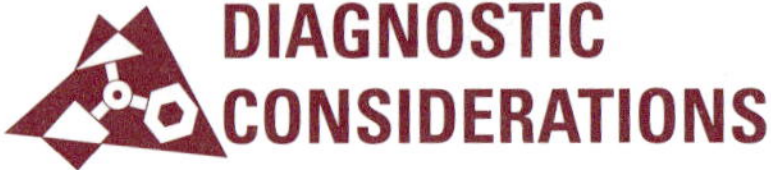

DIAGNOSTIC CONSIDERATIONS

- Pathogens associated with HIV-Associated enteropathy include:
  - *Cryptosporidium*
  - Cytomegalovirus
  - *Entamoeba histolytica*
  - *Giardia lamblia*
  - *Mycobacterium avium-intracellulare*
  - *Salmonella typhimurium*
  - *Shigella*
  - *Campylobacter jejuni*
  - HIV
- Tuberculosis: The pathologic reaction is hypertrophic (causing stenosis and obstruction) or ulcerative (causing abdominal pain, diarrhea, free perforation, fistula formation, or hemorrhage)

RULE OUT

- Noninfectious causes of GI inflammation (pancreatitis, appendicitis)

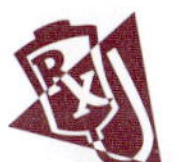

WORK-UP

- CBC count
- Stool for culture
- Plain film or CT scan of the abdomen
- Endoscopy for exam and biopsy

WHEN TO ADMIT

- Perforation
- Obstruction
- Severe bleeding
- Dehydration

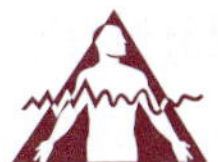

TREATMENT AND MANAGEMENT

SURGERY

- If operation is performed for a diagnosis of appendicitis and the entire distal small bowel is grossly inflamed, appendectomy is usually performed
- Resection is indicated for complications

Indications

- Perforation
- Obstruction
- Bleeding
- Uncertain diagnosis

MEDICATIONS

- Many of these infections are self-limited and require no specific treatment
- Antimicrobial treatment should be aimed at the suspected or confirmed pathogen

COMPLICATIONS

- Perforation
- Hemorrhage

PROGNOSIS

- Overall good prognosis if appropriate antimicrobial treatment is instituted early

RESOURCES

REFERENCES

- Giannella RA. Enteric infections: 50 years of progress. *Gastroenterology.* 1993;104:1589.
- Underwood MJ et al. Presentation of abdominal tuberculosis to general surgeons. *Br J Surg.* 1992;79:1077.

Small Intestine, Obstruction

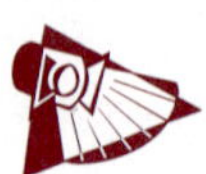

ESSENTIAL FEATURES

Proximal Obstruction

- Vomiting
- Abdominal discomfort
- Abnormal PO contrast x-rays

Mid or Distal Obstruction

- Colicky abdominal pain
- Vomiting
- Abdominal distention
- Constipation-obstipation
- Peristaltic rushes
- Dilated small bowel on x-ray

EPIDEMIOLOGY

- The most common surgical disorder of the small intestine
- Common causes of obstruction:
  - Adhesions: The most common cause of mechanical small bowel obstruction
  - Neoplasms: Intrinsic or extrinsic
  - Hernia: Due to incarceration of bowel
  - Intussusception: Common in children
  - Volvulus: Often results from congenital anomalies or acquired adhesions
  - Foreign bodies: Luminal blockage
  - Gallstone ileus: Passage of a large gallstone through a cholecystenteric fistula
  - Inflammatory bowel disease: Lumen is narrowed by inflammation or fibrosis
  - Stricture-luminal narrowing
  - Cystic fibrosis: Partial obstruction of the distal ileum and right colon
  - Hematoma
  - Paralytic ileus: Neurogenic

CLINICAL FINDINGS

SYMPTOMS AND SIGNS

- Vomiting
- Cramping abdominal pain
- Obstipation
- Distention
  - Minimal in proximal obstruction
  - Pronounced in distal obstruction
- Mild abdominal tenderness
- Audible rushes and high-pitched tinkles

Strangulation Obstruction

- Shock
- High fever
- Abdominal pain: Severe and continuous
- Vomitus may contain blood
- Abdominal tenderness and rigidity

LABORATORY FINDINGS

- Hemoconcentration
- Leukocytosis
- Electrolyte abnormalities that depend on the level of obstruction and the severity of dehydration
- Serum amylase is often elevated

Strangulation Obstruction

- Marked leukocytosis not accounted for by hemoconcentration
- Metabolic acidosis

IMAGING FINDINGS

- **Abdominal x-ray**
  - Dilated bowel
  - Air-fluid levels (minimal in early, proximal, or closed loop obstruction)
- The colon is often devoid of gas
- Intraperitoneal air indicates perforation
- **Contrast upper GI series:** Assesses completeness of obstruction
- **CT scan**
  - Intraperitoneal free fluid
  - Dilated bowel proximal and decompressed distal to the obstruction
  - Point of obstruction may be visualized
- Gas within the bowel wall or portal vein may be seen in strangulation
- Intraperitoneal free air or air-fluid levels indicate perforation

DIAGNOSTIC CONSIDERATIONS

- Classification of small bowel obstruction
- Functional (failure of peristalsis to propel intestinal contents) or mechanical (a physical barrier impedes aboral progress of intestinal contents)
- Complete or partial
- Simple (occludes the lumen only) or strangulated (impaired the blood supply leading to necrosis of the intestine)
- Open loop (the lumen is occluded in 1 place) or closed loop (the lumen is occluded in at least 2 places)
- 33% of strangulation obstructions are unsuspected before operation

RULE OUT

- Acute appendicitis
- Obstruction of the large intestine
- Acute gastroenteritis
- Acute pancreatitis
- Mesenteric vascular occlusion
- Pseudo-obstruction associated with scleroderma, systemic lupus erythematosus, amyloidosis, drug abuse, or radiation
- Intrinsic dysmotility

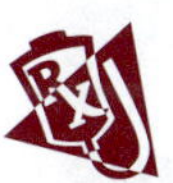

WORK-UP

- Abdominal x-ray
- CBC count
- Serum electrolytes
- ABG measurements (if strangulation suspected)
- Serum amylase and lipase
- Contrast upper GI series or CT scan if diagnosis is in doubt or further information needed

WHEN TO ADMIT

- All cases of acute small bowel obstruction

TREATMENT AND MANAGEMENT

- Partial obstruction can be treated expectantly as long as there is continued passage of stool and flatus; successful in 90% of such patients
- NG decompression

SURGERY

- Details of the operative procedure vary according to the cause of obstruction

Indications

- Persistent incomplete obstruction
- Complete obstruction
- Closed loop obstruction
- Strangulation

Contraindications

- Paralytic ileus
- Abdominal carcinomatosis (relative)
- Inflammatory bowel disease (relative)

MEDICATIONS

- Fluid and electrolyte replacement
- Antibiotics if strangulation is suspected

TREATMENT MONITORING

- Serial abdominal exams
- Serial abdominal x-rays

COMPLICATIONS

- Perforation
- Shock

PROGNOSIS

- Mortality rate in cases of nonstrangulating obstruction is about 2%
- Mortality rate in cases of strangulation obstruction is approximately 8–25%

RESOURCES

REFERENCES

- Jenkins JT. Secondary causes of intestinal obstruction: rigorous preoperative evaluation is required. *Am Surg.* 2000;66:662.
- Miller G et al. Natural history of patients with adhesive small bowel obstruction. *Br J Surg.* 2000;87:1240.

Snakebite

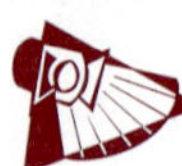

ESSENTIAL FEATURES

- Distinguishing whether the patient has been bitten and envenomed, bitten but not envenomed, or bitten by a nonvenomous snake is critical prior to starting treatments
- Treatments may not only cause discomfort but may also produce serious side effects
- A bite by a venomous snake results in envenomation in only 50–70% of cases
- Degree of envenomation depends on the size of the snake and the duration of contact

VENOMOUS SNAKES

- Indigenous venomous snakes of North America can be placed in 4 groups:
  1. Rattlesnake
  2. Copperhead
  3. Cottonmouth
  4. Coral snake

Pit Vipers

- Include rattlesnakes, copperhead, and cottonmouth
- Can be distinguished from nonvenomous snakes by a round mouth and a pit between the eyes and the nares on each side
- Have retractable canaliculated fangs that can rapidly spring into biting position and deliver venom
- The large venom glands also give the head a triangular or diamond shape
- Have vertically oriented elliptiform irises
- Most deliver a primarily hemotoxic venom
- Hemotoxic effects are mediated by proteolytic enzymes, peptides, and metalloproteins that cause local tissue destruction directly and by intimal injury to blood vessels, followed by thrombosis and necrosis
- Activation of the coagulation cascade can occur at multiple points, resulting in net anticoagulation

Coral Snakes

- Have small mouths, short teeth, and deliver secreted venom into prey through created lacerations
- Bite lacks the characteristic fang marks of bites by pit vipers, sometimes making it hard to detect
- Body coloration pattern is red bands immediately adjacent to yellow bands
- Coral snake venom is primarily neurotoxic
- Neurotoxic venom can cause dysphagia, dysphonia, diplopia, headache, weakness, and respiratory distress

NONVENOMOUS SNAKES

- Most snakebites in the United States are from nonvenomous snakes
- Nonpoisonous snakes such as the red milk snake and the scarlet king snake mimic the bright red, yellow, and black coloration of the coral snake
  - True coral snakes have red bands immediately adjacent to yellow bands
  - The mimics have black bands immediately adjacent to the red bands, thus giving rise to the colloquial mnemonic: "Red on black, venom lack; red on yellow, kill a fellow"

EPIDEMIOLOGY

- About 8000 people are bitten by venomous snakes in the United States each year
- Death from serious envenomation occurs in only 9–15 victims per year in the United States

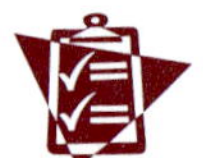

CLINICAL FINDINGS

SYMPTOMS AND SIGNS

- Puncture marks, local ecchymosis and discoloration, vesicles and bullae, and rapid appearance of swelling and edema at the injured area
- Pain of the bite can be quite severe
- Additional signs of hypotension, diaphoresis, nausea, weakness, and faintness are common
- Perioral or peripheral paresthesias, taste changes, and fasciculations
- Signs suggestive of neurotoxic envenomation include dysphagia, dysphonia, diplopia, headache, weakness, and respiratory distress

LABORATORY FINDINGS

- Thrombocytopenia and hypofibrinoginemia
- Myoglobinuria
- Abnormal renal function
- Hemoconcentration initially due to fluid shifts, with later decreases in RBCs and platelets
- UA may show hematuria, glycosuria, and proteinuria
- Prothrombin and partial thromboplastin times are often abnormal

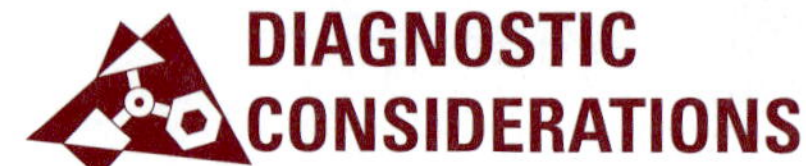

DIAGNOSTIC CONSIDERATIONS

- Distinguish between nonvenomous and venomous snakebite

RULE OUT

- Other or concomitant animal bites

WORK-UP

- Identification of the snake is helpful
- Laboratory evaluation should include blood typing and cross-matching, coagulation studies, a CBC count, serum chemistries, and UA
- Local wound management includes cleansing and disinfection
- Determine degree and manifestations of envenomation as well as time elapsed since the bite
- Determine tetanus prophylaxis status

WHEN TO ADMIT

- Venomous snake bite and its complications: Hemolysis, respiratory failure, paralysis
- Need for additional antivenin administration

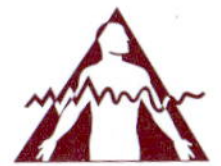

TREATMENT AND MANAGEMENT

- The presence and degree of envenomation dictate treatment
- Wash the bite with soap and water or an antiseptic if available
- Apply a broad, firm compressing bandage over the bite that does not restrict arterial and venous blood flow, and immobilize the bitten area at a level below the heart
- Remove rings and constrictive devices
- Keep patient at rest and warm
- Popular conceptions of first aid measures including tourniquets, wound incision and suction, application of ice, cryotherapy, electrical shock, and ingestion of alcohol are of no proved value and may be hazardous to both the patient and the caregiver
- Bites by nonvenomous snakes are treated as simple puncture wounds, with appropriate use of antitetanus agent
- Systemic measures include administration of antitetanus agent for tetanus prophylaxis and broad-spectrum antibiotic therapy
- Decision to use antivenin is based on identification of the snake as venomous, discernment of the degree and manifestations of envenomation, time elapsed since the bite, and laboratory abnormalities

SURGERY

- Fasciotomy should be reserved for compartment syndrome

Indications

- Elevated compartment pressures or signs suggestive of compartment syndrome require immediate decompression

Contraindications

- Local bite area excision is not usually helpful and should not routinely be done

MEDICATIONS

- Specific antivenins are available for the bites of both pit vipers and Eastern coral snakes
- Crotalidae polyvalent antivenin is effective against all North American pit vipers
- Crotalidae polyvalent antivenin is most effective when given within 4 hours after a bite, of less value after 8 hours, and of questionable value after 30 hours
- North American coral snake antivenin is effective only for the Eastern coral snake
- Coral snake antivenin may be started before any neurologic symptoms manifest if identification is suspected or confirmed
- Antivenin potential side-effects includes both allergic reactions and serum sickness
- Antivenin should ideally be administered early and as a diluted continuous IV infusion; local injection in or around the bite is contraindicated
- Severe envenomations may require over 30 vials; antivenin may be appropriate for moderate envenomation, but the risks outweigh the benefits if envenomation is minimal

TREATMENT MONITORING

- Laboratory evaluation: Coagulation studies, a CBC count, serum chemistry, and UA should be repeated every 8–24 hours

COMPLICATIONS

- Acute hemolytic anemia and acute tubular necrosis
- Bites on extremities may cause subcutaneous tissue destruction and loss of digits
- Myotoxins can cause compromise of muscle compartments from direct myonecrosis
- Systemic effects can include pulmonary edema
- Diffuse bleeding from thrombocytopenia and hypofibrinoginemia (disseminated intravascular coagulation)
- Patients may experience respiratory paralysis, one of the hazards of neurotoxic venom
- Renal failure
- Acute respiratory distress syndrome

PROGNOSIS

- Varies according to the severity of the poisoning, which depends on:
  - Species and size of the snake
  - Location, depth, nature, and number of bites
  - Amount of venom injected
  - Presence of microbes in the snake's mouth
  - Age and size of the patient
  - Patient's sensitivity to the venom
  - Availability of appropriate first-aid treatment and subsequent medical care

RESOURCES

REFERENCES

- Chippaux JP et al. Venoms, antivenoms and immunotherapy. *Toxicon.* 1998;36:823.
- Gold BS et al. Snake venom poisoning in the United States: a review of therapeutic practice. *South Med J.* 1994;87:579.

Soft Tissue Sarcoma

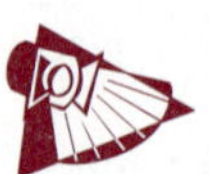

ESSENTIAL FEATURES

- Soft-tissue sarcomas present as asymptomatic large masses in the extremities or retroperitoneum but may also develop occasionally in the neck or within the abdominal viscera
- Originate from a wide variety of mesenchymal cell types and include:
  - Liposarcoma
  - Fibrosarcoma
  - Rhabdomyosarcoma
  - Leiomyosarcoma
  - Desmoid tumors
- Sarcomas tend to behave in a fashion dictated by the tumor grade rather than the cell of origin
- Most soft-tissue sarcomas arise de novo, and rarely do they result from malignant degeneration of a benign lesion
- Sarcomas generally metastasize via a hematogenous route, most commonly to the lung
- Most important prognostic factors include tumor size and grade

EPIDEMIOLOGY

- Account for 1% of all new cancer diagnoses
- 50% of soft-tissue sarcomas arise in the lower extremities, most commonly in the thigh
- There are familial syndromes that genetically predispose patients to the formation of soft-tissue sarcomas:
  - Gardner syndrome: Desmoid tumors
  - Recklinghausen disease: Neurofibrosarcomas
  - Li Fraumeni syndrome
- Risk factors include:
  - Irradiation
  - Chronic extremity lymphedema

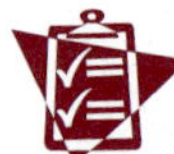

CLINICAL FINDINGS

SYMPTOMS AND SIGNS

- Asymptomatic large soft-tissue mass
- Nerve compression/invasion may result in pain, parasthesias, or neuropathy
- Venous compression/invasion may result in deep venous thrombosis (DVT) formation

IMAGING FINDINGS

- **Chest film:** May demonstrate evidence of metastases
- **CT scan:** Demonstrates a homogenous soft-tissue density mass and differentiate between hematoma or abscess
- **MRI**
  - Accurately defines the extent of the sarcoma and invasion of surrounding structures
  - Probably the best imaging test in the evaluation of an extremity sarcoma

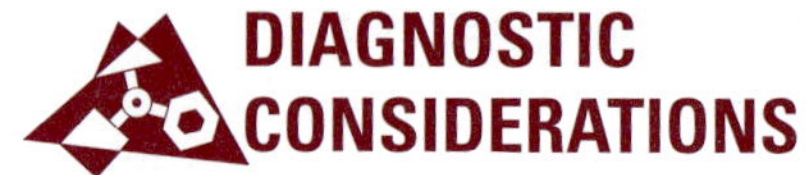

DIAGNOSTIC CONSIDERATIONS

- Soft-tissue sarcoma
- Traumatic injury
- Hematoma
- Cutaneous neoplasm/metastasis
- Desmoid tumor
- Subcutaneous or intramuscular lipoma
- Abscess

RULE OUT

- Other cutaneous malignancy or metastasis
- Hematoma
- Abscess

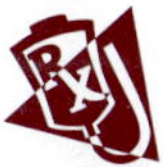

WORK-UP

- Thorough history and physical exam
- Core needle or incisional biopsy to establish diagnosis
- CT or MRI (preferred) to define extent of tumor and invasion of surrounding structures
- Chest film or CT to evaluate for evidence of pulmonary metastases

WHEN TO ADMIT

- Extremity sarcoma work-up can be performed as an outpatient

WHEN TO REFER

- A multidisciplinary approach is essential to ensure optimal outcomes, including an oncology surgeon, medical oncology, and radiation-oncology

TREATMENT AND MANAGEMENT

- Establish diagnosis histologically with a core needle biopsy or incisional biopsy
- Radiographically define extent of tumor and invasion of surrounding structures
- Evaluate for pulmonary metastases
- Surgical wide local excision with a 2 cm margin
- Postoperative radiation therapy for all high-grade sarcomas and those > 2 cm
- Sometimes adjuvant chemotherapy
- Preoperative radiation therapy for patients with tumors larger than 10 cm or to facilitate limb-sparing procedures

SURGERY

Indications

- Initial incisional biopsy to establish diagnosis (always orientate extremity incision longitudinally)
- Therapeutic wide local excision, ideally with 2 cm margin vs amputation in patients whose tumors cannot be resected adequately by wide excision
- Resection of pulmonary metastases in patients who have achieved local control and have fewer than 4 lesions
- Resection of local recurrences in patients without evidence of metastases

MEDICATIONS

- Results of clinical trials using adjuvant chemotherapy in soft-tissue sarcomas are conflicting and no clear survival benefit has been demonstrated

TREATMENT MONITORING

- Physical exam with or without radiographic evaluation to detect local recurrence
- Serial chest films to evaluate for pulmonary metastases

COMPLICATIONS

- Local recurrence
- Systemic disease
- Resection of vital local structures

PROGNOSIS

- More than 50% of all people with soft-tissue sarcoma will eventually die of the cancer
- Most local recurrences occur in the first 2 years after resection

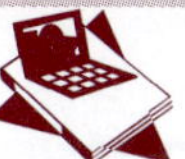

RESOURCES

PREFERENCES

- Brennan MF et al. The role of multimodality therapy in soft-tissue sarcoma. *Ann Surg.* 1991;214:328.
- Gadd MA et al. Development and treatment of pulmonary metastases in adult patients with extremity soft tissue sarcoma. *Ann Surg.* 1993;218:705.

PRACTICE GUIDELINES

- The National Comprehensive Cancer Network http://www.nccn.org

CANCER STAGING

- See Soft Tissue Sarcoma Staging Table on page 755.

STAGE GROUPING

Stage I	T1a, 1b, 2a, 2b	N0	M0
	G1-2	G1	Low
Stage II	T1a, 1b, 2a	N0	M0
	G3-4	G2-3	High
Stage III	T2b	N0	M0
	G3-4	G2-3	High
Stage IV	Any T	N1	M0
	Any G	Any G	High or Low
	Any T	N0	M1
	Any G	Any G	High or Low

Somatostatinoma

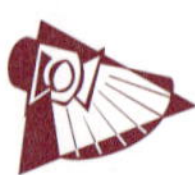

ESSENTIAL FEATURES

- Diabetes mellitus (usually mild)
- Diarrhea
- Malabsorption
- Dilation of the gallbladder (usually with cholelithiasis)
- Hypochlorhydria
- Weight loss

EPIDEMIOLOGY

- Account for 1–2% of pancreatic islet cell tumors
- The syndrome results from secretion of somatostatin by an islet cell tumor of the pancreas
- Most tumors are malignant and accompanied by hepatic, regional lymph node, and bone metastases
- Mean age of presentation is 50 years
- Men and women are affected equally
- The lesion is usually large and readily demonstrated by CT scan

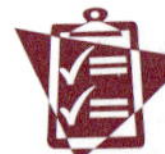

CLINICAL FINDINGS

SYMPTOMS AND SIGNS

- Diarrhea
- Steatorrhea
- Weight loss

LABORATORY FINDINGS

- Increased plasma level of somatostatin

IMAGING FINDINGS

- The lesion is usually large and readily demonstrated by CT scan
- Abdominal US may show gallbladder dilation with cholelithiasis

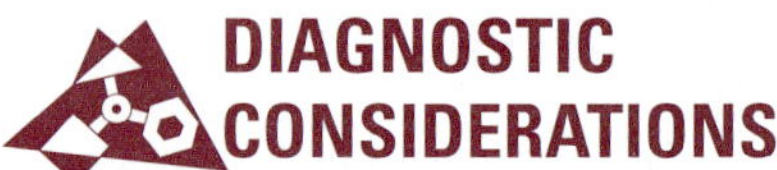

DIAGNOSTIC CONSIDERATIONS

- The diagnosis may be made by recognizing the clinical syndrome and measuring increased concentrations of somatostatin in the serum
- Small somatostatin-rich tumors of the duodenum or ampulla of Vater have also been reported, but none of these lesions have been associated with high serum levels of somatostatin or the clinical syndrome

RULE OUT

- Other islet cell tumors of the pancreas
- Other causes of diarrhea and malabsorption

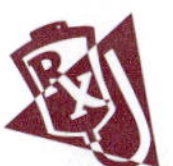

WORK-UP

- Serum somatostatin level
- CT scan for localization and staging

WHEN TO ADMIT

- Severe symptoms

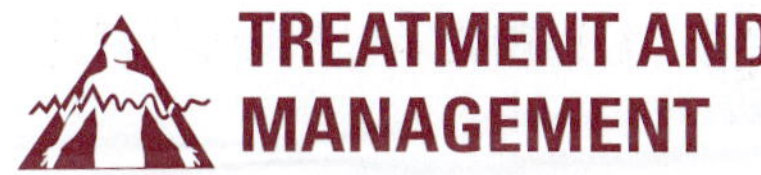

TREATMENT AND MANAGEMENT

SURGERY

- Enucleation is inappropriate for these tumors and a pancreaticoduodenectomy should be performed for lesions located in the head of the pancreas

Indications

- All patients with technically resectable lesions
- Debulking of hepatic metastases is indicated for relief of symptoms

Contraindications

- Technically unresectable

MEDICATIONS

- Chemotherapy with streptozocin, dacarbazine, or doxorubicin for unresectable tumors

PROGNOSIS

- When the disease is localized, resection is able to cure about 50% of patients

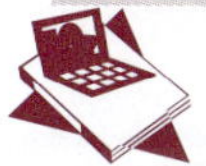

RESOURCES

REFERENCES

- Soga J, Yakuwa Y. Somatostatinoma/inhibitory syndrome: a statistical evaluation of 173 reported cases as compared to other pancreatic endocrinomas. *J Exp Clin Cancer Res.* 1999;18:13.

Spherocytosis

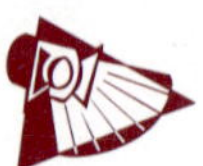

ESSENTIAL FEATURES

- Malaise, abdominal discomfort
- Jaundice, anemia, splenomegaly
- Increased osmotic fragility of red cells, negative Coombs test

EPIDEMIOLOGY

- The most common congenital hemolytic anemia, affecting 1:5000 persons
- Transmitted as an autosomal dominant trait
- Caused by deficiency of spectrin and ankyrin, erythrocyte membrane proteins, which maintain cellular osmotic stability and prevent splenic destruction
- The normal shape of the erythrocyte is changed from a biconcave disk into a sphere, which causes a lack of deformability and delays passage through the channels of the splenic red pulp
- Significant cell destruction occurs only in the presence of the spleen
- Usually diagnosed in the first 3 decades; in occasional instances the diagnosis is not made until later in adult life

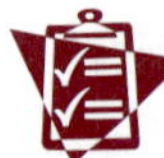

CLINICAL FINDINGS

SYMPTOMS AND SIGNS

- Mild to moderate anemia
- Jaundice
- Easy fatigability
- Discomfort in the left upper quadrant
- Splenomegaly

LABORATORY FINDINGS

- Decreased RBC count and hemoglobin
- Negative Coombs test
- Spherocytes on a Wright-stained smear
- Increased reticulocyte count (5–20%)
- Elevated indirect serum bilirubin and stool urobilinogen
- Decreased or absent serum haptoglobin
- Increased osmotic fragility, best demonstrated by the cryohemolysis test

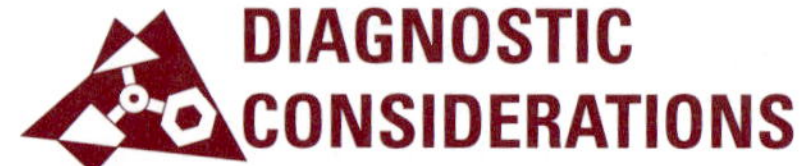

DIAGNOSTIC CONSIDERATIONS

- Periodic exacerbations of hemolysis can occur
- The rare hypoplastic crises, which often follow acute viral illnesses, may be associated with profound anemia, headache, nausea, abdominal pain, pancytopenia, and hypoactive marrow
- Pigment gallstones occur in about 85% of adults with spherocytosis but are uncommon under age 10
  - Gallstones in a child should suggest congenital spherocytosis

RULE OUT

- Spherocytes in large numbers may occur in autoimmune hemolytic anemias, in which osmotic fragility and autohemolysis may be increased
- Spherocytes are also seen in hemoglobin C disease, in some alcoholics, and in some severe burns

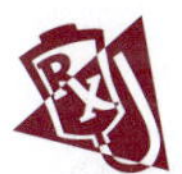

WORK-UP

- CBC count
- Wright stain peripheral smear
- Coombs test
- Tests of osmotic fragility: Cryohemolysis test

WHEN TO ADMIT

- Hemolytic crisis

WHEN TO REFER

- Should be managed in conjunction with a hematologist

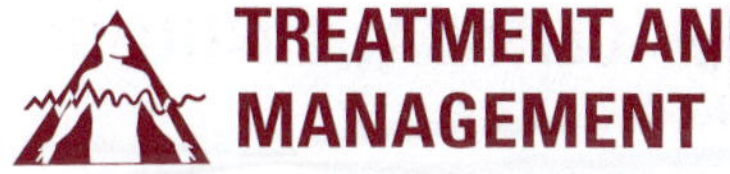

TREATMENT AND MANAGEMENT

SURGERY

- Splenectomy
- When there is associated cholelithiasis, cholecystectomy should be performed along with the splenectomy

Indications

- All patients older than 6 years, even if asymptomatic

Contraindications

- Children younger than 6 years: High risk of infection; if high transfusion requirements, partial splenectomy

TREATMENT MONITORING

- CBC count
- Haptoglobin level
- Serum bilirubin

COMPLICATIONS

- Pigment gallstones
- Chronic leg ulcers

PROGNOSIS

- Splenectomy cures anemia and jaundice; the membrane abnormality, and increased osmotic fragility persist, but RBC life span is almost normal

RESOURCES

REFERENCES

- Marchetti M et al. Prophylactic splenectomy and cholecystectomy in mild hereditary spherocytosis: analyzing the decision in different clinical scenarios. *J Intern Med.* 1998;244:217.

Splenic Abscess

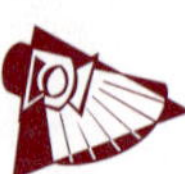

ESSENTIAL FEATURES

- Abdominal pain, tenderness, peritonitis, and sepsis may be present
- CT scan demonstrates fluid-filled lesion, possibly containing gas
- May be caused by:
  - Hematogenous seeding of the spleen with bacteria from remote septic focus (endocarditis, intra-abdominal infection)
  - Direct spread of infection from adjacent structures (pancreatic or perinephric abscess, diverticulitis, colon or gastric perforation)
  - Splenic trauma or infarction with secondarily infected hematoma or necrotic parenchyma
- Complication of injection drug abuse and immunosuppression (AIDS, chemotherapy, transplant, corticosteroid use)

EPIDEMIOLOGY

- 65% of cases are solitary and unilocular; 8% are solitary and multiloculated
- Multiple abscesses are present in 27% of cases
- *Staphylococcus* species, 20%; *Salmonella,* 15%; anaerobic bacteria, 15%; *E coli,* 10–15%; *Streptococcus* species, 10%; *Enterococcus* species, 5–10%

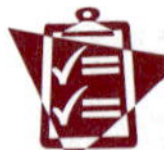

CLINICAL FINDINGS

SYMPTOMS AND SIGNS

- Abdominal pain
- Fever
- Left upper quadrant abdominal tenderness
- Peritonitis with guarding and rebound tenderness
- Palpable spleen

LABORATORY FINDINGS

- Leukocytosis

IMAGING FINDINGS

- **Abdominal x-ray:** Soft-tissue mass in left upper quadrant, displaced gastric bubble, extraluminal gas, elevated left hemidiaphragm
- **Chest film:** Basilar atelectasis, left pleural effusion
- **CT scan:** Nonenhancing, low-density lesion containing gas and fluid levels

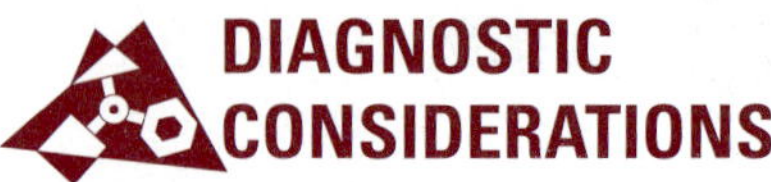

DIAGNOSTIC CONSIDERATIONS

- A left pleural effusion combined with unexplained leukocytosis in a septic patient suggests a splenic abscess
- In some patients, unexplained sepsis, progressive splenic enlargement, and abdominal pain are the presenting manifestations
- Gas in the spleen on radiographic imaging is pathognomonic of splenic abscess
- Most splenic abscesses remain localized, but spontaneous rupture and peritonitis may occur

RULE OUT

- Subphrenic abscess
- Perinephric abscess
- Splenic tumor or cyst

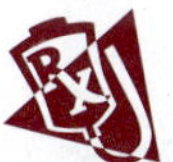

WORK-UP

- CT scan
- CBC count
- Blood cultures
- Culture of abscess fluid

WHEN TO ADMIT

- Peritonitis
- Sepsis

TREATMENT AND MANAGEMENT

- Broad-spectrum antibiotics

SURGERY

- Splenectomy is essential for cure if sepsis is localized to the spleen
- Percutaneous drainage of large, solitary juxtacapsular abscesses may be feasible

Indications

- All abscesses

MEDICATIONS

- Broad-spectrum antibiotics

COMPLICATIONS

- Spontaneous rupture and peritonitis

PROGNOSIS

- 85–95% of cases treated successfully with splenectomy
- 75% treated successfully with percutaneous drainage

RESOURCES

REFERENCES

- Phillips GS et al. Splenic abscess: another look at an old disease. *Arch Surg.* 1997;132:1331.

Splenic Cysts & Tumors

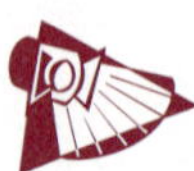

ESSENTIAL FEATURES

- Many discovered incidentally on CT scan or during laparotomy or laparoscopy
- Splenomegaly and left upper quadrant abdominal pain may be present
- CT scan shows evidence of splenic mass
- Low diagnostic yield by percutaneous needle aspiration or core needle biopsy

EPIDEMIOLOGY

- **Malignant primary tumors**
  - Non-Hodgkin lymphoma (NHL): Most common; disease limited to the spleen
  - Angiosarcomas: Rapid growth and early metastases; may rupture
- **Malignant metastatic tumors:** Usually represent widespread dissemination
- **Benign splenic tumors**
  - Hemangiomas: Most common; splenomegaly uncommon; may rupture
  - Lymphangiomas: Typically affect children and young adults
  - Inflammatory pseudotumor: Infiltrative; may mimic a malignant process
- **Splenic cysts**
  - True parasitic cysts (5%); usually hydatid—*Echinococcus granulosus*
  - True nonparasitic cysts (20%); epidermoid is most common
  - Pseudocysts (80%); post-trauma or infarction

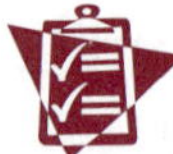

CLINICAL FINDINGS

SYMPTOMS AND SIGNS

- NHL: Splenomegaly, constitutional symptoms
- Angiosarcomas: Abdominal pain, palpable abdominal mass
- Metastatic tumors: Splenomegaly
- Hemangiomas: Usually asymptomatic
- Lymphangiomas: Usually asymptomatic
- Inflammatory pseudotumor: Fever, malaise, weight loss
- True parasitic cysts: Abdominal pain
- True nonparasitic cysts: Abdominal pressure or pain
- Pseudocysts: Abdominal pain, splenomegaly

LABORATORY FINDINGS

- NHL: Anemia, thrombocytopenia, leukopenia due to hypersplenism
- Angiosarcoma: Angiopathic hemolytic anemia
- Hemangioma: May cause consumptive coagulopathy, thrombocytopenia, microangiopathic anemia, disseminated intravascular coagulation
- True parasitic cysts: Positive serologic test for *E granulosus*

IMAGING FINDINGS

- **CT scan:** Splenic mass
- NHL: Splenomegaly with solitary mass (> 5 cm) or multiple masses
- Angiosarcoma: Solitary mass with central tumor necrosis
- Hemangioma: Well circumscribed nodules with enhancement; cystic changes and calcifications
- Lymphangiomas: Cystic with multiple septations
- True parasitic cysts: Unilocular, calcified splenic mass with daughter cysts
- Pseudocysts: Round, well circumscribed unilocular cyst; may have a calcified rim

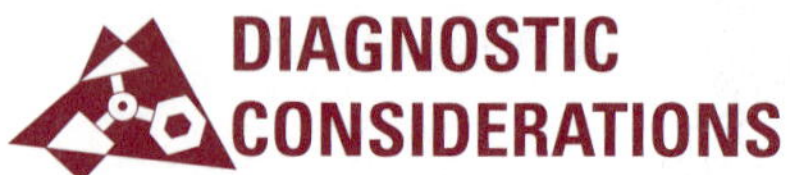

DIAGNOSTIC CONSIDERATIONS

- Some clinicians advocate splenectomy for all splenic masses in order to avoid undertreatment of potential malignancy
- Poor diagnostic yield with percutaneous needle aspiration or core needle biopsy
- NHL: Peripheral adenopathy and bone marrow involvement occur late in the disease
- Rupture of splenic parasitic cysts can cause dissemination of scoleces and anaphylaxis

RULE OUT

- Malignant splenic tumor

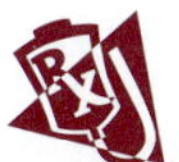

WORK-UP

- CT scan
- CBC count to evaluate for hypersplenism
- Serologic test for *E granulosus* if suspected
- Biopsy not usually indicated

WHEN TO ADMIT

- Severe abdominal pain
- Secondary splenic infection
- High risk of rupture

TREATMENT AND MANAGEMENT

SURGERY

- Splenectomy for all primary malignant tumors and parasitic cysts
- Partial or complete splenectomy for benign tumors and cysts if symptomatic, risk for rupture, or otherwise indicated

Indications

- Symptomatic: Abdominal pain, splenomegaly, hypersplenism with cytopenia
- Metastatic tumors: If solitary
- Pseudocyst: Symptoms or > 10 cm

MEDICATIONS

- NHL: Chemotherapy with or without radiation
- Albendazole for infection with *E granulosus*

COMPLICATIONS

- Tumors: Splenic rupture, bleeding
- Cysts: Splenic or cyst rupture, bacterial superinfection
- Parasitic cyst: Anaphylaxis if rupture

PROGNOSIS

- NHL: Similar to other forms of NHL
- Angiosarcomas: Poor
- Benign tumors and cysts: Cured with splenectomy

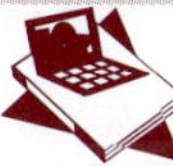

RESOURCES

REFERENCES

- Du Plessis DG et al. Mucinous epithelial cysts of the spleen associated with pseudomyxoma peritonei. *Histopathology.* 1999;35:551.
- Dawes LG et al. Cystic masses of the spleen. *Am Surg.* 1986;52:333.

Splenic Neoplasms

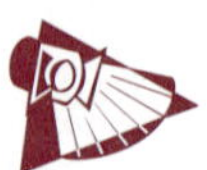

ESSENTIAL FEATURES

- Splenic involvement (splenomegaly and hypersplenism) due to infiltration of lymphocytes or mast cells or initiation of extramedullary hematopeosis
- Splenomegaly and hypersplenism, resulting in anemia, thrombocytopenia, and/or neutropenia
- Splenectomy may be indicated for hypersplenism, for diagnosis, or for primary surgical removal of the predominant or only site of disease

EPIDEMIOLOGY

Chronic Lymphocytic Leukemia (CLL)

- Neoplasm of B cells characterized by bone marrow and splenic infiltration of lymphocytes that are mature morphologically but functionally incompetent

Hairy Cell Leukemia (HCL)

- A low-grade lymphoproliferative disorder with characteristic "hairy cells" that infiltrate the bone marrow and spleen
- Patients are typically middle aged men

Idiopathic Myelofibrosis

- Results in extensive bone marrow fibrosis and extramedullary hematopoiesis in the spleen and liver

Mast Cell Disease (MCD)

- Rare condition characterized by mast cell infiltration of a number of tissues, including the spleen

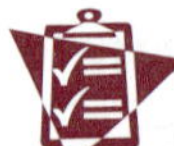

CLINICAL FINDINGS

SYMPTOMS AND SIGNS

CLL

- Fatigue
- Splenomegaly
- Lymphadenopathy
- Bleeding

HCL

- Splenomegaly
- Infections
- Bleeding
- Fatigue

Idiopathic Myelofibrosis

- Weakness and fatigue
- Dyspnea
- Splenomegaly
- Abdominal fullness and pain
- Bleeding
- Infection

MCD

- Splenomegaly
- Bleeding

LABORATORY FINDINGS

CLL

- Lymphocytosis
- Thrombocytopenia and anemia

HCL

- Pancytopenia
- Hairy cells on bone marrow biopsy and peripheral smear

Idiopathic Myelofibrosis

- Anemia
- Leukocytosis or leukopenia
- Thrombocytosis or thrombocytopenia
- Leukoerythroblastic peripheral smear with teardrop poikilocytosis
- Giant abnormal platelets

MCD

- Thrombocytopenia

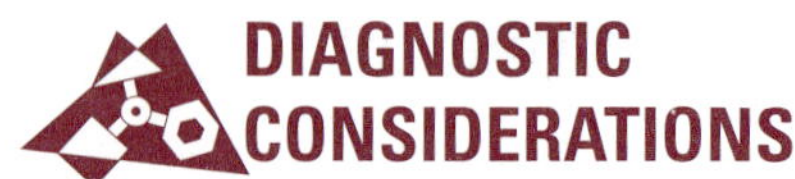

DIAGNOSTIC CONSIDERATIONS

CLL, HCL, and MCD

- Cytopenias due to a combination of bone marrow and splenic infiltration with secondary hypersplenism

Idiopathic Myelofibrosis

- Pain over the spleen from splenic infarcts is common
- Portal hypertension develops in some cases as a result of fibrosis of the liver, greatly increased splenic blood flow, or both

RULE OUT

- Other causes of hypersplenism and cytopenias (Waldenstrom macroglobulinemia, non-Hodgkin lymphoma, Hodgkin disease, chronic myelogenous leukemia)

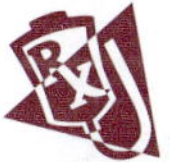

WORK-UP

- CBC count
- Peripheral blood smear
- Bone marrow biopsy and aspiration (may be a dry tap in idiopathic myelofibrosis due to bone marrow fibrosis)

WHEN TO ADMIT

- Severe anemia, leukemia, thrombocytopenia
- Bleeding

WHEN TO REFER

- All disorders should be managed in conjunction with an hematologist

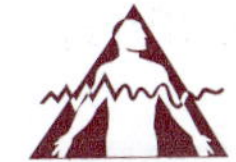

TREATMENT AND MANAGEMENT

SURGERY

- Splenectomy

Indications

- Splenomegaly with abdominal pain
- Hypersplenism with cytopenias
- Adjunct to medical treatment
- Failure of medical treatment
- Portal hypertension (idiopathic myelofibrosis)

MEDICATIONS

CLL

- Chlorambucil, prednisone

HCL

- Cladribine, pentostatin

Idiopathic Myelofibrosis

- Androgens

TREATMENT MONITORING

- CBC count

PROGNOSIS

- Splenectomy relieves symptoms of splenomegaly in most cases; cytopenias are corrected in 50–75% of cases.
- 80–95% of patients with HCL respond to medical therapy

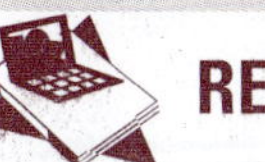

RESOURCES

REFERENCES

- Thiruvengadam R et al. Splenectomy in advanced chronic lymphocytic leukemia. *Leukemia.* 1990;4:758.
- Pettit AR et al. Hairy-cell leukemia: biology and management. *Br J Hematol.* 1999;106:2.
- Austen KF. Systemic mastocytosis. *N Engl J Med.* 1992;326:639.

Splenic Vein Thrombosis

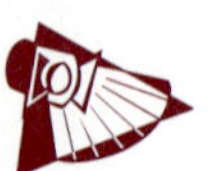

ESSENTIAL FEATURES

- Upper GI hemorrhage with evidence of gastric varices without esophageal varices
- History of pancreatic or gastric disease
- Splenectomy is curative

EPIDEMIOLOGY

- Isolated thrombosis in the splenic vein, diverting the splenic venous outflow to the short gastric vessels as collaterals
- Increased pressure in the short gastric (left-sided or sinistral portal hypertension) veins causes dilation of the submucosal venous plexus in the gastric cardia and fundus, leading to gastric varices
- 50% of cases due to pancreatitis or pancreatic pseudocyst
- Pancreatic cancer with splenic vein invasion is the second most common cause
- Penetrating posterior gastric ulcer and retroperitoneal fibrosis are less common causes

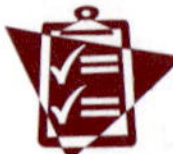

CLINICAL FINDINGS

SYMPTOMS AND SIGNS

- Upper GI hemorrhage
- Splenomegaly may be present

LABORATORY FINDINGS

- Anemia if bleeding is present

IMAGING FINDINGS

- **Gastroscopy:** Bleeding from isolated gastric varices, without evidence of esophageal varices
- **Conventional or magnetic resonance angiography:** Absence of flow through splenic vein, with collateralization through the short gastric veins

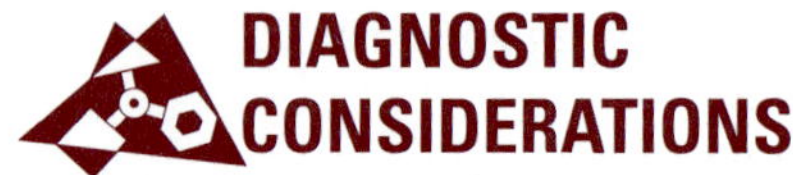

DIAGNOSTIC CONSIDERATIONS

- Splenic vein thrombosis should be suspected in any patient with upper GI hemorrhage and isolated gastric, without esophageal varices at endoscopy

RULE OUT

- Portal hypertension
- Other sources of upper GI bleeding

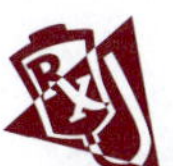

WORK-UP

- Upper GI endoscopy
- Conventional or magnetic resonance angiography (if indicated to make a definitive diagnosis)

WHEN TO ADMIT

- Active bleeding

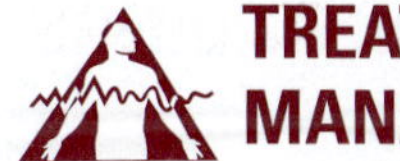

TREATMENT AND MANAGEMENT

SURGERY

- Splenectomy is curative
- Even if the patient is asymptomatic and has not experienced an upper GI bleed, splenectomy should be performed electively

Indications

- All cases

COMPLICATIONS

- Upper GI bleeding

PROGNOSIS

- Splenectomy is curative

RESOURCES

REFERENCES

- Loftus JP et al. Sinistral portal hypertension. Splenectomy or expectant management. *Ann Surg.* 1993;217:35.

Splenosis

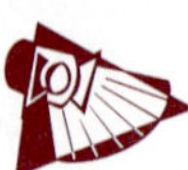

ESSENTIAL FEATURES

- Multiple small implants of splenic tissue disseminated throughout the abdomen following traumatic splenic rupture
- By themselves, splenic implants are of little clinical significance
- Multiple small implants of splenic tissue grow in scattered areas on the peritoneal surfaces throughout the abdomen arising from dissemination and autotransplantation of splenic fragments following traumatic rupture of the spleen
- Usually an incidental finding discovered much later during laparotomy for an unrelated problem
- Splenic implants are capable of cell culling and some immunologic function
- The implants stimulate formation of adhesions and may be a cause of intestinal obstruction

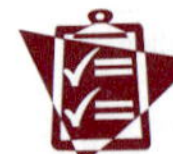

CLINICAL FINDINGS

SYMPTOMS AND SIGNS

- Asymptomatic

LABORATORY FINDINGS

- Absence of Howell-Jolly bodies: Characteristic post-splenectomy RBC nuclear remnants that are typically removed by the spleen

IMAGING FINDINGS

- **CT scan:** May be visualized as small peritoneal or mesenteric nodules

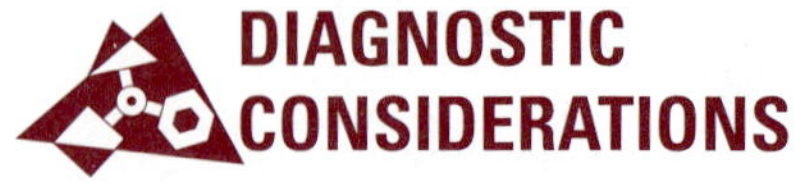

DIAGNOSTIC CONSIDERATIONS

RULE OUT

- Splenosis must be distinguished from peritoneal nodules of metastatic carcinoma and from accessory spleens
- Histologically, they differ from accessory spleens by the absence of elastic or smooth muscle fibers in the delicate capsule

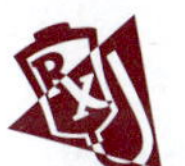

WORK-UP

- None needed

WHEN TO ADMIT

- If complicated by bowel obstruction

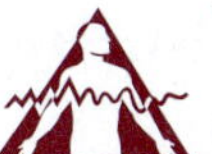

TREATMENT AND MANAGEMENT

- No treatment warranted for uncomplicated splenosis

COMPLICATIONS

- Bowel obstruction

PROGNOSIS

- Usually an incidental finding of little significance

RESOURCES

REFERENCES

- Pisters PWT et al. Autologous splenic transplantation for splenic trauma. *Ann Surg.* 1994;219:225.
- Timens W et al. Splenic autotransplantation and the immune system. *Ann Surg.* 1993;215:256.

Stress Ulcer

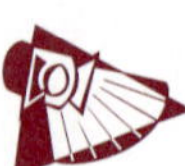

ESSENTIAL FEATURES

- Physiologically stressful illness
- Upper GI bleeding
- Acute gastric or duodenal ulcers
- 4 major etiologic factors
  1. Shock
  2. Sepsis
  3. Burns (Curling ulcers)
  4. CNS tumors or trauma (Cushing ulcers)

EPIDEMIOLOGY

- Clinically apparent ulcers develop in about 20% of susceptible patients
- Perforation occurs in 10% of cases
- Most stress ulcers develop in the stomach; 30% in the duodenum; sometimes both are involved
- Decreased mucosal resistance is the first step, which may involve the effects of ischemia and circulating toxins, followed by decreased mucosal renewal, decreased production of endogenous prostanoids, and thinning of the surface mucus layer
- Acute ulcers associated with CNS tumors or injuries differ from other stress ulcers with elevated serum gastrin and gastric acid secretion

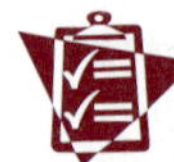

CLINICAL FINDINGS

SYMPTOMS AND SIGNS

- Hemorrhage is nearly always the first manifestation
- Pain rarely occurs
- Physical exam is not contributory except to reveal gross or occult fecal blood or signs of shock
- Clinically evident bleeding is usually seen 3–5 days after the injury, and massive bleeding generally does not appear until 4–5 days later

LABORATORY FINDINGS

- Anemia
- Elevated gastrin and gastric acid secretion with Cushing ulcers

IMAGING FINDINGS

- **Gastroduodenal endoscopy:** Shows shallow, discreet ulcers in the stomach, duodenum, or both

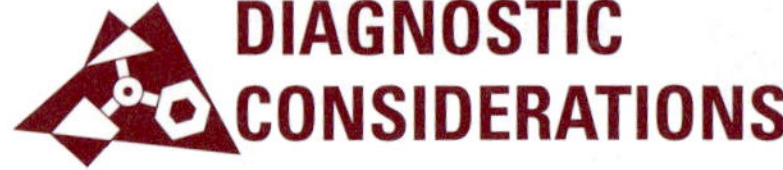

DIAGNOSTIC CONSIDERATIONS

- Any patient with recent history of shock, sepsis, burns, or CNS tumors or trauma and upper GI bleeding should undergo gastroduodenal endoscopy to evaluate for stress ulcers
- All patients at risk for stress ulcers should receive pharmacologic ulcer prophylaxis

RULE OUT

- Other causes of GI hemorrhage

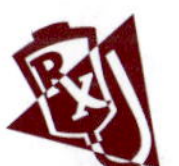

WORK-UP

- Evidence of GI bleeding
  - NG aspiration of blood confirms upper GI source
- Endoscopy to confirm bleeding ulcer as source

WHEN TO ADMIT

- Patients with antecedent physiologic stress necessary for development of stress ulcer will already be hospitalized

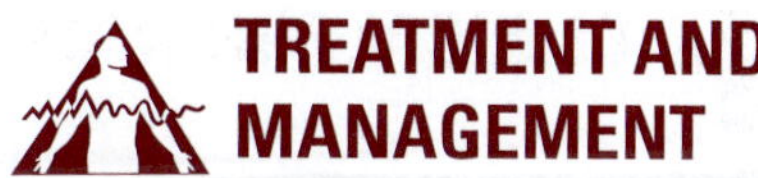

TREATMENT AND MANAGEMENT

SURGERY

- Gastric lavage
- Endoscopic treatment of bleeding ulcers
- Suture the bleeding points, vagotomy, and antrectomy or pyloroplasty
- Rarely, total gastrectomy is necessary
- Infusion of vasopressin into the left gastric artery through a percutaneously placed catheter may be useful

Indications

- Failure of nonoperative treatment

MEDICATIONS

- H_2-receptor blockers may decrease the rate of rebleeding
- Blood and/or crystalloid infusion as indicated

TREATMENT MONITORING

- Monitor clinical signs of ongoing bleeding, such as bloody NG aspirate and decreasing Hct

COMPLICATIONS

- Rebleeding
- Perforation
- Obstruction

PROGNOSIS

- Overall mortality determined largely by underlying disease

PREVENTION

- H_2-receptor antagonists or sulcrate given prophylactically to critically ill patients

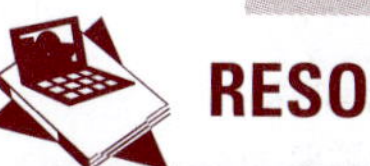

RESOURCES

REFERENCES

- Felig DM, Carafa CJ. Stress ulcers of the stomach. *Gastrointest Endosc.* 2000;51:596.

Superior Mesenteric Artery Obstruction of the Duodenum

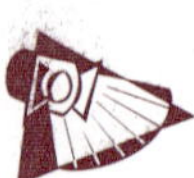

ESSENTIAL FEATURES

- Obstruction of the third portion of the duodenum by compression between the superior mesenteric vessels and the aorta

EPIDEMIOLOGY

- Most commonly appears after rapid weight loss following injury or burns
- Acute loss of mesenteric fat is thought to permit the artery to drop posteriorly, trapping the bowel like in a pair scissors
- Often the patient is a thin, nervous woman whose complaints of dyspepsia and occasional emesis are more properly explained on a functional basis

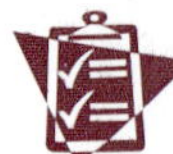

CLINICAL FINDINGS

SYMPTOMS AND SIGNS

- Epigastric bloating
- Crampy pain relieved by vomiting
- Symptoms may remit in the prone position
- Anorexia and postprandial pain lead to additional malnutrition and weight loss

IMAGING FINDINGS

- **Upper GI contrast radiography**
  - Demonstrates a widened duodenum proximal to a sharp obstruction where the artery crosses the third portion of the duodenum, as well as increased duodenal peristalsis proximal to the arterial blockage
  - When the patient moves to the knee-chest position, the passage of contrast material is suddenly unimpeded
- **Angiography**
  - Shows an angle of 25 degrees or less between the superior mesenteric artery and the aorta
  - Not recommended for routine evaluation of obvious cases

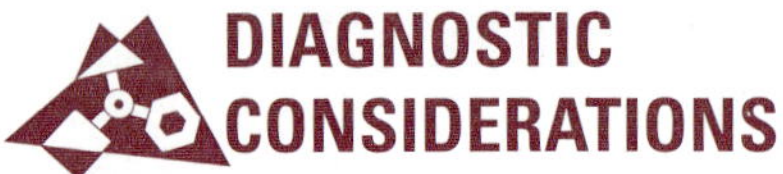

DIAGNOSTIC CONSIDERATIONS

- Onset of epigastric bloating and crampy pain relieved by vomiting following rapid weight loss should be evaluated by upper GI contrast radiography

RULE OUT

- Intestinal malrotation with duodenal obstruction by congenital bands
- Involvement of the duodenum by scleroderma with diminished duodenal peristalsis

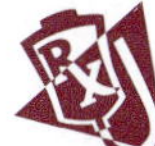

WORK-UP

- Signs and symptoms consistent with duodenal obstruction, particularly in the setting of rapid weight loss should prompt upper GI contrast radiography
- Upper GI contrast radiography will confirm the diagnosis in most cases

WHEN TO ADMIT

- High-grade obstruction with vomiting and inability to tolerate enteral nutrition
- Severe abdominal pain

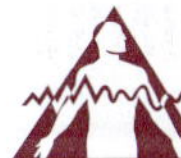

TREATMENT AND MANAGEMENT

- Postural therapy may suffice
  - The patient should be placed prone in the knee-chest position when symptomatic or in anticipation of postprandial difficulties

SURGERY

Indications

- Chronic obstruction: Division of suspensory ligament and mobilization of duodenum, or duodenojejunostomy
- Malrotation: Mobilization of the duodenojejunal flexure

PROGNOSIS

- Surgical correction produces good long-term results

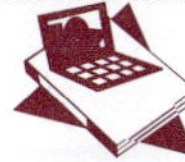

RESOURCES

REFERENCES

- Diwakaran HH et al. Superior mesenteric artery syndrome. *Gastroenterology.* 2001;121:516, 746.
- Richardson WS, Surowiec WJ. Laparoscopic repair of superior mesenteric artery syndrome. *Am J Surg.* 2001;181:377.

Superior Vena Cava (SVC) Syndrome

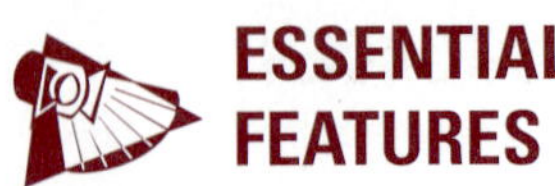

ESSENTIAL FEATURES

SVC Syndrome

- 80–90% caused by malignant tumors
  - Lung cancer (90%)
  - Thymoma
  - Hodgkin disease
  - Lymphosarcoma
  - Metastatic melanoma
  - Breast or thyroid cancer
- Benign tumors unusual
  - Substernal goiter
  - Large benign mediastinal masses
  - Atrial myxoma
- The following thrombotic conditions are unusual causes:
  - Polycythemia
  - Mediastinal infection
  - Indwelling catheters
- Trauma may produce acute obstruction
- Clinical presentation varies with: abruptness of onset, extend of occlusion, collateral pathways
- Venous pressure in arms/head: 200– 500 mm H_2O
- Severity of symptoms correlates with pressure
- Cerebral edema can occur with complete obstruction
- Symptoms milder with patent azygous vein
- Azygous venous flow can increase to 35% of venous return (normal is 11%)
- Thrombus can propagate proximally to innominate and axillary veins

EPIDEMIOLOGY

- 80–90% caused by malignant tumors
- Lung cancer 90% of malignant tumors
- Incidence is 3–5% in lung cancer patients
- Male:female ratio is 5:1
- Malignant SVC obstruction: 35% have thrombosis of innominate or axillary vein, 15% have complete caval obstruction without thrombosis, 50% have partial SVC obstruction

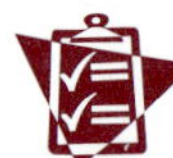

CLINICAL FINDINGS

SYMPTOMS AND SIGNS

- Nasal congestion often earliest symptom
- Swelling in face, arms, shoulders
- Blue/purple discoloration of skin
- Headache, nausea, dizziness, vomiting, vision changes, drowsiness, stupor
- Cough, hoarseness, dyspnea (edema of vocal cords)
- Symptoms may be worse when patient lies on back or bends forward
- Esophageal varices may develop: GI bleeding
- Neck, arm veins may be visibly distended
- Fibrosing mediastinitis: Early morning edema of face and head
- Unilateral symptoms suggest ipsilateral occlusion
- Effort thrombosis or axillary vein and innominate vein obstruction from elongation and buckling of innominate artery in unilateral cases

IMAGING FINDINGS

- **Chest film:** May show right upper lobe lung lesion or right paratracheal mass
- **Venography:** Determines location and extent of obstruction
- **Interosseous azygography:** Useful to determine patency of azygous vein
- **Aortography or CT scan:** Excludes aortic aneurysm

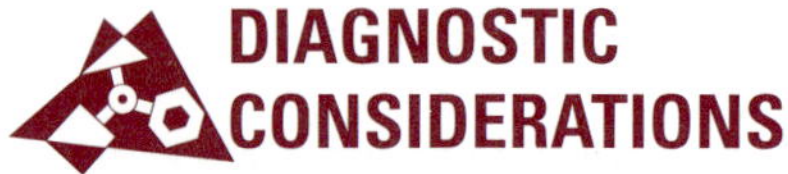

DIAGNOSTIC CONSIDERATIONS

- Measure upper extremity venous pressure: > 350 mm H_2O
- Location/extent of obstruction determined by venography

RULE OUT

- Angioneurotic edema
- Congestive heart failure
- Constrictive pericarditis

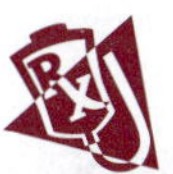

WORK-UP

- Physical exam
- Chest film
- Chest CT scan
- Venography

TREATMENT AND MANAGEMENT

- Etiology of obstruction determines treatment

Cancer

- Diuretics, restriction, head elevation prompt radiation or chemotherapy
- Often subsides at 7–10 days of treatment
- Fibrinolytics or anticoagulation can be considered but rule out metastatic cerebral metastases with CT/MRI
- Percutaneous stents allows good immediate drainage; long-term results unknown
- Tissue diagnosis often needed for therapy (via fine-needle aspiration, bronchoscopy, mediastinoscopy, or thoracotomy)
- Avoid operation if acutely obstructed due to high bleeding rate

Benign Tumors

- Surgical excision for incomplete obstruction
- **For complete obstruction:** Many improve without treatment, others require SVC bypass

COMPLICATIONS

- **Partial SVC obstruction:** Thrombosis may suddenly worsen mild symptoms
- Bleeding esophageal varices rare except in long-standing cases

PROGNOSIS

- Radiotherapy for incomplete SVC obstruction most effective
- **Lung cancer with SVC obstruction:** Mean survival, 6–8 mos
- Death rate from SVC obstruction, 1–2%

RESOURCES

REFERENCES

- Doty DB et al. Bypass of superior vena cava: fifteen years' experience with spiral vein graft for obstruction of superior vena cava caused by benign disease. *J Thorac Cardiovasc Surg.* 1990;99:889.

Surgical Site Infections

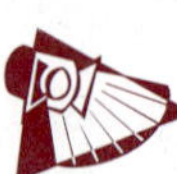

ESSENTIAL FEATURES

- Postoperative wound infections resulting from bacterial contamination during or after a surgical procedure
- Infection usually is confined to the subcutaneous tissues
- Site infections are more likely if:
  - Excessive tissue trauma
  - Undrained hamartomas
  - Retained foreign bodies
  - Excessively tight ligatures
  - Allowing wound to become desiccated
  - Contaminated
  - Poor perfusion
  - Poor oxygenation
  - Dead space
- Degree of intraoperative contamination can be divided into 4 categories which correlate with risk of postoperative wound infection
  1. Clean: No gross contamination from exogenous or endogenous sources
  2. Clean-contaminated: For example, with gastric or biliary surgery
  3. Heavily contaminated: Operations on the unprepared colon or emergency operations for intestinal bleeding or perforation
  4. Infected
- Classification of surgical site infection:
  - Incisional: Superficial (skin and subcutaneous tissues) and deep incisional (deep soft tissue of the incision)
  - Organ/space infection: Any part of the anatomy other than body wall
- WounBd infections usually appear between the fifth and tenth postoperative days, but they may appear as early as the first postoperative day

EPIDEMIOLOGY

- Surgical site infections are the third most frequently reported nosocomial infection, accounting for 14–16% of all nosocomial infections in acutely hospitalized patients
- Among surgical patients, surgical site infections are the most frequent nosocomial infections, accounting for 38% of the total
- Infection rate per degree of contamination:
  - Clean: 1.5%
  - Clean-contaminated: 2–5%
  - Heavily contaminated: 5–30%
  - Infected: 100%
- Patient risk factors include:
  - Diabetes mellitus
  - Nicotine use
  - Corticosteroids
  - Malnutrition
  - Poor hygiene

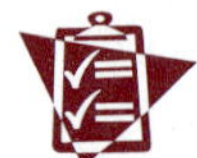

CLINICAL FINDINGS

SYMPTOMS AND SIGNS

- Fever
- Erythema
- Pain
- Swelling, induration
- Palpation of the wound may disclose an abscess
- Palpation may reveal areas of firmness, fluctuance, crepitus, or tenderness
- Drainage from the wound may be free flowing or expressible

LABORATORY FINDINGS

- Leukocytosis
- Increased ESR and C-reactive protein (CRP)
- Bacteremia in complex deep wound infections
- Wound culture may reveal source of infection

IMAGING FINDINGS

- Imaging may reveal abscess, soft-tissue swelling/edema, subcutaneous air (US or CT)

DIAGNOSTIC CONSIDERATIONS

- Differential diagnosis includes all other causes of postoperative fever
  - Atelectasis
  - Urinary tract infection
  - Deep venous thrombosis
  - Medications
- Wound dehiscence
- Wound herniation
- Necrotizing infection
- Drug reaction

RULE OUT

- Necrotizing wound infection (high fever early postoperative, crepitus)

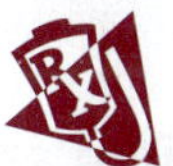

WORK-UP

- Postoperative fever requires inspection of the wound
- Palpation of the wound may disclose an abscess
- Palpation may reveal areas of firmness, fluctuance, crepitus, or tenderness
- Culture should be performed to help locate the source
- Culture blood, urine, sputum to evaluate for other sources of fever and infection
- Ensure adequate oxygenation/perfusion status

WHEN TO ADMIT

- High fever, sepsis, dehydration
- Failure to respond to opening of wound and/or oral antibiotics
- Need for operative drainage

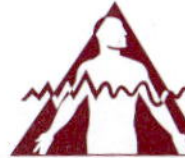

TREATMENT AND MANAGEMENT

- Mild superficial wound infections may be treated successfully with IV antibiotics
- Deep wound infections require drainage, usually by removing a few staples or stitches and breaking-up the abscess with a sterile cotton-tip swab
- Basic treatment of wound infection is to open the wound and allow it to drain
- If no pus is present, the wound may be closed or packed and left open

SURGERY

Indications

- Undrained abscess
- Evidence of necrotizing infection

MEDICATIONS

- Prophylactic antibiotics are indicated whenever wound contamination during the operation can be predicted to be high (eg, operations on the colon)
- Antibiotic treatment of surgical wound infection should ideally be tailored to the pathogenic organism(s)

TREATMENT MONITORING

- Exam of wound following drainage or addition of antibiotics

COMPLICATIONS

- Sepsis
- Incisional hernia
- Tissue necrosis

PROGNOSIS

- Most wound infections make illness more severe
- Wound infection correlates positively with death rates but is not often the cause of death

PREVENTION

- Wise use of isolation techniques, preoperative antibiotics, and delayed primary closure will keep rates of surgical site infections within acceptable limits
- Susceptibility to infection can be reduced by such simple methods as rapid infusion of additional fluids, warming, better pain control, and oxygen administration
- Careful, gentle, clean surgery
- Reduction of contamination
- Thorough hand washing
- Support of the patient's defenses, including use of prophylactic antibiotics when appropriate
- Using skin tapes instead of skin sutures or staples lowers infection rates, especially in contaminated wounds
- Severely contaminated wounds in which subcutaneous infection is likely to develop are best left open initially and managed by delayed primary closure
- The principles of antibiotic prophylaxis are:
  1. Choose antibiotics effective against the expected type of contamination
  2. Use antibiotics only if the risk of infection justifies doing so
  3. Give antibiotics in appropriate doses and at appropriate times
  4. Stop dosing before the risk of side effects outweighs benefits
- A first-generation cephalosporin (eg, cefazolin) is preferred for most procedures since it is effective against common gram-positive and gram-negative bacteria
- Agents with better gram-negative and anaerobic bacterial activity (eg, cefoxitin, cefotetan) are preferred for colorectal and gynecologic procedures
- A single dose of antibiotic given 30 minutes prior to making the skin incision is sufficient
- Postoperative doses of prophylactic antibiotics are usually not necessary

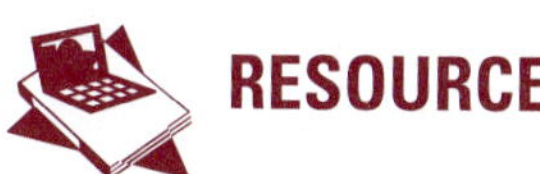

RESOURCES

REFERENCES

- Culver DH et al. Surgical wound infection rates by wound class, operative procedure, and patient risk index. National Nosocomial Infections Surveillance System. *Am J Med.* 1991;91:152S.

WEB SITES

- http://www.cdc.gov/ncidod/hip/

Tetanus

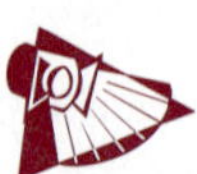

ESSENTIAL FEATURES

- Anaerobic infection mediated by a neurotoxin that causes nervous irritability and tetanic muscular contraction
- Causative organism, *Clostridium tetani*
- Wounds contaminated with soil or feces (eg, deep puncture from stepping on a nail)
- Tetanus-prone wound is usually a puncture wound or one containing devitalized tissue or a foreign body
- Tetanus-prone wounds are characterized by:
  - Elapsed time from injury (more than 6 hrs)
  - Deeper than 1 cm
  - Contaminated by soil, feces, rust
  - Stellate configuration
  - Caused by missile, crush, burn, or frostbite
  - Characterized by devitalized or denervated tissue
  - Cause by animal or human bite

EPIDEMIOLOGY

- Occurrence of tetanus in United States has dropped over the last 5 decades
- Improvement is attributed to the increasingly widespread use of tetanus toxoid and improved wound management
- Tetanus continues to be a severe disease primarily of older adults who are unvaccinated or inadequately vaccinated
- Disproportionately high number of cases (35%) was reported in persons aged 60 or older

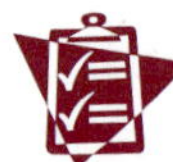

CLINICAL FINDINGS

SYMPTOMS AND SIGNS

- Tetanus is a clinical diagnosis, as confirmatory laboratory tests are not routinely available
- Symptoms of tetanus may occur as soon as 1 day following exposure or as long as several months later
- First symptoms are usually pain or tingling in the area of injury
- "Lockjaw" (limitation of movements of the jaw)
- Spasms of the facial muscles (risus sardonicus)
- Neck stiffness
- Dysphagia
- Laryngospasm
- Chest and diaphragm spasms occur, longer and longer periods of apnea follow
- Temperature is normal or slightly elevated

LABORATORY FINDINGS

- Wound isolation of the organism is neither sensitive nor specific

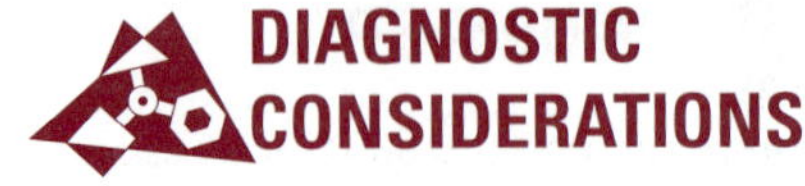

DIAGNOSTIC CONSIDERATIONS

RULE OUT

- Associated animal bites
- Associated injuries

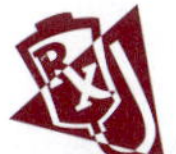

WORK-UP

- History and physical exam
- Careful exam of wound
- Determine tetanus prophylaxis status

WHEN TO ADMIT

- Complications of tetanus: Paralysis, respiratory compromise

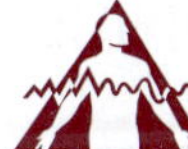

TREATMENT AND MANAGEMENT

- Imperative that all patients with traumatic wounds be asked about previous tetanus prophylaxis
- Neutralization of the toxin with tetanus immune globulin (TIG)
- IV high-dose penicillin
- Ventilator support if indicated
- Surgical wound debridement

SURGERY

Indications

- If tetanus is suspected, perform excision and debridement of the wound

MEDICATIONS

- IV high-dose penicillin
- Tetanus-diphtheria (Td) booster (active immunization for clean wounds)
- TIG (passive immunization for contaminated wounds)

TREATMENT MONITORING

- An attack of tetanus does not confer lasting immunity, and patients who have recovered from the disease require active immunization according to the usual recommended schedules

COMPLICATIONS

- Respiratory embarrassment
- Paralysis
- Death

PROGNOSIS

- Mortality approximately 18% in established tetanus

PREVENTION

- Each person should be actively immunized with tetanus toxoid, beginning with routine childhood immunization and continuing with booster injections every 10 years

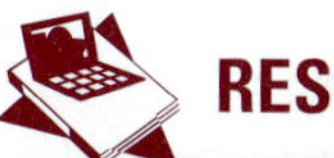

RESOURCES

PRACTICE GUIDELINES

- Available at http://www.cdc.gov/nip/publications/pink/tetanus.pdf

WEB SITES

- www.cdc.gov/nip

Tetralogy of Fallot

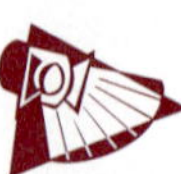

ESSENTIAL FEATURES

- A congenital heart lesion that decreases pulmonary arterial blood flow resulting in a right-to-left shunt
- Cyanosis and decreased oxygen delivery causes compensatory polycythemia (Hct > 70%) and spontaneous thrombosis
- Exercise, acidosis, pain worsens cyanosis, can cause hypoxic spells
- Squatting increases systemic resistance, causing increased pulmonary flow and oxygen saturation
- β-Blockers (decreases spasm), fluid intake, HCO_3 administration, norepinephrine (increases systemic resistance) may help decrease hypoxia
- Clubbing due to proliferation of capillaries and AV fistulas in extremities
- Bronchial and mediastinal arteries enlarge
- Ductus arteriosus maintains flow to lungs during fetal development
- Alprostadil early can allow time for optimization before definitive treatment
- 4 anomalies:
  1. Ventricular septal defect (VSD)
  2. Pulmonary stenosis or atresia
  3. Overriding aorta
  4. RV hypertrophy
- Pulmonary stenosis may involve infundibulum, valve, or main pulmonary artery (PA)
- Extent of pulmonary atresia/stenosis has wide spectrum of severity
- Pulmonary flow depends on aortopulmonary collaterals, can be extensive enough to cause congestive heart failure
- Spasm of infundibular muscle may cause unconciousness and death

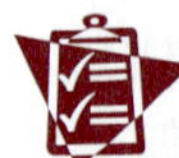

CLINICAL FINDINGS

SYMPTOMS AND SIGNS

- Symptoms related to amount of pulmonary blood flow
- With close of ductus, cyanosis and acidosis may be severe
- Hypoxic spells and cyanosis may lead to cerebral hypoxia and death
- Squatting and clubbing
- Prominent RV impulse, single S2
- Ejection murmur, left third intercostal space
- Murmur softens during cyanotic spell

LABORATORY FINDINGS

- **ECG:** RV hypertrophy

IMAGING FINDINGS

- **Chest film:** Small heart size + cyanosis + decreased pulmonary flow
- **Echocardiography:** Confirms diagnosis
- **Catheterization:** Necessary to define size of pulmonary arteries and identify aortopulmonary arteries

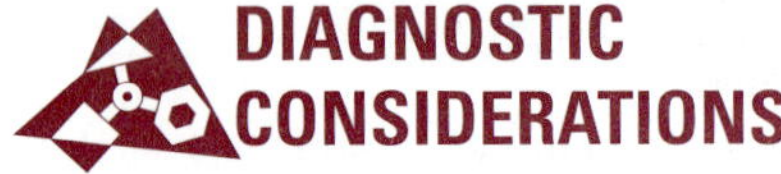

DIAGNOSTIC CONSIDERATIONS

- Consider other congenital anomalies
- Diminutive PA can lead to right heart failure with operative repair
- **McGoon ratio:** Diameter of PAs normalized to diameter of aorta > 2.0

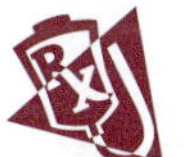

WORK-UP

- Chest film, ECG
- Echocardiography, cardiac catheterization

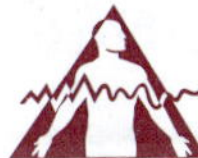

TREATMENT AND MANAGEMENT

- Most symptomatic at diagnosis
- Alprostadil, HCO_3, oxygen
- **One stage correction:** Patch repair of VSD, patch to infundibulum to widen outflow tract, pulmonary insufficiency tolerated in child, may not be long-term
- **Two stage:** Initial systemic-PA shunt, later stage definitive correction
- **Tetralogy of Fallot with pulmonary atresia:** Connect large aortopulmonary shunts to RV outflow or to shunt; induces growth of vasculature

SURGERY

- Operative options to increase pulmonary flow:
  - Blalock-Taussig shunt: Subclavian artery to ipsilateral PA end to side fashion
  - Modified Blalock-Taussig shunt: Subclavian to PA using PTFE
  - Glenn: Superior vena cava (SVC) to PA shunt
  - Fontan: SVC and inferior vena cava (IVC) rerouted to PA
  - Excision of obstructive muscle, patch enlargement of infundibulum, and valve replacement

Indications

- Once diagnosed, repair

PROGNOSIS

- RV dysfunction common
- Mortality < 5% in stenosis; 30–45% in atresia
- Reoperation on outflow tract: 10-15% at 10 years
- Those reaching adulthood: > 90% employed, > 50% exercise, > 20% need cardiac medications
- Late pulmonary valve replacement now beginning to occur

RESOURCES

REFERENCES

- Fraser CD et al. Tetralogy of Fallot: surgical management individualized to the patient. *Ann Thorac Surg.* 2001;71:1556.
- Knott-Craig CJ et al. A 26-year experience with surgical management of tetralogy of Fallot: risk analysis for mortality or late reintervention. *Ann Thorac Surg.* 1998;66:506.
- Norgaard MA et al. Twenty-to-thirty-seven-year follow-up after repair for tetralogy of Fallot. *Eur J Cardiothorac Surg.* 1999;16:125.

Thoracic Aortic Aneurysms

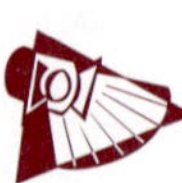

ESSENTIAL FEATURES

- Can be saccular, fusiform
- Common etiologies include:
  - Atherosclerosis
  - Medial degeneration of aortic wall
  - Marfan syndrome (defect in fibrillin gene)
  - Trauma and infection
- Increased aneurysm rupture rate depend on:
  - Size
  - Marfan syndrome
  - Family history of rupture or dissection
  - Advancing age
  - Chronic obstructive pulmonary disease
  - Growth rate > 0.1 cm yearly
- Affect the ascending, arch, or descending aorta (descending is most common)

EPIDEMIOLOGY

- More common in men
- History of hypertension usual

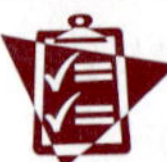

CLINICAL FINDINGS

SYMPTOMS AND SIGNS

- Symptoms, if present, are due to local pressure or obstruction of adjacent structures
- **Ascending aorta**
  - Aortic regurgitation
  - Superior vena cava obstruction
  - Chest pain
- **Aortic arch:** Tracheal compression
- **Descending aorta**
  - Recurrent laryngeal nerve compression
  - Phrenic paralysis
  - Dysphagia
  - Stridor

IMAGING FINDINGS

- **Chest film:** May show convex right cardiac border in ascending aneurysms, prominent aortic knob in arch aneurysms, posterior lateral thoracic mass in descending aneurysms
- **CT scans or magnetic resonance angiography (MRA):** Define anatomy and extent of aneurysm
- **Aortography:** Occasionally useful

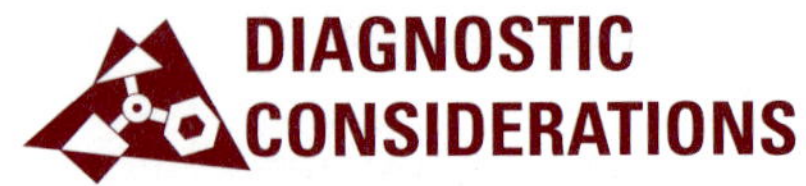

DIAGNOSTIC CONSIDERATIONS

- Evaluate for peripheral aneurysms

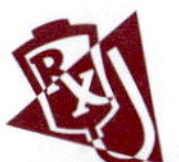

WORK-UP

- Chest CT/MRA: Diagnostic
- Consider aortography
- **Stress test:** Examine for coronary artery disease

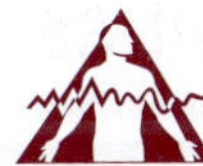

TREATMENT AND MANAGEMENT

- Primary determinants for repair: Aneurysm size, etiology, and symptoms
- For asymptomatic aneurysms measuring ≤ 5.5 cm, aggressive blood pressure control with β-blockers
- Consider repair when aneurysm measures > 5.5 cm, especially if symptoms are present
- Dacron replacement is standard

SURGERY

- **Ascending aorta**
  - Cardiopulmonary bypass via RA and right femoral artery cannulation
  - If extends proximal toward sinuses of Valsalva, need composite prosthetic valve-ascending aortic graft conduit (patients with Marfan syndrome)
  - Isolated ascending aortic aneurysm, replace with Dacron graft
- **Arch**
  - Provide cerebral protection during repair via hypothermic circulatory arrest
  - Dacron graft, anastomose great vessels as single button
- **Descending aorta**
  - Dacron replacement via left thoracotomy with spinal cord protection via replacement of large intercostals, drainage of CSF
  - Percutaneous stent grafts now being used

Indications

- Aneurysm > 5.5 cm, consider repair especially if symptoms are present
- Marfan syndrome: Aneurysm > 5 cm

COMPLICATIONS

- Spinal cord ischemia in descending aortic repair 5–15%

PROGNOSIS

- Operative mortality, 5–15%
- 10-year survival: Ascending = 50%, descending = 38%

RESOURCES

REFERENCES

- Coady MA et al. Natural history, pathogenesis, and etiology of thoracic aortic aneurysms and dissections. *Cardiol Clin.* 1999;17:615.
- Coady MA et al. Surgical intervention criteria for thoracic aortic aneurysms: a study of growth rates and complications. *Ann Thorac Surg.* 1999;67:1922.
- Umana JP, Mitchell RS. Endovascular treatment of aortic dissections and thoracic aortic aneurysms. *Semin Vasc Surg.* 2000;13:290.

Thoracic Aortic Dissection

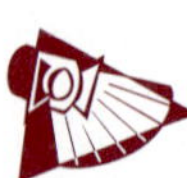

ESSENTIAL FEATURES

- Often lethal event
- Degeneration of aortic media is hallmark of disease
- Pathogenesis controversial
  1. Medial degeneration leads to rupture of vasa vasorum
  2. Intimal tears allows blood to shear weakened media
- Location of intimal tear: Ascending aorta, 62%; arch, 10%; isthmus, 16%; rest in distal aorta
- Risk factors include:
  - Hypertension
  - Atherosclerosis
  - Iatrogenic injury (catheter or open heart surgery)
  - Closed chest trauma
  - Marfan syndrome
  - Aortic coarctation

Classification

- Debakey type I
  - Originate in ascending aorta
  - Extend beyond left subclavian (Stanford type A)
- Debakey type II
  - Involve ascending aorta only
  - Often chronic
  - Associated with aortic valve incompetence (Stanford type A)
- Debakey type III
  - Occur distal to left subclavian artery
  - Often extend into abdominal aorta (Stanford type B)

EPIDEMIOLOGY

- Most common cause of aortic rupture
- 2000 cases yearly
- Men affected more often than women
- Usually occurs in fifth to seventh decades of life

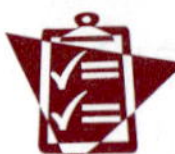

CLINICAL FINDINGS

SYMPTOMS AND SIGNS

- Most common
  - Severe, tearing chest pain often signifies intimal tear and formation of false lumen
  - Ascending: Pain anterior
  - Descending: Pain posterior between scapulas
- Hypotension with blood loss, leak into pericardium
- Sudden death if extends into pericardium or down a coronary artery
- If involves aortic valve or root, aortic insufficiency and acute congestive heart failure
- Obstruction of aortic branch vessels:
  - Stroke
  - Asymmetric extremity pulses
  - Paraplegia
  - Renal failure
  - Acute mesenteric ischemia
  - Lower extremity occlusion

LABORATORY FINDINGS

- ECG: Useful to rule out myocardial infarction (MI)
- Cardiac enzymes: Rule out MI

IMAGING FINDINGS

- **Chest film**
  - 50% have widened mediastinum
  - Cardiomegaly if in failure or with pericardial effusion
  - Left pleural effusion if contained rupture
- **Chest CT:** Diagnostic procedure of choice
- **Transesophageal echocardiography (TEE)**
  - Information about myocardial function
  - Aortic valve competence
  - Diagnostic
  - Limited in evaluation of arch and descending dissections
- **Magnetic resonance angiography (MRA):** Useful but time-consuming

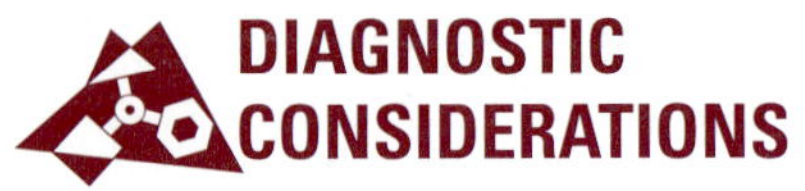

DIAGNOSTIC CONSIDERATIONS

RULE OUT

- MI

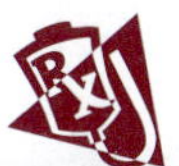

WORK-UP

- Physical exam
- ECG
- Chest film
- Chest CT scan
- TEE
- MRA if stable

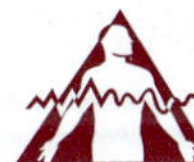

TREATMENT AND MANAGEMENT

- Aggressive blood pressure control critical; esmolol commonly used (decreases dP/dT and aortic shear force)

Ascending

- Death occurs from cardiac tamponade, acute coronary occlusion, acute atrial regurgitation
- Replacement of ascending aorta with resection of intimal tear
- Resuspension of aortic valve commissures restores valve competence

Descending

- Majority have benign course
- Medical therapy treatment of choice
- 20% require surgery for rupture or organ ischemia
- 20% develop aneurysmal dilation of aorta requiring surgery
- Endovascular stent procedure and fenestration are new approaches being studied

MEDICATIONS

- β-Blockers (esmolol)
- Vasodilators if still hypertensive after β-blockade

COMPLICATIONS

- Untreated type A
  - 3% sudden death
  - 27% die within 24 hrs
  - 70% die within 1 wk

PROGNOSIS

- Repair of ascending aorta: Operative mortality, 5%; 5-yr survival, 55%
- Emergent repair of descending aorta: Operative mortality, 15%

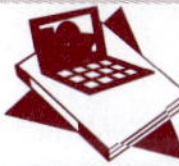

RESOURCES

REFERENCES

- Elefteriades JA et al. Management of descending aortic dissection. *Ann Thorac Surg.* 1999;67:2002.
- Meszaros I et al. Epidemiology and clinicopathology of aortic dissection. *Chest.* 2000;117:1271.
- Sabik JF et al. Long-term effectiveness of operations for ascending aortic dissections. *J Thorac Cardiovasc Surg.* 2000;119:946.

Thoracic Injuries

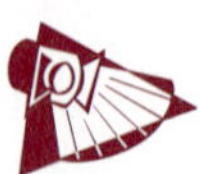

ESSENTIAL FEATURES

- Simple rib fracture is most common thoracic injury
- Spectrum from simple rib fracture to fracture with hemothorax to flail chest with associated pulmonary contusion
- Flail chest occurs when a portion of the chest wall becomes separated from the rib cage by multiple fractures and moves opposite to the rib cage with rib inspiration and expiration decreasing respiratory efficiency
- Early deaths commonly due to:
  - Airway obstruction
  - Flail chest
  - Open pneumothorax
  - Massive hemothorax
  - Tension pneumothorax
  - Cardiac tamponade
- Late deaths are due to:
  - Respiratory failure
  - Sepsis
  - Unrecognized injuries
- 85% of chest injuries do NOT require open thoracotomy

EPIDEMIOLOGY

- Accounts directly or contributes to 50% of deaths from trauma
- 80% of blunt thoracic injuries are related to motor vehicle accidents
- Penetrating injury nearly as frequent as blunt injury

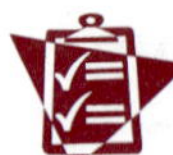

CLINICAL FINDINGS

SYMPTOMS AND SIGNS

- Pain on inspiration
- Decreased ventilation
- Cyanosis, ashen or gray facies may indicate upper airway obstruction
- Stridor
- Poor respiratory excursion
- Retraction of supraclavicular, suprasternal, intercostal, or epigastric regions
- Paradoxic chest wall movement indicates flail chest
- Tracheal shift, dullness to percussion and absence of breath sounds unilaterally with flat neck veins can indicate massive hemothorax
- Tracheal shift, tympany to percussion and absence of breath sounds unilaterally with distended neck veins may indicate tension pneumothorax

LABORATORY FINDINGS

- Hypoxemia
- Hypercapnea

IMAGING FINDINGS

- **Chest film or CT scan:**
  - Rib fractures
  - Pneumothorax
  - Hemothorax
  - Tension pneumothorax (does not need chest film to diagnose)
  - Wide mediastinum

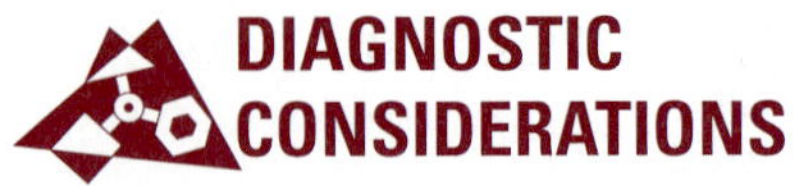

DIAGNOSTIC CONSIDERATIONS

- Associated injuries in abdomen may dictate therapy

RULE OUT

- Airway obstruction
- Tension pneumothorax
- Flail chest
- Massive hemothorax
- Cardiac tamponade
- Open pneumothorax

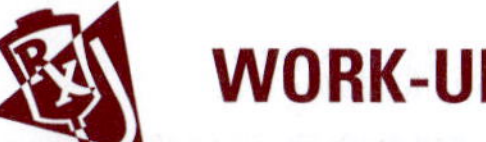

WORK-UP

- Physical exam
- Chest film

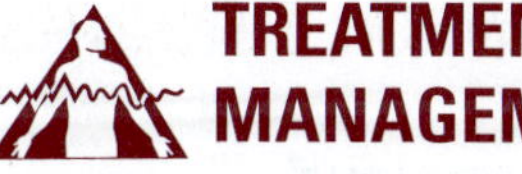

TREATMENT AND MANAGEMENT

- Adequate analgesia
- Intubation and mechanical ventilation as needed

SURGERY

- Rarely, external fixation of chest wall
- Operative repair specific for injury

TREATMENT MONITORING

- Serial ABG measurements

COMPLICATIONS

- Atelectasis
- Hypercapnea
- Hypoxia

PROGNOSIS

- Hospital mortality of isolated thoracic injury is 4–8%, but rises to 10–15% with 1 other organ system involved and to 35% if multiple organs involved

PREVENTION

- Seatbelt use

RESOURCES

REFERENCES

- Enoch S et al. Tube thoracostomy. *Arch Surg.* 1995;130:521.
- Pape HC et al. Appraisal of early evaluation of chest trauma: development of a standardized scoring system for initial clinical decision-making. *J Trauma.* 2000;49:496.
- Feliciano DV et al. Advances in the diagnosis and treatment of thoracic trauma. *Surg Clin North Am.* 1999;79:1417.

Thoracic Outlet Syndrome

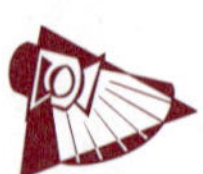

ESSENTIAL FEATURES

- Variety of disorders caused by arterial, venous, or neural compression at base of neck
- Mechanical causes for compression include:
  - Cervical rib
  - Anomalous ligaments
  - Anterior scalene hypertrophy
  - Positional changes with relation to first rib
- Patients may describe history of cervical trauma
- Symptoms rare prior to adulthood, suggesting alteration of normal structure with age is cause
- Subclavian artery stenosis: Arterial stenosis and poststenotic dilation
- Subclavian vein compression: Can lead to effort thrombosis (Paget-Schroetter)

EPIDEMIOLOGY

- Prolonged hyperabduction in hairdressers, painters, truck drivers

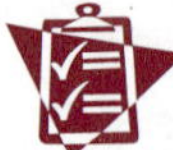

CLINICAL FINDINGS

SYMPTOMS AND SIGNS

- Neurologic symptoms predominate
- Pain, paresthesias, numbness in brachial plexus trunks (ulnar most common)
- Hand numbness often wakes patients from sleep
- Motor deficits indicate long duration
- Muscular atrophy of hand may be present
- May be reproducible on exam with various maneuvers of shoulder girdle
- **Adson test:** Weakened radial pulse with arm abduction and head rotated to opposite side
- **Tinel test:** Light percussion in supraclavicular fossa produces peripheral sensations
- Venous compression and arterial compression less common
- **Subclavian artery compression:** Bruit, distal emboli, or arterial occlusion
- **Subclavian vein compression:** Thrombosis of vein leading to extremity pain and swelling (effort thrombosis called Paget-Schroetter syndrome)

IMAGING FINDINGS

- Cervical x-ray may identify cervical rib

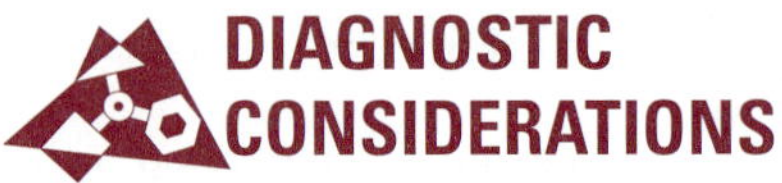

DIAGNOSTIC CONSIDERATIONS

- No objective study to confirm diagnosis of neurogenic thoracic outlet syndrome

RULE OUT

- Carpal tunnel syndrome
- Cervical disk disease

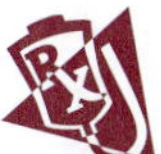

WORK-UP

- Cervical x-ray and electromyography to rule out other causes of neurologic syndrome
- Arterial syndrome: Angiography
- Venous syndrome: Venography

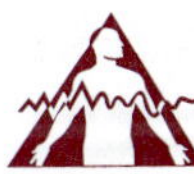

TREATMENT AND MANAGEMENT

- Postural correction and physical therapy
- If surgical repair warranted, thoracic outlet decompression
- 2 approaches possible
  1. Supraclavicular
  2. Transaxillary
- Goals:
  – Excise anterior scalene and fibrous bands
  – Rib resection
- Arterial disease: Thoracic decompression and arterial reconstruction
- Venous disease: First treat with thrombolytics or anticoagulation, then thoracic outlet decompression, may need venous reconstruction (open or endovascular)

SURGERY

Indications

- Arterial disease
- Venous disease
- Neurologic symptoms not attributable to other disease and failure of conservative therapy after 3–6 months

RESOURCES

REFERENCES

- Sharp WJ et al. Long-term follow-up and patient satisfaction after surgery for thoracic outlet syndrome. *Ann Vasc Surg.* 2001;15:32.
- Wilbourn AJ. Thoracic outlet syndrome. *Neurol Clin.* 1999;17:477.
- Kreienberg PB et al. Long-term results in patients treated with thrombolysis, thoracic inlet decompression, and subclavian vein stenting for Paget-Schroetter syndrome. *J Vasc Surg.* 2001;33:5100.

Thrombophlebitis, Superficial

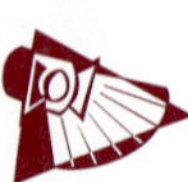

ESSENTIAL FEATURES

- Can occur spontaneously in varicose veins, pregnant or postpartum women, thromboangiitis obliterans, Behçet disease
- Most common after IV therapy, area of local trauma
- Superficial migratory phlebitis (Trousseau): Suggests abdominal carcinoma
- Pulmonary embolism (PE) is rare without deep venous thrombosis (DVT)

EPIDEMIOLOGY

- Saphenous vein most common vein affected
- 20% of patients have simultaneous DVT

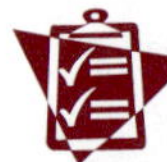

CLINICAL FINDINGS

SYMPTOMS AND SIGNS

- Local extremity pain, redness
- Indurated, erythematous, tender areas = thrombosed superficial veins; tends to be well localized over superficial vein
- Firm cord may develop with time
- Generalized edema absent unless deep veins involved
- Fever or chills suggests septic or suppurative phlebitis (complication of IV cannulation)

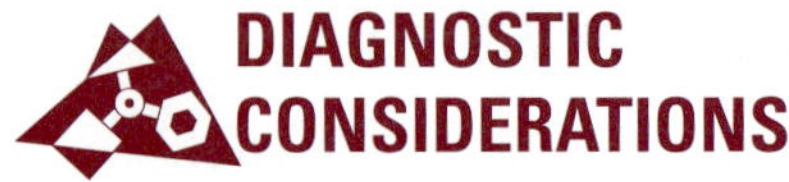

DIAGNOSTIC CONSIDERATIONS

RULE OUT

- Ascending lymphangitis
- Cellulitis
- Erythema nodosum
- Erythema induratum
- Panniculitis

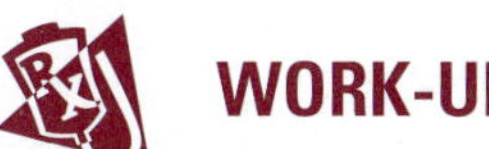

WORK-UP

- Physical exam
- CBC count

TREATMENT AND MANAGEMENT

- Primary treatment: NSAIDs, heat, elevation, support stockings, elastic wrap
- Ambulation encouraged
- Anticoagulation with monthly venous duplex can be attempted to avoid surgery

SURGERY

- Excision of vein if persists > 2 wks or recurrent
- Ligate and resection vein at junction of saphenofemoral or cephalic-subclavian junction
- Septic thrombophlebitis: Broad-spectrum antibiotics; if patient is septic, immediate excision of infected vein

Indications

- > 2 wks duration or local recurrence
- Septic patient

TREATMENT MONITORING

- Usually resolves in 7–10 days; is self-limited

PROGNOSIS

- **Uncomplicated superficial thrombophlebitis:** Responds well to conservative therapy
- Extension into DVT associated with PE

RESOURCES

REFERENCES

- Belcaro G et al. Superficial thrombophlebitis of the legs: a randomized, controlled, follow-up study. *Angiology.* 1999;50:523.

Thrombotic Thrombocytopenia Purpura

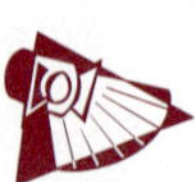

ESSENTIAL FEATURES

- Fever
- Thrombocytopenic purpura
- Hemolytic anemia
- Neurologic abnormalities
- Renal failure

EPIDEMIOLOGY

- Cause is unknown: Believed to be autoimmune response to endothelial cell antigen in small vessels
- It is most common between ages 20 and 50 years
- The thrombocytopenia is probably due to a shortened platelet lifespan
- The microangiopathic hemolytic anemia is produced by passage of RBCs over damaged small blood vessels containing fibrin strands
- The anemia is often severe, and it may be aggravated by hemorrhage secondary to thrombocytopenia

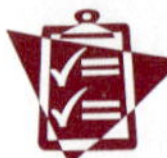

CLINICAL FINDINGS

SYMPTOMS AND SIGNS

- Fever
- Purpura and ecchymosis
- Neurologic changes
  - Headache
  - Confusion
  - Aphasia
  - Lethargy
  - Hemiparesis
  - Seizures
  - Coma
- Hepatomegaly
- Splenomegaly
- Bleeding

LABORATORY FINDINGS

- Thrombocytopenia
- Anemia
- Increased lactate dehydrogenase (LDH)
- Normal prothrombin time (PT), partial thromboplastin time (PTT), international normalized ratio (INR)
- Reticulocytosis
- Increased bilirubin
- Decreased haptoglobin
- Negative Coombs test
- Fragmented RBCs on peripheral smear

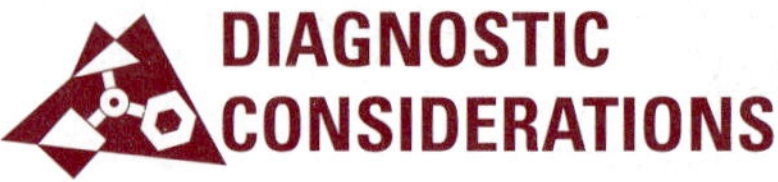

DIAGNOSTIC CONSIDERATIONS

- End-organ damage (renal failure, neurologic changes) due to occlusion of arteries and capillaries by hyaline membranes composed of platelets and fibrinogen

RULE OUT

- Other causes of thrombocytopenia and anemia
  - Disseminated intravascular coagulation
  - Evan syndrome
  - Endocarditis
  - Vasculitis

WORK-UP

- CBC count
- PT, PTT, INR
- LDH
- Reticulocyte count
- Serum bilirubin
- Serum haptoglobin
- Coombs test
- Peripheral blood smear

WHEN TO ADMIT

- Severe thrombocytopenia
- Bleeding
- Neurologic changes
- Acute renal failure

WHEN TO REFER

- All patients should be managed in consultation with a hematologist

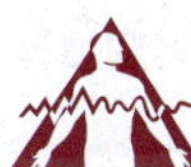

TREATMENT AND MANAGEMENT

- Plasmapheresis with plasma exchange, corticosteroids, antiplatelet agents
- Splenectomy can be used as an adjunct to medical treatment in order to reduce platelet and RBC loss

SURGERY

Indications

- As an adjunct to medical treatment

MEDICATIONS

- Corticosteroids
- Antiplatelet drugs (aspirin and dipyridamole)

TREATMENT MONITORING

- Platelet count

COMPLICATIONS

- Renal failure
- Neurologic changes

PROGNOSIS

- 65% remission with splenectomy alone
- With combined therapy, prolonged remission can be achieved in most patients

RESOURCES

REFERENCES

- Allford SL et al. Current understanding of the pathophysiology of thrombotic thrombocytopenic purpura. *J Clin Path.* 2000;53:497.
- Rock GA. Management of thrombotic thrombocytopenic purpura. *Br J Hematol.* 2000;109:496.

Thymic Carcinoma

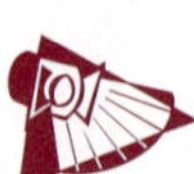

ESSENTIAL FEATURES

- Rare variant of thymic lesions (< 15%)
- Biologically different from malignant thymoma
- Tend to be very invasive and aggressive

EPIDEMIOLOGY

- Young men (< 50-years-old, typically)

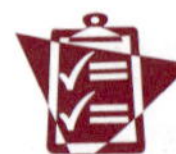

CLINICAL FINDINGS

SYMPTOMS AND SIGNS

- 50% of asymptomatic cases identified on chest film
- Chest pain dysphagia, dyspnea, or superior vena cava syndrome most common if symptomatic

IMAGING FINDINGS

- **Chest film:** Anterior mediastinal mass
- **CT scan:** Useful in assessing extent of lesion
- **MRI:** Can assess vascular invasion

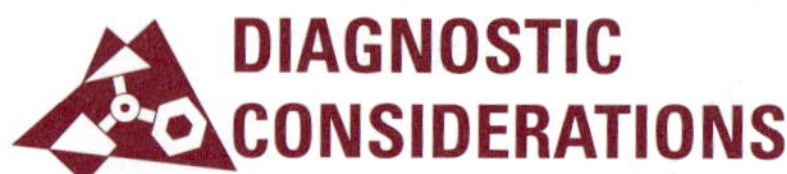

DIAGNOSTIC CONSIDERATIONS

- **Definitive diagnosis:** Histologic tissue analysis
- Do not biopsy small, well-encapsulated mediastinal masses-
- Do complete excision, otherwise risk tumor seeding

RULE OUT

- Lymphoma
  - Can be difficult to differentiate histologically from thymoma
- Thymoma
  - Very aggressive variant of thymic lesions

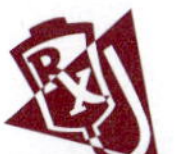

WORK-UP

- Chest CT
- Biopsy

TREATMENT AND MANAGEMENT

- Attempt complete resection

MEDICATIONS

- Induction chemotherapy
- Postoperative chemoradiation

PROGNOSIS

- High recurrence locally and at distant sites
- After thymectomy, 75% with myasthenia gravis are improved; 30% complete remission
- Younger patients (< 40 years) do better after thymectomy

RESOURCES

REFERENCES

- Rea F et al. Chemotherapy and operation for invasive thymoma. *J Thorac Cardiovasc Surg.* 1993;106:543.

Thymoma & Myasthenia Gravis

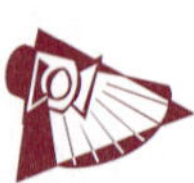

ESSENTIAL FEATURES

- Thymic tumors occur in anterior mediastinum and include thymomas, lymphomas, Hodgkin lymphoma

Thymomas

- Most common type often difficult to distinguish from lymphoma
- 3 predominant cell types
  - Lymphocytic (25%)
  - Epithelial (25%)
  - Lymphoepithelial (50%)

Myasthenia Gravis (MG)

- Neuromuscular disorder characterized by weakness and fatigability of voluntary muscles
- Decreased number of acetylcholine receptors at neuromuscular junctions
- Believed to be autoimmune process

EPIDEMIOLOGY

- 30% of patients with thymoma have MG
- Thymoma develops in 15% of patients with MG
- Thymomas associated with paraneoplastic syndromes including:
  - Cytopenias
  - Red cell aplasias
  - Hypogammaglobulinemias
  - Autoimmune diseases, such as rheumatoid arthritis and lupus
- MG is more commonly associated with lymphocytic variety

CLINICAL FINDINGS

SYMPTOMS AND SIGNS

- 50% of asymptomatic cases identified on chest film
- Chest pain dysphagia, MG, dyspnea, or superior vena cava syndrome most common if symptomatic
- Easy fatigability in patients with MG

LABORATORY FINDINGS

- MG
  - 90% have serum antibodies against acetylcholine receptors
  - 70% have germinal center formation on thymic biopsy

IMAGING FINDINGS

- **Chest film:** Anterior mediastinal mass
- **CT scan:** Useful in assessing extent of lesion
- **MRI:** Can assess vascular invasion

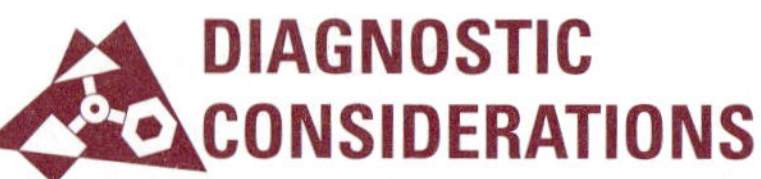

DIAGNOSTIC CONSIDERATIONS

- **MG:** Decremental response in muscular contraction to repeated stimulation with improvement after edrophonium administration (short-acting anticholinesterase)
- **Definitive diagnosis:** Histologic tissue analysis
- Do not biopsy small, well-encapsulated mediastinal masses
- Do complete excision, otherwise risk tumor seeding

RULE OUT

- Lymphoma
  - Can be difficult to differentiate histologically from thymoma
- Thymic carcinoma
  - Very aggressive variant of thymic lesions

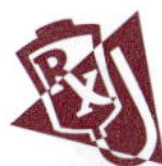

WORK-UP

- Tissue histology necessary to make diagnosis

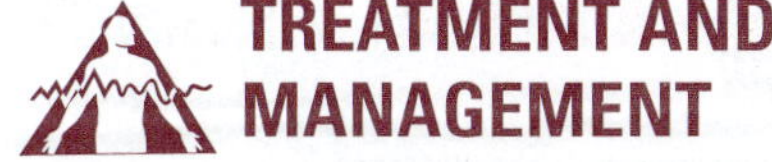

TREATMENT AND MANAGEMENT

SURGERY

- Treatment of choice for thymoma is total thymectomy
- Performed via median sternotomy, trap door, or clamshell approach
- Cervical incision not useful for malignant disease, only for benign disease

Indications

- Stages I, II, III should be aggressively resected
- En bloc resection with associated structures is warranted if complete resection is possible
- Large (> 5 cm) neoadjuvant chemotherapy may shrink tumor
- Large lesions with gross invasion-biopsy to confirm histologic diagnosis, then neoadjuvant therapy prior to resection
- MG indication for early thymectomy

Contraindications

- Lymphoma not indication for thymectomy

MEDICATIONS

- Postoperative radiation therapy indicated for stage II

MG

- Anticholinesterase drugs initial treatment and used aggressively in postoperative period
- Corticosteroids used in select cases
- Plasmapheresis can minimize need for anticholinesterase agents
- Avoid muscle relaxants and atropine

TREATMENT MONITORING

- Response rate exceeds 70% with chemotherapy
- 75% of patients with MG improve after thymectomy

COMPLICATIONS

- Thymyectomy complications are low, except in extensive tumors
- Anticholinesterase drugs minimize respiratory difficulties postoperatively in patients with MG

PROGNOSIS

- For thymomas, stage and histologic type determine survival
- Poorer prognosis if aneuploidy and presence of epithelial cells resembling thymic carcinoma
- Presence of MG no bearing on prognosis
- 10-year survival
  - Stage I: 100%
  - Stage II: 75%
  - Stage III: 25%
  - Stage IV: Poor

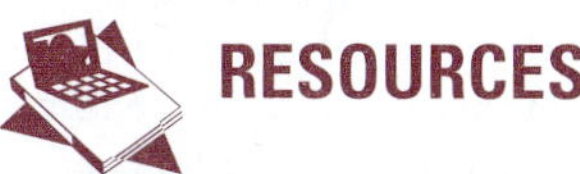

RESOURCES

REFERENCES

- Park HS et al. Thymoma. A retrospective study of 87 cases. *Cancer.* 1994;73:2491.
- Cooper JD. Current therapy for thymoma. (Review.) *Chest.* 1993;103(4 Suppl):3345.

PRACTICE GUIDELINES

- The National Comprehensive Cancer Network http://www.nccn.org

Thyroglossal Cyst

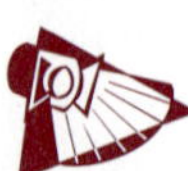

ESSENTIAL FEATURES

- Thyroid develops from an evagination of the floor of the primitive pharynx (during fourth week of gestation)
- Abnormal movement of the thyroid anlage can lead to a lingual thyroid or appear as a mass anywhere in the neck midline
- Persistence of the thyroglossal duct leaves an epithelial lined tract that forms a cyst that communicates with the foramen cecum at the base of the tongue
- Tract of a persistent thyroglossal duct extends through the hyoid bone

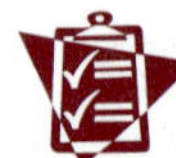

CLINICAL FINDINGS

SYMPTOMS AND SIGNS

- Lingual thyroid (dysphagia, dysphonia, dyspnea, hemorrhage, pain)
- Rounded, cystic mass in the midline of the neck (just below hyoid bone)
- Cephalad-caudad movement of mass with deglutition and protrusion of tongue

IMAGING FINDINGS

- Lingual thyroid lights up on thyroid scintigraphy

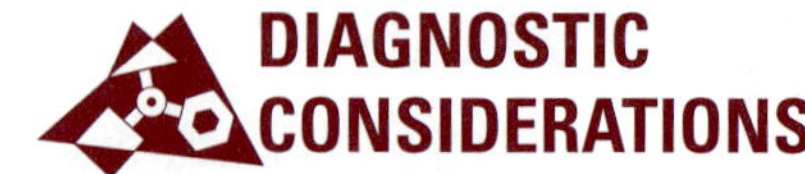

RULE OUT

- Dermoid cyst
- Enlarged lymph nodes (especially Delphian)

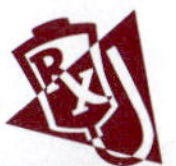

WORK-UP

- Physical exam
- Cervical ultrasound
- Thyroid scintigraphy

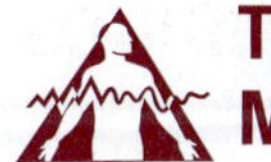

TREATMENT AND MANAGEMENT

SURGERY

- Lingual or ectopic thyroid should be excised
- Acute thyroglossal tract infections should be treated with heat, antibiotics, and incision and drainage (if indicated)
  - Complete tract excision (en bloc with middle of hyoid bone—Sistrunk procedure) once inflammation has subsided

COMPLICATIONS

- Thyroglossal cysts are prone to infection
- Excision of lingual or ectopic thyroid can lead to permanent hypothyroidism
- Carcinoma develops more frequently in ectopic thyroid tissue than normal thyroid tissue

PROGNOSIS

- Recurrence of thyroglossal cyst is 6–9% and is more common following infection

RESOURCES

REFERENCES

- Housawa M et al. Anatomical reconstruction of the thyroglossal duct. *J Pediatr Surg.* 1991;26:766.
- Roback SA, Telander RL. Thyroglossal duct cysts and branchial cleft anomalies. *Semin Pediatr Surg.* 1994;3:142.

Thyroid Cancer, Anaplastic

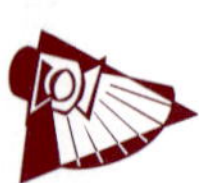

ESSENTIAL FEATURES

- History of irradiation to the neck (in some patients)
- Painless or enlarging nodule, dysphagia or hoarseness
- Firm or hard, fixed thyroid nodule; cervical lymphadenopathy
- Family history of thyroid cancer
- Appears later in life
- Invasive, nonencapsulated tumor
- Patients often die of local recurrence, pulmonary metastases, or both
- Microscopically, has 3 different types:
  1. Giant cell
  2. Spindle cell
  3. Small cell

EPIDEMIOLOGY

- Occurs principally in women beyond middle life (peak incidence in the seventh decade of life)
- 1% of all thyroid cancers
- 50% have clinically positive cervical lymph nodes at presentation
- 30% have distant metastases at presentation

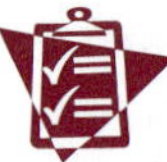

CLINICAL FINDINGS

SYMPTOMS AND SIGNS

- Hard, irregular anterior neck mass
- Quickly enlarging mass
- May be tender
- Dyspnea or stridor
- Dysphagia or odynophagia

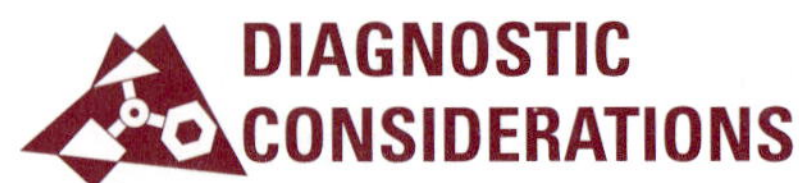

DIAGNOSTIC CONSIDERATIONS

- These tumors are reliably diagnosed by fine-needle aspiration biopsy

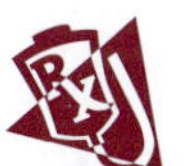

WORK-UP

- History and physical exam
- Fine-needle aspiration biopsy

TREATMENT AND MANAGEMENT

- Complete surgical resection is the best chance for cure
- Local recurrence after surgical treatment is the rule
- Combination therapy with chemotherapy and external beam radiation offers the best palliation, but is rarely curative

SURGERY

Indications

- All tumors should be excised as completely as possible
- Tracheostomy below the tumor may be helpful for patients with actual or impending airway compromise

Contraindications

- Advanced metastatic disease

MEDICATIONS

- Radioiodine ablation 6 weeks after surgery
- Thyroid-stimulating hormone suppression with thyroid hormone (may have little effect since cells are undifferentiated)

TREATMENT MONITORING

- Monthly physical exam for local recurrence

PROGNOSIS

- Almost all patients have recurrence and die of the disease
- Life expectancy after diagnosis is typically about 6 months
- 1-year survival is 5–15%

RESOURCES

REFERENCES

- Ordonez NG et al. Anaplastic thyroid carcinoma. *Am J Clin Pathol.* 1991;96:15.

PRACTICE GUIDELINES

- The National Comprehensive Cancer Network http://www.nccn.org

CANCER STAGING

- See Thyroid Staging Table on page 756.

Thyroid Cancer, Follicular

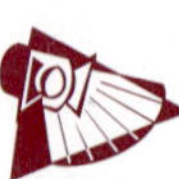

ESSENTIAL FEATURES

- History of radiation to the neck in some patients
- Painless or enlarging nodule, dysphagia, or hoarseness
- Firm or hard, fixed thyroid nodule; cervical lymphadenopathy
- Normal thyroid function; nodule stippled with calcium (x-ray), solid (US), cold (radioiodine scan), positive or suspicious cytologic studies
- Family history of thyroid cancer

EPIDEMIOLOGY

- Accounts for approximately 10% of all malignant thyroid tumors
- Appears later in life than papillary thyroid cancers, with peak incidence in fifth decade
- 3 times more common in women than in men
- Incidence decreasing as the intake of dietary iodine has increased
- 80% of encapsulated follicular tumors > 4 cm are malignant

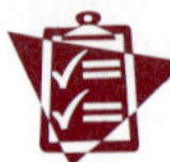

CLINICAL FINDINGS

SYMPTOMS AND SIGNS

- Thyroid nodule: Hard, rubbery, or soft
- Enlarged or hard cervical lymph nodes
- Pain in the thyroid or paralaryngeal neck
- Hoarseness
- Dyspnea
- Stridor
- Dysphagia

LABORATORY FINDINGS

- Normal thyroid-stimulating hormone (TSH) levels

IMAGING FINDINGS

- **US:** Solid or cystic nodule
- **Radioiodine scans:** Nonfunctioning (cold)

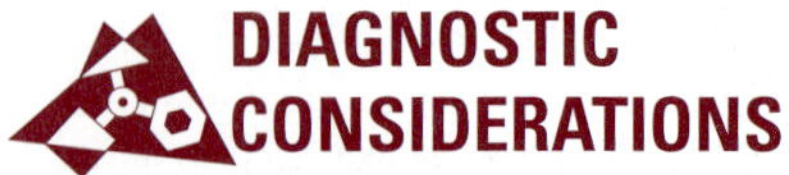

DIAGNOSTIC CONSIDERATIONS

- Fine-needle aspiration is unable to reliably differentiate the atypical cells of invasive follicular adenocarcinoma from its counterpart benign adenoma
- Follicular carcinoma distinguished from follicular adenoma by capsular and vascular invasion
- 7% spread lymphatically; most spread hematogenously (to lungs, skeleton, liver, and CNS)
- Skeletal metastases may appear 10 years after resection of primary tumor

RULE OUT

- Concurrent hyperparathyroidism (so that it can be treated at the same operation if necessary)

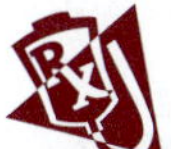

WORK-UP

- Complete history and physical exam, with attention to risk factors, family history, palpable characteristics of the nodule or lymphadenopathy
- Measurement of serum TSH and calcium
- Fine-needle aspiration biopsy

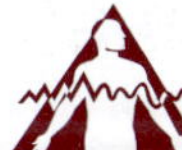

TREATMENT AND MANAGEMENT

- Treatment starts with operative removal
- External beam radiation may palliate nonresectable metastases that are resistant to radioiodine

SURGERY

Indications

- All follicular thyroid cancers should be excised
- Bulky or palpable nodal recurrences

MEDICATIONS

- Suppressive doses of thyroid hormone after thyroid ablation or thyroidectomy
- Radioactive iodine therapy for remnant, recurrent, or metastatic disease

TREATMENT MONITORING

- Semiannual or yearly neck exams, serum thyroglobulin, thyroglobulin antibodies, and whole body radioiodine scan

COMPLICATIONS

- Neck hematoma
- Superior laryngeal nerve injury
- Recurrent laryngeal nerve injury
- Transient or permanent hypoparathyroidism
- Wound infection

PROGNOSIS

- Worse prognosis predicted by extensive angioinvasion, older age, and presence of distant metastases
- 10-year survival nearly 100% with only microinvasion
- 10-year survival about 72% with angioinvasion

RESOURCES

REFERENCES

- Kebebew E et al. Differentiated thyroid cancer: "complete" rational approach. *World J Surg.* 2000;24:942.

PRACTICE GUIDELINES

- The National Comprehensive Cancer Network http://www.nccn.org

CANCER STAGING

- See Thyroid Staging Table on page 756.

Thyroid Cancer, Medullary

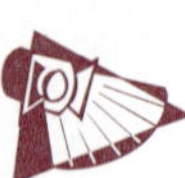

ESSENTIAL FEATURES

- Aggressive form of thyroid cancer that can be either sporadic or familial
- Arises from parafollicular or C cells

EPIDEMIOLOGY

- 5% of malignant tumors of the thyroid
- 35% of medullary thyroid cancer (MTC) is familial
- 65% of MTC is sporadic
- Peak incidence of familial MTC is second to third decade of life
- Peak incidence of sporadic MTC is fifth to sixth decade of life

CLINICAL FINDINGS

SYMPTOMS AND SIGNS

- Hard thyroid nodule
- Enlarged or hard cervical lymph nodes
- Pain in the thyroid or paralaryngeal area
- Hoarseness
- Dyspnea
- Stridor
- Dysphagia
- Diarrhea

LABORATORY FINDINGS

- Normal thyroid-stimulating hormone (TSH) levels
- Elevated calcitonin level (basal or calcium/pentagastrin stimulated)

IMAGING FINDINGS

- **US:** Demonstrates extent of tumor and can detect enlarged lymph nodes
- Plain films of neck may reveal irregular dense calcifications of the MTC lesion

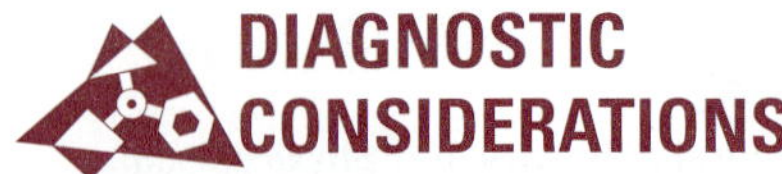

DIAGNOSTIC CONSIDERATIONS

- Tumors contain amyloid
- Resistant to radioiodine uptake
- Growth not stimulated by TSH
- Spread is lymphatic
- Familial tumors are often multifocal and bilateral (vs unilateral in sporadic disease)

RULE OUT

- Multiple endocrine neoplasia type 2A or 2B

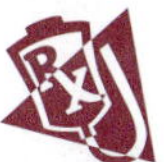

WORK-UP

- Complete history and physical exam, with special consideration to family history and exam of the neck and cervical lymph nodes
- Fine-needle aspiration biopsy
- Serum calcitonin
- Screen for *Ret* mutations (10% of patients without a family history have de novo mutations)

TREATMENT AND MANAGEMENT

- Prophylactic total thyroidectomy before age 5 recommended for patients without symptoms and if detected by family genetic screening
- Surgical treatment represents the only chance for cure
- Nonresectable recurrence of MTC may respond to external beam radiation or multidrug chemotherapy regimen

SURGERY

Indications

- All MTCs should be removed, with central neck dissection, as completely as possible

MEDICATIONS

- Postoperative thyroid hormone replacement

TREATMENT MONITORING

- Calcitonin level and neck palpation every 3–6 months

COMPLICATIONS

- Neck hematoma
- Superior laryngeal nerve injury
- Recurrent laryngeal nerve injury
- Transient or permanent hypoparathyroidism

PROGNOSIS

- Outcome correlates directly with completeness of tumor resection and degree of extrathyroidal spread
- 10-year survival about 30–40%

RESOURCES

REFERENCES

- Moley JF et al. Reoperation for recurrent or persistent medullary thyroid cancer. *Surgery.* 1993;114:1090.
- Bergholm U et al. Clinical characteristics in sporadic and familial medullary thyroid carcinoma. *Cancer.* 1989;63:1196.
- Chi DD, Moley JF. Medullary thyroid carcinoma. Genetic advances, treatment recommendations, and the approach to the patient with persistent hypercalcitoninemia. *Surg Oncol Clin North Am.* 1998;7:681.
- Rieu M et al. Prevalence of sporadic medullary thyroid carcinoma: the importance of routine measurement of serum calcitonin in the diagnostic evaluation of thyroid nodules. *Clin Endocrinol.* 1995;42:453.

PRACTICE GUIDELINES

- The National Comprehensive Cancer Network
  http://www.nccn.org

CANCER STAGING

- See Thyroid Staging Table on page 756.

Thyroid Cancer, Papillary

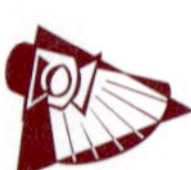

ESSENTIAL FEATURES

- History of radiation to the neck in some patients
- Painless or enlarging nodule, dysphagia, or hoarseness
- Firm or hard, fixed thyroid nodule; cervical lymphadenopathy
- Normal thyroid function; nodule stippled with calcium (x-ray), solid (US), cold (radioiodine scan), positive or suspicious cytologic studies
- Family history of thyroid cancer

EPIDEMIOLOGY

- Usually occurs in young adults
- 80–85% of all thyroid cancers
- 80% of children and 20% of adults present with clinically positive lymph node metastases
- Psammoma bodies are seen on pathologic analysis in 60% of cases

CLINICAL FINDINGS

SYMPTOMS AND SIGNS

- Solitary thyroid nodule
- Enlarged or hard cervical lymph nodes
- Pain in the thyroid or paralaryngeal neck
- Hoarseness
- Dyspnea
- Stridor
- Dysphagia

LABORATORY FINDINGS

- Normal thyroid-stimulating hormone (TSH) level

IMAGING FINDINGS

- **US:** Solid or cystic nodule
- **Radioiodine scan:** Nonfunctioning (cold)

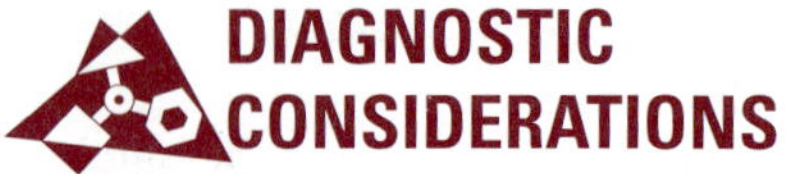

DIAGNOSTIC CONSIDERATIONS

- Grows slowly, and metastasizes through lymph nodes
- Rate of growth may be stimulated by TSH
- Often multifocal or bilobar

RULE OUT

- Concurrent hyperparathyroidism (so that it can be treated at the same operation if necessary)

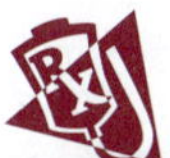

WORK-UP

- Complete history and physical, with attention to risk factors, family history, palpable characteristics of the nodule or lymphadenopathy
- Measurement of serum TSH and calcium levels
- Fine-needle aspiration biopsy

TREATMENT AND MANAGEMENT

- Treatment starts with operative removal
- External beam radiation may palliate nonresectable metastases that are resistant to radioiodine

SURGERY

Indications

- All papillary thyroid cancers should be excised
- Bulky or palpable nodal recurrences

MEDICATIONS

- Suppressive doses of thyroid hormone after thyroid ablation or thyroidectomy
- Radioactive iodine therapy for remnant, recurrent, or metastatic disease

TREATMENT MONITORING

- Semiannual or yearly serum thyroglobulin, thyroglobulin antibodies, and whole body radioiodine scan

COMPLICATIONS

- Neck hematoma
- Superior laryngeal nerve injury
- Recurrent laryngeal nerve injury
- Transient or permanent hypoparathyroidism
- Wound infection

PROGNOSIS

- Very good even in the presence of metastases
- 10-year survival rate after operation for papillary cancer is over 80%

RESOURCES

REFERENCES

- Gagel RF et al. Changing concepts in the pathogenesis and management of thyroid carcinoma. *CA Cancer J Clin.* 1996;46:261.
- Jossart G et al. Well differentiated thyroid cancer. *Curr Probl Surg.* 1994;31:933.
- Kebebew E et al. Differentiated thyroid cancer: "complete" rational approach. *World J Surg.* 2000;24:942.
- Loree TR. Therapeutic implications of prognostic factors in differentiated carcinoma of the thyroid gland. *Semin Surg Oncol.* 1995;11:246.

PRACTICE GUIDELINES

- The National Comprehensive Cancer Network
  http://www.nccn.org

CANCER STAGING

- See Thyroid Staging Table on page 756.

Thyroid Lymphoma

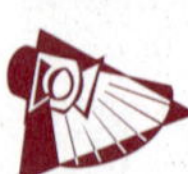

ESSENTIAL FEATURES

- Often history of hypothyroidism, specifically Hashimoto thyroiditis

EPIDEMIOLOGY

- 2.2–2.6% of all cases of non-Hodgkin lymphoma
- Incidence of 0.5–1/100,000
- Approximately 2% of all thyroid malignancies
- Strong female prevalence
- Median age of onset is late seventh decade
- Hashimoto thyroiditis is frequent precursor
- Vast majority are B-cell type
- 42–60% of patients present with stage IE disease

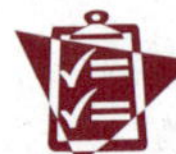

CLINICAL FINDINGS

SYMPTOMS AND SIGNS

- Rapidly enlarging neck mass
- Hoarseness
- Stridor
- Dysphagia, odynophagia
- Thyroid is firm and fixed

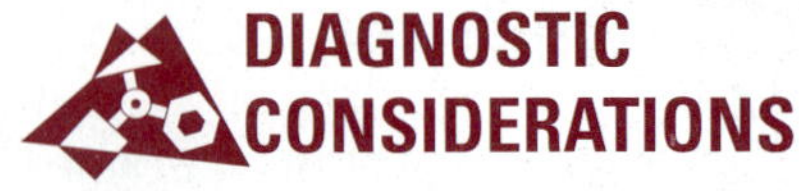

DIAGNOSTIC CONSIDERATIONS

RULE OUT

- Anaplastic thyroid carcinoma

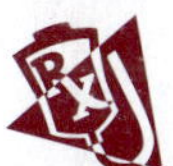

WORK-UP

- History and physical exam
- Needle biopsy/open biopsy
- Full staging with neck, chest, abdomen, and pelvis CT or MRI

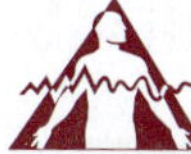

TREATMENT AND MANAGEMENT

- Little role for surgical therapy except for incisional biopsy
- Multiple agent chemotherapy and radiation therapy are the mainstays
- Radiation therapy can abrogate airway compromise

SURGERY

Indications

- Tracheostomy if airway compromise

MEDICATIONS

- Multiple agent chemotherapy

PROGNOSIS

- Poor; predicted by dysphagia, hoarseness, initial tumor size > 10 cm, and stage at presentation beyond IE
- 5-year survival for stage IE is 80%
- 5-year survival for stage IIE is 50%

RESOURCES

PRACTICE GUIDELINES

- The National Comprehensive Cancer Network
  http://www.nccn.org

CANCER STAGING

- Stage IE: Disease within the thyroid gland
- Stage IIE: Disease confined to the thyroid and regional lymph nodes
- Stage IIIE: Disease on both sides of the diaphragm
- Stage IV: Disseminated disease

Thyroid Metastasis

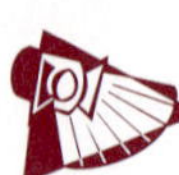

ESSENTIAL FEATURES

- Thought to be due to the rich vascularity of the thyroid gland
- Primary tumor types include:
  - Renal
  - Lung
  - Breast
  - Melanoma
  - Head and neck tumors

EPIDEMIOLOGY

- Secondary metastases to the thyroid account for 1–2% of all thyroid malignancies

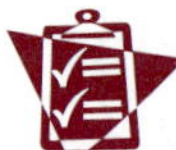

CLINICAL FINDINGS

LABORATORY FINDINGS

- Fine-needle aspiration biopsy demonstrates metastatic carcinoma

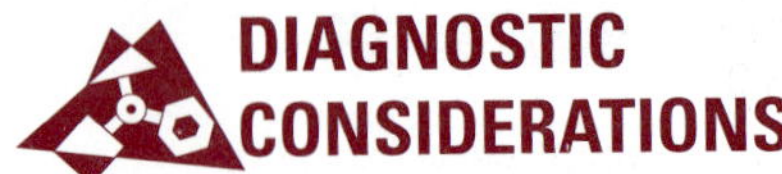

DIAGNOSTIC CONSIDERATIONS

- Must evaluate for primary thyroid tumors
- If tumor is proved metastatic, then must identify primary and other sites of metastatic disease to make a comprehensive plan

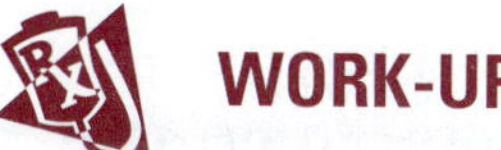

WORK-UP

- Detection of mass
- Needle biopsy

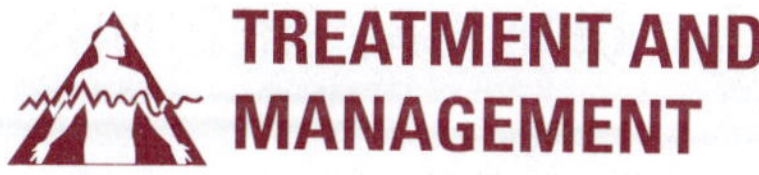

TREATMENT AND MANAGEMENT

SURGERY

Indications

- Inconclusive biopsy
- Occult primary tumor
- Negative metastatic work-up, thus leaving the thyroid mass as the only site of recurrence of a distant primary tumor

PROGNOSIS

- Poor; one series had 11 of 12 patients die in 9 months from diagnosis

RESOURCES

REFERENCES

- Haugen BR. Secondary malignancy of the thyroid gland: a case report and review of the literature. *Thyroid.* 1994;4:297.
- Lin JD et al. Clinical and pathologic characteristics of secondary thyroid cancer. *Thyroid.* 1998;2:149.
- Nakhjavani MK et al. Metastasis to the thyroid gland: a report of 43 cases. *Cancer.* 1997;79:574.
- McCabe DP et al. Clinical and pathologic correlations in disease metastatic to the thyroid gland. *Am J Surg.* 1985;150:519.

Thyroid Nodule

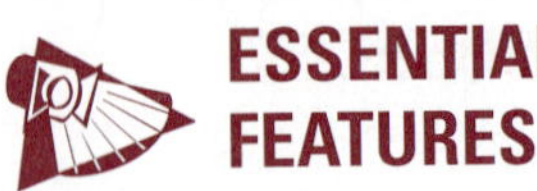

ESSENTIAL FEATURES

- Very common and most are not cancer
- Central diagnostic question is whether the lesion is benign or malignant

EPIDEMIOLOGY

- Present in about 5% of the population
- 5% of nodules represent thyroid cancer
- 2-fold more common in females, although malignant nodules slightly more common in males
- Risk of malignancy greater in persons older than 60 or in children younger than 15
- 20% of cold nodules on thyroid scintigraphy are malignant

CLINICAL FINDINGS

SYMPTOMS AND SIGNS

- Often asymptomatic, and discovered as a nodule on routine physical exam or exam for another head/neck pathology
- Occasional pain
- Hoarseness

LABORATORY FINDINGS

- Serum thyroid-stimulating level (TSH) level (low in solitary toxic nodule, normal or elevated in nonfunctioning nodules)
- Fine-needle aspiration biopsy can have the following results:
  - Malignant
  - Benign
  - Indeterminate
  - Inadequate

IMAGING FINDINGS

- **US**
  - Can distinguish size of nodules and assess for presence of nonpalpable nodules
  - Also can distinguish solid from cystic nodules
- **Thyroid scintigraphy:** Demonstrates functional nodules to be warm/hot and nonfunctioning nodules to be cold

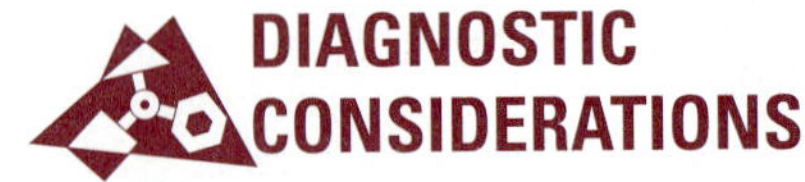

DIAGNOSTIC CONSIDERATIONS

RULE OUT

- Thyroid cancer

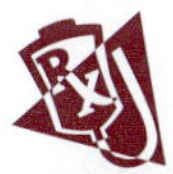

WORK-UP

- Complete history and physical exam
  - Focus on duration of swelling, recent growth, local symptoms (dysphagia, pain, voice changes), and systemic symptoms (hyperthyroidism, hypothyroidism); the patient's age, sex, place of birth, family history, and history of head/neck irradiation are most important
- Thyroid function tests
- Thyroid US
- Fine-needle aspiration biopsy
- Observation, medical therapy, or surgery
- Thyroid scintigraphy only if patient hyperthyroid

TREATMENT AND MANAGEMENT

SURGERY

Indications

- Obstruction of the aerodigestive tract
- FNA biopsy with malignant or indeterminate result
- 3 successive inadequate biopsies
- Recurrence of cyst after 2 aspirations

MEDICAL

- TSH suppression with L-thyroxine if patient hypothyroid; may arrest nodule growth

RESOURCES

REFERENCES

- Mazzaferri EL. Management of a solitary thyroid nodule. *N Engl J Med.* 1993;328:553.
- Wong CK et al. Thyroid nodules: Rational management. *World J Surg.* 2000;24:934.

Thyroiditis, Acute Suppurative

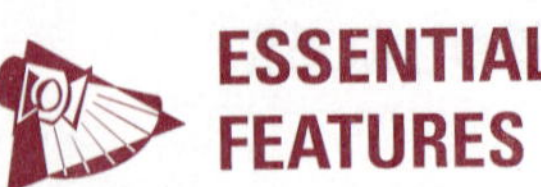

ESSENTIAL FEATURES

- Sudden onset
- Often follows an upper respiratory tract infection

EPIDEMIOLOGY

- Rare condition
- 50% of patients have preexisting thyroid disease
- Peak incidence in childhood or young and middle-age adults

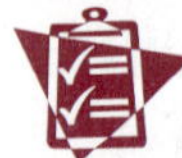

CLINICAL FINDINGS

SYMPTOMS AND SIGNS

- Acute neck pain, exacerbated by neck extension
- Dysphagia
- Fever, chills
- Neck enlargement
- Warmth and erythema
- Hemoptysis
- Cervical lymphadenopathy

LABORATORY FINDINGS

- Leukocytosis
- Normal thyroid function

IMAGING FINDINGS

- Barium swallow (if suspect piriform sinus) demonstrates fistulous tract
- Areas of decreased uptake on thyroid scan (if associated abscess)
- Partially cystic mass seen on thyroid US

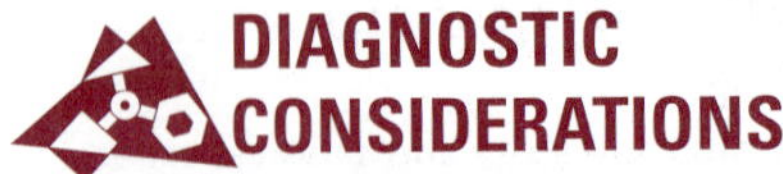

DIAGNOSTIC CONSIDERATIONS

- Percutaneous aspiration, with Gram stain and culture often yields diagnosis
- Most common organisms are:
  - Streptococci
  - Staphylococci
  - Pneumococci
  - Coliforms
- May be associated with a piriform sinus fistula
- Extremely rare causes include:
  - TB
  - Actinomycoses
  - Echinococcosis
  - Aspergillosis
  - Syphilis
- Infection usually arises from drainage from local structures but can also be hematogenously spread or after direct trauma
- Blood-tinged sputum suggest tracheal involvement

RULE OUT

- Chronic suppurative thyroiditis
- De Quervain thyroiditis

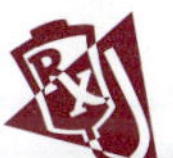

WORK-UP

- History and physical exam
- Needle aspiration, with Gram stain and culture of aspirate

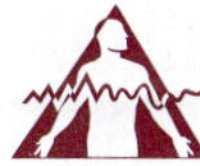

TREATMENT AND MANAGEMENT

- Primary treatment is antibiotics

SURGERY

- Thyroid abscess should be operatively drained

Indications

- Thyroid abscess
- Cysts communicating with the piriform sinus or trachea (surgery to excise this fistula should be done after the infection has been completely eradicated)

MEDICATIONS

- Antibiotics are indicated in all cases

TREATMENT MONITORING

- Improvement should occur within 48–72 hours of starting antibiotics, with complete resolution after 2–4 weeks

RESOURCES

REFERENCES

- Miyauchi A et al. Piriform sinus fistula: an underlying abnormality common in patients with autosuppurative thyroiditis. *World J Surg.* 1990;14:400.
- Altemeier WA. Acute pyogenic thyroiditis. *Arch Surg.* 1950;61:76.
- Hagan AD et al. Acute streptococcal thyroiditis. *JAMA.* 1969;202:829.

Thyroiditis, De Quervain, Subacute

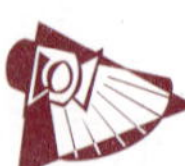

ESSENTIAL FEATURES

- Also known as subacute or giant-cell thyroiditis
- Noninfectious disorder
- Can be present without pain (silent thyroiditis)
- Self-limited disorder
- Often follows upper respiratory infection, and thus postulated to have a viral etiology

EPIDEMIOLOGY

- 1% of all cases of thyroid disease
- One-eighth the incidence of Graves disease
- Most common cause of an anterior neck mass and pain in the thyroid
- Uncommon in children
- Most common in the third to fifth decade
- Male:female ratio of 5:1

CLINICAL FINDINGS

SYMPTOMS AND SIGNS

- Thyroid swelling
- Head and chest pain
- Weakness, fever, malaise
- Palpitations
- Weight loss
- Dysphagia
- Odynophagia

LABORATORY FINDINGS

- Elevated ESR
- Elevated serum gamma globulin
- Increased or normal thyroid hormone function tests
- Decreased thyroid-stimulating hormone (TSH) levels
- Decreased radioactive iodine uptake
- Increased thyroglobulin

IMAGING FINDINGS

- Decreased uptake on radioiodine thyroid scan

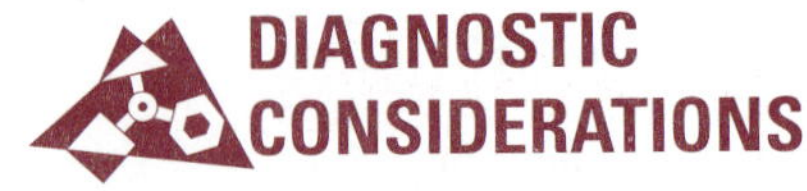

DIAGNOSTIC CONSIDERATIONS

RULE OUT

- Graves disease
- Thyroid cancer
- Acute suppurative thyroiditis

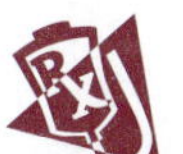

WORK-UP

- Physical exam
- Thyroid function tests
- Radioiodine thyroid scan

TREATMENT AND MANAGEMENT

- Illness is usually self-limited

MEDICATIONS

- Aspirin, ibuprofen, or corticosteroids relieve symptoms

TREATMENT MONITORING

- Monitor thyroid function

PROGNOSIS

- Patients are usually left euthyroid
- 10% of patients have permanent hypothyroidism

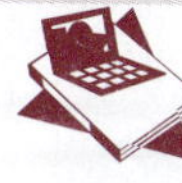

RESOURCES

REFERENCES

- Singer PA. Thyroiditis: acute, subacute and chronic. *Med Clin North Am.* 1991;75:61.

Thyroiditis, Riedel

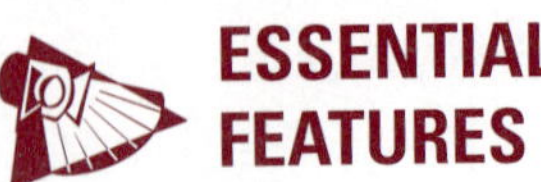

ESSENTIAL FEATURES

- Rare condition
- Invasive fibrosis of the thyroid gland
- Symptoms appear gradually

EPIDEMIOLOGY

- Extremely rare
- Usually presents in middle-aged women

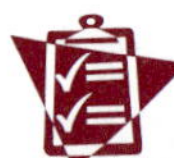

CLINICAL FINDINGS

SYMPTOMS AND SIGNS

- Large, nontender, woody mass in the thyroid region
- Stridor
- Dysphagia
- Hoarse voice

LABORATORY FINDINGS

- Biopsy shows marked fibrosis and chronic inflammation
- Hypothyroid (late stage)
- Absent or low titers of antithyroid antibodies

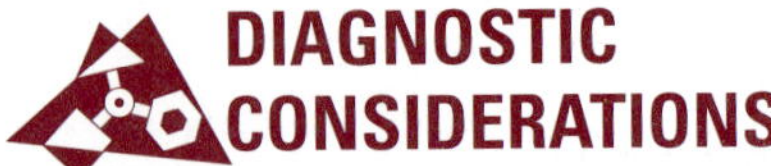

DIAGNOSTIC CONSIDERATIONS

- Inflammatory process involves surrounding muscles and causes tracheal compression or esophageal obstruction
- Etiology is unknown
- May be associated with fibrosis of other organ systems, such as the retroperitoneum

RULE OUT

- Thyroid carcinoma

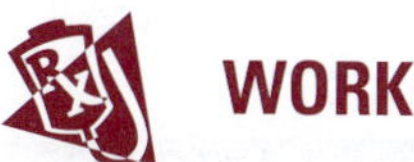

WORK-UP

- Physical exam
- Thyroid function tests

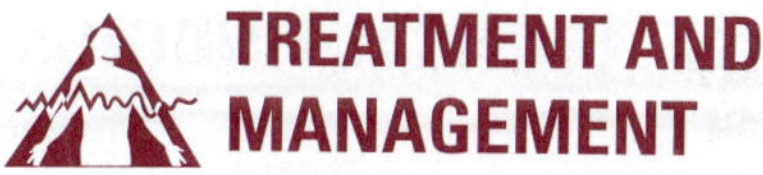

TREATMENT AND MANAGEMENT

- Corticosteroid therapy is first-line and often requires long-term maintenance therapy
- Low-dose radiation may be beneficial if corticosteroids or surgery is unsuccessful

SURGERY

Indications

- Esophageal or tracheal compression

MEDICATIONS

- Corticosteroid therapy
- Thyroid hormone replacement if hypothyroid

PROGNOSIS

- Multifocal fibrosis may develop in a few patients as many as 10 years after diagnosis with Reidel thyroiditis; this may be life-threatening

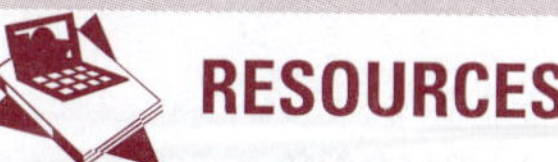

RESOURCES

REFERENCES

- Girod DA et al. Riedel's thyroiditis: Report of a lethal case and review of the literature. *Otolaryngol Head Neck Surg.* 1992;107:591.
- Turner-Wawick R et al. Riedel's thyroiditis and retroperitoneal fibrosis. *Proc R Soc Med.* 1966;59:596.
- Woolner LB et al. Invasive fibrous thyroiditis. *J Clin Endocrinol.* 1957;17:201.

Tietze Syndrome

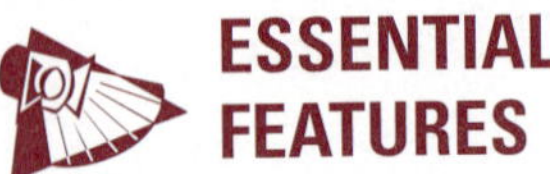

ESSENTIAL FEATURES

- Painful, nonsuppurative inflammation of costochondral cartilage
- Unknown cause
- May represent seronegative rheumatic disease
- Often self-limited
- Unilateral or bilateral
- Involves second–fourth costal cartilages

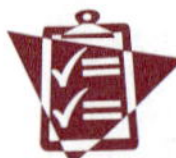

CLINICAL FINDINGS

SYMPTOMS AND SIGNS

- Local swelling, tenderness in parasternal area

IMAGING FINDINGS

- **Bone scan:** Can localize inflamed costochondral junctions
- **Chest CT:** Can localize, but less sensitive than bone scan
- **Transthoracic echocardiography:** May demonstrate pathologic cartilage hyperechogenicity

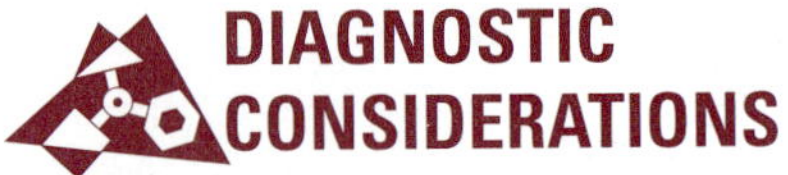

DIAGNOSTIC CONSIDERATIONS

RULE OUT

- Costochondral neoplasm: if symptoms last longer than 3 wks
- Breast pain/causes

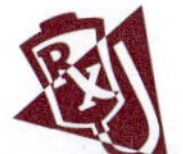

WORK-UP

- Physical exam
- Consider chest CT or bone scan; usually not needed

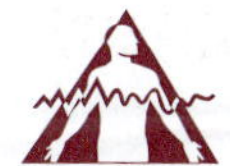

TREATMENT AND MANAGEMENT

- If symptomatic, NSAIDs, local or systemic corticosteroids

SURGERY

Indications

- If symptoms longer than 3 wks and mass is present, consider neoplasm and excise

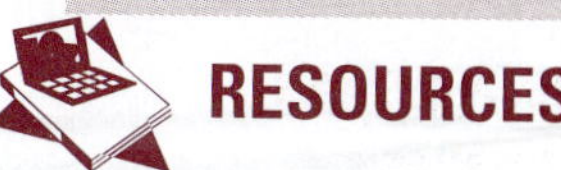

RESOURCES

REFERENCES

- Aeschlimann A, Kahn MF. Tietze's syndrome: a critical review. *Clin Exper Rheumatol.* 1990;8:407.

Tracheobronchial Injuries

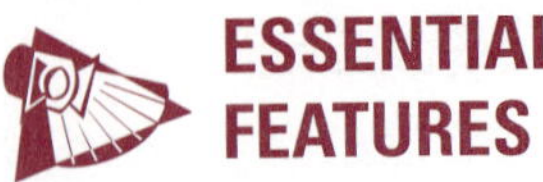

ESSENTIAL FEATURES

- Blunt tracheobronchial injuries are often the result of compression of the airway between the sternum and the vertebral column
- Blunt injury usually involves distal trachea or mainstem bronchi
- Penetrating tracheobronchial injuries may occur at any location
- Tracheobronchial injury should be suspected with massive air leak or when there is poor reexpansion after chest tube placement

EPIDEMIOLOGY

- Trauma patients

CLINICAL FINDINGS

SYMPTOMS AND SIGNS

- Most patients have pneumothorax, subcutaneous emphysema, and hemoptysis
- Penetrating injuries usually cause massive hemoptysis

IMAGING FINDINGS

- Pneumothorax
- Pneumomediastinum
- Subcutaneous air
- Pneumothorax that persists after chest tube placement

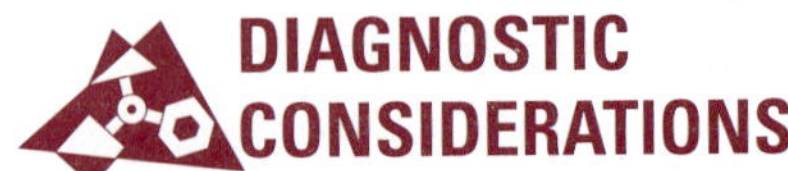

DIAGNOSTIC CONSIDERATIONS

- Associated abdominal injuries may dictate care

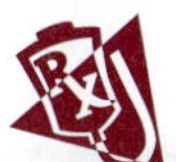

WORK-UP

- Physical exam
- ABG measurements
- Chest film
- Late presenting injuries may require bronchoscopy

TREATMENT AND MANAGEMENT

- Resuscitation and stabilization
- Chest tube
- Intubation and mechanical ventilation

SURGERY

- Immediate primary repair is indicated for tracheobronchial laceration

Indications

- Tracheobronchial laceration

TREATMENT MONITORING

- Serial chest film
- Serial ABG measurements

RESOURCES

REFERENCES

- Feliciano DV et al. Advances in the diagnosis and treatment of thoracic trauma. *Surg Clin North Am.* 1999;79:1417.

Transposition of the Great Arteries

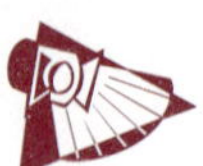

ESSENTIAL FEATURES

- A congenital heart lesion that decreases pulmonary arterial blood flow
- Cyanosis and decreased oxygen delivery causes compensatory polycythemia (Hct > 70%) and spontaneous thrombosis
- Exercise, acidosis, pain worsens cyanosis, can cause hypoxic spells
- β-Blockers (decreases spasm), fluid intake, HCO_3 administration, norepinephrine (increases systemic resistance) may help decrease hypoxia
- Bronchial and mediastinal arteries enlarge
- Ductus arteriosus maintains flow to lungs during fetal development
- Early administration of alprostadil can allow time for optimization before definitive treatment

Transposition of Great Arteries (TGA)

- Normal ventricular arrangement (D-transposition)
- Terminology often confusing:
  - Dextrocardia: Right-sided heart, no relation to "looping" (levocardia is normal)
  - Levo- and dextro- (normal): Refers to ventricular looping; levo-: Right-sided morphologic LV, left-sided RV
  - D-, L-, A-: Indicates malposition of great vessels; letter designates relationship of aorta to pulmonary artery (PA) (D- to the right, normal; L-, to left; A-, anterior)
- **Aorta connected to morphologic RV is most common (D-transposition)**
  - Normal looping, rightward aorta connected to RV, left-sided PA connected to LV, 2 independent circulations requiring mixing of blood for survival
  - Atrial septal defect (ASD), patent ductus arteriosus (PDA) common
  - Ventricular septal defect (VSD) in 25%; more common in unusual arrangements
  - LV outflow obstruction may occur
  - Coronary arteries still arise from aortic sinuses facing pulmonary valve, but origin and course may vary and make repair more difficult
  - Cyanosis proportional to mixing of blood
  - In VSD, more risk for pulmonary hypertension due to large left-to-right shunting
  - Normally, LV increases in size at 2–3 wks of life; in TGA, however, RV increases instead due to increased work load

Corrected Transposition of Great Arteries (CTGA)

- Referred to as L-transposition (true)
- Right-sided morphologic LV connected to PA, left-sided morphologic RV connected to aorta
- L- refers to aorta being to left of PA, does not refer to levo- loop
- Blood flow in series through right and left side, so oxygenated blood reaches systemic
- VSD in > 75%, subpulmonary obstruction in 50%
- Coronary pattern reversed to correspond to ventricular arrangement
- Conduction passes to right side of ventricular septum, superior to VSD
- Mitral valve = right-sided, tricuspid valve = left-sided

CLINICAL FINDINGS

SYMPTOMS AND SIGNS

TGA

- Cyanosis at birth
  - Deterioration with duct closure
  - Worsening hypoxia and acidosis
- In VSD or large shunt, symptoms may be minimal in first few weeks of life
- Progressive heart failure
- Murmurs variable, nondiagnostic

CTGA

- Uncommon in infancy
- Congestive failure eventually develops due to pulmonary stenosis, tricuspid insufficiency
- Heart block (first, second, third) in infancy or later

LABORATORY FINDINGS

- **ECG:** RV hypertrophy

IMAGING FINDINGS

- **Chest film:** Enlarged heart, increased pulmonary circulation
- **Echocardiography:** Diagnostic
- **Catheterization:** Assess pressures and suitability of LV for switch

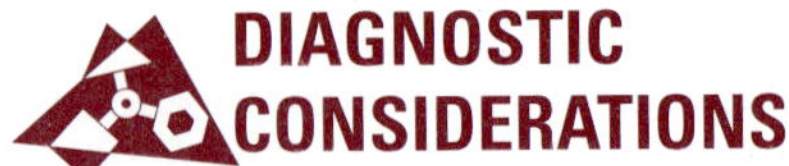

DIAGNOSTIC CONSIDERATIONS

- Evaluate for other cardiac or extracardiac anomalies

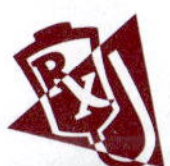

WORK-UP

- Echocardiogram and catheterization

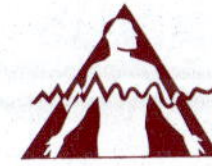

TREATMENT AND MANAGEMENT

TGA

- Without treatment, 50% die within 1 mo, 90% die within 1 yr
- Once diagnosed, atrial septostomy
- **Mustard and Senning procedures:** Intra-atrial channels direct systemic venous return to LV, pulmonary to RV
- **Arterial switch procedure:** Done with hypothermic cardiopulmonary bypass or hypothermic circulatory arrest; switches aorta and PA onto correct ventricles; coronaries also switched with aorta
- Timing important; if in first 2 wks of life, primary switch procedure performed
- If done later than 2 wks old, 2 stage:

1. Modified Blalock-Taussig shunt with PA band (provides pulmonary flow, conditions LV)
2. After 2 wks, shunt and band removed, switch performed

- VSD and ASD can be closed during switch procedure
- **Rastelli procedure (used if VSD and LV outflow obstruction):** Enlarge VSD, place intraventricular baffle to allow an unobstructed LV outflow tract; main PA divided and oversewn, pulmonary homograft sewn to infundibulotomy and distal main PA

CTGA

- VSD closure via aorta or LA
- Tricuspid insufficiency via RA or LA
- **Double switch (atrial and arterial):** Advocated by some

SURGERY

Indications

- Diagnosis warrants repair

COMPLICATIONS

- Complications with coronary transfer contribute to postoperative cardiac dysfunction

PROGNOSIS

- Switch procedure: < 2% mortality
- Infrequently require further intervention
- **Mustard/Senning:** Tricuspid insufficiency, arrhythmias, venous obstruction, right heart failure occur in older patients
- 10-year survival 50% for CTGA

RESOURCES

REFERENCES

- Kirlin JW et al. Clinical outcomes after the arterial switch operation for transposition: patient, support, procedural, and institutional risk factors. *Circulation.* 1992;86:1501.
- Wernovsky G et al. Factors influencing early and late outcome of the arterial switch operation for transposition of the great arteries. *J Thorac Cardiovasc Surg.* 1995;109:289.
- Alva C et al. The feasibility of complete anatomical correction in the setting of discordant atrioventricular connections. *Br Heart J.* 1999;81:539.

Trauma Evaluation

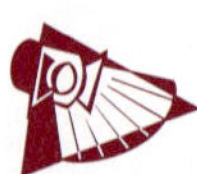

ESSENTIAL FEATURES

- Primary survey attempts to identify and treat immediate life-threatening conditions
- Identification of life-threatening injuries
- Resuscitation
- Response to treatment evaluated
- Primary evaluation includes:
  - Airway
  - Breathing
  - Circulation
  - Deficit
  - Exposure
- Secondary survey evaluates for additional injuries
- Rapid and complete history and physical exam are essential for patients with serious or multiple injuries
- Progressive changes in clinical findings are often the key to correct diagnosis
- Certain types of trauma should prompt directed evaluation for associated injuries

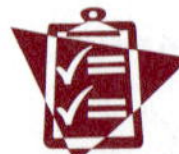

CLINICAL FINDINGS

LABORATORY FINDINGS

- Blood should be immediately drawn for Hct, WBC count, creatinine, blood urea nitrogen, and blood typing and crossmatch
- ABG measurement if any sign of respiratory compromise
- Liver panel if any indication of liver disease
- UA should be obtained, checking especially for hematuria

IMAGING FINDINGS

- Films of the chest and abdomen are required in all major injuries
- Cervical spine films should be obtained in patients at risk for this kind of injury
- CT scan of head and abdomen may be considered in patients with altered mental status and hemodynamic stability
- Intravenous pyelogram is critical in abdominal injuries and pelvic fractures

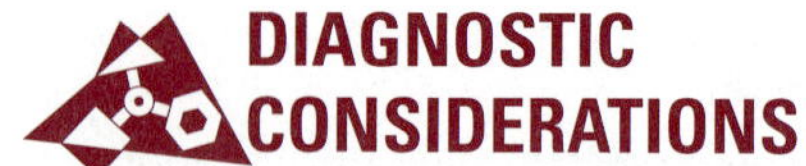

DIAGNOSTIC CONSIDERATIONS

- Multiple injuries may be identified and should be addressed by the A-B-C (Airway-Breathing-Circulation) approach

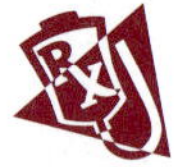

WORK-UP

Airway

- The establishment of an adequate airway has the highest priority in the primary survey
- Cervical spine injury is always assumed until proved otherwise
- Orotracheal intubation can be attempted if second person maintains in-line cervical stabilization
- If necessary, cricothyroidotomy should be performed as quickly as possible

Breathing

- Ensure that ventilation is adequate; examine chest rise, breath sounds, tachypnea, crepitus, and subcutaneous emphysema, presence of open or penetrating wounds
- Identify immediately life-threatening conditions:
  - Tension pneumothorax
  - Open pneumothorax
  - Massive hemothorax
  - Flail chest

Circulation

- Gross hemorrhage from accessible surface wounds is usually obvious and can most often be controlled with direct pressure and elevation
- Firm pressure on the major arteries in the axilla, groin, antecubital space, wrist, popliteal space, or ankle may suffice for temporary control of arterial hemorrhage distal to these points
- When other measures have failed, a tourniquet may rarely be necessary to control major hemorrhage from an extremity
- Tourniquets must be released for 1–2 minutes every 20 minutes until definitive care is provided
- All patients with significant trauma should have 2 large caliber IV catheters inserted immediately for the administration of drugs and fluids

- If any degree of shock present, a large bore venous catheter should be placed in the femoral vein to monitor central venous pressure (CVP)
- As soon as IV access is gained, rapid crystalloid infusion should begin
- Adults should receive 2 L of normal saline or lactated Ringer's with an additional 2 L given for transient or no response
- For children, 20 mL/kg should be initial volume administered
- If additional fluid is necessary, it should include administration of blood products

Neurologic Disability

- Various degrees of coma due to a number of causes may accompany trauma and require treatment
- Most common causes:
  - Alcohol
  - Cerebrovascular accident
  - Diabetic ketoacidosis
  - Barbiturate poisoning
  - Narcotic overdose
  - Hypovolemic shock
- Less common:
  - Epilepsy
  - Eclampsia
  - Electrolyte imbalance
- Differential depends on careful history, careful and complete physical exam, laboratory tests, CT scan

Exposure

- All clothing should be removed at once
- All surfaces must be examined to identify injuries not readily apparent

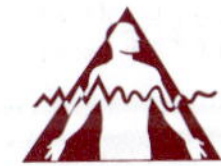

TREATMENT AND MANAGEMENT

Hypovolemic Shock

- Keep patient recumbent
  - Balanced salt solutions should be given rapidly until signs of shock abate and urinary output normalizes
- Blood pressure and pulse are less reliable than urinary output
- Successful resuscitation is indicated by by warm dry, well-perfused skin, urinary output 30–60 mL/hr, and an alert sensorium
- If patient requires ongoing fluid, further investigation is warranted

Neurogenic Shock

- Due to the pooling of blood in autonomically denervated venules and is usually due to spinal cord injury NOT isolated head injury
- Patient should be placed in Trendelenburg position and given 2 L crystalloid IV followed by another bolus if suboptimal response
- Phenylephrine or another vasopressor should be given IV drip and titrated to blood pressure

Cardiac Compressive Shock

- Caused by compression of the thin-walled chambers of the heart (atria, RV) or by compression or distortion of the great veins (superior vena cava, inferior vena cava)
- Usual causes in trauma are pericardial tamponade, tension pneumothorax, massive hemothorax, diaphragmatic rupture, or elevated diaphragm from massive abdominal bleeding
- Treatment is urgent decompression depending on cause

Cardiogenic Shock

- Caused by decreased myocardial contractility and is usually caused by myocardial infarction or arrhythmia
- Rarely caused by massive cardiac contusion
- Treatment is supportive, with volume replacement and use of inotropes

Treatment Priorities

- If signs of hypovolemic shock, coma likely due to cerebral ischemia; resuscitation and blood volume replacement have first priority
- Coma absent signs of shock indicates likely head injury
- Deepening stupor in patients under observation should arouse suspicion of expanding intracranial lesion
- Cerebral injuries take precedence in care only when there is rapidly deepening coma
- In most cases, skull fractures are low priority
- Most urologic injuries are managed at the time of intra-abdominal injury management
- Long bone fractures can be splinted and treated urgently except when there is associated vascular injury with limb ischemia
- Open fractures should be cleaned and debrided as soon as possible
- Hand injuries require early treatment to avoid infection
- Tetanus prophylaxis should be given in all instances of open contaminated wounds, puncture wounds, and burns

SURGERY

Indications

- Emergency thoracotomy is indicated for cardiopulmonary arrest in the emergency department as a result of penetrating trauma
- Emergency left anterolateral thoracotomy is performed in the fourth or fifth intercostals space and the pericardium opened anterior to the phrenic nerve
- Open cardiac massage, cross-clamping of descending thoracic aorta, repair of cardiac injuries and internal defibrillation all can be performed as appropriate

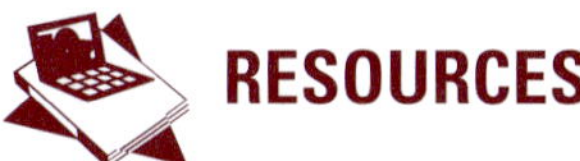

REFERENCES

- *ATLS Student Manual,* 7e. American College of Surgeons, Chicago, Ill. 2003.

Tricuspid Atresia

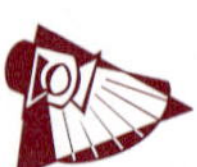

ESSENTIAL FEATURES

- A congenital heart lesion that decreases pulmonary arterial blood flow resulting in a right-to-left shunt
- Cyanosis and decreased oxygen delivery cause compensatory polycythemia (Hct > 70%) and spontaneous thrombosis
- Exercise, acidosis, pain worsens cyanosis, can cause hypoxic spells
- Squatting increases systemic resistance, causing increased pulmonary flow and oxygen saturation
- β-Blockers (decreases spasm), fluid intake, HCO_3 administration, norepinephrine (increases systemic resistance) may help decrease hypoxia
- Clubbing due to proliferation of capillaries and AV fistulas in extremities
- Bronchial and mediastinal arteries enlarge
- Ductus arteriosus maintains flow to lungs during fetal development
- Early administration of alprostadil can allow time for optimization before definitive treatment
- Operative options to increase pulmonary flow:
  - Blalock-Taussig shunt: Subclavian artery to ipsilateral pulmonary artery (PA) end to side fashion
  - Modified Blalock-Taussig shunt: Subclavian to PA using PTFE
  - Glenn: Superior vena cava (SVC) to PA shunt
  - Fontan: SVC and inferior vena cava (IVC) rerouted to PA
  - Excision of obstructive muscle, patch enlargement of infundibulum, and valve replacement

Tricuspid Atresia

- Lack of communication between RA and RV
- Usually RV small
- Ventricular septal defect (VSD) common, usually restrictive
- Connections of great arteries to ventricles abnormal in 30%
- Degree of obstruction correlates to systemic and pulmonary blood flow

Ebstein Anomaly

- Septal and posterior leaflets of tricuspid valve small displaced toward RV apex
- Portion of RV thin and atrialized
- Associated atrial septal defect (ASD) and patent foramen ovale (PFO)

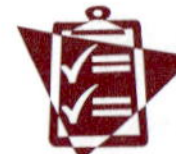

CLINICAL FINDINGS

SYMPTOMS AND SIGNS

Tricuspid Atresia

- Symptoms relate to degree of ASD/VSD restriction, great vessels anatomy
- Clinical presentation can vary
- Majority have some degree of cyanosis no obstruction to systemic output

Ebstein Anomaly

- Cyanosis, arrhythmias common
- 50% develop right heart failure, hypoxia, hepatomegaly, dysrhythmias

IMAGING FINDINGS

- **Echocardiography:** Diagnostic
- **Catheterization:** Determine suitability for repair and potential correction of ASD

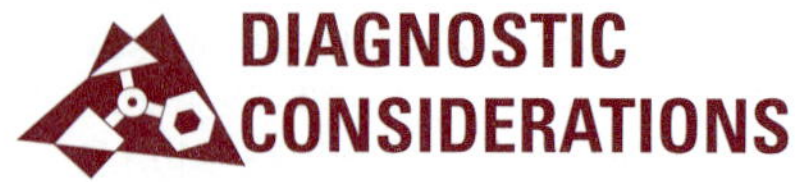

DIAGNOSTIC CONSIDERATIONS

- Echocardiography and catheterization

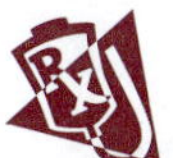

WORK-UP

- Echocardiography and catheterization

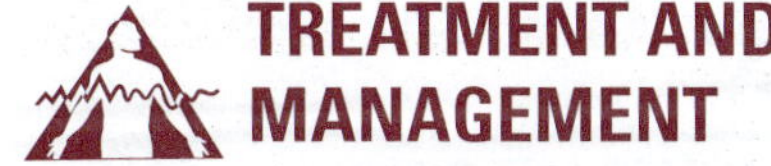

TREATMENT AND MANAGEMENT

Tricuspid Atresia

- ASD balloon septoplasty: If restrictive
- Blalock-Taussig often done initially, provide pulmonary flow
- Glenn followed by Fontan to complete 3 stage repairs
- Goal: To provide adequate, not excessive pulmonary flow, minimize RV overload

Ebstein Anomaly

- Oversew atrialized portion of RV, correct tricuspid valve incompetence (successful in 50% of cases)
- Newer techniques involve correction of RV and tricuspid valve
- Some cases, irreparable

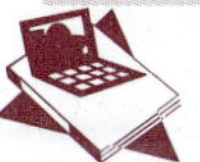

RESOURCES

REFERENCES

- Castaneda AR. From Glenn to Fontan: a continuing evolution. *Circulation.* 1992;86(5 Suppl):II80.
- Dearani JA et al. Congenital Heart Surgery Nomenclature and Database Project: Ebstein's anomaly and tricuspid valve disease. *Ann Thorac Surg.* 2000;69:S106.
- Knott-Craig CJ et al. Neonatal repair of Ebstein's anomaly: indications, surgical technique and medium-term follow-up. *Ann Thorac Surg.* 2000;69:1505.

Tricuspid Valve Disease

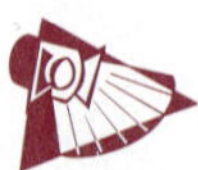

ESSENTIAL FEATURES

- Tricuspid valve (TV) has 3 leaflets:
  1. Anterior
  2. Posterior
  3. Septal
- Anterior commonly largest, posterior smallest
- Papillary muscles often multiple, grouped into 3 (anterior, inferior, septal) and contribute chordae to multiple leaflets
- Functional tricuspid disease:
  - Secondary to RV dilation causing enlargement of free-wall tricuspid annulus
  - Reflects RV failure and further worsens RV failure
- Organic regurgitation: Infective endocarditis
- Tricuspid stenosis (TS): Rheumatic usually (significant in 5% of patients)
- Carcinoid involvement of tricuspid valve: Deposits on leaflets
- RA myxomas rarely cause obstruction of tricuspid orifice
- TS and tricuspid regurgitation (TR): RA hypertension, systemic venous engorgement, hepatic congestion, edema
- Can lead to hepatic failure, cardiac cirrhosis, anasarca, and renal failure

EPIDEMIOLOGY

- Causes of valve disease:
  - Rheumatic carditis (most common)
  - Valve collagen degeneration
  - Infection
- Less common causes:
  - Collagen-vascular disease
  - Tumors
  - Carcinoid
  - Marfan syndrome
- Valvular heart disease: 89,000 hospital discharges in 1998
- Etiology of TV disease:
  - Mitral valve disease
  - Cor pulmonale
  - Primary pulmonary hypertension
  - RV infarction
  - Congenital heart disease

CLINICAL FINDINGS

SYMPTOMS AND SIGNS

- **TS and TR**
  - Related to degree of systemic venous hypertension
  - Fatigue, weakness; without signs of pulmonary congestion
- **TR with mitral valve disease**
  - Pulmonary hypertension
  - RV failure
  - Rapid deterioration
- **TS:** Prominent a wave if in sinus
- **TR:** Accentuated jugular v wave
- Liver enlarged, may be firm and fibrotic
- Ascites and edema without pulmonary congestion
- Murmurs similar to mitral valve counterparts; usually located more toward left lower sternal border, less at apex; enhanced by inspiration

LABORATORY FINDINGS

- ECG
  - In sinus rhythm: tricuspid valve disease suggested if P wave amplitude > 0.25mV on lead II

IMAGING FINDINGS

- **Chest film:** Cardiomegaly with prominent RA shadow, absence of pulmonary congestion
- **Echocardiography:** Information on anatomy and severity of regurgitation, RV function, etiology
- **Cardiac catheterization:** Diagnosis and identification of etiology

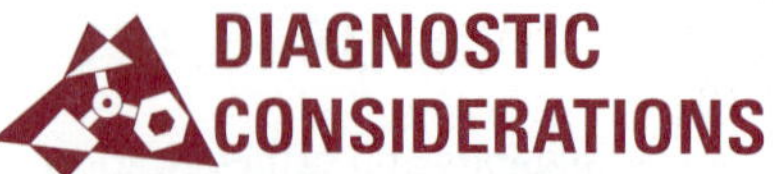

DIAGNOSTIC CONSIDERATIONS

- The findings may be subtle, and tricuspid disease is often overlooked
- Distended neck veins or the absence of pulmonary congestion
- Murmurs may be hard to distinguish

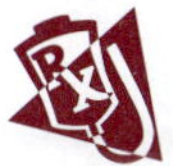

WORK-UP

- Cardiac catheterization
  - TS: Demonstrates diastolic pressure gradient between RA and RV (mean diastolic gradient of 5 mm Hg is significant
  - TR: Prominent v wave by catheterization (ventricularization of atrial pressure)
  - Pulmonary hypertension suggests functional cause; absence indicates organic cause of tricuspid disease

TREATMENT AND MANAGEMENT

- Rheumatic TS: Commissurotomy or valve replacement (residual gradients tolerated poorly); bioprosthetic valve or allografts preferred for TV due to risk of thromboembolism in low flow right heart
- Symptomatic carcinoid: Replace valve
- Tricuspid endocarditis: Many have septic pulmonary emboli; antibiotics, replace valve with allograft (resistant to infection)
- TR: Mitral valve disease (if present) + tricuspid ring annuloplasty

SURGERY

Indications

- Mitral valve disease requiring operation
- Symptomatic disease

RESOURCES

REFERENCES

- Bonow RO et al. Guidelines for the management of patients with valvular heart disease: executive summary. A report of the American College of Cardiology/American Heart Association Task Force on Practice Guidelines (Committee on Management of Patients with Valvular Heart Disease). *Circulation.* 1998;98:1949.

Truncus Arteriosus

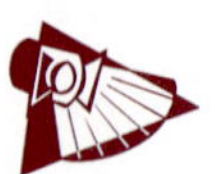

ESSENTIAL FEATURES

- A congenital heart lesion that increases pulmonary arterial blood flow
- Results in left-to-right shunt, results in lung infection, pulmonary vascular congestion, pulmonary artery (PA) hypertension, right heart failure, pulmonary vasoconstriction, pulmonary vascular obstructive disease
- **Eisenmenger syndrome:** Increased pulmonary hypertension such that left-to-right shunt ceases and shunt becomes right-to-left, requiring heart-lung transplant
- Inhaled nitric oxide, oxygen, or IV tolazoline reverses PA vasoconstriction
- PA band is palliative and can reduce PA flow to alleviate RV failure and progression of pulmonary hypertension
- Single large truncal vessel overrides ventricular septum and distributes all blood ejected from heart
- Truncal root bifurcates into pulmonary trunk and aorta
- Ventricular septal defect (VSD) present usually direct beneath truncal valve
- Atrial septal defect (ASD) (> 40%), interrupted aortic arch (10%), abnormal origins of coronary artery
- In most cases, pulmonary flow is increased

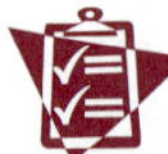

CLINICAL FINDINGS

SYMPTOMS AND SIGNS

- Heart failure in most
- Pulmonary vascular disease early

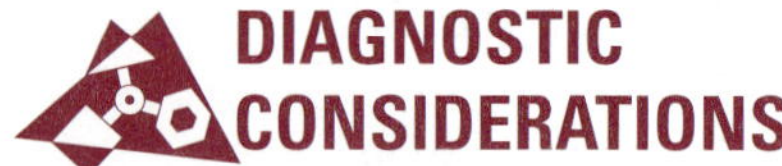

DIAGNOSTIC CONSIDERATIONS

- Evaluate for associated cardiac and extracardiac anomalies

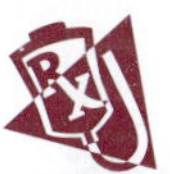

WORK-UP

- Echocardiography: Diagnostic
- Catheterization: Assess coronary arteries or truncal valve, or if age > 3 mos to assess for pulmonary hypertension

TREATMENT AND MANAGEMENT

- Surgical repair: Closure of VSD, separation pulmonary arteries from truncal root, placing pulmonary allograft valve from RV, correct truncal insufficiency

SURGERY

Indications

- Warranted once diagnosis made

Contraindications

- Eisenmenger physiology (irreversible)

PROGNOSIS

- Operative mortality 5–30% (related to truncal valve insufficiency, interrupted arch, coronary anomalies, and pulmonary hypertension)
- Survivors often need future repair or replacement of truncal or pulmonary valve

RESOURCES

REFERENCES

- Jahangiri M et al. Repair of the truncal valve and associated interrupted arch in neonates with truncus arteriosus. *J Thorac Cardiovasc Surg.* 2000;119:508.

Tuberculosis: Pulmonary

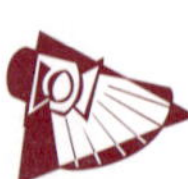

ESSENTIAL FEATURES

- Gram-positive rods, often dormant but remain alive for the life of the host
- Initial infection affects midzone of lungs, causing caseation in a few weeks
- Regional hilar lymph nodes become enlarged; most cases arrest at this stage
- If progresses, giant cells produce a typical tubercle
- Latent disease occurs when dormant tubercles reactivate in elderly or immunocompromised patients
- Apical segments of upper lobes most often affected in latent disease
- Extrapulmonary disease may involve pericardium, bones, joints, urinary tract, meninges, lymph nodes, pleural space

EPIDEMIOLOGY

- Had markedly declined from 1953 until 1984 due to anti-TB drugs
- Since 1984, has increased due to emergence of HIV
- 25,000 new cases annually
- < 20% of population in the United States is tuberculin-positive
- 95% of cases are due to infection with *Mycobacterium tuberculosis, Mycobacterium bovis,* and *Mycobacterium avium-intracellulare*

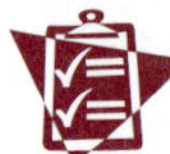

CLINICAL FINDINGS

SYMPTOMS AND SIGNS

- Minimal symptoms in many
- Fever, cough
- Anorexia, weight loss
- Night sweats, excessive perspiration
- Chest pain
- Lethargy, fatigue
- Dyspnea
- Erythema nodosum seen in active disease

LABORATORY FINDINGS

- Purified protein derivative (PPD): False-negative due to improper testing, anergy
- Anergy due to disseminated disease, sarcoidosis, lymphomas, immunosuppressive drugs (used in HIV, transplant patients)
- Sputum culture for mycobacterium

IMAGING FINDINGS

- **Chest film**
  - Involvement of apical and posterior upper lobes (85%)
  - 10% of cases affect superior lower lobes and seen most often in women, blacks and diabetics
  - Variations: Cavitation, acute TB pneumonia, miliary TB, bronchiectasis, tuberculoma

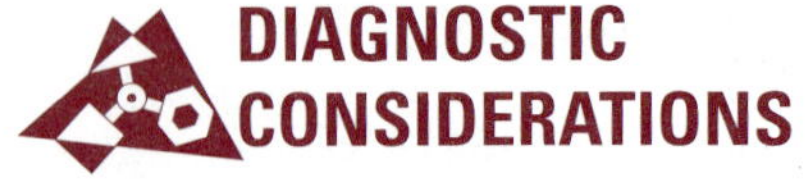

DIAGNOSTIC CONSIDERATIONS

RULE OUT

- Bronchogenic carcinoma
- Fungal infections, such as histoplasmosis

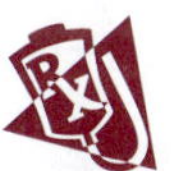

WORK-UP

- PPD
- Sputum culture
- Gastric aspirate, tracheal washing culture
- Pleural fluid culture; pleural and lung biopsies may be needed for diagnosis

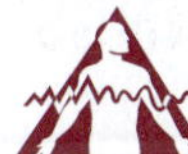

TREATMENT AND MANAGEMENT

- Multidrug regimens including isoniazid, rifampin, pyrazinamide, and ethambutol

SURGERY

- Role of surgery diminished dramatically

Indications

- Failure of medical therapy
- Performance of diagnostic procedures
- Destroyed lung, cavitary lesions
- Postoperative complications
- Persistent bronchopleural fistula
- Intractable hemorrhage

MEDICATIONS

- Isoniazid
- Streptomycin
- Ethambutol
- Rifampin

COMPLICATIONS

- TB empyema: Treated by pulmonary decortication, or drainage if associated with pyogenic infection or bronchopleural fistula

PROGNOSIS

- Mortality 10% with medical treatment
- Perioperative mortality: 1–10%
- Relapse rate is 4%

RESOURCES

REFERENCES

- Pomerantz M et al. Surgical management of resistant mycobacterial tuberculosis and other mycobacterial pulmonary infections. *Ann Thorac Surg.* 1991;52:1108.
- Reed CE et al. Surgical resection for complications of pulmonary tuberculosis. *Ann Thorac Surg.* 1989;48:165.
- Bass JB Jr et al. Treatment of tuberculosis and tuberculosis infection in adults and children. *Am J Respir Crit Care Med.* 1994;149:1359.

Umbilical Hernia

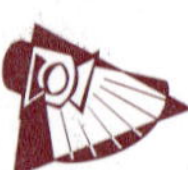

ESSENTIAL FEATURES

- Bulge elicited by the Valsalva maneuver at the umbilicus
- Main complaint associated with umbilical hernias is the cosmetic appearance
- Patients may note discomfort or a heaviness sensation associated with the hernia bulge
- The hernia sac usually contains only pre-peritoneal fat although small bowel or other abdominal viscera may be present
- Classification of incisional hernias
  - Reducible: Visceral contents of the hernia sac able to retract into the abdominal cavity
  - Incarcerated: Visceral contents cannot be returned to the abdominal cavity
  - Strangulated: Incarcerated hernia where the blood flow to the entrapped viscera is compromised

EPIDEMIOLOGY

- Common in children (especially blacks), where spontaneous umbilical hernia closure by age 3 is the norm
- Develop not infrequently in cirrhotic patients with uncontrolled ascites

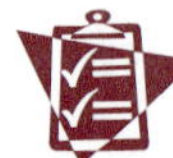

CLINICAL FINDINGS

SYMPTOMS AND SIGNS

- Asymptomatic umbilical bulge most common presentation
- Patients may complain of a discomfort, fullness or heaviness associated with the hernia bulge
- Progressive enlargement of the defect is common
- Hernia bulge may or may not be reducible
- Incarcerated hernias are exquisitely painful to palpation
- Patients with a strangulated hernia may present with an acute abdomen
- Small bowel obstructive symptoms may be present with incarcerated umbilical hernias

IMAGING FINDINGS

- Plain films are typically normal
- US can be used to detect fascial defects as well as differentiate between an incarcerated umbilical hernia and a solid mass
- Abdominal pelvic CT scan is excellent in the detection of umbilical hernias and characterization of involved viscera; CT is particularly useful in diagnosing acute incarceration in the morbidly obese where physical exam is difficult and unreliable

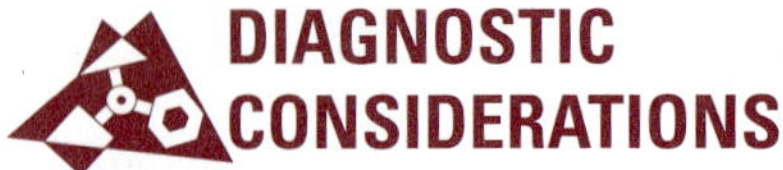

- Epigastric hernia
- Urachal cyst
- Primary or metastatic abdominal wall neoplasm

RULE OUT

- Incarcerated or strangulated hernia
- Abdominal wall tumor

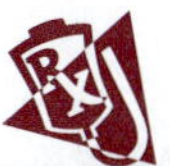

WORK-UP

- Thorough history and physical exam usually will accurately diagnosis umbilical hernia
- Abdominal CT scan when diagnosis is in doubt or to anatomically define the adjacent intestinal viscera in complicated cases

WHEN TO ADMIT

- Depends on magnitude of repair and comorbidities; patients may require postoperative hospitalization

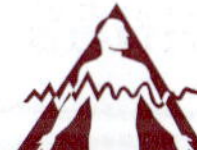

TREATMENT AND MANAGEMENT

- Minimize or eliminate medications deleterious to wound healing such as corticosteroids
- Weight loss in obese patients
- Ascitic control in cirrhotic patients

SURGERY

- Repair can be performed laparoscopically or open

Indications

- Umbilical hernias should be fixed in all patients without medical contraindications

Contraindications

- Cirrhotic patients with uncontrolled ascites

TREATMENT MONITORING

- Clinical evidence of recurrence

COMPLICATIONS

- Postoperative wound or mesh infection
- Recurrence

RESOURCES

REFERENCES

- Deveney K. Hernias & Other Lesions of the Abdominal Wall. In: Way LW, Doherty GM (editors). *Current Surgical Diagnosis & Treatment,* 11e. New York: McGraw-Hill; 2003:791.
- Albanese CT et al. Pediatric Surgery. In: Way LW, Doherty GM (editors). *Current Surgical Diagnosis & Treatment,* 11e. New York: McGraw-Hill; 2003: 1339.

Ureteral or Renal Calculi

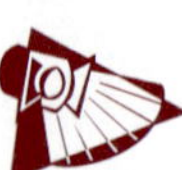

ESSENTIAL FEATURES

- Costovertebral angle/ flank pain
- Pain may radiate to the ipsilateral lower abdominal quadrant
- Hematuria
- Nausea, vomiting, intestinal ileus
- Radiographic evidence of renal or ureteral calculus
- Fever, if proximal infection present

EPIDEMIOLOGY

- Many affected patients have history of prior renal calculi
  - Roughly 50% chance of developing second stone within 5 years of the first calculi
- Hypercalcuria is a metabolic risk factor for stone formation, seen in:
  - Hyperparathyroidism
  - Excess calcium and vitamin D intake
  - Immobilization osteoporosis
  - Paget disease
  - Sarcoidosis
  - Dehydration
- Urea-splitting bacteria create magnesium-ammonium phosphate (struvite) stones
- Metabolic stones form from the hypersecretion of uric acid or cystine
- Other metabolic risk factors include:
  - Hyperuricosuria
  - Hypocitraturia
  - Hypomagnesuria
  - Hyperoxaluria

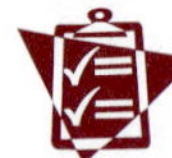

CLINICAL FINDINGS

SYMPTOMS AND SIGNS

- Moderate to severe costovertebral angle/flank pain that does not improve with change in position
- Pain may radiate to ipsilateral lower abdominal quadrant depending on location of calculus
- Often nausea and vomiting, associated with an intestinal ileus
- Gross hematuria occurs more often than microscopic
- Symptoms of pyelonephritis with proximal infection (costovertebral angle tenderness, high fever, chills, dysuria)
- Nonobstructive calculi are typically asymptomatic

LABORATORY FINDINGS

- Evidence of hematuria
- Pyuria, bacturia, and leukocytosis with secondary infection
- Urine pH > 7.6 suggests presence of urea-splitting organisms
- Urine pH < 5.5 suggests metabolic stone formation (uric acid and cystine)
- Hypercalcemia and hypophosphatemia consistent with hyperparathyroidism
- Hyperchloremic metabolic acidosis consistent with renal tubular acidosis with secondary renal calcifications

IMAGING FINDINGS

- 90% of stones are radiopaque (calcium, cystine, and struvite) and seen on plain films
- Uric acid stones are non-radiopaque, but can be seen on spiral CT
- Spiral CT without contrast demonstrates entire urinary tract and can distinguish between stones, tumor, and blood clots
- Excretory urography will verify stone location and provides qualitative information on renal function

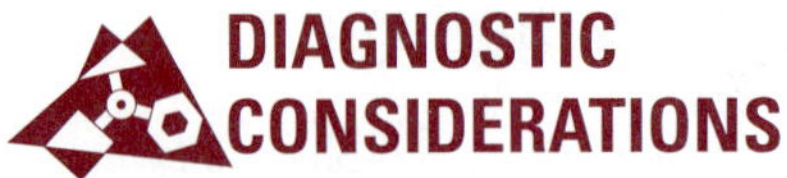

DIAGNOSTIC CONSIDERATIONS

- Acute pyelonephritis
- Renal adenocarcinoma (hematuria)
- Transitional cell tumors (obstruction)
- Renal papillary necrosis
- Renal infarction
- Acute pancreatitis
- Psoas abscess
- Symptomatic abdominal aortic aneurysm (AAA)
- Acute appendicitis
- Acute salpingitis
- Herpes zoster

RULE OUT

- Symptomatic/ruptured AAA
- Proximal infection
- Presence of a urologic neoplasm

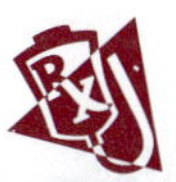

WORK-UP

- CBC count
- Basic chemistries
- UA
- Urine culture and sensitivities
- Qualitative urine cystine
- Abdominal x-ray
- Spiral CT without contrast ("stone protocol") has become diagnostic test of choice in urgent setting
- Calculi composition analysis if recovered

WHEN TO ADMIT

- Fever and leukocytosis
- Severe ureterorenal colic requiring parenteral analgesics
- Inability to tolerate PO fluids or analgesia
- Obstruction complicated by infection, requiring percutaneous nephrostomy tube or ureteral stent for drainage

WHEN TO REFER

- All patients should be managed by a urologist

TREATMENT AND MANAGEMENT

- 80% of ureteral stones pass spontaneously
  - Passage depends on stone size and location—a 5 mm distally located calculus more likely to pass than a large proximally located calculus
- Extracorporeal shock-wave lithotripsy (ESWL) for renal pelvis calculi
- For most proximal and midureteral calculi < 1 cm, ureteroscopic treatment with laser or other lithotripsy device is now first-line treatment
- Percutaneous extraction or pulverization for large pelvic stones or staghorn calculi
- Endoureteroscopic basket extraction of selected distal stones
- Open surgical approach rarely required
- Metabolic work-up should be performed for patients with > 1 calculi, family history of calculi, recurrent urinary tract infections or other risk factors

SURGERY

Indications

- Persistent intractable pain, uncontrolled by PO analgesics
- Progressive hydronephrosis
- Evidence of pyelonephritis
- Staghorn calculi
- Large stone burden or stones that are unlikely to pass spontaneously based on size and location
- Patient considerations (eg, job)
- Failure of medical management

MEDICATIONS

- Medical management of acute ureteral or renal calculi includes PO narcotic analgesics, NSAIDs, and nifedipine XL
- Thiazide diuretics or orthophosphates to decrease urine calcium
- Urinary alkalinization with citrate for metabolic stones
- Allopurinol for uric acid stones
- Penicillamine for cystine stones

TREATMENT MONITORING

- Serial plain films to follow progression of stones managed conservatively
- Interval US to assess degree of hydronephosis

COMPLICATIONS

- Renal impairment
- Ureteral stricture
- Hydronephrosis
- Recurrence

PROGNOSIS

- 80% of ureteral stones pass spontaneously
- Increased recurrence of renal stones unless preventive measures taken

PREVENTION

- Increase fluid intake
- Combat urinary infections
- Minimize calcium/vitamin D intake for calcium-based stones
- Metabolic stones as described above

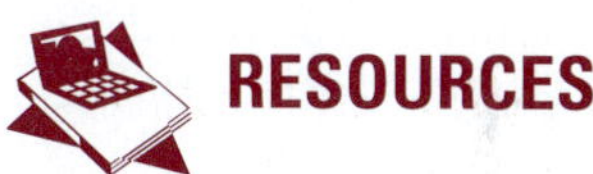

RESOURCES

REFERENCES

- Pak CYC. Southwestern Internal Medicine Conference: medical management of nephrolithiasis—a new, simplified approach for general practice. *Am J Med Sci.* 1997;313:215.
- Ramakumar S et al. Renal calculi: percutaneous management. *Urol Clin North Am.* 2000;27:617.
- Spencer BA et al. Helical CT and ureteral colic. *Urol Clin North Am.* 2000;27:231.

Varicose Veins

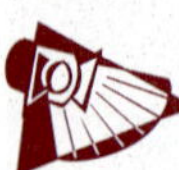

ESSENTIAL FEATURES

- Dilated, tortuous superficial veins in lower extremities, usually bilateral
- Pigmentation, ulceration, edema suggest concomitant venous stasis disease
- Classified as primary or secondary
- Risk factors for varicose veins (VV) include:
  - Female gender
  - Pregnancy
  - Family history
  - Prolonged standing
  - History of phlebitis

Primary

- Due to genetic or developmental defects in vein wall causing valvular incompetence
- Most cases of isolated superficial venous insufficiency are primary

Secondary

- Destruction or dysfunction of valves caused by trauma, deep venous thrombosis (DVT), AV fistula, proximal venous obstruction (pregnancy, pelvic tumor, etc)
- Disruption of valves results in chronic venous stasis changes
- Long-standing venous dysfunction leads to chronic skin changes leading to infection

EPIDEMIOLOGY

- 10–20% of population affected
- Highest incidence in women 40- to 50-years-old

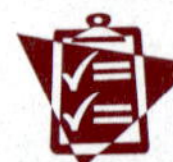

CLINICAL FINDINGS

SYMPTOMS AND SIGNS

- Variable presentation
- Many patients are asymptomatic
- Localized pain (ache or heaviness with prolonged standing), phlebitis
- Predominantly located medially (saphenous vein)
- Small, flat blue-green reticular and spider veins indicates venous dysfunction
- Secondary VV can cause edema, hyperpigmentation, dermatitis, ulcers

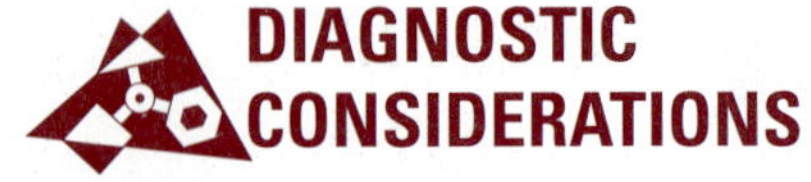

DIAGNOSTIC CONSIDERATIONS

RULE OUT

- Chronic deep venous insufficiency
- Klippel-Trénaunay syndrome: Unilateral VV, limb hypertrophy, cutaneous birthmark (port wine stain/venous malformation)
  - Therapy: Graduated support stockings, avoid saphenous vein stripping as deep veins often absent

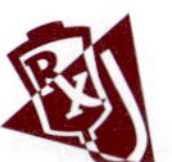

WORK-UP

- Brodie-Trendelenburg test
  - Identifies saphenofemoral dysfunction: Elevate leg until varicosities collapse, place tourniquet around mid thigh to occlude reflux from saphenofemoral incompetence
  - If veins fill, implies perforator incompetence
  - If veins remain collapsed, implies saphenofemoral dysfunction
- Duplex US is test of choice

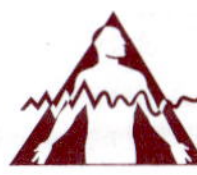

TREATMENT AND MANAGEMENT

- First manage venous insufficiency: Elastic stockings, leg elevation, exercise
- Avoid prolonged sitting/standing

SURGERY

- Operative therapy:
  1. Remove entire saphenous vein (for incompetent saphenofemoral junction, varicosities along entire length)
  2. Selective VV removal with stab-avulsion technique
  3. Combined technique
- Inject small volume of sclerosing solution (0.2% sodium tetradecyl sulfate) into varix, telangiectasia, spider vein; maintain direct pressure for 1 wk with stockings

Indications

- Persistent or disabling pain
- Recurrent superficial thrombophlebitis
- Erosion of overlying skin with bleeding

COMPLICATIONS

- Hematoma formation
- Infection
- Saphenous nerve irritation

PROGNOSIS

- 10% recurrence after treatment

RESOURCES

REFERENCES

- Belcaro G et al. Endovascular sclerotherapy, surgery, and surgery plus sclerotherapy in superficial venous incompetence: a randomized, 10 year follow-up trial—final results. *Angiology.* 2000;51:529.

Vascular Lesions, Congenital

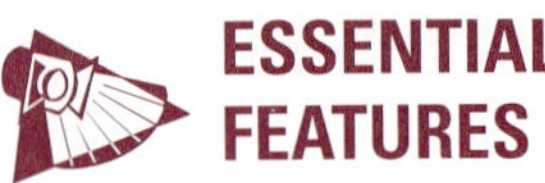

ESSENTIAL FEATURES

- 2 main processes: AV malformations and vascular rings

AV Malformations

- Uncommon, abnormal capillary formation during canalicular phase of development, mostly from pulmonary artery, rarely coronary artery
- Coronary AV fistulas drain into RV (40%) and RA (25%) of time

Vascular Rings

- Abnormal development of aortic arches and branches with compression of trachea and esophagus
- Normal fetal development: A dual system of 6 aortic arches regresses so that the left fourth arch persists as main left aorta; the left sixth arch remains as the ductus arteriosus; and the right fourth arch becomes the right innominate and subclavian arteries
- Most associated with right-sided aortic arch
- Classified as complete or incomplete (arterial sling)
- **Common complete rings:** Double aortic arch (67%), right aortic arch with left subclavian and ductus arteriosus (30%)
- **Incomplete rings:** Aberrant right subclavian originating from left side, and left pulmonary artery arising from right pulmonary artery (pulmonary artery sling)

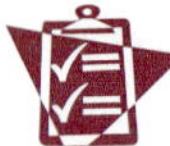

CLINICAL FINDINGS

SYMPTOMS AND SIGNS

AV Malformations

- Asymptomatic, otherwise dyspnea, congestive heart failure, angina
- Continuous murmur and signs of rapid aortic runoff on physical exam

Vascular Rings

- Symptoms of tracheal or esophageal compression
- **Dysphagia lusoria:** Swallowing symptoms from anomalous right subclavian
- **Complete ring and pulmonary artery slings:** Present within 6 mos with respiratory distress, poor feeding

IMAGING FINDINGS

AV Malformation

- Echocardiogram with Doppler often diagnostic

Vascular Rings

- Barium esophagogram may be diagnostic
  - Bilateral indentations imply double aortic arch
  - Posterior indentation implies aberrant right subclavian artery
  - Right indentation implies right aortic arch
  - Anterior impression: Pulmonary artery sling
- Echocardiography can confirm diagnosis
- CT and aortography may be required for diagnosis

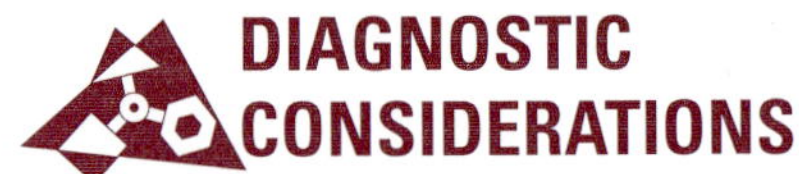

DIAGNOSTIC CONSIDERATIONS

- Shunt fraction calculation via angiography is definitive for diagnosis

WORK-UP

- Physical exam
- Echocardiography
- Barium esophagogram for vascular rings
- Occasionally angiography

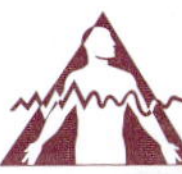

TREATMENT AND MANAGEMENT

- Once diagnosed, symptomatic vascular rings should be repaired
- **Vascular rings:** If double aortic arch, divide smaller of 2 arches
- **Complete rings:** Divide ligamentum arteriosum
- **Pulmonary artery slings:** Reimplantation of left pulmonary artery

SURGERY

Indications

- AV malformations: Symptomatic patients or if large shunts
- Vascular rings: Should be repaired via left thoracotomy

RESOURCES

REFERENCES

- van Son JA et al. Surgical treatment of vascular rings: The Mayo Clinic Experience. *Mayo Clin Proc.* 1993;68:1056.

Vascular Occlusive Disease, Peripheral (PVOD)

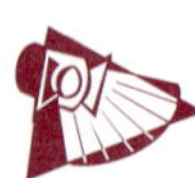

ESSENTIAL FEATURES

- Predominantly disease of lower extremities
- In arms, subclavian and axillary mostly affected, radial and ulnar if diabetic
- In legs, femoropopliteal disease more common than aortoiliac disease
- Indicator for early death (from myocardial infarction [MI] and strokes) and imminent limb loss
- Single arterial segment obstruction limits walking to half to 1 block on average prior to onset of claudication pain
- Also known as peripheral artery insufficiency

EPIDEMIOLOGY

- Affects 20% of population > age 70
- Indicates atherosclerotic disease; high risk of death from MI or stroke
- 20% die of nonatherosclerotic causes

CLINICAL FINDINGS

SYMPTOMS AND SIGNS

- Intermittent claudication
  - Pain, fatigue, cramping in leg muscles (most often calf) with walking; relieved by 2–5 min rest
  - Is reproducible and does not occur at rest
  - Thigh pain if occlusion proximal to profunda femoral, gluteal pain if proximal to hypogastric arteries
  - Leriche syndrome: Aortoiliac disease— claudication of hip, thigh, buttock, atrophy of leg muscles, impotence, and diminished femoral pulses
  - Sensation usually intact except in cases of peripheral neuropathy (diabetes)
- Ischemic rest pain
  - Severe, burning pain in forefoot aggravated by leg elevation, improved with leg in dependent position
  - Grave symptom caused by ischemic neuritis and tissue necrosis
  - Indicates advanced arterial insufficiency
  - Without treatment, results in gangrene and amputation
  - Often preceded by claudication
- Nonhealing wounds ulcers
  - Trivial trauma may cause wounds in pts with PVOD
  - Commonly located on toes, or distal foot
  - Usually painful with eventual gangrene
- Erectile dysfunction
  - Due to obstructed blood flow through hypogastric and/or terminal aorta
  - Less common than other causes of erectile dysfunction
- Diminished pulses, bruits (may be present at stenosis), pallor, reactive hyperemia, rubor, decreased temperature in foot, ulceration, tissue necrosis of toes, muscle atrophy, loss of hair on foot, thickening of toenails (slow keratin turnover), skin atrophy

LABORATORY FINDINGS

- Noninvasive vascular tests: ABIs (ankle to brachial index)
- ABI < 1.0 indicates occlusive disease, rest pain typically ABI < 0.4
- Calcified vessels may not be compressed and suspected when ABI > 1.2 and does not correlate to clinical status (diabetics often elevated ABI, measure toe-brachial index (TBI)
- Segmental limb pressures: Measure pressure and pulsatile wave forms from thigh to foot to identify location of occlusive disease
- Exercise ABI done within 1 min of exercise may help diagnose occlusive disease

IMAGING FINDINGS

- **Color duplex:** Can identify arterial lesions but is operator dependent
- **Arteriography:** Provides anatomic information for location of disease (complications of arteriography: hematoma, pseudoaneurysm, contrast allergy, contrast nephropathy)
- **Magnetic resonance angiography (MRA):** Can delineate arteries without contrast, but overestimates disease

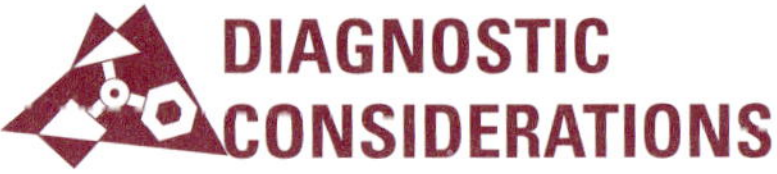

DIAGNOSTIC CONSIDERATIONS

- Intermittent claudication
- Ischemic rest pain
- Decreased pulses
- Nonhealing ulcers/wounds
- Necrosis and atrophy
- Low ABI

RULE OUT

- Osteoarthritis
- Neurospinal compression (spinal stenosis)
- Venous claudication
- Vasculitis
- Aortic coarctation
- Popliteal entrapment
- Popliteal cysts
- Persistent sciatic arteries
- External iliac dysplasias
- Primary vascular tumors
- Diabetic neuropathy pain

Vascular Occlusive Disease, Peripheral (PVOD)

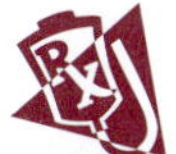

WORK-UP

- ABIs, segmental limb pressures
- Arteriography or MRA
- Evaluate cardiac status, often patients have ischemic heart disease or chronic obstructive pulmonary disease

TREATMENT AND MANAGEMENT

- Objectives are symptom relief and limb salvage

MEDICAL

- Risk reduction
  - Smoking cessation
  - Blood pressure control
  - Lower cholesterol (low-density lipoprotein goal < 100 mg/dL)
  - Control of diabetes
- Exercise program increases claudication distance
- Maintain foot care and hygiene
- Aspirin, clodiprogel: Decrease cardiovascular events
- Pentoxyphylline, cilastazol may improve claudication symptoms

ENDOVASCULAR TREATMENT

- Used alone or in conjunction with surgery
- Percutaneous transluminal angioplasty and stenting results in plaque rupture and stretching of media
- 1-year success: 85% in common iliac, 50% in femoropopliteal disease

SURGERY

- β-Blockers prior to surgery if patient tolerates

Aortoiliofemoral

- Aortofemoral bypass or endarterectomy
- Mortality, 5%; 5- to 10-year patency, 80%
- Risks: infection, aortointestinal fistula, pseudoaneurysms, limb occlusion, erectile dysfunction
- Femorofemoral or iliofemoral can be used in high risk patients
- Axillofemoral in high risk patients or those with infected aortic graft

Femoropopliteal

- If disease affects aortoiliac and femoral, consider aortofemoral bypass with profundaplasty
- If isolated disease in femoral/popliteal region: femoropopliteal bypass used
- Saphenous vein best graft, PTFE may be used if above knee
- Mortality, 2%; 5-year patency, 60–80%
- 5-year mortality, 50% (strokes, MIs)

Distal Arterial Reconstruction

- Performed primarily for limb salvage
- Saphenous vein is best graft material, otherwise composite arm or lesser saphenous vein used
- Mortality, 5%; 5-year 50% survival; 25% fail within 1 month

Amputation

- More likely with with poor medical treatment or noncompliance with medical therapy, ie, continue smoking
- 5% with rest pain require amputation as primary therapy

Indications

- Incapacitating claudication
- Limb salvage

PROGNOSIS

- Nondiabetics + PVOD: 5-year survival = 70%
  - If patients also have cerebrovascular or ischemic heart disease: 5-year survival = 60%
- PVOD + renal failure: 2-year survival < 50%

RESOURCES

REFERENCES

- Donnelly R et al. ABC of arterial and venous disease: vascular complications of diabetes. *BMJ.* 2000;320:1062.
- Gordon IL et al. Three-year outcome of endovascular treatment of superficial femoral artery occlusion. *Arch Surg.* 2001;136:221.
- Johnson WC et al. A comparative evaluation of polytetrafluoroethylene, umbilical vein, and saphenous vein bypass grafts for femoral-popliteal above-knee revascularization: a prospective randomized Department of Veterans Affairs cooperative study. *J Vasc Surg.* 2000;32:268.
- Strandness DE Jr et al. Peripheral vascular disease. *Circulation.* 2000;102 (Suppl 4):46.

Vasoconstrictive Disorders

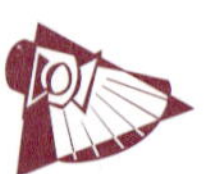

ESSENTIAL FEATURES

- Characterized by abnormal lability of sympathetic nervous system
- Affects arterial and venous side of capillary bed to reduce cutaneous blood flow
- Sluggish flow of deoxygenated blood causes cutaneous cyanosis, coldness, numbness, pain

Raynaud Syndrome

- Precipitated by exposure to cold or stress
- May follow virulent or benign course

Acrocyanosis

- Persistent cyanosis of hands and feet
- Occurs in young females

Scleroderma

- Connective tissue disease: Fibrosis due to increased collagen and elastin, arterial intimal thickening
- Affects lung, kidney, GI, muscle, CNS

Reflex Sympathetic Dystrophy

- Post-traumatic pain syndrome
- Poorly understood
- Initial injury: Fracture, laceration, crush
- Unendurable burning pain of entire extremity, extreme sensitivity
- Increased sympathetic activity is cause
- Vasoconstriction prominent feature

EPIDEMIOLOGY

Raynaud Syndrome

- Associated with immunologic and connective tissue disorders (scleroderma, lupus, polymyositis, diabetic arterial disease, trauma, etc)
- Association with *Helicobacter* infection reported

Scleroderma

- More common in women, 25- to 50-years old

Reflex Sympathetic Dystrophy

- Equally common in men and women; upper = lower extremity

CLINICAL FINDINGS

SYMPTOMS AND SIGNS

Raynaud Syndrome

- Sequence of pallor, cyanosis, rubor (white-blue-red color changes)

Acrocyanosis

- Cyanosis, numbness, and pain
- Changes disappear when warm
- Examine in cold room: Diffuse cyanosis, coldness, and hyperhidrosis symmetrically
- Allen test may be delayed in cold
- Pulses normal when warm, absent when cold

Scleroderma

- First skin and vasculature of hands
- Skin thick and taut, limited finger flexion
- Forearm muscles: Woody induration
- Progressive finger coldness/numbness
- Painful ulceration of terminal phalanges
- Allen test: Uneven color return to fingers

Reflex Sympathetic Dystrophy

- Exquisite pain to minimal stimuli
- Progressive atrophy

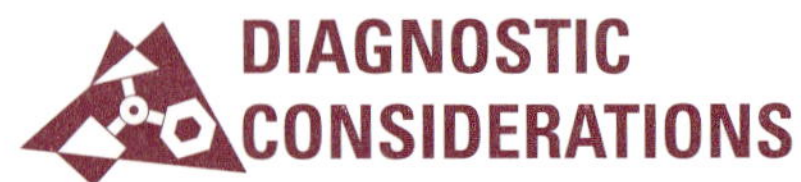

DIAGNOSTIC CONSIDERATIONS

Reflex Sympathetic Dystrophy

- Sympathetic block often diagnostic

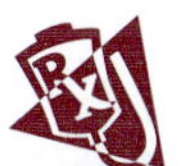

WORK-UP

Raynaud Syndrome

- Helpful to differentiate occlusive lesion from transient vasconstrictive variety

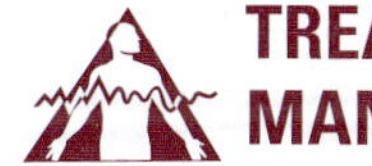

TREATMENT AND MANAGEMENT

Raynaud Syndrome

- Avoid cold, tobacco, oral contraceptives, β-blockers
- Calcium channel blockers, prostaglandins, ketanserin, dilastazol may be helpful
- Cervical sympathectomy if cause is transient

Scleroderma

- Palliative, sympathectomy rarely helps
- Corticosteroids slows progression
- Amputation if gangrene develops

Reflex Sympathetic Dystrophy

- Sympathetic block
- Surgical sympathectomy
- Spinal cord stimulation, intrathecal baclofen-temporary pain relief

SURGERY

Indications

- Amputation if gangrene develops

MEDICATIONS

- Corticosteroids for scleroderma may slow disease

RESOURCES

REFERENCES

- Knapid-Kordecka M et al. Clinical spectrum of Raynaud's phenomenon in patients referred to a vascular clinic. *Cardiovasc Surg.* 2000;8:457.
- Schwartzman RJ. New treatments for reflex sympathetic dystrophy. *N Engl J Med.* 2000;343:654.

Venous Insufficiency, Chronic

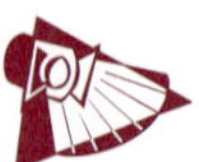

ESSENTIAL FEATURES

- Chronic venous insufficiency (CVI) caused by chronic elevation in venous pressure
- 3 factors
  1. Calf muscle pump dysfunction
  2. Valvular reflux
  3. Outflow obstruction
- Venous outflow obstruction results in "venous claudication" pain during exercise
- Valvular incompetence
  - Congenital or secondary to phlebitis
  - Varicose veins
  - Deep venous thrombosis (DVT)
- Venous stasis changes centered in "gaiter areas" around ankles: commonly affected perforator veins, region of sparse soft-tissue support
- Local inflammation, hemosiderin deposits, leakage of plasma fluid results in fibrosis and ulceration
- Isolated saphenous vein incompetence & DVT can lead to chronic venous stasis changes
- May-Thurner syndrome: Compression of left iliac vein by right iliac artery causing venous stasis, CVI

EPIDEMIOLOGY

- Venous reflux demonstrable in 17% of extremities 1 wk after thrombosis and in 66% 1-year after thrombosis

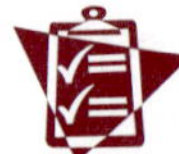

CLINICAL FINDINGS

SYMPTOMS AND SIGNS

- First symptom usually ankle and calf edema, worse at end of day, improves with leg elevation
- Involvement of foot and toes suggests lymphedema
- Long-lasting disease:
  - Stasis dermatitis
  - Hyperpigmentation
  - Brawny induration
- Venous stasis ulcers: Large, painless, irregular, located in medial or lateral gaiter area

IMAGING FINDINGS

- **Duplex US:** Can identify location of incompetent perforating veins, does not assess calf muscle function/proximal obstruction
- **Venography**
  - Determines functional outflow obstruction
  - Descending phlebography tests valves and identifies reflux

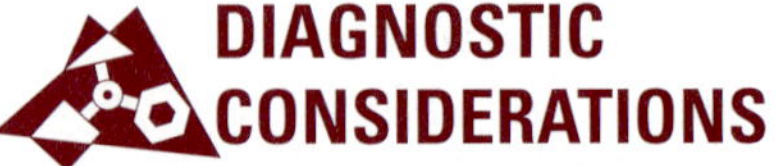

DIAGNOSTIC CONSIDERATIONS

- **Air plethysmography:** Quantitative assessments of venous reflux, calf muscle pump function, overall venous function; can be used to differentiate superficial from deep veins

RULE OUT

- Lymphedema: Nonpitting edema of foot and toes
- Acute DVT
- Congestive heart failure, chronic liver disease, chronic kidney disease
- Arterial insufficiency: Ulcer location is more distal and painful
- Erythema nodosum
- Fungal infections

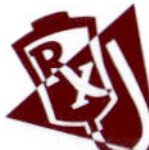

WORK-UP

- Physical exam
- Duplex US
- Occasional venography to define valve function

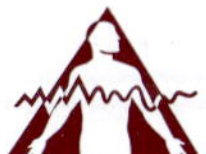

TREATMENT AND MANAGEMENT

- Incurable disease
- Conservative: Leg elevation, graduated compression stockings, exercise
- Venous ulcers improve with leg elevation, compression, and wound care
- Unna's boot or occlusive wound dressing can be used for compression

SURGERY

- 2 categories of procedures

Antireflux Procedures

- Perforating vein ligation: Incompetent perforating veins
- Valvuloplasty, venous segment transposition, valvular transplantation; popliteal vein valve may be most important valve for CVI

Bypass Operations for Obstruction

- Palma procedure: Cross-femoral bypass with contralateral proximal saphenous vein; can use prosthetic material
- May-Thurner syndrome: Angioplasty and stenting
- Superficial vein occlusion: May-Husni procedure = saphenopopliteal bypass (75% improvement)

Indications

- Nonhealing ulcers
- Disabling symptoms

PROGNOSIS

- Perforator ligation surgery: Ulcer recurrence 15–20%
- Difficult patient population
- At best, surgical results show 70% improvement in symptoms

RESOURCES

REFERENCES

- Mohr DN et al. The venous stasis syndrome after deep venous thrombosis or pulmonary embolism: a population-based study. *Mayo Clin Proc.* 2000;75:1249.

Ventricular Septal Defect (VSD)

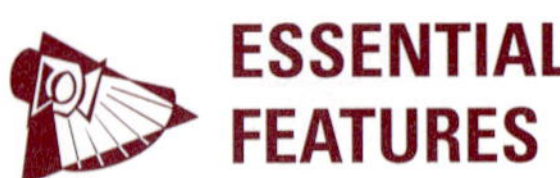

ESSENTIAL FEATURES

Postinfarct VSD

- Infarction of interventricular septum with subsequent VSD formation
- Interval between myocardial infarction (MI) and septal rupture: 1–12 days
- **Histologic findings:** Cardiac muscle degeneration and weakening
- Classically, sudden shock or congestive heart failure develops in a patient after MI
- Defect in anterior apical septum if left anterior descending coronary artery occlusion, posterior basilar septum if right coronary occlusion

LV Aneurysm

- Large MI progresses to thinned-out transmural scar, bulges paradoxically during systole
- 90% of aneurysms involve anteroseptal LV, 10% posterior
- 50% contain mural thrombus

EPIDEMIOLOGY

Postinfarct VSD

- < 1% of patients with acute MI
- Poor prognosis
  - 24% die on first day
  - 65% by 2 weeks
  - 81% by 2 mos

LV Aneurysm

- 2–4% of MI, incidence is decreasing with more aggressive management of MI

CLINICAL FINDINGS

SYMPTOMS AND SIGNS

Postinfarct VSD

- Harsh holosystolic murmur along left sternal border
- 67% have palpable thrill

LV Aneurysm

- Congestive heart failure, angina, embolization, ventricular dysrhythmias
- Prominent apical pulse

LABORATORY FINDINGS

- ECG: Q wave MI with persistent ST segment elevation

IMAGING FINDINGS

Postinfarct VSD

- Echocardiography: Definitive diagnosis
- Catheterization: Also definitive

LV Aneurysm

- **Chest film:** Localized LV bulge
- Echocardiography and catheterization are definitive

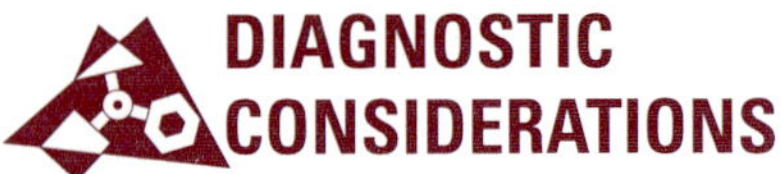

DIAGNOSTIC CONSIDERATIONS

- Echocardiography and catheterization

RULE OUT

- Papillary muscle dysfunction
- Rupture of papillary muscle with acute mitral insufficiency
- Pericardial friction rub after MI (Dressler syndrome)

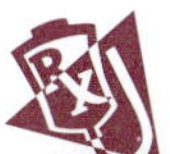

WORK-UP

- Echocardiography: Definitive diagnosis
- Catheterization: Also definitive

TREATMENT AND MANAGEMENT

Postinfarct VSD

- Preoperative intra-aortic balloon pump
- Operation: Patch closure of VSD (using double patch) + coronary artery bypass performed early

LV Aneurysm

- Resect aneurysm (Dor procedure) + coronary revascularization

SURGERY

Indications

Postinfarct VSD

- Indicated in nearly all cases

LV Aneurysm

- Good to moderate operative risk

Contraindications

- **Postinfarct VSD:** Advanced age with multiorgan failure

COMPLICATIONS

Postinfarct VSD

- 50–80% survive operation depending on degree of multiorgan failure

PROGNOSIS

LV Aneurysm

- Improvement in congestive heart failure, angina in 70–85% of survivors
- 70–80% of patients alive 5 years postoperatively, significantly more than those who received medical therapy
- Operative mortality: 5% elective, 20% for emergency procedures
- Subendocardial resection for ventricular tachycardia: 11% mortality

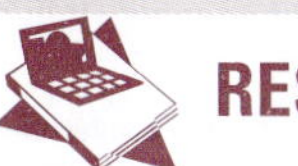

RESOURCES

REFERENCES

- Chaux AC et al. Postinfarction ventricular septal defect. *Semin Thorac Cardiovasc Surg.* 1998;10:93.

Ventricular Septal Defect (VSD), Congenital

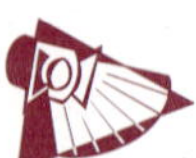

ESSENTIAL FEATURES

- A congenital heart lesion that increases pulmonary arterial blood flow
- Results in left-to-right shunt, results in lung infection, pulmonary vascular congestion, pulmonary artery (PA) hypertension, right heart failure, pulmonary vasoconstriction, pulmonary vascular obstructive disease
- **Eisenmenger syndrome:** Increased pulmonary hypertension such that left-to-right shunt ceases and shunt becomes right-to-left, requiring heart-lung transplant
- Inhaled nitric oxide, oxygen, or IV tolazoline reverses PA vasoconstriction
- PA band is palliative and can reduce PA flow to alleviate RV failure and progression of pulmonary hypertension
- Defects occur in 4 anatomic positions
  - Perimembranous septum (85%), anterior to crista supraventricularis, beneath leaflet of tricuspid valve, or muscular septum
- Often associated with more complex defects: Truncus arteriosus, AV canal defect, tetralogy of Fallot, transposition of great arteries
- Isolated perimembranous defects may have associated patent ductus arteriosus (PDA), aortic coarctation
- Supracristal defects may have aortic regurgitation

EPIDEMIOLOGY

- VSD accounts for 25% of congenital cardiac anomalies
- In infants, 33% of defects are small, many close spontaneously by age 8

CLINICAL FINDINGS

SYMPTOMS AND SIGNS

- If defect small, asymptomatic
- If large, heart failure with dyspnea, frequent respiratory infections, poor growth
- Pansystolic murmur at left lower sternal border
- Loud S with apical diastolic flow murmur and biventricular enlargement
- Dyspnea on exertion, poor weight gain, easy fatigability
- Chronic respiratory difficulties, poor feeding
- Pulmonary vascular disease may develop

IMAGING FINDINGS

- **Chest film:** Enlarged heart, congested lung fields
- **Echocardiography:** Diagnostic
- **Catheterization:** If older defect or young child: Assess pulmonary artery pressure and vascular resistance

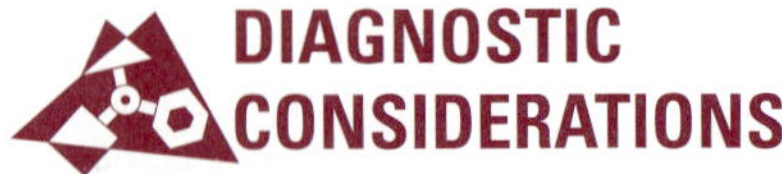

DIAGNOSTIC CONSIDERATIONS

- May be a part of a more complex defect (truncus arteriosus, AV canal defect, tetralogy of Fallot)
- Isolated perimembranous defects may also have PDA or aortic coarctation
- Supracristal defects occasionally have aortic valve regurgitation

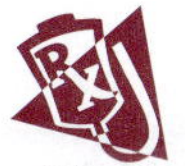

WORK-UP

- Physical exam
- Echocardiography
- Cardiac catheterization selectively

TREATMENT AND MANAGEMENT

- 33% have small defects, often close spontaneously by age 8
- 33% have large defects (symptomatic) require aggressive treatment
- Synthetic patch closure, sutures away from conduction system
- May require deep hypothermic circulatory arrest
- Percutaneous device closure recently used

SURGERY

Indications

- Medically refractory symptoms in infant
- Elevated PA pressure
- Canal-type defect or malaligned conoventricular defect
- Aortic insufficiency (supracristal defect)

COMPLICATIONS

- Risk of damage to conduction system

PROGNOSIS

- Operative mortality rare
- Severe preoperative failure: Mortality, 3–5%
- Symptomatic improvement dramatic
- Pulmonary resistance: No change

RESOURCES

REFERENCES

- Anderson RH et al. The surgical anatomy of ventricular septal defect. *J Card Surg.* 1992;7:17.
- Jacobs JP et al. Congenital Heart Surgery Nomenclature and Database Project: ventricular septal defect. *Ann Thorac Surg.* 2000;69:S25.
- McGrath LB et al. Methods for repair of simple isolated ventricular septal defect. *J Card Surg.* 1991;6:13.

VIPoma

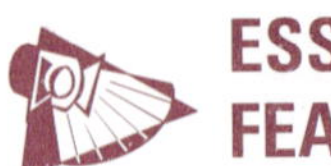

ESSENTIAL FEATURES

- Chronic profuse watery diarrhea
- Massive fecal loss of potassium
- Low serum potassium
- Extreme weakness
- Elevated serum vasoactive intestinal polypeptide (VIP) level

EPIDEMIOLOGY

- A non-beta islet cell tumor of the pancreas that secretes VIP
- VIPomas cause the WDHH syndrome (watery diarrhea, hypokalemia, hypochlorhydria)
- Approximately 80% of the tumors are solitary, located in the body or tail of the pancreas
- About 50% of the lesions are malignant, and 75% of those have metastasized by the time of exploration.
- Mean age of presentation is 47 years; women are affected 3 times as often as men

CLINICAL FINDINGS

SYMPTOMS AND SIGNS

- Profuse watery diarrhea
- Extreme weakness

LABORATORY FINDINGS

- Elevated fasting VIP levels (> 190 pg/mL)
- Low serum potassium
- Severe metabolic acidosis results from loss of HCO in the stool
- Elevated serum calcium, possibly from secretion by the tumor of a parathyroid hormone-like substance
- Mild hyperglycemia
- Hypochlorhydria

IMAGING FINDINGS

- CT scan or MRI is the best initial imaging test for localization and metastases
- Somatostatin receptor scintigraphy is also useful for localization

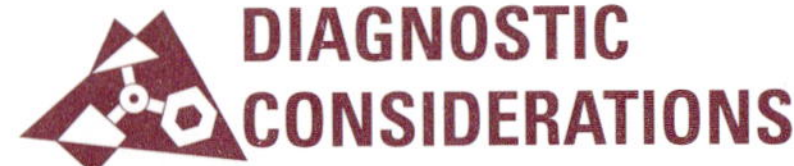

DIAGNOSTIC CONSIDERATIONS

- Severe chronic watery diarrhea along with metabolic acidosis and hypokalemia may prompt investigation for VIPoma
- Severe secretory diarrhea, elevated serum VIP level and pancreatic mass suggests diagnosis

RULE OUT

- Patients who complain of severe diarrhea must be evaluated carefully for other causes before seriously considering the diagnosis of VIPoma
- Gastrinoma
- Carcinoid
- Medullary thyroid tumor

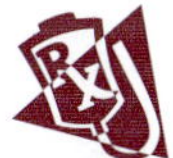

WORK-UP

- Documentation of severe, watery diarrhea (stool volume averages about 5 L/d during acute episodes)
- Serum VIP level
- CT scan or MRI
- Somatostatin receptor scintigraphy if not detected by CT scan or MRI

WHEN TO ADMIT

- Severe metabolic acidosis
- Severe hypokalemia

TREATMENT AND MANAGEMENT

- Octreotide for palliation of symptoms.

SURGERY

- Resection of entire tumor
  - Pancreaticoduodenectomy for tumor on head of pancreas
  - Distal pancreatectomy for tumor on body and tail
- Palliative debulking of metastases

Indications

- All cases in which resection is technically feasible

MEDICATIONS

- Long-acting somatostatin analogs decrease VIP levels, controls diarrhea, and may even reduce tumor size
- Streptozocin if not completely resected

PROGNOSIS

- 1-year survival is 40% in patients whose tumors cannot be completely resected

RESOURCES

REFERENCES

- Jensen RT. Overview of chronic diarrhea caused by functional neuroendocrine neoplasms. *Semin Gastrointest Dis.* 1999;10:156.
- Soga J, Yakuwa Y. Vipoma/diarrheogenic syndrome: a statistical evaluation of 241 reported cases. *J Exp Clin Cancer Res.* 1998;17:389.

Visceral Aneurysms

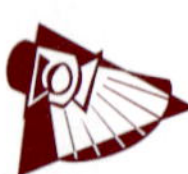

ESSENTIAL FEATURES

- Comprise splenic, hepatic, and superior mesenteric artery (SMA) aneurysms

Splenic Artery Aneurysms (SAA)

- Rupture < 2%, rarely occurs if < 3cm
- Rupture during pregnancy occurs during third trimester: 75% maternal death, 90% fetal death

Hepatic Artery Aneurysms (HAA)

- 20% rupture frequency

SMA Aneurysm (SMAA)

- Aneurysm may involve origin or branches
- Lesion rarely calcified

EPIDEMIOLOGY

SAA

- Second in frequency of abdominal aneurysms after aortoiliac aneurysms
- 60% of visceral artery aneurysms
- More women affected than men (4:1); often during childbearing years
- Arterial fibrodysplasia and portal hypertension predispose to SAA

HAA

- 20% of visceral aneurysms
- More men than women affected (2:1)

SMAA

- < 5% of visceral aneurysms
- 60% are mycotic, rest atherosclerotic

CLINICAL FINDINGS

SYMPTOMS AND SIGNS

SAA

- Often asymptomatic, occasionally abdominal pain, rupture

HAA

- Rupture into peritoneal cavity, viliary tress, or into viscus
- Hemobilia with rupture into biliary tree
- 33% of patients have triad
  - Intermittent abdominal pain
  - GI bleeding
  - Jaundice

SMAA

- Nonspecific abdominal pain
- Mobile pulsatile abdominal mass
- Abdominal apoplexy with rupture

IMAGING FINDINGS

SAA

- Abdominal x-ray: Concentric calcification in left upper quadrant
- CT scan often diagnostic
- Angiogram often diagnostic

HAA

- CT scan helpful
- Angiogram diagnostic

SMAA

- CT scan helpful
- Angiogram diagnostic

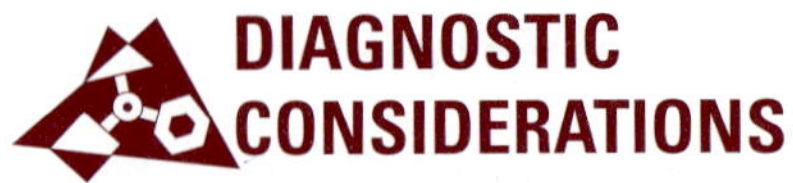

DIAGNOSTIC CONSIDERATIONS

- Angiogram often performed prior to any operative intervention

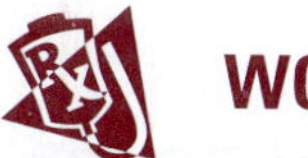

WORK-UP

- Abdominal x-ray
- CT scan
- Angiography

TREATMENT AND MANAGEMENT

SAA

- Aneurysm exclusion with or without splenectomy
- Laparoscopic ligation feasible

HAA

- If common hepatic artery involved, can be ligated
- If other portions of artery, reconstruct

SMAA

- Options include:
  - Ligation
  - Endoaneurysmorrhaphy
  - Replace with autogenous vessel
- For branch aneurysm, consider bowel resection

SURGERY

Indications

- **SAA:** Symptomatic aneurysms, pregnant women, aneuruysm > 3 cm
- **HAA:** Required with ruptures

PROGNOSIS

SAA

- Rupture during pregnancy occurs during third trimester: 75% maternal death, 90% fetal death

HAA

- 35% mortality with rupture

RESOURCES

REFERENCES

- Carr SC et al. Visceral artery aneurysm rupture. *J Vasc Surg.* 2001;33:806.
- Messina LM et al. Visceral artery aneurysms. *Surg Clin North Am.* 1997;77:425.

Volume Overload

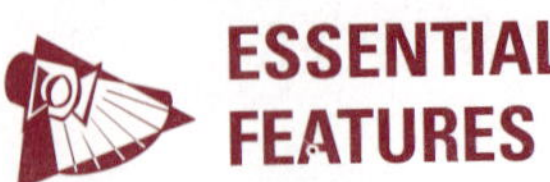

ESSENTIAL FEATURES

- Volume overload

EPIDEMIOLOGY

- Postoperative patients
- Heart failure
- Liver disease
- Renal failure
- Hypoalbuminuria
- Head injury (syndrome of inappropriate antidiuretic hormone [SIADH])
- Burns (SIADH)
- Cancer (SIADH)

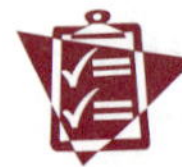

CLINICAL FINDINGS

SYMPTOMS AND SIGNS

- Sacral edema
- Extremity edema
- Jugular venous distention
- Tachypnea
- Increased body weight
- Elevated central pressures
- Gallop rhythm
- Confusion (SIADH)
- Lethargy (SIADH)

LABORATORY FINDINGS

- Hyponatremia (SIADH)
- Concentrated urine (SIADH)
- Elevated urine sodium (SIADH)
- Low urine sodium
- High urine potassium

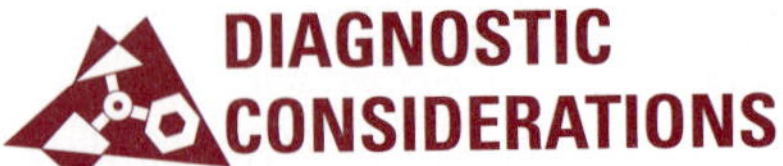

DIAGNOSTIC CONSIDERATIONS

- May be concurrent with myocardial failure or ischemia
- Evaluation should include cardiac evaluation

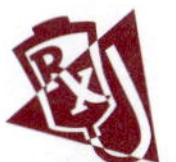

WORK-UP

- Serum electrolytes
- UA (SIADH)

WHEN TO REFER

- Cardiology consult if primary cardiogenic failure

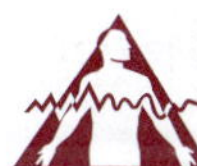

TREATMENT AND MANAGEMENT

- Sodium restriction
- Water restriction if low sodium
- Diuretics if severe
- Diuretics (SIADH)
- IV isotonic saline to match urinary output (SIADH)

MEDICATIONS

- Diuretics

TREATMENT MONITORING

- Serum sodium

COMPLICATIONS

- Pulmonary edema
- Congestive heart failure
- Prerenal azotemia

PROGNOSIS

- Excellent

PREVENTION

- Monitor daily weights
- Judicious IV hydration
- Monitor sodium intake

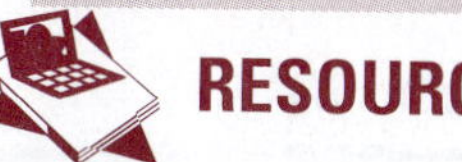

RESOURCES

REFERENCES

- Chang MC et al. Redefining cardiovascular performance during resuscitation: ventricular stroke work, power, and the pressure-volume diagram. *J Trauma.* 1998;45:470.

Volvulus

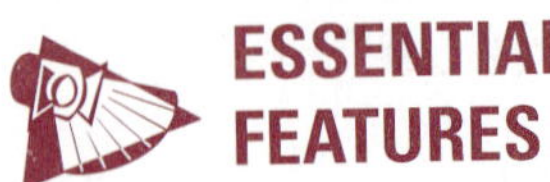

ESSENTIAL FEATURES

- Rotation of a segment of intestine on an axis (bowel twists on its mesentery)
- Most commonly sigmoid colon (65%) and cecum
- May produce large or small bowel obstruction
- Causes closed-loop obstruction
- Predisposes to bowel infarction, perforation

EPIDEMIOLOGY

- Usually in older age groups
- 25% of bowel obstruction in pregnant patients
- 50% of patients > 70 years of age
- Frequently seen in bedridden, debilitated patients
- Associated with high fiber, high residue diet

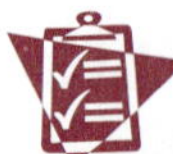

CLINICAL FINDINGS

SYMPTOMS AND SIGNS

- Severe intermittent colicky abdominal pain
- Abdominal distention
- Nausea, vomiting
- Constipation leading to obstipation

LABORATORY FINDINGS

- No specific findings
- Leukocytosis, metabolic acidosis should raise suspicion of bowel compromise, possible perforation

IMAGING FINDINGS

- Abdominal x-ray
  - "Bent inner tube"
  - Signs of intestinal obstruction, including air-fluid levels and dilated loops of bowel
- Barium enema: "Bird's beak" or "ace of spades" deformity

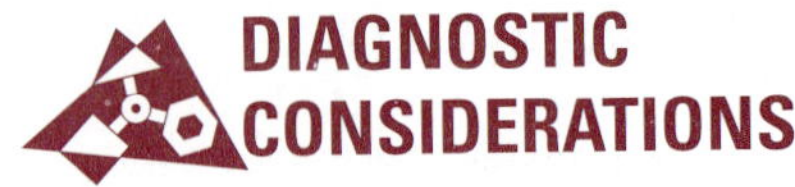

DIAGNOSTIC CONSIDERATIONS

- Functional bowel obstruction
  - Adynamic ileus
  - Pseudo-obstruction
- Other causes of mechanical obstruction
  - Neoplasm
  - Stricture
  - Extrinsic compression
  - Hernia (external or internal)
  - Adhesion
- Intussusception
- Gallstone ileus
- Inflammatory bowel disease

WORK-UP

- Complete history and physical exam, including surgical history, history of malignancy, medications (especially psychotropic)
- Abdominal x-ray
- Barium enema

WHEN TO ADMIT

- Signs and symptoms of bowel obstruction

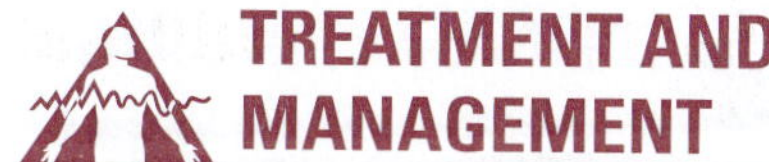

TREATMENT AND MANAGEMENT

SURGERY

- NG decompression
- Endoscopic evaluation and attempt at decompression for sigmoid volvulus
- Placement of rectal tube
- Exploratory laparatomy, untwisting of the bowel, resection of ischemic or necrotic bowel
- Attempts at re-anastomosis vs exteriorization of bowel dependent on absence or presence of perforation, peritoneal soilage, gangrenous bowel

Indications

- Peritoneal findings due to strangulation or perforation
- Failure to resolve volvulus with endoscopic decompression
- Prevention of recurrence even after successful detorsion

Contraindications

- Extremely high-risk patients may have decompression via tube cecostomy
- Signs of perforation or peritonitis preclude endoscopic decompression

COMPLICATIONS

- Bowel infarction

PROGNOSIS

- Mortality rate following emergent operation for cecal volvulus, 12%; if cecum is gangrenous, mortality, 35%
- Mortality rate of perforated sigmoid volvulus, 50%

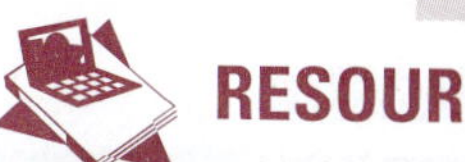

RESOURCES

REFERENCES

- Chang GJ et al. Large Intestine. In: Way LW, Doherty GM (editors). *Current Surgical Diagnosis & Treatment,* 11e. New York: McGraw-Hill; 2003: 738–740.

Wilms Tumor

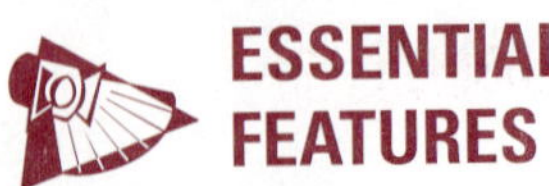

ESSENTIAL FEATURES

- Associated with:
  - Beckwith-Wiedemann syndrome (macroglossia, gigantism, visceromegaly, hypoglycemia, abdominal wall defects)
  - WAGR syndrome (Wilms, aniridia, ambiguous genitalia, mental retardation)
  - Neurofibromatosis
  - Denys-Drash syndrome
  - Perlman familial nephroblastomatosis
  - Other genital abnormalities
- 1–2% incidence of bilateral disease
- As high as 7% multicentricity

EPIDEMIOLOGY

- 6.9% of cancers diagnosed before age 15
- Incidence highest in blacks
- Peak incidence between ages 2 and 3

CLINICAL FINDINGS

SYMPTOMS AND SIGNS

- Abdominal mass
- Pain
- Fever
- Hematuria

IMAGING FINDINGS

- **CT scan:** Shows extent of disease in kidney and extent of distant or nodal disease

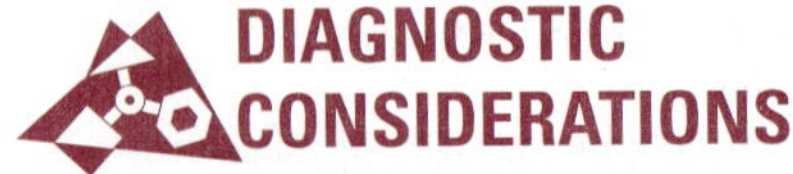

DIAGNOSTIC CONSIDERATIONS

- Stage, bilateral disease, major vessel involvement

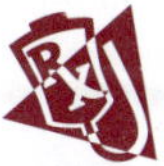

WORK-UP

- History and physical exam
- Abdominal CT scan
- Chest film
- Doppler US when concern of major vessel involvement

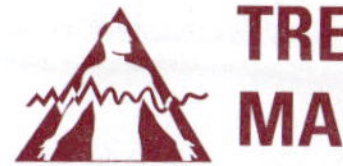

TREATMENT AND MANAGEMENT

SURGERY

- Resection of tumor with inspection of contralateral kidney and sampling of regional nodes
- Resection performed after chemotherapy/radiation therapy if bilateral disease to spare renal function or in presence of major vessel involvement (inferior vena cava, renal veins, etc)

MEDICATIONS

- Chemotherapy (vincristine and actinomycin D with doxorubicin added for stage III and IV)
- Radiation for stage III, pulmonary or hepatic metastases or all stages if unfavorable histology

COMPLICATIONS

- Damage to major neurovascular structures
- Recurrence

PROGNOSIS

- 4-year survival ranging from 78% to 97% (stage dependent)

RESOURCES

REFERENCES

- Capra ML et al. Wilms' tumor: a 25-year review of the role of preoperative chemotherapy. *J Pediatr Surg.* 1999;34:579.
- Haase GM, Ritchey ML. Nephroblastoma. *Semin Pediatr Surg.* 1997;6:11.

Cancer Staging Tables

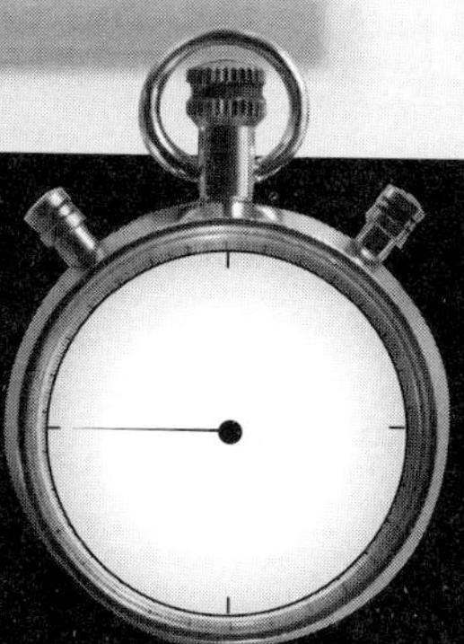

Ampulla of Vater

Primary Tumor (T)

TX	Primary tumor cannot be assessed
T0	No evidence of primary tumor
Tis	Carcinoma *in situ*
T1	Tumor limited to ampulla of Vater or sphincter of Oddi
T2	Tumor invades duodenal wall
T3	Tumor invades pancreas
T4	Tumor invades peripancreatic soft tissues or other adjacent organs or structures

Regional Lymph Nodes (N)

NX	Regional lymph nodes cannot be assessed
N0	No regional lymph node metastasis
N1	Regional lymph node metastasis

Distant Metastasis (M)

MX	Distant metastasis cannot be assessed
M0	No distant metastasis
M1	Distant metastasis

STAGE GROUPING

Stage 0	Tis	N0	M0
Stage IA	T1	N0	M0
Stage IB	T2	N0	M0
Stage IIA	T3	N0	M0
Stage IIB	T1	N1	M0
	T2	N1	M0
	T3	N1	M0
Stage III	T4	Any N	M0
Stage IV	Any T	Any N	M1

AJCC Cancer Staging Manual, 6th ed. Springer, 2002.

Anal Canal

Primary Tumor (T)

TX	Primary tumor cannot be assessed
T0	No evidence of primary tumor
Tis	Carcinoma in situ
T1	Tumor 2 cm or less in greatest dimension
T2	Tumor more than 2 cm but not more than 5 cm in greatest dimension
T3	Tumor more than 5 cm in greatest dimension
T4	Tumor of any size invades adjacent organ(s), e.g., vagina, urethra, bladder*

**Note:* Direct invasion of the rectal wall, perirectal skin, subcutaneous tissue, or the sphincter muscle(s) is not classified as T4.

Regional Lymph Nodes (N)

NX	Regional lymph nodes cannot be assessed
N0	No regional lymph node metastasis
N1	Metastasis in perirectal lymph node(s)
N2	Metastasis in unilateral internal iliac and/or inguinal lymph node(s)
N3	Metastasis in perirectal and inguinal lymph nodes and/or bilateral internal iliac and/or inguinal lymph nodes

Distant Metastasis (M)

MX	Distant metastasis cannot be assessed
M0	No distant metastasis
M1	Distant metastasis

STAGE GROUPING

Stage 0	Tis	N0	M0
Stage I	T1	N0	M0
Stage II	T2	N0	M0
	T3	N0	M0
Stage IIIA	T1	N1	M0
	T2	N1	M0
	T3	N1	M0
	T4	N0	M0
Stage IIIB	T4	N1	M0
	Any T	N2	M0
	Any T	N3	M0
Stage IV	Any T	Any N	M1

AJCC Cancer Staging Manual, 6th ed. Springer, 2002.

Breast

Primary Tumor (T)

Definitions for classifying the primary tumor (T) are the same for clinical and for pathologic classification. If the measurement is made by physical examination, the examiner will use the major headings (T1, T2, or T3). If other measurements, such as mammographic or pathologic measurements, are used, the subsets of T1 can be used. Tumors should be measured to the nearest 0.1 cm increment.

TX	Primary tumor cannot be assessed
T0	No evidence of primary tumor
Tis	Carcinoma *in situ*
Tis (DCIS)	Ductal carcinoma *in situ*
Tis (LCIS)	Lobular carcinoma *in situ*
Tis (Paget)	Paget disease of the nipple with no tumor

Note: Paget disease associated with a tumor is classified according to the size of the tumor.

T1	Tumor 2 cm or less in greatest dimension
T1mic	Microinvasion 0.1 cm or less in greatest dimension
T1a	Tumor more than 0.1 cm but not more than 0.5 cm in greatest dimension
T1b	Tumor more than 0.5 cm but not more than 1 cm in greatest dimension
T1c	Tumor more than 1 cm but not more than 2 cm in greatest dimension
T2	Tumor more than 2 cm but not more than 5 cm in greatest dimension
T3	Tumor more than 5 cm in greatest dimension
T4	Tumor of any size with direction extension to (a) chest wall or (b) skin, only as described below
T4a	Extension to chest wall, not including pectoralis muscle
T4b	Edema (including peau d'orange) or ulceration of the skin of the breast, or satellite skin nodules confined to the same breast
T4c	Both T4a and T4b
T4d	Inflammatory carcinoma

Regional Lymph Nodes (N)

Clinical

NX	Regional lymph nodes cannot be assessed (e.g., previously removed)
N0	No regional lymph node metastasis
N1	Metastasis to movable ipsilateral axillary lymph node(s)
N2	Metastases in ipsilateral axillary lymph nodes fixed or matted, or in clinically apparent* ipsilateral internal mammary nodes in the *absence* of clinically evident axillary lymph node metastasis
N2a	Metastasis in ipsilateral axillary lymph nodes fixed to one another (matted) or to the other structures
N2b	Metastasis only in clinically apparent* ipsilateral internal mammary nodes and in the *absence* of clinically evident axillary lymph node metastasis
N3	Metastasis in ipsilateral infraclavicular lymph node(s) with or without axillary lymph node involvement, or in clinically apparent* ipsilateral internal mammary lymph node(s) and in the *presence* of clinically evident axillary lymph node metastasis; or metastasis in ipsilateral supraclavicular lymph node(s) with or without axillary or internal mammary lymph node involvement
N3	Metastasis in ipsilateral infraclavicular lymph node(s)
N3b	Metastasis in ipsilateral internal mammary lymph node(s) and axillary lymph node(s)
N3c	Metastasis in ipsilateral supraclavicular lymph node(s)

**Clinically apparent* is defined as detected by imaging studies (excluding lymphoscintigraphy) or by clinical examination or grossly visible pathologically.

Pathologic (pN)[a]

pNX	Regional lymph nodes cannot be assessed (e.g., previously removed, or not removed for pathologic study)
pN0	No regional lymph node metastasis histologically, no additional examination for isolated tumor cells (ITC)

Note: Isolated tumor cells (ITC) are defined as single tumor cells or small cell clusters not greater than 0.2 mm, usually detected only by immunohistochemical (IHC) or molecular methods but which may be verified on H&E stains. ITCs do not usually show evidence of malignant activity e.g., proliferation or stromal reaction.

pN0(i-)	No regional lymph node metastasis histologically, negative IHC
pN0(i+)	No regional node metastasis histologically, positive IHC, no IHC cluster greater than 0.2 mm
pN0(mol-)	No regional lymph node metastasis histologically, negative molecular findings (RT-PCR)[b]
pN0(mol+)	No regional lymph node metastasis histologically, positive molecular findings (RT-PCR)[b]

[a]Classification is based on axillary lymph node dissection with or without sentinel lymph node dissection. Classification based solely on sentinel lymph node dissection without subsequent axillary lymph node dissection is designated (sn) for "sentinel node," e.g., pN0(i+)(sn).

[b]RT-PCR: reverse transcriptase/polymerase chain reaction.

pN1	Metastasis in 1 to 3 axillary lymph nodes, and/or in internal mammary nodes with microscopic disease detected by sentinel lymph node dissection but not clinically apparent**
pN1mi	Micrometastasis (greater than 0.2 mm, none greater than 2.0 mm)
pN1a	Metastasis in 1 to 3 axillary lymph nodes
pN1b	Metastasis in internal mammary nodes with microscopic disease detected by sentinel lymph node dissection but not clinically apparent**
pN1c	Metastasis in 1 to 3 axillary lymph nodes and in internal mammary lymph nodes with microscopic disease detected by sentinel lymph node dissection but not clinically apparent.** (If associated with greater than 3 positive axillary lymph nodes, the internal mammary nodes are classified as pN3b to reflect increased tumor burden)
pN2	Metastasis in 4 to 9 axillary lymph nodes, or in clinically apparent* internal mammary lymph nodes in the *absence* of axillary lymph node metastasis
pN2a	Metastasis in 4 to 9 axillary lymph nodes (at least one tumor deposit greater than 2.0 mm)
pN2b	Metastasis in clinically apparent* internal mammary lymph nodes in the *absence* of axillary lymph node metastasis
pN3	Metastasis in 10 or more axillary lymph nodes, or in infraclavicular lymph nodes, or in clinically apparent* ipsilateral internal mammary lymph nodes in the presence of 1 or more positive axillary lymph nodes; or in more than 3 axillary lymph nodes; or in ipsilateral supraclavicular lymph nodes
pN3a	Metastasis in 10 or more axillary lymph nodes (at least one tumor deposit greater than 2.0 m), or metastasis to the infraclavicular lymph nodes
pN3b	Metastasis in clinically apparent* ipsilateral internal mammary lymph nodes in the presence of 1 or more positive axillary lymph nodes; or in more than 3 axillary lymph nodes and in internal mammary lymph nodes with microscopic disease detected by sentinel lymph node dissection but not clinically apparent**
pN3c	Metastasis in ipsilateral supraclavicular lymph nodes

**Clinically apparent* is defined as detected by imaging studies (excluding lymphoscintigraphy) or by clinical examination.

***Not clinically apparent* is defined as not detected by imaging studies (excluding lymphoscintigraphy) or by clinical examination.

Distant Metastasis (M)

MX	Distant metastasis cannot be assessed
M0	No distant metastasis
M1	Distant metastasis

STAGE GROUPING

Stage 0	Tis	N0	M0
Stage I	T1*	N0	M0
Stage IIA	T0	N1	M0
	T1*	N1	M0
	T2	N0	M0
Stage IIB	T2	N1	M0
	T3	N0	M0
Stage IIIA	T0	N2	M0
	T1*	N2	M0
	T2	N2	M0
	T3	N1	M0
	T3	N2	M0

Stage IIIB	T4	N0	M0
	T4	N1	M0
	T4	N2	M0
Stage IIIC	Any T	N3	M0
Stage IV	Any T	Any N	M1

*T1 includes T1mic

Note: Stage designation may be changed if post-surgical imaging studies reveal the presence of distant metastases, provided that the studies are carried out within 4 months of diagnosis in the absence of disease progression and provided that the patient has not received neoadjuvant therapy.

AJCC Cancer Staging Manual, 6th ed. Springer, 2002.

Carcinoma of the Skin

Primary Tumor (T)

- TX Primary tumor cannot be assessed
- T0 No evidence of primary tumor
- Tis Carcinoma *in situ*
- T1 Tumor 2 cm or less in greatest dimension
- T2 Tumor more than 2 cm, but not more than 5 cm, in greatest dimension
- T3 Tumor more than 5 cm in greatest dimension
- T4 Tumor invades deep extradermal structures (i.e., cartilage, skeletal muscle, or bone)

Note: In case of multiple simultaneous tumors, the tumor with the highest T category will be classified and the number of separate tumors will be indicated in parentheses, e.g., T2(5).

Regional Lymph Nodes (N)

- NX Regional lymph nodes cannot be assessed
- M0 No regional lymph node metastasis
- N1 Regional lymph node metastasis

Distant Metastasis (M)

- MX Distant metastasis cannot be assessed
- M0 No distant metastasis
- M1 Distant metastasis

STAGE GROUPING

Stage 0	Tis	N0	M0
Stage I	T1	N0	M0
Stage II	T2	N0	M0
	T3	N0	M0
Stage III	T4	N0	M0
	Any T	N1	M0
Stage IV	Any T	Any N	M1

AJCC Cancer Staging Manual, 6th ed. Springer, 2002.

Colon and Rectum

Primary Tumor (T)

- TX Primary tumor cannot be assessed
- T0 No evidence of primary tumor
- Tis Carcinoma in situ: intraepithelial or invasion of lamina propria*
- T1 Tumor invades submucosa
- T2 Tumor invades muscularis propria
- T3 Tumor invades through the muscularis propria into the subserosa, or into nonperitonealized pericolic or perirectal tissues
- T4 Tumor directly invades other organs or structures, and/or perforates visceral peritoneum**,***

**Note:* Tis includes cancer cells confined within the glandular basement membrane (intraepithelial) or lamina propria (intramucosal) with no extension through the muscularis mucosae into the submucosa.

***Note:* Direct invasion in T4 includes invasion of other segments of the colorectum by way of the serosa; for example, invasion of the sigmoid colon by a carcinoma of the cecum.

***Tumor that is adherent to other organs or structures, macroscopically, is classified T4. However, if no tumor is present in the adhesion, microscopically, the classification should be pT3. The V and L substaging should be used to identify the presence of vascular or lymphatic invasion.

Regional Lymph Nodes (N)

- NX Regional lymph nodes cannot be assessed
- N0 No regional lymph node metastasis
- N1 Metastasis in 1 to 3 regional lymph nodes
- N2 Metastasis in 4 or more regional lymph nodes

Note: A tumor nodule in the pericolorectal adipose tissue of a primary carcinoma without histologic evidence of residual lymph node in the nodule is classified in the pN category as a regional lymph node metastasis if the nodule has the form and smooth contour of a lymph node. If the nodule has an irregular contour, it should be classified in the T category and also coded as V1 (microscopic venous invasion) or as V2 (if it was grossly evident), because there is a strong likelihood that it represents venous invasion.

Distant Metastasis (M)

MX	Distant metastasis cannot be assessed
M0	No distant metastasis
M1	Distant metastasis

STAGE GROUPING

Stage	T	N	M	Dukes*	MAC*
0	Tis	N0	M0	-	-
I	T1	N0	M0	A	A
	T2	N0	M0	A	B1
IIA	T3	N0	M0	B	B2
IIB	T4	N0	M0	B	B3
IIIA	T1-T2	N1	M0	C	C1
IIIB	T3-T4	N1	M0	C	C2/C3
IIIC	Any T	N2	M0	C	C1/C2/C3
IV	Any T	Any N	M1	-	D

*Dukes B is a composite of better (T3 N0 M0) and worse (T4 N0 M0) prognostic groups, as is Dukes C (Any TN1 M0 and Any T N2 M0). MAC is the modified Astler-Coller classification.

Note: The y prefix is to be used for those cancers that are classified after pretreatment, whereas the r prefix is to be used for those cancers that have recurred.

AJCC Cancer Staging Manual, 6th ed. Springer, 2002.

Esophagus

Primary Tumor (T)

TX	Primary tumor cannot be assessed
T0	No evidence of primary tumor
Tis	Carcinoma in situ
T1	Tumor invades lamina propria or submucosa
T2	Tumor invades muscularis propria
T3	Tumor invades adventitia
T4	Tumor invades adjacent structures

Regional Lymph Nodes (N)

NX	Regional lymph nodes cannot be assessed
N0	No regional lymph node metastasis
N1	Regional lymph node metastasis

Distant Metastasis (M)

MX	Distant metastasis cannot be assessed
M0	No distant metastasis
M1	Distant metastasis

Tumors of the lower thoracic esophagus:

M1a	Metastasis in celiac lymph nodes
M1b	Other distant metastasis

Tumors of the midthoracic esophagus:

M1a	Not applicable
M1b	Nonregional lymph nodes and/or other distant metastasis

Tumors of the upper thoracic esophagus:

M1a	Metastasis in cervical nodes
M1b	Other distant metastasis

STAGE GROUPING

Stage 0	Tis	N0	M0
Stage I	T1	N0	M0
Stage IIA	T2	N0	M0
	T3	N0	M0
Stage IIB	T1	N1	M0
	T2	N1	M0
Stage III	T3	N1	M0
	T4	Any N	M0
Stage IV	Any T	Any N	M1
Stage IVA	Any T	Any N	M1a
Stage IVB	Any T	Any N	M1b

AJCC Cancer Staging Manual, 6th ed. Springer, 2002.

Exocrine Pancreas

Primary Tumor (T)

TX Primary tumor cannot be assessed

T0 No evidence of primary tumor

Tis Carcinoma *in situ**

T1 Tumor limited to the pancreas, 2 cm or less in greatest dimension

T2 Tumor limited to the pancreas, more than 2 cm in greatest dimension

T3 Tumor extends beyond the pancreas but without involvement of the celiac axis or the superior mesenteric artery

T4 Tumor involves the celiac axis or the superior mesenteric artery (unresectable primary tumor)

Regional Lymph Nodes (N)

NX Regional lymph nodes cannot be assessed

N0 No regional lymph node metastasis

N1 Regional lymph node metastasis

Distant Metastasis (M)

MX Distant metastasis cannot be assessed

M0 No distant metastasis

M1 Distant metastasis

*This also includes the "PanInIII" classification

STAGE GROUPING

Stage 0	Tis	N0	M0
Stage IA	T1	N0	M0
Stage IB	T2	N0	M0
Stage IIA	T3	N0	M0
Stage IIB	T1	N1	M0
	T2	N1	M0
	T3	N1	M0
Stage III	T4	Any N	M0
Stage IV	Any T	Any N	M1

AJCC Cancer Staging Manual, 6th ed. Springer, 2002.

Extrahepatic Bile Ducts

Primary Tumor (T)

TX Primary tumor cannot be assessed

T0 No evidence of primary tumor

Tis Carcinoma *in situ*

T1 Tumor confined to the bile duct histologically

T2 Tumor invades beyond the wall of the bile duct

T3 Tumor invades the liver, gallbladder, pancreas, and/or unilateral branches of the portal vein (right or left) or hepatic artery (right or left)

T4 Tumor invades any of the following: main portal vein or its branches bilaterally, common hepatic artery, or other adjacent structures, such as the colon, stomach, duodenum, or abdominal wall

Regional Lymph Nodes (N)

NX Distant metastasis cannot be assessed

M0 No distant metastasis

M1 Distant metastasis

STAGE GROUPING

Stage 0	Tis	N0	M0
Stage IA	T1	N0	M0
Stage IB	T2	N0	M0
Stage IIA	T3	N0	M0
Stage IIB	T1	N1	M0
	T2	N1	M0
	T3	N1	M0
Stage III	T4	Any N	M0
Stage IV	Any T	Any N	M1

AJCC Cancer Staging Manual, 6th ed. Springer, 2002.

Gallbladder

Primary Tumor (T)

TX Primary tumor cannot be assessed

T0 No evidence of primary tumor

Tis Carcinoma *in situ*

T1 Tumor invades lamina propria or muscle layer (Fig. 15.1)

T1a Tumor invades lamina propria

T1b Tumor invades muscle layer

T2 Tumor invades perimuscular connective tissue; no extension beyond serosa or into liver

T3 Tumor perforates the serosa (visceral peritoneum) and/or directly invades the liver and/or one other adjacent organ or structure, such as the stomach, duodenum, colon, or pancreas, omentum or extrahepatic bile ducts

T4 Tumor invades main portal vein or hepatic artery or invades multiple extrahepatic organs or structures

Regional Lymph Nodes (N)

NX Regional lymph nodes cannot be assessed

N0 No regional lymph node metastasis

N1 Regional lymph node metastasis

Distant Metastasis (M)

MX Distant metastasis cannot be assessed

M0 No distant metastasis

M1 Distant metastasis

STAGE GROUPING

Stage 0	Tis	N0	M0
Stage IA	T1	N0	M0
Stage IB	T2	N0	M0
Stage IIA	T3	N0	M0
Stage IIB	T1	N1	M0
	T2	N1	M0
	T3	N1	M0
Stage III	T4	Any N	M0
Stage IV	Any T	Any N	M1

AJCC Cancer Staging Manual, 6th ed. Springer, 2002.

Larynx

Primary Tumor (T)

TX	Primary tumor cannot be assessed
T0	No evidence of primary tumor
Tis	Carcinoma *in situ*

Supraglottis

T1	Tumor limited to one subsite of supraglottis with normal vocal cord mobility
T2	Tumor invades mucosa of more than one adjacent subsite of supraglottis or glottis or region outside the supraglottis (e.g., mucosa of base of tongue, vallecula, medial wall of pyriform sinus) without fixation of the larynx
T3	Tumor limited to larynx with vocal cord fixation and/or invades any of the following: postcricoid area, pre-epiglottic tissues, paraglottic space, and/or minor thyroid cartilage erosion (e.g., inner cortex)
T4a	Tumor invades through the thyroid cartilage and/or invades tissues beyond the larynx (e.g., trachea, soft tissues of neck including deep extrinsic muscle of the tongue, strap muscles, thyroid, or esophagus)
T4b	Tumor invades prevertebral space, encases carotid artery, or invades mediastinal structures

Glottis

T1	Tumor limited to the vocal cord(s) (may involve anterior or posterior commissure) with normal mobility
T1a	Tumor limited to one vocal cord
T1b	Tumor involves both vocal cords
T2	Tumor extends to supraglottis and/or subglottis and/or with impaired vocal cord mobility
T3	Tumor limited to the larynx with vocal cord fixation and/or invades paraglottic space, and/or minor thyroid cartilage erosion (e.g., inner cortex)
T4a	Tumor invades through the thyroid cartilage and/or invades tissues beyond the larynx (e.g., trachea, soft tissues of neck including deep extrinsic muscle of the tongue, strap muscles, thyroid, or esophagus)
T4b	Tumor invades prevertebral space, encases carotid artery, or invades mediastinal structures

Subglottis

T1	Tumor limited to the subglottis
T2	Tumor extends to vocal cord(s) with normal or impaired mobility
T3	Tumor limited to larynx with vocal cord fixation
T4a	Tumor invades cricoid or thyroid cartilage and/or invades tissues beyond the larynx (e.g., trachea, soft tissues of neck including deep extrinsic muscles of the tongue, strap muscles, thyroid or esophagus)
T4b	Tumor invades prevertebral space, encases carotid artery, or invades mediastinal structures

Regional Lymph Nodes (N)

NX	Regional lymph nodes cannot be assessed
N0	No regional lymph node metastasis
N1	Metastasis in a single ipsilateral lymph node, 3 cm or less in greatest dimension
N2	Metastasis in a single ipsilateral lymph node, more than 3 cm but not more than 6 cm in greatest dimension, or in multiple ipsilateral lymph nodes, none more than 6 cm in greatest dimension, or in bilateral or contralateral lymph nodes, none more than 6 cm in greatest dimension
N2a	Metastasis in a single ipsilateral lymph node, more than 3 cm but not more than 6 cm in greatest dimension
N2b	Metastasis in bilateral or contralateral lymph nodes, none more than 6 cm in greatest dimension
N2c	Metastasis in bilateral or contralateral lymph nodes, none more than 6 cm in greatest dimension
N3	Metastasis in a lymph node, more than 6 cm in greatest dimension

Distant Metastasis (M)

MX	Distant metastasis cannot be assessed
M0	No distant metastasis
M1	Distant metastasis

STAGE GROUPING

Stage 0	Tis	N0	M0
Stage I	T1	N0	M0
Stage II	T2	N0	M0
Stage III	T3	N0	M0
	T1	N1	M0
	T2	N1	M0
	T3	N1	M0
Stage IVA	T4a	N0	M0
	T4a	N1	M0
	T1	N2	M0
	T2	N2	M0
	T3	N2	M0
	T4a	N2	M0
Stage IVB	T4b	Any N	M0
	Any T	N3	M0
Stage IVC	Any T	Any N	M1

AJCC Cancer Staging Manual, 6th ed. Springer, 2002.

Lip and Oral Cavity

Primary Tumor (T)

TX	Primary tumor cannot be assessed
T0	No evidence of primary tumor
Tis	Carcinoma *in situ*
T1	Tumor 2 cm or less in greatest dimension
T2	Tumor more than 2 cm but not more than 4 cm in greatest dimension
T3	Tumor more than 4 cm in greatest dimension
T4(lip)	Tumor invades through cortical bone, inferior alveolar nerve, floor of mouth, or skin of face, i.e., chin or nose
T4a	(oral cavity) Tumor invades adjacent structures (e.g., through cortical bone, into deep [extrinsic] muscle of tongue [genioglossus, hyoglossus, palatoglossus, and styloglossus], maxillary sinus, skin of face)
T4b	Tumor invades masticator space, pterygoid plates, or skull base and/or encases internal carotid artery

Note: Superficial erosion alone of bone/tooth socket by gingival primary is not sufficient to classify a tumor as T4.

Regional Lymph Nodes (N)

NX	Regional lymph nodes cannot be assessed
N0	***No regional lymph node metastasis***
N1	Metastasis in a single ipsilateral lymph node, 3 cm or less in greatest dimension
N2	Metastasis in a single ipsilateral lymph node, more than 3 cm but not more than 6 cm in greatest dimension; or in multiple ipsilateral lymph nodes, none more than 6 cm in greatest dimension; or in bilateral or contralateral lymph nodes, none more than 6 cm in greatest dimension
N2a	Metastasis in single ipsilateral lymph node more than 3 cm but not more than 6 cm in greatest dimension
N2b	Metastasis in multiple ipsilateral lymph nodes, none more than 6 cm in greatest dimension
N2c	Metastasis in bilateral or contralateral lymph nodes, none more than 6 cm in greatest dimension
N3	Metastasis in a lymph node more than 6 cm in greatest dimension

Distant Metastasis (M)

MX	Distant metastasis cannot be assessed
M0	No distant metastasis
M1	Distant metastasis

STAGE GROUPING

Stage 0	Tis	N0	M0
Stage I	T1	N0	M0
Stage II	T2	N0	M0
Stage III	T3	N0	M0
	T1	N1	M0
	T2	N1	M0
	T3	N1	M0
Stage IVA	T4a	N0	M0
	T4a	N1	M0
	T1	N2	M0
	T2	N2	M0
	T3	N2	M0
	T4a	N2	M0
Stage IVB	Any T	N3	M0
	T4b	Any N	M0
Stage IVC	Any T	Any N	M1

AJCC Cancer Staging Manual, 6th ed. Springer, 2002.

Liver (Including Intrahepatic Bile Ducts)

Primary Tumor (T)

TX	Primary tumor cannot be assessed
T0	No evidence of primary tumor
T1	Solitary tumor without vascular invasion
T2	Solitary tumor with vascular invasion or multiple tumors none more than 5 cm
T3	Multiple tumors more than 5 cm or tumor involving a major branch of the portal or hepatic vein(s)
T4	Tumor(s) with direct invasion of adjacent organs other than the gallbladder or with perforation of visceral peritoneum

Regional Lymph Nodes (N)

NX	Regional lymph nodes cannot be assessed
N0	No regional lymph node metastasis
N1	Regional lymph node metastasis

Distant Metastasis (M)

MX	Distant metastasis cannot be assessed
M0	No distant metastasis
M1	Distant metastasis

STAGE GROUPING

Stage I	T1	N0	M0
Stage II	T2	N0	M0
Stage IIIA	T3	N0	M0
IIIB	T4	N0	M0
IIIC	Any T	N1	M0
Stage IV	Any T	Any N	M1

AJCC Cancer Staging Manual, 6th ed. Springer, 2002.

Lung

Primary Tumor (T)

Note: All categories may be subdivided: (a) solitary tumor, (b) multifocal tumor (the largest determines the classification).

TX	Primary T cannot be assessed, or tumor proven by the presence of malignant cells in sputum or bronchial washings but not visualized by imaging or bronchoscopy
T0	No evidence of primary T
Tis	Carcinoma *in situ*
T1	T 3 cm or less in greatest dimension, surrounded by lung or visceral pleura, without bronchoscopic evidence of invasion more proximal than the lobar bronchus,* (i.e., not in the main bronchus)
T2	T with any of the following features of size or extent: > 3cm in greatest dimension Involves main bronchus, 2 cm or more distal to the carina Invades the visceral pleura Associated with atelectasis or obstructive pneumonitis that extends to the hilar region but does not involve the entire lung
T3	T of any size that directly invades any of the following: chest wall (including superior sulcus tumors), diaphragm, mediastinal pleura, parietal pericardium; or tumor in the main bronchus < 2cm distal to the carina, but without involvement of the carina; or associated atelectasis or obstructive pneumonitis of the entire lung
T4	T of any size that invades any of the following: mediastinum, heart, great vessels, trachea, esophagus, vertebral body, carina; or separate tumor nodules in the same lobe; or tumor with malignant pleural effusion**

**Note:* The uncommon superficial tumor of any size with its invasive component limited to the bronchial wall, which may extend proximal to the bronchial wall, which may extend proximal to the main bronchus, is also classified T1.

***Note:* Most pleural effusions associated with lung cancer are due to tumor. However, there are a few patients in whom multiple cytopathologic examinations of pleural fluid are negative for tumor. In these cases, fluid is nonbloody and is not an exudate. Such patients may be further evaluated by the videothoracoscopy (VATS) and direct pleural biopsies. When these elements and clinical judgment dictate that the effusion is not related to the tumor, the effusion should be excluded as a staging element and the patient should be staged T1, T2, or T3.

Regional Lymph Nodes (N)

NX	Regional lymph nodes cannot be assessed.
N0	No regional lymph node metastasis
N1	Metastasis to ipsilateral peribronchial and/or ipsilateral hilar lymph nodes, and intrapulmonary nodes including involvement by direct extension of the primary T
N2	Metastasis to ipsilateral mediastinal and/or subcarinal lymph nodes(s)
N3	Metastasis to contralateral mediastinal, contralateral hilar, ipsilateral or contralateral scalene, or supraclavicular lymph nodes(s)

Distant Metastasis (M)

MX	Distant metastasis cannot be assessed
M0	No distant metastasis
M1	Distant metastasis present

Note: M1 includes separate tumor nodule(s) in a different lobe (ipsilateral or contralateral).

STAGE GROUPING

Occult Carcinoma	TX	N0	M0
Stage 0	Tis	N0	M0
Stage IA	T1	N0	M0
Stage IB	T2	N0	M0
Stage IIA	T1	N1	M0
Stage IIB	T2	N1	M0
	T3	N0	M0
Stage IIIA	T1	N2	M0
	T2	N2	M0
	T3	N1	M0
	T3	N2	M0
Stage IIIB	Any T	N3	M0
	T4	Any N	M0
Stage IV	Any T	Any N	M1

Melanoma of the Skin

Primary Tumor (T)

TX	Primary tumor cannot be assessed (e.g., shave biopsy or regressed melanoma)
T0	No evidence of primary tumor
Tis	Melanoma *in situ*
T1	Melanoma ≤ 1.0 mm in thickness with or without ulceration
T1a	Melanoma ≤ 1.0 mm in thickness and level II or III, no ulceration
T1b	Melanoma ≤ 1.0 mm in thickness and level IV or V or with ulceration
T2	Melanoma 1.01-2 mm in thickness with or without ulceration
T2a	Melanoma 1.01-2.0 mm in thickness, no ulceration
T2b	Melanoma 1.01-2.0 mm in thickness, with ulceration
T3	Melanoma 2.01-4 mm in thickness with or without ulceration
T3a	Melanoma 2.01-4.0 mm in thickness, no ulceration
T3b	Melanoma 2.01-4.0 mm in thickness, with ulceration
T4	Melanoma greater than 4.0 mm in thickness with or without ulceration
T4a	Melanoma > 4.0 mm in thickness, no ulceration
T4b	Melanoma > 4.0 mm in thickness, with ulceration

Regional Lymph Nodes (N)

NX	Regional lymph nodes cannot be assessed
N0	No regional lymph node metastasis
N1	Metastasis in one lymph node
N1a	Clinically occult (microscopic) metastasis
N1b	Clinically apparent (macroscopic) metastasis
N2	Metastasis in two to three regional nodes or intralymphatic regional metastasis without model metastases
N2a	Clinically occult (microscopic) metastasis
N2b	Clinically apparent (macroscopic) metastasis

N2c	Metastasis in two to three regional nodes or intralymphatic regional metastasis without nodal metastases
N3	Metastasis in four or more regional nodes, or matted metastatic nodes, or in-transit metastasis or satellite(s) *with* metastasis in regional node(s)

Distant Metastasis (M)

MX	Distant metastasis cannot be assessed
M0	No distant metastasis
M1	Distant metastasis
M1a	Metastasis to skin, subcutaneous tissues or distant lymph nodes
M1b	Metastasis to lung
M1c	Metastasis to all other visceral sites or distant metastasis at any site associated with an elevated serum lactic dehydrogenase (LDH)

AJCC Cancer Staging Manual, 6th ed. Springer, 2002.

Nasal Cavity and Paranasal Sinuses

Primary Tumor (T)

TX	Primary tumor cannot be assessed
T0	No evidence of primary tumor
Tis	Carcinoma *in situ*

Maxillary Sinus

T1	Tumor limited to maxillary sinus mucosa with no erosion or destruction of bone
T2	Tumor causing bone erosion or destruction including extension into the hard palate and/or middle nasal meatus, except extension to posterior wall of maxillary sinus and pterygoid plates
T3	Tumor invades any of the following: bone of the posterior wall of maxillary sinus, subcutaneous tissues, floor or medial wall of orbit, ptergoid fossa, ethmoid sinuses
T4a	Tumor invades anterior orbital contents, skin of cheek, pterygoid plates, intratemporal fossa, cribriform plate, sphenoid or frontal sinuses
T4b	Tumor invades any of the following: orbital apex, dura, brain, middle cranial fossa, cranial nerves other than maxillary division of trigeminal nerve (V_2), nasopharynx, or clivus

Nasal Cavity and Ethmoid Sinus

T1	Tumor restricted to any one subsite, with or without bony invasion
T2	Tumor invading two subsites in a single region or extending to involve an adjacent region within the nasoethmoidal complex, with or without bony invasion
T3	Tumor extends to invade the medial wall or floor of the orbit, maxillary sinus, palate, or cribriform plate
T4a	Tumor invades any of the following: anterior orbital contents, skin of nose or cheek, minimal extension to anterior cranial fossa, pterygoid plates, sphenoid or frontal sinuses
T4b	Tumor invades any of the following: orbital apex, dura, brain, middle cranial fossa, cranial nerves other than (V_2), nasopharynx, or clivus

Regional Lymph Nodes (N)

NX	Regional lymph nodes cannot be assessed
N0	No regional lymph node metastasis
N1	Metastasis in a single ipsilateral lymph node, 3 cm or less in greatest dimension
N2	Metastasis in a single ipsilateral lymph node, more than 3 cm but not more than 6 cm in greatest dimension, or in multiple ipsilateral lymph nodes, none more than 6 cm in greatest dimension, or in bilateral or contralateral lymph nodes, none more than 6 cm in greatest dimension
N2a	Metastasis in a single ipsilateral lymph node, more than 3 cm but not more than 6 cm in greatest dimension
N2b	Metastasis in multiple ipsilateral lymph nodes, none more than 6 cm in greatest dimension
N2c	Metastasis in bilateral or contralateral lymph nodes, none more than 6 cm in greatest dimension
N3	Metastasis in a lymph node, more than 6 cm in greatest dimension

Distant Metastasis (M)

MX	Distant metastasis cannot be assessed
M0	No distant metastasis
M1	Distant metastasis

STAGE GROUPING

Stage 0	Tis	N0	M0
Stage I	T1	N0	M0
Stage II	T2	N0	M0
Stage III	T3	N0	M0
	T1	N1	M0
	T2	N1	M0
	T3	N1	M0
Stage IVA	T4a	N0	M0
	T4a	N1	M0
	T1	N2	M0
	T2	N2	M0
	T3	N2	M0
	T4a	N2	M0
Stage IVB	T4b	Any N	M0
	Any T	N3	M0
Stage IVC	Any T	Any N	M1

AJCC Cancer Staging Manual, 6th ed. Springer, 2002.

Pharynx (Including Base of Tongue, Soft Palate, and Uvula)

Primary Tumor (T)

TX	Primary tumor cannot be assessed
T0	No evidence of primary tumor
Tis	Carcinoma *in situ*

Nasopharynx

T1	Tumor confined to the nasopharynx
T2	Tumor extends to soft tissues T2a Tumor extends to the oropharynx and/or nasal cavity without parapharyngeal extension
T3	Tumor involves bony structures and/or paranasal sinuses
T4	Tumor with intracranial and/or involvement of cranial nerves, infratemporal fossa, hypopharynx, orbit, or masticator space

**Note:* Parapharyngeal extension denotes posterolateral infiltration of tumor beyond the pharyngobasilar fascia.

Oropharynx

T1	Tumor 2 cm or less in greatest dimension
T2	Tumor more than 2 cm but not more than 4 cm in greatest dimension
T3	Tumor more than 4 cm in greatest dimension
T4a	Tumor invades the larynx, deep/extrinsic muscle of tongue, medial pterygoid, hard palate, or mandible
T4b	Tumor invades lateral pterygoid muscle, pterygoid plates, lateral nasopharynx, or skull base or encases carotid artery

Hypopharynx

T1	Tumor limited to one subsite of hypopharynx and 2 cm or less in greatest dimension
T2	Tumor invades more than one subsite of hypopharynx or an adjacent site, or measures more than 2 cm but not more than 4 cm in greatest diameter without fixation of hemilarynx
T3	Tumor more than 4 cm in greatest dimension or with fixation of hemilarynx
T4a	Tumor invades thyroid/cricoid cartilage, hyoid bone, thyroid gland, esophagus, or central compartment soft tissue*
T4b	Tumor invades prevertebral fascia, encases carotid artery, or involves mediastinal structures

**Note:* Central compartment soft tissue includes prelaryngeal strap muscles and subcutaneous fat.

Regional Lymph Nodes (N)

Nasopharynx

The distribution and the prognostic impact of regional lymph node spread from nasopharynx cancer, particularly of the undifferentiated type, are different from those of other head and neck mucosal cancers and justify the use of a different N classification scheme.

NX	Regional lymph nodes cannot be assessed
N0	No regional lymph node metastasis
N1	Unilateral metastasis in lymph node(s), 6 cm or less in greatest dimension, above the supraclavicular fossa*
N2	Bilateral metastasis in lymph node(s), 6 cm or less in greatest dimension, above the supraclavicular fossa*
N3	Metastasis in a lymph node(s)* >6 cm and/or to supraclavicular fossa
	N3a Greater than 6 cm in dimension
	N3b Extension to the supraclavicular fossa**

**Note:* Midline nodes are considered ipsilateral nodes.

**Supraclavicular zone or fossa is relevant to the staging of nasopharyngeal carcinoma and is the triangular region originally described by Ho. It is defined by three points: (1) the superior margin of the sternal end of the clavicle, (2) the superior margin of the lateral end of the clavicle, (3) the point where the neck meets the shoulder. Note that this would include caudal portions of Levels IV and V. All cases with lymph nodes (whole or part) in the fossa are considered N3b.

Oropharynx and Hypopharynx

NX	Regional lymph nodes cannot be assessed
N0	No regional lymph node metastasis
N1	Metastasis in a single ipsilateral lymph node, 3 cm or less in greatest dimension
N2	Metastasis in a single ipsilateral lymph node, more than 3 cm but not more than 6 cm in greatest dimension, or in multiple ipsilateral lymph nodes, none more than 6 cm in greatest dimension, or in bilateral or contralateral lymph nodes, none more than 6 cm in greatest dimension
N2a	Metastasis in a single ipsilateral lymph node more than 3 cm but not more than 6 cm in greatest dimension
N2b	Metastasis in multiple ipsilateral lymph nodes, none more than 6 cm in greatest dimension
N2c	Metastasis in bilateral or contralateral lymph nodes, none more than 6 cm in greatest dimension
N3	Metastasis in a lymph node more than 6 cm in greatest dimension

Distant Metastasis (M)

MX	Distant metastasis cannot be assessed
M0	No distant metastasis
M1	Distant metastasis

STAGE GROUPING: NASOPHARYNX

Stage 0	Tis	N0	M0
Stage I	T1	N0	M0
Stage IIA	T2a	N0	M0
Stage IIB	T1	N1	M0
	T2	N1	M0
	T2a	N1	M0
	T2b	N0	M0
	T2b	N1	M0
Stage III	T1	N2	M0
	T2a	N2	M0
	T2b	N2	M0
	T3	N0	M0
	T3	N1	M0
	T3	N2	M0
Stage IVA	T4	N0	M0
	T4	N1	M0
	T4	N2	M0
Stage IVB	Any T	N3	M0
Stage IVC	Any T	Any N	M1

STAGE GROUPING: OROPHARYNX, HYPOPHARYNX

Stage 0	Tis	N0	M0
Stage I	T1	N0	M0
Stage II	T2	N0	M0
Stage III	T3	N0	M0
	T1	N1	M0
	T2	N1	M0
	T3	N1	M0

Stage IVA	T4a	N0	M0
	T4a	N1	M0
	T1	N2	M0
	T2	N2	M0
	T3	N2	M0
	T4a	N2	M0
Stage IVB	T4b	Any N	M0
	Any T	N3	M0
Stage IVC	Any T	Any N	M1

AJCC Cancer Staging Manual, 6th ed. Springer, 2002.

Salivary Glands, Major

Primary Tumor (T)

TX Primary tumor cannot be assessed

T0 No evidence of primary tumor

T1 Tumor 2 cm or less in greatest dimension without extraparenchymal extension*

T2 Tumor more than 2 cm but not more than 4 cm in greatest dimension without extraparenchymal extension*

T3 Tumor more than 4 cm and/or tumor having extraparenchymal extension*

T4a Tumor invades skin, mandible, ear canal, and/or facial nerve

T4b Tumor invades skull base and/or pterygoid plates and/or encases carotid artery

**Note:* Extraparenchymal extension is clinical or macroscopic evidence of invasion of soft tissues. Microscopic evidence alone does not constitute extraparenchymal extension for classification purposes.

Regional Lymph Nodes (N)

NX Regional lymph nodes cannot be assessed

N0 No regional lymph node metastasis

N1 Metastasis in a single ipsilateral lymph node, 3 cm or less in greatest dimension

N2 Metastasis in a single ipsilateral lymph node, more than 3 cm but not more than 6 cm in greatest dimension, or in multiple ipsilateral lymph nodes, none more than 6 cm in greatest dimension, or in bilateral or contralateral lymph nodes, none more than 6 cm in greatest dimension

N2a Metastasis in a single ipsilateral lymph node, more than 3 cm but not more than 6 cm in greatest dimension, or in bilateral or contralateral lymph nodes, none more than 6 cm in greatest dimension

N2b Metastasis in multiple ipsilateral lymph nodes, none more than 6 cm in greatest dimension

N2c Metastasis in bilateral or contralateral lymph nodes, none more than 6 cm in greatest dimension

N3 Metastasis in a lymph node, more than 6 cm in greatest dimension

Distant Metastasis (M)

MX Distant metastasis cannot be assessed

M0 No distant metastasis

M1 Distant metastasis

STAGE GROUPING

Stage I	T1	N0	M0
Stage II	T2	N0	M0
Stage III	T3	N0	M0
	T1	N1	M0
	T2	N1	M0
	T3	N1	M0
Stage IVA	T4a	N0	M0
	T4a	N1	M0
	T1	N2	M0
	T2	N2	M0
	T3	N2	M0
	T4a	N2	M0
Stage IVB	T4b	Any N	M0
	Any T	N3	M0
Stage IVC	Any T	Any N	M1

AJCC Cancer Staging Manual, 6th ed. Springer, 2002.

Small Intestine

Primary Tumor (T)

TX	Primary tumor cannot be assessed
T0	No evidence of primary tumor
Tis	Carcinoma *in situ*
T1	Tumor invades lamina propria or submucosa
T2	Tumor invades muscularis propria
T3	Tumor invades through the muscularis propria into the subserosa or into the nonperitonealized perimuscular tissue (mesentery or retroperitoneum) with extension 2 cm or less*
T4	Tumor perforates the visceral peritoneum or directly invades other organs or structures (includes other loops of small intestine, mesentery, or retroperitoneum more than 2 cm, and abdominal wall by way of serosa; for duodenum only, invasion of pancreas)

**Note:* The nonperitonealized perimuscular tissue is, for jejunum and ileum, part of the mesentery and, for duodenum in areas where serosa is lacking, part of the retroperitoneum.

Regional Lymph Nodes (N)

NX	Regional lymph nodes cannot be assessed
N0	No regional lymph node metastasis
N1	Regional lymph node metastasis

Distant Metastasis (M)

MX	Distant metastasis cannot be assessed
M0	No distant metastasis
M1	Distant metastasis

STAGE GROUPING

Stage 0	Tis	N0	M0
Stage I	T1	N0	M0
	T2	N0	M0
Stage II	T3	N0	M0
	T4	N0	M0
Stage III	Any T	N1	M0
Stage IV	Any T	Any N	M1

AJCC Cancer Staging Manual, 6th ed. Springer, 2002.

Soft Tissue Sarcoma

Primary Tumor (T)

TX	Primary tumor cannot be assessed
T0	No evidence of primary tumor
T1	Tumor 5 cm or less in greatest dimension
	T1a superficial tumor
	T1b deep tumor
T2	Tumor more than 5 cm in greatest dimension
	T2a superficial tumor
	T2b deep tumor

Note: Superficial tumor is located exclusively above the superficial fascia without invasion of the fascia; deep tumor is located either exclusively beneath the superficial fascia, superficial to the fascia with invasion of or through the fascia, or both superficial yet beneath the fascia. Retroperitoneal, mediastinal, and pelvic sarcomas are classified as deep tumors.

Regional Lymph Nodes (N)

NX	Regional lymph nodes cannot be assessed
N0	No regional lymph node metastasis
N1*	Regional lymph node metastasis

**Note:* Presence of positive nodes (N1) is considered Stage IV.

Distant Metastasis (M)

MX	Distant metastasis cannot be assessed
M0	No distant metastasis
M1	Distant metastasis

STAGE GROUPING

Stage I	T1a, 1b, 2a, 2b	N0	M0
	G1-2	G1	Low
Stage II	T1a, 1b, 2a	N0	M0
	G3-4	G2-3	High
Stage III	T2b	N0	M0
	G3-4	G2-3	High
Stage IV	Any T	N1	M0
	Any G	Any	High or Low
	Any T	N0	M1
	Any G	Any G	High or Low

AJCC Cancer Staging Manual, 6th ed. Springer, 2002.

Stomach

Primary Tumor (T)

TX	Primary tumor cannot be assessed
T0	No evidence of primary tumor
Tis	Carcinoma in situ: intraepithelial tumor without invasion of the lamina propria
T1	Tumor invades lamina propria or submucosa
T2	Tumor invades muscularis propria or subserosa*
T2a	Tumor invades muscularis propria
T2b	Tumor invades subserosa
T3	Tumor penetrates serosa (visceral peritoneum) without invasion of adjacent structures**, ***
T4	Tumor invades adjacent structures**, ***

**Note:* A tumor may penetrate the muscularis propria with extension into the gastrocolic or gastrohepatic ligaments, or into the greater or lesser omentum, without perforation of the visceral peritoneum covering these structures. In this case, the tumor is classified T2. If there is perforation of the visceral peritoneum covering the gastric ligaments or the omentum, the tumor should be classified T3.

***Note:* The adjacent structures of the stomach include the spleen, transverse colon, liver, diaphragm, pancreas, abdominal wall, adrenal gland, kidney, small intestine, and retroperitoneum.

****Note:* Intramural extension of the duodenum or esophagus is classified by the depth of the greatest invation in any of these sites, including the stomach.

Regional Lymph Nodes (N)

NX	Regional lymph node(s) cannot be assessed
N0	No regional lymph node metastasis*
N1	Metastasis in 1 to 6 regional lymph nodes
N2	Metastasis in 7 to 15 regional lymph nodes
N3	Metastasis in more than 15 regional lymph nodes

**Note:* A designation of pN0 should be used if all examined lymph nodes are negative, regardless of the total number removed and examined.

Distant Metastasis (M)

MX	Distant metastasis cannot be assessed
M0	No distant metastasis
M1	Distant metastasis

STAGE GROUPING

Stage 0	Tis	N0	M0
Stage IA	T1	N0	M0
Stage IB	T1	N1	M0
	T2a/b	N0	M0
Stage II	T1	N2	M0
	T2a/b	N1	M0
	T3	N0	M0
Stage IIIA	T2a/b	N2	M0
	T3	N1	M0
	T4	N0	M0
Stage IIIB	T3	N2	M0
Stage IV	T4	N1-3	M0
	T1-3	N3	M0
	Any T	Any N	M1

AJCC Cancer Staging Manual, 6th ed. Springer, 2002.

Thyroid

Primary Tumor (T)

Note: All categories may be subdivided: (a) solitary tumor, (b) multifocal tumor (the largest determines the classification).

TX	Primary T cannot be assessed
T0	No evidence of primary T
T1	T < 2cm in greatest dimension limited to the thyroid
T2	T > 2cm but not > 4cm in greatest dimension limited to the thyroid
T3	T > 4cm in greatest dimension limited to the thyroid or any T with minimal extrathyroid ext (e.g., ext. to sternothyroid muscle or perithyroid soft tissues)
T4a	T of any size extending beyond the thyroid capsule to invade subcutaneous soft tissues, larynx, trachea, esophagus, or recurrent laryngeal nerve
T4b	T invades prevertebral fascia or encases carotid artery or mediastinal vessels

All anaplastic carcinomas are considered T4 tumors.

T4a	Intrathyroidal anaplastic carcinoma – surgically resectable.
T4b	Extrathyroidal anaplastic carcinoma – surgically unresectable.

Regional Lymph Nodes (N)

Regional lymph nodes are the central compartment, lateral cervical, and upper mediastinal lymph nodes.

NX	Regional lymph nodes cannot be assessed.
N0	No regional lymph node metastasis
N1	Regional lymph node metastasis
N1a	Metastasis to Level VI (pretracheal, paratracheal, and prelaryngeal/Delphian lymph nodes)
N1b	Metastasis to unilateral, bilateral, or contralateral cervical or superior mediastinal lymph nodes

Distant Metastasis (M)

MX	Distant metastasis cannot be assessed
M0	No distant metastasis
M1	Distant metastasis

STAGE GROUPING

Separate stage groupings are recommended for papillary or follicular, medullary, and anaplastic (undifferentiated) carcinoma.

Papillary or Follicular			
UNDER 45 YEARS			
Stage I	Any T	Any N	M0
Stage II	Any T	Any N	M1
Papillary or Folicular			
45 YEARS AND OLDER			
Stage I	T1	N0	M0
Stage II	T2	N0	M0
Stage III	T3	N0	M0
	T1	N1a	M0
	T2	N1a	M0
	T3	N1a	M0
Stage IVA	T4a	N0	M0
	T4a	N1a	M0
	T1	N1b	M0
	T2	N1b	M0
	T3	N1b	M0
	T4a	N1b	M0
Stage IVB	T4b	Any N	M0
Stage IVC	Any T	Any N	M1
Medullary Carcinoma			
Stage I	T1	N0	M0
Stage II	T2	N0	M0
Stage III	T3	N0	M0
	T1	N1a	M0
	T2	N1a	M0
	T3	N1a	M0
Stage IVA	T4a	N0	M0
	T4a	N1a	M0
	T1	N1b	M0
	T2	N1b	M0
	T3	N1b	M0
	T4a	N1b	M0
Stage IVB	T4b	Any N	M0
Stage IVC	Any T	Any N	M1
Anaplastic Carcinoma			
All anaplastic carcinomas are considered Stage IV			
Stage IVA	T4a	Any N	M0
Stage IVB	T4b	Any N	M0
Stage IVC	Any T	Any N	M1

AJCC Cancer Staging Manual, 6th ed. Springer, 2002.

Index